Williams'
Basic Nutrition
and Diet Therapy

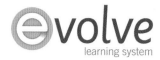
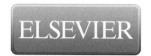
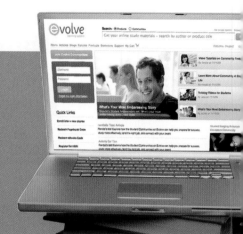

DIETARY REFERENCE INTAKES (DRIs): RECOMMENDED DIETARY ALLOWANCES AND ADEQUATE INTAKES, ELEMENTS
Food and Nutrition Board, Institute of Medicine, National Academies

Life Stage Group	Calcium (mg/d)	Chromium (µg/d)	Copper (µg/d)	Fluoride (mg/d)	Iodine (µg/d)	Iron (mg/d)	Magnesium (mg/d)	Manganese (mg/d)	Molybdenum (µg/d)	Phosphorus (mg/d)	Selenium (µg/d)	Zinc (mg/d)	Potassium (g/d)	Sodium (g/d)	Chloride (g/d)
Infants															
0 to 6 mo	200*	0.2*	200*	0.01*	110*	0.27*	30*	0.003*	2*	100*	15*	2*	0.4*	0.12*	0.18*
6 to 12 mo	260*	5.5*	220*	0.5*	130*	11	75*	0.6*	3*	275*	20*	3	0.7*	0.37*	0.57*
Children															
1-3 y	**700**	11*	**340**	0.7*	**90**	**7**	**80**	1.2*	**17**	**460**	**20**	**3**	3.0*	1.0*	1.5*
4-8 y	**1,000**	15*	**440**	1*	**90**	**10**	**130**	1.5*	**22**	**500**	**30**	**5**	3.8*	1.2*	1.9*
Males															
9-13 y	**1,300**	25*	**700**	2*	**120**	**8**	**240**	1.9*	**34**	**1,250**	**40**	**8**	4.5*	1.5*	2.3*
14-18 y	**1,300**	35*	**890**	3*	**150**	**11**	**410**	2.2*	**43**	**1,250**	**55**	**11**	4.7*	1.5*	2.3*
19-30 y	**1,000**	35*	**900**	4*	**150**	**8**	**400**	2.3*	**45**	**700**	**55**	**11**	4.7*	1.5*	2.3*
31-50 y	**1,000**	35*	**900**	4*	**150**	**8**	**420**	2.3*	**45**	**700**	**55**	**11**	4.7*	1.5*	2.3*
51-70 y	**1,000**	30*	**900**	4*	**150**	**8**	**420**	2.3*	**45**	**700**	**55**	**11**	4.7*	1.3*	2.0*
>70 y	**1,200**	30*	**900**	4*	**150**	**8**	**420**	2.3*	**45**	**700**	**55**	**11**	4.7*	1.2*	1.8*
Females															
9-13 y	**1,300**	21*	**700**	2*	**120**	**8**	**240**	1.6*	**34**	**1,250**	**40**	**8**	4.5*	1.5*	2.3*
14-18 y	**1,300**	24*	**890**	3*	**150**	**15**	**360**	1.6*	**43**	**1,250**	**55**	**9**	4.7*	1.5*	2.3*
19-30 y	**1,000**	25*	**900**	3*	**150**	**18**	**310**	1.8*	**45**	**700**	**55**	**8**	4.7*	1.5*	2.3*
31-50 y	**1,000**	25*	**900**	3*	**150**	**18**	**320**	1.8*	**45**	**700**	**55**	**8**	4.7*	1.5*	2.3*
51-70 y	**1,200**	20*	**900**	3*	**150**	**8**	**320**	1.8*	**45**	**700**	**55**	**8**	4.7*	1.3*	2.0*
>70 y	**1,200**	20*	**900**	3*	**150**	**8**	**320**	1.8*	**45**	**700**	**55**	**8**	4.7*	1.2*	1.8*
Pregnancy															
14-18 y	**1,300**	29*	**1,000**	3*	**220**	**27**	**400**	2.0*	**50**	**1,250**	**60**	**12**	4.7*	1.5*	2.3*
19-30 y	**1,000**	30*	**1,000**	3*	**220**	**27**	**350**	2.0*	**50**	**700**	**60**	**11**	4.7*	1.5*	2.3*
31-50 y	**1,000**	30*	**1,000**	3*	**220**	**27**	**360**	2.0*	**50**	**700**	**60**	**11**	4.7*	1.5*	2.3*
Lactation															
14-18 y	**1,300**	44*	**1,300**	3*	**290**	**10**	**360**	2.6*	**50**	**1,250**	**70**	**13**	5.1*	1.5*	2.3*
19-30 y	**1,000**	45*	**1,300**	3*	**290**	**9**	**310**	2.6*	**50**	**700**	**70**	**12**	5.1*	1.5*	2.3*
31-50 y	**1,000**	45*	**1,300**	3*	**290**	**9**	**320**	2.6*	**50**	**700**	**70**	**12**	5.1*	1.5*	2.3*

NOTE: This table (taken from the DRI reports, see www.nap.edu) presents Recommended Dietary Allowances (RDAs) in **bold type** and Adequate Intakes (AIs) in ordinary type followed by an asterisk (*). An RDA is the average daily dietary intake level; sufficient to meet the nutrient requirements of nearly all (97-98 percent) healthy individuals in a group. It is calculated from an Estimated Average Requirement (EAR).

If sufficient scientific evidence is not available to establish an EAR, and thus calculate an RDA, an AI is usually developed. For healthy breastfed infants, an AI is the mean intake. The AI for other life stage and gender groups is believed to cover the needs of all healthy individuals in the groups, but lack of data or uncertainty in the data prevent being able to specify with confidence the percentage of individuals covered by this intake.

SOURCES: *Dietary Reference Intakes for Calcium, Phosphorous, Magnesium, Vitamin D, and Fluoride* (1997); *Dietary Reference Intakes for Thiamin, Riboflavin, Niacin, Vitamin B₆, Folate, Vitamin B₁₂, Pantothenic Acid, Biotin, and Choline* (1998); *Dietary Reference Intakes for Vitamin C, Vitamin E, Selenium, and Carotenoids* (2000); and *Dietary Reference Intakes for Vitamin A, Vitamin K, Arsenic, Boron, Chromium, Copper, Iodine, Iron, Manganese, Molybdenum, Nickel, Silicon, Vanadium, and Zinc* (2001); *Dietary Reference Intakes for Water, Potassium, Sodium, Chloride, and Sulfate* (2005); and *Dietary Reference Intakes for Calcium and Vitamin D* (2011). These reports may be accessed via www.nap.edu.

DIETARY REFERENCE INTAKES (DRIs): RECOMMENDED DIETARY ALLOWANCES AND ADEQUATE INTAKES, TOTAL WATER AND MACRONUTRIENTS

Food and Nutrition Board, Institute of Medicine, National Academies

Life Stage Group	Total Water^a (L/d)	Total Fiber (g/d)	Linoleic Acid (g/d)	α-Linolenic Acid (g/d)	Protein^b (g/d)
Infants					
0 to 6 mo	0.7*	ND	4.4*	0.5*	9.1*
6 to 12 mo	0.8*	ND	4.6*	0.5*	**11.0**
Children					
1-3 y	1.3*	19*	7*	0.7*	**13**
4-8 y	1.7*	25*	10*	0.9*	**19**
Males					
9-13 y	2.4*	31*	12*	1.2*	**34**
14-18 y	3.3*	38*	16*	1.6*	**52**
19-30 y	3.7*	38*	17*	1.6*	**56**
31-50 y	3.7*	38*	17*	1.6*	**56**
51-70 y	3.7*	30*	14*	1.6*	**56**
>70 y	3.7*	30*	14*	1.6*	**56**
Females					
9-13 y	2.1*	26*	10*	1.0*	**34**
14-18 y	2.3*	26*	11*	1.1*	**46**
19-30 y	2.7*	25*	12*	1.1*	**46**
31-50 y	2.7*	25*	12*	1.1*	**46**
51-70 y	2.7*	21*	11*	1.1*	**46**
>70 y	2.7*	21*	11*	1.1*	**46**
Pregnancy					
14-18 y	3.0*	28*	13*	1.4*	**71**
19-30 y	3.0*	28*	13*	1.4*	**71**
31-50 y	3.0*	28*	13*	1.4*	**71**
Lactation					
14-18	3.8*	29*	13*	1.3*	**71**
19-30 y	3.8*	29*	13*	1.3*	**71**
31-50 y	3.8*	29*	13*	1.3*	**71**

NOTE: This table (take from the DRI reports, see www.nap.edu) presents Recommended Dietary Allowances (RDA) in **bold type** and Adequate Intakes (AI) in ordinary type followed by an asterisk (*). An RDA is the average daily dietary intake level; sufficient to meet the nutrient requirements of nearly all (97-98 percent) healthy individuals in a group. It is calculated from an Estimated Average Requirement (EAR).

If sufficient scientific evidence is not available to establish an EAR, and thus calculate an RDA, an AI is usually developed. For healthy breastfed infants, an AI is the mean intake. The AI for other life stage and gender groups is believed to cover the needs of all healthy individuals in the groups, but lack of data or uncertainty in the data prevent being able to specify with confidence the percentage of individuals covered by this intake.

^{a}*Total* water includes all water contained in food, beverages, and drinking water.

^{b}Based on g protein per kg of body weight for the reference body weight, e.g., for adults 0.8 g/kg body weight for the reference body weight.

SOURCE: *Dietary Reference Intakes for Energy, Carbohydrate, Fiber, Fat, Fatty Acids, Cholesterol, Protein, and Amino Acids* (2002/2005) and *Dietary Reference Intakes for Water, Potassium, Sodium, Chloride, and Sulfate* (2005). The report may be accessed via www.nap.edu.

DIETARY REFERENCE INTAKES (DRIs): ACCEPTABLE MACRONUTRIENT DISTRIBUTION RANGES

Food and Nutrition Board, Institute of Medicine, National Academies

Macronutrient	RANGE (PERCENT OF ENERGY)		
	Children, 1-3 y	Children, 4-18 y	Adults
Fat	30-40	25-35	20-35
n-6 polyunsaturated fatty acids^a (linoleic acid)	5-10	5-10	5-10
n-3 polyunsaturated fatty acids^a (α-linolenic acid)	0.6-1.2	0.6-1.2	0.6-1.2
Carbohydrate	45-65	45-65	45-65
Protein	5-20	10-30	10-35

^{a}Approximately 10 percent of the total can come from longer-chain n-3 or n-6 fatty acids.

SOURCE: *Dietary Reference Intakes for Energy, Carbohydrate, Fiber, Fat, Fatty Acids, Cholesterol, Protein, and Amino Acids* (2002/2005). The report may be accessed via www.nap.edu.

DIETARY REFERENCE INTAKES (DRIs): ACCEPTABLE MACRONUTRIENT DISTRIBUTION RANGES

Food and Nutrition Board, Institute of Medicine, National Academies

Macronutrient	Recommendation
Dietary cholesterol	As low as possible while consuming a nutritionally adequate diet
Trans fatty Acids	As low as possible while consuming a nutritionally adequate diet
Saturated fatty acids	As low as possible while consuming a nutritionally adequate diet
Added sugars^a	Limit to no more than 25 % of total energy

^{a}Not a recommended intake. A daily intake of added sugars that individuals should aim for to achieve a healthful diet was not set.

SOURCE: *Dietary Reference Intakes for Enemy, Carbohydrate, Fiber, Fat, Fatty Acids, Cholesterol, Protein, and Amino Acids* (2002/2005). The report may be accessed via www.nap.edu.

DIETARY REFERENCE INTAKES (DRIs): TOLERABLE UPPER INTAKE LEVELS, VITAMINS
Food and Nutrition Board, Institute of Medicine, National Academies

Life Stage Group	Vitamin A (µg/d)[a]	Vitamin C (mg/d)	Vitamin D (µg/d)	Vitamin E (mg/d)[b,c]	Vitamin K	Thiamin	Riboflavin	Niacin (mg/d)[c]	Vitamin B6 (mg/d)	Folate (µg/d)[c]	Vitamin B12	Pantothenic Acid	Biotin	Choline (g/d)	Carotenoids[d]
Infants															
0 to 6 mo	600	ND[e]	25	ND	ND	ND	ND	ND	ND	ND	ND	ND	ND	ND	ND
6 to 12 mo	600	ND	38	ND	ND	ND	ND	ND	ND	ND	ND	ND	ND	ND	ND
Children															
1-3 y	600	400	63	200	ND	ND	ND	10	30	300	ND	ND	ND	1.0	ND
4-8 y	900	650	75	300	ND	ND	ND	15	40	400	ND	ND	ND	1.0	ND
Males															
9-13 y	1,700	1,200	100	600	ND	ND	ND	20	60	600	ND	ND	ND	2.0	ND
14-18 y	2,800	1,800	100	800	ND	ND	ND	30	80	800	ND	ND	ND	3.0	ND
19-30 y	3,000	2,000	100	1,000	ND	ND	ND	35	100	1,000	ND	ND	ND	3.5	ND
31-50 y	3,000	2,000	100	1,000	ND	ND	ND	35	100	1,000	ND	ND	ND	3.5	ND
51-70 y	3,000	2,000	100	1,000	ND	ND	ND	35	100	1,000	ND	ND	ND	3.5	ND
>70 y	3,000	2,000	100	1,000	ND	ND	ND	35	100	1,000	ND	ND	ND	3.5	ND
Females															
9-13 y	1,700	1,200	100	600	ND	ND	ND	20	60	600	ND	ND	ND	2.0	ND
14-18 y	2,800	1,800	100	800	ND	ND	ND	30	80	800	ND	ND	ND	3.0	ND
19-30 y	3,000	2,000	100	1,000	ND	ND	ND	35	100	1,000	ND	ND	ND	3.5	ND
31-50 y	3,000	2,000	100	1,000	ND	ND	ND	35	100	1,000	ND	ND	ND	3.5	ND
51-70 y	3,000	2,000	100	1,000	ND	ND	ND	35	100	1,000	ND	ND	ND	3.5	ND
>70 y	3,000	2,000	100	1,000	ND	ND	ND	35	100	1,000	ND	ND	ND	3.5	ND
Pregnancy															
14-18 y	2,800	1,800	100	800	ND	ND	ND	30	80	800	ND	ND	ND	3.0	ND
19-30 y	3,000	2,000	100	1,000	ND	ND	ND	35	100	1,000	ND	ND	ND	3.5	ND
31-50 y	3,000	2,000	100	1,000	ND	ND	ND	35	100	1,000	ND	ND	ND	3.5	ND
Lactation															
14-18 y	2,800	1,800	100	800	ND	ND	ND	30	80	800	ND	ND	ND	3.0	ND
19-30 y	3,000	2,000	100	1,000	ND	ND	ND	35	100	1,000	ND	ND	ND	3.5	ND
31-50 y	3,000	2,000	100	1,000	ND	ND	ND	35	100	1,000	ND	ND	ND	3.5	ND

NOTE: A Tolerable Upper Intake Level (UL) is the highest level of daily nutrient intake that is likely to pose no risk of adverse health effects to almost all individuals in the general population. Unless otherwise specified, the UL represents total intake from food, water, and supplements. Due to a lack of suitable data, ULs could not be established for vitamin K, thiamin, riboflavin, vitamin B12, pantothenic acid, biotin, and carotenoids. In the absence of a UL, extra caution may be warranted in consuming levels above recommended intakes. Members of the general population should be advised not to routinely exceed the UL. The UL is not meant to apply to individuals who are treated with the nutrient under medical supervision or to individuals with predisposing conditions that modify their sensitivity to the nutrient.

[a] As preformed vitamin A only.

[b] As α-tocopherol; applies to any form of supplemental α-tocopherol.

[c] The ULs for vitamin E, niacin, and folate apply to synthetic forms obtained from supplements, fortified foods, or a combination of the two.

[d] β-Carotene supplements are advised only to serve as a provitamin A source for individuals at risk of vitamin A deficiency.

[e] ND = Not determinable due to lack of data of adverse effects in this age group and concern with regard to lack of ability to handle excess amounts. Source of intake should be from food only to prevent high levels of intake.

SOURCES: *Dietary Reference Intakes for Calcium, Phosphorous, Magnesium, Vitamin D, and Fluoride* (1997); *Dietary Reference Intakes for Thiamin, Riboflavin, Niacin, Vitamin B6, Folate, Vitamin B12, Pantothenic Acid, Biotin, and Choline* (1998); *Dietary Reference Intakes for Vitamin C, Vitamin E, Selenium, and Carotenoids* (2000); *Dietary Reference Intakes for Vitamin A, Vitamin K, Arsenic, Boron, Chromium, Copper, Iodine, Iron, Manganese, Molybdenum, Nickel, Silicon, Vanadium, and Zinc* (2001); and *Dietary Reference Intakes for Calcium and Vitamin D* (2011). These reports may be accessed via www.nap.edu.

DIETARY REFERENCE INTAKES (DRIs): TOLERABLE UPPER INTAKE LEVELS, ELEMENTS

Food and Nutrition Board, Institute of Medicine, National Academies

Life Stage Group	Arsenic[a]	Boron (mg/d)	Calcium (mg/d)	Chromium	Copper (μg/d)	Fluoride (mg/d)	Iodine (μg/d)	Iron (mg/d)	Magnesium (mg/d)[b]	Manganese (mg/d)	Molybdenum (μg/d)	Nickel (mg/d)	Phosphorus (g/d)	Selenium (μg/d)	Silicon[c]	Vanadium (mg/d)[d]	Zinc (mg/d)	Sodium (g/d)	Chloride (g/d)
Infants																			
0 to 6 mo	ND[e]	ND	1,000	ND	ND	0.7	ND	40	ND	ND	ND	ND	ND	45	ND	ND	4	ND	ND
6 to 12 m0	ND	ND	1,500	ND	ND	0.9	ND	40	ND	ND	ND	ND	ND	60	ND	ND	5	ND	ND
Children																			
1-3 y	ND	3	2,500	ND	1,000	1.3	200	40	65	2	300	0.2	3	90	ND	ND	7	1.5	2.3
4-8 y	ND	6	2,500	ND	3,000	2.2	300	40	110	3	600	0.3	3	150	ND	ND	12	1.9	2.9
Males																			
9-13 y	ND	11	3,000	ND	5,000	10	600	40	350	6	1,100	0.6	4	280	ND	ND	23	2.2	3.4
14-18 y	ND	17	3,000	ND	8,000	10	900	45	350	9	1,700	1.0	4	400	ND	ND	34	2.3	3.6
19-30 y	ND	20	2,500	ND	10,000	10	1,100	45	350	11	2,000	1.0	4	400	ND	1.8	40	2.3	3.6
31-50 y	ND	20	2,500	ND	10,000	10	1,100	45	350	11	2,000	1.0	4	400	ND	1.8	40	2.3	3.6
51-70 y	ND	20	2,000	ND	10,000	10	1,100	45	350	11	2,000	1.0	4	400	ND	1.8	40	2.3	3.6
>70 y	ND	20	2,000	ND	10,000	10	1,100	45	350	11	2,000	1.0	3	400	ND	1.8	40	2.3	3.6
Females																			
9-13 y	ND	11	3,000	ND	5,000	10	600	40	350	6	1,100	0.6	4	280	ND	ND	23	2.2	3.4
14-18 y	ND	17	3,000	ND	8,000	10	900	45	350	9	1,700	1.0	4	400	ND	ND	34	2.3	3.6
19-30 y	ND	20	2,500	ND	10,000	10	1,100	45	350	11	2,000	1.0	4	400	ND	1.8	40	2.3	3.6
31-50 y	ND	20	2,500	ND	10,000	10	1,100	45	350	11	2,000	1.0	4	400	ND	1.8	40	2.3	3.6
51-70 y	ND	20	2,000	ND	10,000	10	1,100	45	350	11	2,000	1.0	4	400	ND	1.8	40	2.3	3.6
>70 y	ND	20	2,000	ND	10,000	10	1,100	45	350	11	2,000	1.0	3	400	ND	1.8	40	2.3	3.6
Pregnancy																			
14-18 y	ND	17	3,000	ND	8,000	10	900	45	350	9	1,700	1.0	3.5	400	ND	ND	34	2.3	3.6
19-30 y	ND	20	2,500	ND	10,000	10	1,100	45	350	11	2,000	1.0	3.5	400	ND	ND	40	2.3	3.6
61-50 y	ND	20	2,500	ND	10,000	10	1,100	45	350	11	2,000	1.0	3.5	400	ND	ND	40	2.3	3.6
Lactation																			
14-18 y	ND	17	3,000	ND	8,000	10	900	45	350	9	1,700	1.0	4	400	ND	ND	34	2.3	3.6
19-30 y	ND	20	2,500	ND	10,000	10	1,100	45	350	11	2,000	1.0	4	400	ND	ND	40	2.3	3.6
31-50 y	ND	20	2,500	ND	10,000	10	1,100	45	350	11	2,000	1.0	4	400	ND	ND	40	2.3	3.6

NOTE: A Tolerable Upper Intake Level (UL) is the highest level of daily nutrient intake that is likely to pose no risk of adverse health effects to almost all individuals in the general population. Unless otherwise specified, the UL represents total intake from food, water, and supplements. Due to a lack of suitable data, ULs could not be established for vitamin K, thiamin, riboflavin, vitamin B_{12}, pantothenic acid, biotin, and carotenoids. In the absence of a UL, extra caution may be warranted in consuming levels above recommended intakes. Members of the general population should be advised not to routinely exceed the UL. The UL is not meant to apply to individuals who are treated with the nutrient under medical supervision or to individuals with predisposing conditions that modify their sensitivity to the nutrient.

[a]Although the UL was not determined for arsenic, there is no justification for adding arsenic to food or supplements.

[b]The ULs for magnesium represent intake from a pharmacological agent only and do not include intake from food and water.

[c]Although silicon has not been shown to cause adverse effects in humans, there is no justification for adding silicon to supplements.

[d]Although vanadium in food has not been shown to cause adverse effects in humans, there is no justification for adding vanadium to food and vanadium supplements should be used with caution. The UL is based on adverse effects in laboratory animals and this data could be used to set a UL for adults but not children and adolescents.

[e]ND = Not determinable due to lack of data of adverse effects in this age group and concern with regard to lack of ability to handle excess amounts. Source of intake should be from food only to prevent high levels of intake.

SOURCES: *Dietary Reference Intakes for Calcium, Phosphorous, Magnesium, Vitamin D, and Fluoride* (1997); *Dietary Reference Intakes for Thiamin, Riboflavin, Niacin, Vitamin B₆, Folate, Vitamin B₁₂, Pantothenic Acid, Biotin, and Choline* (1998); *Dietary Reference Intakes for Vitamin C, Vitamin E, Selenium, and Carotenoids* (2000); *Dietary Reference Intakes for Vitamin A, Vitamin K, Arsenic, Boron, Chromium, Copper, Iodine, Iron, Manganese, Molybdenum, Nickel, Silicon, Vanadium, and Zinc* (2001); *Dietary Reference Intakes for Water, Potassium, Sodium, Chloride, and Sulfate* (2005); and *Dietary Reference Intakes for Calcium and Vitamin D* (2011). These reports may be accessed via www.nap.edu.

Williams'
Basic Nutrition and Diet Therapy

Staci Nix, MS, RD, CD
Assistant Professor
Division of Nutrition
College of Health
University of Utah
Salt Lake City, Utah

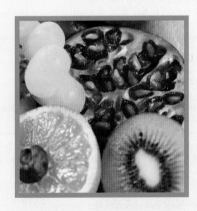

14th Edition

ELSEVIER

3251 Riverport Lane
St. Louis, Missouri 63043

WILLIAMS' BASIC NUTRITION & DIET THERAPY

ISBN: 978-0-323-08347-8

**Copyright © 2013, 2009, 2005, 2001, 1995, 1992, 1988, 1984, 1980,
1975, 1969, 1966, 1962, 1958 by Mosby, Inc., an affiliate of Elsevier Inc.**

Notices

Knowledge and best practice in this field are constantly changing. As new research and experience broaden our understanding, changes in research methods, professional practices, or medical treatment may become necessary.

Practitioners and researchers must always rely on their own experience and knowledge in evaluating and using any information, methods, compounds, or experiments described herein. In using such information or methods they should be mindful of their own safety and the safety of others, including parties for whom they have a professional responsibility.

With respect to any drug or pharmaceutical products identified, readers are advised to check the most current information provided (i) on procedures featured or (ii) by the manufacturer of each product to be administered, to verify the recommended dose or formula, the method and duration of administration, and contraindications. It is the responsibility of practitioners, relying on their own experience and knowledge of their patients, to make diagnoses, to determine dosages and the best treatment for each individual patient, and to take all appropriate safety precautions.

To the fullest extent of the law, neither the Publisher nor the authors, contributors, or editors, assume any liability for any injury and/or damage to persons or property as a matter of products liability, negligence or otherwise, or from any use or operation of any methods, products, instructions, or ideas contained in the material herein.

Library of Congress Cataloging-in-Publication Data
Nix, Staci.
   Williams' basic nutrition & diet therapy / Staci Nix.—14th ed.
      p. ; cm.
   Williams' basic nutrition and diet therapy
   Basic nutrition & diet therapy
   Includes bibliographical references and index.
   ISBN 978-0-323-08347-8 (pbk. : alk. paper)
   I. Williams, Sue Rodwell. Basic nutrition & diet therapy.   II. Title.   III. Title: Williams' basic nutrition and diet therapy.   IV. Title: Basic nutrition & diet therapy.
   [DNLM: 1. Diet Therapy.   2. Food Habits.   3. Nutritional Physiological Phenomena.   4. Nutritional Requirements.   WB 400]
   615.8′54—dc23

2011043887

Senior Content Strategist: Yvonne Alexopoulos
Senior Content Development Specialist: Lisa P. Newton
Publishing Services Manager: Deborah L. Vogel
Project Manager: John W. Gabbert
Design Direction: Karen Pauls

Printed in Canada

Last digit is the print number: 9   8   7   6   5   4   3

Contributors and Reviewers

CONTRIBUTORS

Kelli Boi, MS, RD
Adjunct Nutrition Instructor
Weber State University
Ogden, Utah

Sara O. Harcourt, MS, RD
Assistant Professor and Extension Agent
Utah State University
Logan, Utah

Jennifer Schmidt, MS, RD Candidate
Division of Nutrition
University of Utah
Salt Lake City, Utah

REVIEWERS

Pat Floro, RN
PN Instructor
Nancy J. Knight School of Nursing
Ohio Hi-Point Career Center
Bellefontaine, Ohio

Debra Hodge, RN, MSN
Clinical and Theory Instructor
ACT School of PN
Beckley, West Virginia
Assistant Adjunct Professor
Mountain State University
School of Nursing
Beckley, West Virginia

Sharon Hunt, MS, RD, LD
Department of Family and Consumer Sciences
Fort Valley State University
Fort Valley, Georgia

Debra A. Indorato, RD, LDN, CLT
APPROACH Nutrition
Food Allergy Management LLC
Virginia Beach, Virginia

Karla Kennedy-Hagan, PhD, RD, LDN
Assistant Chair, School of Family & Consumer Sciences
Graduate Dietetic Coordinator
Eastern Illinois University
Charleston, Illinois

Elizabeth Betty Kenyon, RD, LMNT
Adjunct Faculty, Western Nebraska Community
  College
Community Action Partnership of Western Nebraska
Scottsbluff, Nebraska

Lauralee Krabill, RN, C, CNOR, MBA
Director, Practical Nursing Program
Sandusky Career Center
2130 Hayes Avenue
Sandusky, Ohio

Diane T. Kupensky, RN, MSN, CNS
Trauma—Advanced Practice Nurse
  St. Elizabeth Health Center
Masury, Ohio

Dennis McClure, MS, Ph D
Instructor
Nursing Certificate Programs
Division of Workforce Development and Lifelong
  Learning
Community College of the District of Columbia
Member, University System of the District of Columbia
Washington, DC

Linda Kautz Osterkamp PhD, RD, FADA
Nutrition Consultant
Tucson, Arizona

Jessie Pavlinac, MS, RD, CSR, LD
Director, Clinical Nutrition
Food & Nutrition Services
Oregon Health & Science University
Portland, Oregon

Janet Peterson, RN, MSN, CNS
Clinical Coordinator
Kent State University
East Liverpool Campus
400 East Fourth Street
East Liverpool, Ohio

Toni Pritchard, BSN, MSN, Ed D
Professor
Central Louisiana Technical College—Lamar Salter
  Campus
Leesville, Lousiana

Rena Quinton, PhD, RD, LDN
Director Dietetic Internship
Assistant Professor
Immaculata University
Immaculata, Pennsylvania

Beth Wolfgram MS, RD, CSSD, CSCS
Sports Dietitian, University of Utah Athletic Department
  Adjunct Faculty, Division of Nutrition
University of Utah
Salt Lake City, Utah

*Dedicated to my mentor and friend, **Dr. Nina Marable.***

Preface to the Instructor

The field of nutrition is a dynamic human endeavor that is continuously expanding and evolving. Three main factors continue to change the modern face of nutrition. First, the science of nutrition continues to grow rapidly with exciting research. New knowledge in any science challenges some traditional ideas and lends to the development of new ones. Instead of primarily focusing on nutrition in the treatment of disease, we are expanding the search for disease prevention and general enhancement of life through nutrition and healthy lifestyles. Thus was the spirit during the establishment of the current Dietary Reference Intakes. Second, the rapidly increasing multiethnic diversity of the United States population enriches our food patterns and presents a variety of health care opportunities and needs. Third, the public is more aware and concerned about health promotion and the role of nutrition, largely because of the media's increasing attention. Clients and patients seek more self-directed involvement in their health care, and an integral part of that care is nutrition.

This new edition continues to reflect upon the evolving face of nutrition science. Its guiding principle is our own commitment, along with that of our publisher, to the integrity of the material. Our basic goal is to produce a new book for today's needs, with updated content, and to meet the expectations and changing needs of students, faculty, and practitioners of basic health care.

AUDIENCE

This text is primarily designed for students in licensed practical or vocational nursing (LPN/LVN) programs and associate degree programs (ADN/RN), as well as for diet technicians or aides. It is also appropriate for programs in various professions related to health care.

Conceptual Approach

The general purpose of this text is to introduce the basic scientific principles of nutrition and their applications in person-centered care. As in previous editions, basic concepts are carefully explained when introduced. In addition, our personal concerns are ever present, as follows: (1) that this introduction to the science and practice we love will continue to lead students and readers to enjoy learning about nutrition in the lives of people and stimulate further reading in areas of personal interest; (2) that caretakers will be alert to nutrition news and questions raised by their increasingly diverse clients and patients; and (3) that contact and communication with professionals in the field of nutrition will help build a strong team approach to clinical nutrition problems in all patient care.

Organization

In keeping with the previous format, I have updated content areas to meet the needs of a rapidly developing science and society.

In **Part 1,** *Introduction to Basic Principles of Nutrition Science*, Chapter 1 focuses on the directions of health care and health promotion, risk reduction for disease prevention, and community health care delivery systems, with emphasis on team care and the active role of clients in self-care. Descriptions and illustrations accompany the new Healthy People 2020 Objectives, the Dietary Guidelines for Americans 2010, and MyPlate guidelines. The Dietary Reference Intakes (DRIs) are incorporated throughout chapter discussions in Part 1 as well as throughout the rest of the text. New and improved illustrations for the visual learner are in this edition of the text for complicated metabolic pathways such as the renin-angiotensin-aldosterone system, the antidiuretic system, and iron metabolism. Current research updates all the basic nutrient and energy chapters in the remainder of Part 1.

In **Part 2,** *Nutrition throughout the Life Cycle*, Chapters 10, 11, and 12 reflect current material on human growth and development needs in different parts of the life cycle. Current National Academy of Science guidelines for positive weight gain to meet the metabolic demands of pregnancy and lactation are reinforced. Positive growth support for infancy, childhood, and adolescence is emphasized. The expanding health maintenance needs of a growing adult population through the aging process focus on building a healthy lifestyle to reduce disease risks. In all cases, statistics represent the most recent publications available at the time of print.

In **Part 3,** *Community Nutrition and Health Care*, a strong focus on community nutrition is coordinated with an emphasis on weight management and physical fitness as they pertain to health care benefits and risk reduction. The Nutrition Labeling and Education Act is discussed in terms of its current regulations and helpful label format as well as its effects on food marketing. Issues of malnutrition and the cycle of despair are discussed and illustrated in Chapter 13. Highlights of foodborne diseases reinforce concerns about food safety in a changing marketplace. Chapter 14 and Appendix F highlight information on America's multiethnic cultural food patterns and various religious dietary practices. New information on the topics of obesity and genetics, along with the use of alternative weight loss methods, is included in Chapter 15. Chapter 16 discusses aspects of athletics, the proliferation of sports drinks, and the performance benefits of a well hydrated and nourished athlete.

In **Part 4**, *Clinical Nutrition*, chapters are updated to reflect current medical nutrition therapy and approaches to nutrition education and management. As with previous editions, Drug-Nutrient Interaction boxes in this section address specific concerns with nutrition and medication interactions. The fourteenth edition includes new Drug-Nutrient Interaction boxes throughout. Special areas include developments in gastrointestinal disease, heart disease, diabetes mellitus, renal disease, surgery, cancer, and AIDS.

Content and Features

- **Book format and design.** The chapter format and use of color continue to enhance the book's appeal. Basic chapter concepts and overview, illustrations, tables, boxes, definitions, headings, and subheadings make the content easier and more interesting to read.
- **Learning supplements.** Educational aids have been developed to assist both students and instructors in the teaching and learning process. Please see the *Ancillaries* section on the next page for more detailed information.
- **Illustrations.** Color illustrations, including artwork, graphs, charts, and photographs, help students and practitioners better understand the concepts and clinical practices presented.
- **Content threads.** This book shares a number of features—reading level; Key Concepts; Key Terms; Critical Thinking Questions; Chapter Challenge Questions; References; Further Reading and Resources; Glossary; and Cultural Considerations, For Further Focus, Drug-Nutrient Interactions, and Clinical Applications boxes—with other Elsevier books intended for students in demanding and fast-paced nursing curricula. These common threads help promote and hone the skills these students must master. (See the Content Threads page after this preface for more detailed information on these learning features.)

LEARNING AIDS

As indicated, this new edition is especially significant because of its use of many learning aids throughout the text.

- **Part openers.** To provide the "big picture" of the book's overall focus on nutrition and health, the four main sections are introduced as successive developing parts of that unifying theme.
- **Chapter openers.** To immediately draw students into the topic for study, each chapter opens with a short list of the basic concepts involved and a brief chapter overview leading into the topic to "set the stage."
- **Chapter headings.** Throughout each chapter, the major headings and subheadings in special type or color indicate the organization of the chapter material, providing easy reading and understanding of the key ideas. Main concepts and terms also are highlighted with color or bold type and italics.
- **Special boxes.** The inclusion of For Further Focus, Cultural Considerations, Drug-Nutrient Interactions, and Clinical Applications boxes leads students a step further on a given topic or presents a case study for analysis. These boxes enhance understanding of concepts through further exploration or application.
- **Case studies.** In clinical care chapters, case studies are provided in **Clinical Applications** boxes to focus students' attention on related patient care problems. Each case is accompanied by questions for case analysis. Students can use these examples for similar patient care needs in their own clinical assignments.
- **Diet therapy guides.** In clinical chapters, medical nutrition therapy guides provide practical help in patient care and education.
- **Definitions of terms.** Key terms important to students' understanding and application of the material in patient care are presented in two ways. They are identified in the body of the text and are listed in a glossary at the back of the book for quick reference.
- **Summaries.** A brief summary in bulleted format reviews chapter highlights and helps students see how the chapter contributes to the book's "big picture." Students then can return to any part of the material for repeated study and clarification of details as needed.
- **Critical Thinking Questions.** To help students understand key parts of the chapter or apply it to patient care problems, critical thinking questions are posed after each chapter summary for review and analysis of the material presented. Thorough answers for the questions are provided on the accompanying Evolve Resource website for students to check their work.

- **Chapter Challenge Questions.** In addition, self-test questions in true-false, multiple choice, and matching formats are provided at the end of each chapter to allow students to test their basic knowledge of the chapter's contents.
- **References.** Background references throughout the text provide resources used in each chapter for students who may want to probe a particular topic of interest.
- **Further Reading and Resources.** To encourage further reading of useful materials, expand students' knowledge of key concepts, and help students apply material in practical ways for patient care and education, a brief list of annotated resources—including books, journals, and Web sites—is provided at the end of each chapter.
- **Appendixes.** The numerous appendixes include information on the cholesterol, dietary fiber, sodium, and potassium content of food and on cultural and religious dietary patterns, along with the Eating Well with Canada's Food Guide.

ANCILLARIES

Teaching and Learning Package for the Instructors

TEACH Instructor Resources on Evolve: available at www.evolve.elsevier.com/Williams/basic/ provides a wealth of material to help you make your Nutrition instruction a success. In addition to all of the Student Resources, the following are provided for faculty:

- **TEACH Lesson Plans:** Based on textbook chapter Learning Objectives, serve as ready-made, modifiable lesson plans and a complete roadmap to link all parts of the educational package. These concise and straightforward lesson plans can be modified or combined to meet your particular scheduling and teaching needs.
- Examview **Test Bank:** Contains approximately 700 multiple-choice and alternate-format questions for the NCLEX Examination. Each question is coded for correct answer, rationale, page reference, Nursing Process Step, NCLEX Client Needs Category, and Cognitive Level.
- **Image Collection:** These images can be used in a unique presentation or as visual aids.
- **PowerPoint Presentations** with incorporated **Audience Response Questions** and unfolding **Case Study** to accompany each chapter guide classroom lectures.
- **Nutrition Concepts Online** is an online course available to supplement your classroom learning or allow you to work at your own pace! Used in conjunction with your Elsevier textbook, this dynamic online course integrates illustrations, animations, interactive exercises, and quizzes to reinforce your comprehension

of key nutrition concepts and provide an exciting interactive learning experience. Ask your sales representative for more information.

For Students

- ***Nutritrac Nutrition Analysis Program, Version 5.0 (Online):*** The new edition of this popular tool is designed to allow the user to calculate and analyze food intake and energy expenditure, taking the guesswork out of nutrition planning. The new version features comprehensive databases containing more than 5000 foods organized into 18 different categories and more than 175 common/daily recreational, sporting, and occupational activities. The *Personal Profile* feature allows users to enter and edit the intake and output of an unlimited number of individuals, and the *Weight Management Planner* helps outline healthy lifestyles tailored to various personal profiles. In addition to foods and activities, new program features include an ideal body weight (IBW) calculator, a Harris-Benedict calculator to estimate total daily energy needs, and the complete *Exchange Lists for Meal Planning*.
- **Evolve Resources**
  - **Study Questions:** More than 350 self-assessment questions that provide students practice questions and immediate feedback to help them prepare for exams.

    Infant and Child Growth Charts, United States, Centers for Disease Control and Prevention and the ADA Nutrition Care Process are available as useful handouts to encourage use of these valuable resources inside and outside of the classroom.
  - **Case Studies** engage students with the opportunity to apply the knowledge they have learned in real-life situations.
  - **Answers to Critical Thinking and Chapter Challenge Questions** are provided for students to check their work and get additional feedback on questions at the end of each chapter.
  - **WebLinks** offer direct links to a wealth of Web sites on nutrition-related topics above and beyond information covered in the book.
- **Nutrition Resource Center Web site:** This informative Web site is available at *http://nutrition.elsevier.com* to provide the reader access to information about all Elsevier nutrition texts in one convenient location.

ACKNOWLEDGMENTS

Throughout this process, various staff members from Elsevier have kindly provided guidance and assistance, and I am grateful to all of them. I would like to especially acknowledge the professionalism, fortitude, and diligence of Yvonne Alexopoulos, Senior Content Strategist; Lisa P. Newton, Senior Content Development Specialist; Kit Blanke, Content Coordinator; Johnny Gabbert, Project Manager; and Jen Gann, Copyeditor. Your vision for this text is the true power behind the print.

I would like to acknowledge the hard work and dedication of Elsevier's Nursing Marketing Department for supporting this book through its many editions. Their ability to bridge the gap between a product and the end point—students who will hopefully learn from and enjoy this text—is integral to the success of this project. In addition, I am grateful to the many reviewers who have provided constructive feedback on this edition. Your involvement provides the strength and thoroughness that no author can accomplish alone.

Finally, I want to thank my family and friends who have compassionately dealt with me and "the book." Your abundant support sustains me.

Staci Nix

Content Threads

The fourteenth edition of Williams' Basic Nutrition & Diet Therapy shares a number of learning features with other Elsevier titles used in nursing programs. These user-friendly Content Threads are designed to streamline the learning process among the variety of books and content areas included in this fast-paced and demanding curriculum.

Shared elements included in Williams' Basic Nutrition & Diet Therapy, fourteenth edition, include the following:

- **Reading level**: The easy-to-read and user-friendly format, as well as the often personal writing style, engage the reader and help unfold the information simply and effectively.
- **Cover design**: Graphic similarities help readers to instantly recognize the book as containing content and features relevant to today's nursing curricula.
- Bulleted lists of **Key Concepts** on each chapter opening page help focus the student on the "big picture" content presented.
- **Key Terms** presented in color are readily apparent throughout the book. In addition, key terms boxes presented on the book pages in which the terms are discussed provide complete definitions to help with memory association.
- **Critical Thinking Questions** presented after each chapter's summary encourage the student to recall the information as well as analyze its implications and uses. Answers are provided on the Evolve website.
- **Chapter Challenge Questions** presented in true-false, multiple-choice, and matching formats help students test their comprehension of various content areas. Answers are provided on Evolve.
- A complete list of **References** is accompanied by **Further Reading and Resources**, a section that includes a wealth of resources—books, journal articles, and Web sites—that supplement the information provided in the textbook.
- Four types of boxes—**Cultural Considerations, For Further Focus, Clinical Applications, and Drug-Nutrient Interaction**—explore current hot topics in nutrition today and provide insight beyond the information presented in the chapter text.

Preface to the Student

Williams' Basic Nutrition & Diet Therapy is a market leader in nutrition textbooks for support personnel in health care. It provides careful explanations of the basic principles of scientific nutrition and presents their applications in person-centered care in health and disease.

The author, Staci Nix, provides this important information in an easy-to-read, user-friendly format by including helpful learning tools throughout the text. Check out the following features to familiarize yourself with the book and help you get the most value out of this text:

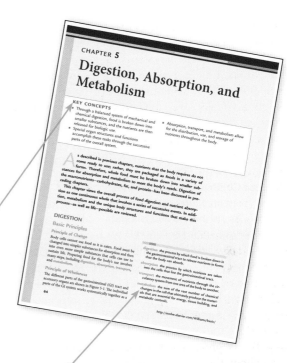

A short list of **Key Concepts** and a brief **Chapter Overview** begin each chapter to immediately draw you into the subject at hand.

Key Terms Boxes throughout the text identify and define key terms important to your understanding and application of the material.

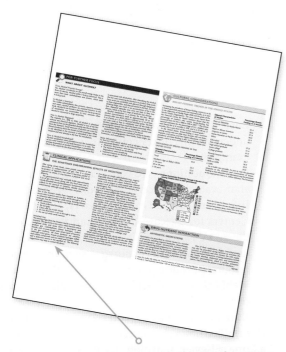

For Further Focus, **Cultural Considerations**, **Clinical Applications**, and **Drug-Nutrient Interaction boxes** take you one step further in the discussion of a given topic, enhancing your understanding of concepts through further exploration or application.

A bulleted **Summary** is included at the end of every chapter to review content highlights and help you see how particular chapters contribute to the book's overall focus.

Critical Thinking Questions and **Chapter Challenge Questions** are presented after each chapter summary for review and analysis and allow you to apply key concepts to patient care problems.

References and **Further Reading and Resources** complete the chapter with lists of relevant citations that provide a wealth of nutrition-related information above and beyond the book's content.

Nutritrac Nutrition Analysis Program, Version 5.0 (Online): The new edition of this popular tool is designed to allow the user to calculate and analyze food intake and energy expenditure, taking the guesswork out of nutrition planning. The new version features comprehensive databases containing more than 5000 foods organized into 18 different categories and more than 175 common/daily recreational, sporting, and occupational activities. The *Personal Profile* feature allows users to enter and edit the intake and output of an unlimited number of individuals, and the *Weight Management Planner* helps outline healthy lifestyles tailored to various personal profiles. In addition to foods and activities, new program features include an ideal body weight (IBW) calculator, a Harris-Benedict calculator to estimate total daily energy needs, and the complete *Exchange Lists for Meal Planning.*

Be sure to visit our two Web sites of interest.

1. An **Evolve** web site has been created specifically for this book at http://evolve.elsevier.com/Williams/basic/ (See the Evolve page at the beginning of this text for more information.) The following exciting features are available:

- **Case Studies** are an integral tool to reinforce your understanding of key concepts and provide real-life examples.
- **Study Questions** give you a chance to practice for your exams and receive immediate feedback.
- **Infant and Child Growth Charts, United States, Centers for Disease Control and Prevention** and the ADA Nutrition Care Process are available as useful handouts to encourage use of these valuable resources inside and outside of the classroom.
- **WebLinks** offer direct links to a wealth of nutrition-related Web sites.

2. A **Nutrition Resource Center** Web site is available at *http://nutrition.elsevier.com* to provide you access to all the Elsevier nutrition texts in one convenient location.

We are pleased that you have included *Williams' Basic Nutrition & Diet Therapy* as a part of your nutrition education. Be sure to check out our Web site at *www.elsevierhealth.com* for all your health science educational needs!

Contents

CHAPTER 1

Food, Nutrition, and Health

KEY CONCEPTS

- Optimal personal and community nutrition are major components of health promotion.
- Certain nutrients in food are essential to our health and well-being.
- Food and nutrient guides help us to plan a balanced diet that is in accordance with our individual needs and goals.

We live in a world of rapidly changing elements, including our environment, food supply, population, and scientific knowledge. Within different environments, our bodies, emotional responses, needs, and goals change. To be realistic within the concepts of change and balance, the study of food, nutrition, and health care must focus on health promotion. Although we may define health and disease in a variety of ways, the primary basis for promoting health and preventing disease must start with a balanced diet and the nutrition it provides. The study of nutrition is of primary importance in the following two ways: it is fundamental for our own health, and it is essential for the health and well-being of our patients and clients.

HEALTH PROMOTION

Basic Definitions

Nutrition and Dietetics

Nutrition is the food people eat and how their bodies use it. Nutrition science comprises the body of scientific knowledge that governs food requirements for maintenance, growth, activity, reproduction, and lactation. Dietetics is the health profession responsible for applying nutrition science to promote human health and treat disease. The registered dietitian (RD), who is also referred to as the *clinical nutrition specialist* or the *public health nutritionist,* is the nutrition authority on the health care team; this health care professional carries the major responsibility of nutrition care for patients and clients.

Health and Wellness

High-quality nutrition is essential to good health throughout life, beginning with prenatal life and continuing through old age. In its simplest terms, the word *health* is defined as the absence of disease. However, life experience shows that the definition of health is much more complex. It must include extensive attention to the roots of health for the meeting of basic needs (e.g., physical, mental, psychologic, and social well-being). This approach recognizes the individual as a whole and relates health to both internal and external environments. The concept of *wellness* broadens this approach one step further. Wellness seeks the full development of potential for all people within their given environments. It implies a balance between activities and goals: work versus leisure, lifestyle choices versus health risks, and personal needs versus others' expectations. The term *wellness* implies a positive dynamic state that motivates a person to seek a higher level of functioning.

National Health Goals

The ongoing wellness movement continues to be a fundamental response to the health care system's emphasis on illness and disease and the rising costs of medical care. Since the 1970s, holistic health and health promotion have focused on lifestyle and personal choice when it comes to helping individuals and families develop plans for maintaining health and wellness. The U.S. national health goals continue to reflect this wellness philosophy. The most recent report in the *Healthy People* series published by the U.S. Department of Health and Human Services, *Healthy People 2020,* continues to focus on the nation's main objective of positive health promotion and disease prevention[1] (Figure 1-1). The guidelines encompass four overarching goals with the ultimate vision of a "society in which all people live long, healthy lives."[1]

A major theme throughout the report is the encouragement of healthy choices in diet, weight control, and other risk factors for disease, especially in the report's specific nutrition objectives. Community health agencies continue to implement these goals and objectives in local, state, public, and private health programs, particularly in areas where malnutrition and poverty exist. Programs such as the Special Supplemental Nutrition Program for Women, Infants, and Children (WIC) and school lunch programs are well established throughout the United States. Each effort recognizes personal nutrition as an integral component of health and health care for all people.

Traditional and Preventive Approaches to Health

The preventive approach to health involves identifying risk factors that increase a person's chances of developing a particular health problem. Knowing these factors, people can choose behaviors that will prevent or minimize their risks for disease. Alternatively, the traditional approach to health only attempts change when symptoms of illness or disease already exist, at which point those who are ill seek a physician to diagnose, treat, and "cure" the condition (see the Drug-Nutrient Interaction box, "Introduction to Drug-Nutrient Interactions"). The traditional approach has little value for lifelong positive health. Major chronic problems (e.g., heart disease, cancer, diabetes) may develop long before signs become apparent.

Importance of a Balanced Diet

Food and Health

Food is a necessity of life. However, many people are only concerned with food insofar as it relieves their hunger or satisfies their appetite and not with whether it supplies their bodies with all of the components of proper nutrition. The six essential nutrients in human nutrition are the following:

1. Carbohydrates
2. Proteins
3. Fats
4. Vitamins
5. Minerals
6. Water

The core practitioners of the health care team (i.e., physician, dietitian, and nurse) are all aware of the important part that food plays in maintaining good health and recovering from illness. Therefore, assessing a patient's nutritional status and identifying his or her nutrition needs are primary activities in the development of a health care plan.

---

health promotion the active engagement in behaviors or programs that advance positive well-being.

nutrition the sum of the processes involved with the intake of nutrients as well as assimilating and using them to maintain body tissue and provide energy; a foundation for life and health.

nutrition science the body of science, developed through controlled research, that relates to the processes involved in nutrition internationally, clinically, and in the community.

dietetics the management of the diet and the use of food; the science concerned with nutrition planning and the preparation of foods.

registered dietitian (RD) a professional dietitian accredited with an academic degree from an undergraduate or graduate study program who has passed required registration examinations administered by the Commission on Dietetic Registration.

health a state of optimal physical, mental, and social well-being; relative freedom from disease or disability.

metabolism the sum of all chemical changes that take place in the body by which it maintains itself and produces energy for its functioning; products of the various reactions are called *metabolites*.

Healthy People 2020

A society in which all people live long, healthy lives

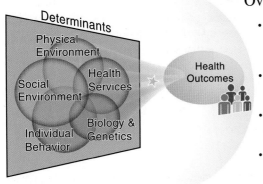

Overarching Goals:

- Attain high quality, longer lives free of preventable disease, disability, injury, and premature death
- Achieve health equity, eliminate disparities, and improve the health of all groups
- Create social and physical environments that promote good health for all
- Promote quality of life, healthy development and healthy behaviors across all life stages

Figure 1-1 Healthy People 2020 **Goals.** (From the U.S. Department of Health and Human Services. *Healthy People 2020*, Washington, DC: U.S. Government Printing Office; 2010.)

DRUG-NUTRIENT INTERACTION

INTRODUCTION TO DRUG-NUTRIENT INTERACTIONS

Part of the traditional approach to medicine is "curing" the condition or disease. This often includes a physician's prescription for a medication to alleviate symptoms or to treat the condition. Drug regimens should be strictly followed. Many medications have potentially dangerous side effects, such as heart arrhythmias, hypertension, dizziness, and tingling in the hands and feet when they are consumed inappropriately.

Some medications may interact with nutrients in food or dietary supplements, thereby creating a drug-nutrient interaction. The presence of food in the stomach may increase or decrease drug absorption, thus potentially enhancing or diminishing the effects of the intended medication. Dietary supplements that contain vitamins and minerals can be especially dangerous if they are consumed at the same time as a drug. Knowing which drugs are influenced by nutrients and how to work with a patient's diet is essential to the development of a complete medical plan.

In the following chapters of this book, look for the Drug-Nutrient Interaction boxes to learn about some of the more common interactions that may be encountered in the health care setting.

Sara Harcourt

Signs of Good Nutrition

A lifetime of good nutrition is evidenced by a well-developed body, the ideal weight for height and body composition (i.e., the ratio of muscle mass to fat mass), and good muscle development. In addition, a healthy person's skin is smooth and clear, the hair is glossy, and the eyes are clear and bright. Appetite, digestion, and elimination are normal. Well-nourished people are more likely to be mentally and physically alert and to have a positive outlook on life. They are also more able to resist infectious diseases as compared with undernourished people. This is particularly important with our current trends of population growth and ever-increasing life expectancy. National vital statistics reports published in 2010 stated that life expectancy in the United States reached a high of 75.4 years for men and 80.4 for women.[2]

FUNCTIONS OF NUTRIENTS IN FOOD

To sustain life, the nutrients in foods must perform the following three basic functions within the body:

1. Provide energy
2. Build tissue
3. Regulate metabolic processes

Metabolism refers to the sum of all body processes that accomplish the basic life-sustaining tasks. Intimate metabolic relations exist among all nutrients and their metabolic products. This is the fundamental principle of *nutrient interaction,* which involves two concepts. First, the individual nutrients have many specific metabolic functions, including primary and supporting roles. Second, no nutrient ever works alone; this key principle of nutrient interaction is demonstrated more clearly in the following chapters. Although the nutrients may be separated for study purposes, remember that they do not exist that way in the human body. They always interact as a dynamic whole to produce and maintain the body.

Energy Sources

Carbohydrates

Dietary carbohydrates (e.g., starches, sugars) provide the body's primary and preferred source of fuel for energy. They also maintain the body's backup store of quick energy as glycogen (see Chapter 2). Human energy is measured in heat units called *kilocalories,* which is abbreviated as *kcalories* or *kcal* (see Chapter 6). Each gram of carbohydrate consumed yields 4 kcal of body energy. In a well-balanced diet, carbohydrates from all sources should provide approximately 45% to 65% of the total kilocalories.

Fats

Dietary fats from both animal and plant sources provide the body's secondary or storage form of energy. This form is more concentrated, yielding 9 kcal for each gram consumed. In a well balanced diet, fats should provide no more than 20% to 35% of the total kilocalories. Approximately two thirds of this amount should be from plant sources, which provide monounsaturated and polyunsaturated fats, and no more than 10% of kcals should come from saturated fat (see Chapter 3).

Proteins

Ideally protein would not be used for energy by the body. Rather, it should be preserved for other critical functions, such as structure, enzyme and hormone production, fluid balance, and so on. However, in the event that necessary energy from carbohydrates and fat is insufficient, the body may draw from dietary or tissue protein to obtain required energy. When this occurs, protein yields 4 kcal per gram. In a well-balanced diet, protein should provide approximately 10% to 35% of the total kilocalories (see Chapter 4).

Thus, the recommended intake of each energy-yielding nutrient, as a percent of total calories, is as follows (Figure 1-2):

- Carbohydrate: 45% to 65%
- Fat: 20% to 35%
- Protein: 10% to 35%

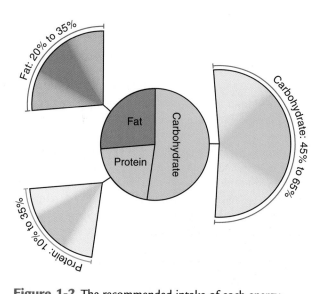

Figure 1-2 The recommended intake of each energy-yielding nutrient as a percentage of total energy intake.

Tissue Building

Proteins

The primary function of protein is tissue building. Dietary protein provides amino acids, which are the building blocks that are necessary for constructing and repairing body tissues (e.g., organs, muscle, cells, blood proteins). Tissue building is a constant process that ensures the growth and maintenance of a strong body structure as well as the creation of vital substances for cellular functions.

glycogen a polysaccharide; the main storage form of carbohydrate in the body, which is stored primarily in the liver and to a lesser extent in muscle tissue.

kilocalorie the general term *calorie* refers to a unit of heat measure, and it is used alone to designate the small calorie; the calorie that is used in nutrition science and the study of metabolism is the large Calorie or kilocalorie, which avoids the use of large numbers in calculations; a kilocalorie, which is composed of 1000 calories, is the measure of heat that is necessary to raise the temperature of 1000 g (1 L) of water by 1° C.

amino acids the nitrogen-bearing compounds that form the structural units of protein; after digestion, amino acids are available for the synthesis of required proteins.

Other Nutrients

Several other nutrients contribute to the building and maintenance of tissues.

Vitamins and Minerals. Vitamins and minerals are nutrients that help to regulate many body processes. An example of the use of a vitamin in tissue building is that of vitamin C in developing collagen. Collagen is the protein found in fibrous tissues such as cartilage, bone matrix, skin, and tendons. Two major minerals, calcium and phosphorus, participate in building and maintaining bone tissue. Another example is the mineral iron, which contributes to building the oxygen carrier hemoglobin in red blood cells. Several other vitamins and minerals are discussed in greater detail in Chapters 7 and 8 with regard to their functions, which include tissue building.

Fatty Acids. Fatty acids, which are derived from fat metabolism, help to build the central fat substance that is necessary in all cell membranes, and they promote the transport of fat-soluble nutrients throughout the body.

Regulation and Control

The multiple chemical processes in the body that are necessary for providing energy and building tissue are carefully regulated and controlled to maintain a constant dynamic balance among all body parts and processes. Several of these regulatory functions involve essential nutrients.

Vitamins

Many vitamins function as coenzyme factors, which are components of cell enzymes, in the governing of chemical reactions during metabolism. For example, this is true for most of the B-complex vitamins.

Minerals

Many minerals also serve as coenzyme factors with enzymes in cell metabolism. For example, cobalt, which is a central constituent of vitamin B_{12} (cobalamin), functions with this vitamin in the synthesis of heme for hemoglobin formation.

Water and Fiber

Water and fiber also function as regulatory agents. In fact, water is the fundamental agent for life itself, providing the essential base for all metabolic processes. The adult body is approximately 50% to 70% water. Dietary fiber helps to regulate the passage of food material through the gastrointestinal tract, and it influences the absorption of nutrients.

NUTRITIONAL STATES

Optimal Nutrition

Optimal nutrition means that a person receives and uses substances obtained from a varied and balanced diet of carbohydrates, fats, proteins, minerals, vitamins, and water in appropriate amounts. The desired amount of each essential nutrient should be balanced to cover variations in health and disease and to provide reserve supplies without unnecessary excesses.

Malnutrition

Malnutrition refers to a condition that is caused by an improper or insufficient diet. Both undernutrition and overnutrition are forms of malnutrition. Dietary surveys have shown that approximately one third of the U.S. population lives on suboptimal diets. That does not necessarily mean that all of these Americans are undernourished. Some people can maintain health on somewhat less than the optimal amounts of various nutrients in a state of borderline nutrition. However, on average, someone who is receiving less than the desired amounts of nutrients has a greater risk for physical illness and compromised immunity as compared with someone who is receiving the appropriate amounts.[3] Such nutritionally deficient people are limited with regard to their physical work capacity, immune system function, and mental activity. They lack the nutritional reserves to meet any added physiologic or metabolic demands from injury or illness or to sustain fetal development during pregnancy or proper growth during childhood. This state may result from poor eating habits or a continuously stressful environment with little or no available food.

Undernutrition

Signs of more serious malnutrition appear when nutritional reserves are depleted and nutrient and energy intake are not sufficient to meet day-to-day needs or added metabolic stress. Many malnourished people live in conditions of poverty or illness. Such conditions influence the health of all involved but especially that of the most vulnerable populations: pregnant women, infants, children, and elderly adults. In the United States, which is one of the wealthiest countries in the world, widespread hunger and malnutrition among the poor still exist, which indicates that food security problems involve urban development issues, economic policies, and more general poverty issues (see the Cultural Considerations box, "Food Insecurity").

CULTURAL CONSIDERATIONS

FOOD INSECURITY

Food insecurity is defined by the U.S. Department of Agriculture as the limited or uncertain availability of nutritious and adequate food. Using this definition, the Food Assistance and Nutrition Research Program of the U.S. Department of Agriculture reported that 17 million households (i.e., 14.6% of all U.S. households) qualified as having food insecurity in 2008. Furthermore, homes with children report double the rate of food insecurity as compared with homes without children (21% and 11.3%, respectively).[1] Many studies document widespread hunger and malnutrition among the poor, especially among the growing number of homeless, including mothers with young children. Such problems can manifest themselves as physical, psychologic, and sociofamilial disturbances in all age groups, with a significant negative impact on health status (including mental health) and the risk of chronic disease. Data from the National Health and Nutrition Examination Study (NHANES) demonstrated an increased incidence of cardio-vascular risk factors such as hypertension and hyperlipidemia among food-insecure adults.[2]

Feeding America, which is the nation's largest organization of emergency food providers, estimated that 14 million children in the United States receive emergency food services each year.[3] Malnourished children are at an increased risk for stunted growth and episodes of infection and disease, which often have lasting effects on their intellectual development. Hunger is a chronic issue (i.e., persisting 8 months or more per year) among most households that report food insecurity. The prevalence of food insecurity is substantially higher among households that are headed by single mothers and in African-American and Hispanic households.[1] A variety of federal and nonfederal programs are available to address hunger issues in all cultural and age groups. The U.S. Department of Agriculture's Food and Nutrition Service provides detailed information about such programs on its Web site at www.fns.usda.gov/fns.

1. Nord M, Andrews M, Carlson S. *Household food security in the United States, 2008 (Economic research report 83).* Alexandria, Va: U.S. Department of Agriculture, Economic Research Services; 2009.
2. Seligman HK, Laraia BA, Kushel MB. Food insecurity is associated with chronic disease among low-income NHANES participants. *J Nutr.* 2010;140:304-310.
3. Mabli J, Cohen R, Potter F, Zhao Z. *Hunger in America 2010; National Report Prepared for Feeding America.* Chicago: Feeding America; 2010.

Malnutrition sometimes occurs in hospitals as well. For example, acute trauma or chronic illness, especially among older people, places added stress on the body, and the daily nutrient and energy intake may be insufficient to meet the needs of these patients.

Overnutrition

Some people are in a state of overnutrition, which results from excess nutrient and energy intake over time. Overnutrition is another form of malnutrition, especially when excess caloric intake produces harmful body weight (i.e., morbid obesity; see Chapter 15). Harmful overnutrition can also occur among people who consistently use excessive (e.g., "megadose") amounts of nutrient supplements, which can result in vitamin or mineral toxicities (see Chapters 7 and 8).

NUTRIENT AND FOOD GUIDES FOR HEALTH PROMOTION

Nutrient Standards

Most of the developed countries of the world have established nutrient standard recommendations. These standards serve as a reference for intake levels of the essential nutrients to meet the known nutrition needs of most healthy population groups. Although these standards are similar in most countries, they vary according to the philosophies of the scientists and practitioners with regard to the purpose and use of such standards. In the United States, these standards are referred to as the *Dietary Reference Intakes (DRIs)*.

U.S. Standards: Dietary Reference Intakes

Since 1941, the Recommended Dietary Allowances (RDAs), which are published by the National Academy of Sciences, have been the authoritative source for setting standards for the minimum amounts of nutrients necessary to protect almost all people against the risk for nutrient deficiency. The U.S. RDA standards were first published during World War II as a guide for planning and obtaining food supplies for national defense and for providing population standards as a goal for good nutrition. These standards are revised and expanded every 5 to 10 years to reflect increasing scientific knowledge and social concerns about nutrition and health.

Both public awareness and research attention have shifted to reflect an increasing emphasis on nutrient requirements for maintaining optimal health within the general population as opposed to only preventing deficiency. This change of emphasis resulted in the DRIs project. The creation of the DRIs involved distinguished

1. Calcium, vitamin D, phosphorous, magnesium, and fluoride
2. Folate and other B vitamins
3. Antioxidants
4. Macronutrients
5. Trace elements
6. Electrolytes and water

U.S. and Canadian scientists, who were divided into six functional panels (Box 1-1) and who have examined thousands of nutrition studies addressing the health benefits of nutrients and the hazards of consuming too much of a nutrient. The working group of nutrition scientists responsible for these standards forms the Food and Nutrition Board of the Institute of Medicine. The DRI recommendations were published over several years in a series of six volumes.[4-9]

The DRIs include recommendations for each gender and age group as well as recommendations for pregnancy and lactation (see the inside front cover of this book). For the first time, excessive amounts of nutrients were identified as tolerable upper intakes. The new DRIs incorporate and expand on the well-established RDAs. The DRIs encompass the following four interconnected categories of nutrient recommendations:

1. *RDA.* This is the daily intake of a nutrient that meets the needs of almost all (i.e., 97.5%) healthy individuals of a specific age and gender. Individuals should use the RDA as a guide to achieve adequate nutrient intake to decrease the risk of chronic disease. RDAs are established only when enough scientific evidence exists about a specific nutrient.
2. *Estimated Average Requirement.* This is the intake level that meets the needs of half of the individuals in a specific group. This quantity is used as the basis for the development of the RDA.
3. *Adequate Intake.* The Adequate Intake is used as a guide when not enough scientific evidence is available to establish the RDA. Both the RDA and the Adequate Intake may be used as goals for individual intake.
4. *Tolerable Upper Intake Level.* This indicator is not a recommended intake. Rather, it sets the maximal intake that is unlikely to pose adverse health risks in almost all healthy individuals. For most nutrients, the Tolerable Upper Intake Level refers to the daily intake from food, fortified food, and nutrient supplements combined.

Other Standards

Historically, Canadian and British standards have been similar to the U.S. standards. In less-developed countries, where factors such as the quality of available protein foods must be considered, individuals look to standards such as those set by the Food and Agriculture Organization and World Health Organization. Nonetheless, all standards provide a guideline to help health care workers who work with a variety of population groups to promote good health and prevent disease through sound nutrition.

Food Guides and Recommendations

To interpret and apply nutrient standards, health care workers need practical food guides to use for nutrition education and food planning with individuals and families. Such tools include the U.S. Department of Agriculture's MyPlate system and the *Dietary Guidelines for Americans.*

MyPlate

The MyPlate food guidance system (Figure 1-3), which was released in June 2011 by the U.S. Department of Agriculture, provides the public with a valuable nutrition education tool. The goal of this food guide is to promote variety, proportionality, moderation, gradual improvements, and physical activity.[10] Participants are encouraged to personalize their own plans via the public Web site www.choosemyplate.gov by entering their age, gender, weight, height, and activity level. The system will create a plan with individualized calorie levels and specific recommendations for serving amounts from each food group. In addition, the MyPlate site provides participants with individualized meal-tracking worksheets, tips, resources, and sample menus as well as access to the Choose MyPlate Tracker, an online dietary and physical activity assessment tool.

Dietary Reference Intakes (DRIs) the nutrient recommendations for each gender and age group that can be used for assessing and planning diets for healthy populations.

Recommended Dietary Allowances (RDAs) the recommended daily allowances of nutrients and energy intake for population groups according to age and gender with defined weight and height.

MyPlate a visual pattern of the current basic five food groups—grains, vegetables, fruits, dairy, and protein—arranged on a plate to indicate proportionate amounts of daily food choices.

choose MyPlate

10 **tips** to a great plate

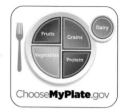

ChooseMyPlate.gov

Making food choices for a healthy lifestyle can be as simple as using these 10 Tips.
Use the ideas in this list to *balance your calories*, to choose foods to *eat more often*, and to cut back on foods to *eat less often*.

1 balance calories
Find out how many calories YOU need for a day as a first step in managing your weight. Go to www.ChooseMyPlate.gov to find your calorie level. Being physically active also helps you balance calories.

2 enjoy your food, but eat less
Take the time to fully enjoy your food as you eat it. Eating too fast or when your attention is elsewhere may lead to eating too many calories. Pay attention to hunger and fullness cues before, during, and after meals. Use them to recognize when to eat and when you've had enough.

3 avoid oversized portions
Use a smaller plate, bowl, and glass. Portion out foods before you eat. When eating out, choose a smaller size option, share a dish, or take home part of your meal.

4 foods to eat more often
Eat more vegetables, fruits, whole grains, and fat-free or 1% milk and dairy products. These foods have the nutrients you need for health—including potassium, calcium, vitamin D, and fiber. Make them the basis for meals and snacks.

5 make half your plate fruits and vegetables
Choose red, orange, and dark-green vegetables like tomatoes, sweet potatoes, and broccoli, along with other vegetables for your meals. Add fruit to meals as part of main or side dishes or as dessert.

6 switch to fat-free or low-fat (1%) milk
They have the same amount of calcium and other essential nutrients as whole milk, but fewer calories and less saturated fat.

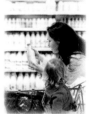

7 make half your grains whole grains
To eat more whole grains, substitute a whole-grain product for a refined product—such as eating whole-wheat bread instead of white bread or brown rice instead of white rice.

8 foods to eat less often
Cut back on foods high in solid fats, added sugars, and salt. They include cakes, cookies, ice cream, candies, sweetened drinks, pizza, and fatty meats like ribs, sausages, bacon, and hot dogs. Use these foods as occasional treats, not everyday foods.

9 compare sodium in foods
Use the Nutrition Facts label to choose lower sodium versions of foods like soup, bread, and frozen meals. Select canned foods labeled "low sodium," "reduced sodium," or "no salt added."

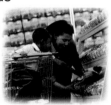

10 drink water instead of sugary drinks
Cut calories by drinking water or unsweetened beverages. Soda, energy drinks, and sports drinks are a major source of added sugar, and calories, in American diets.

USDA
Center for Nutrition
Policy and Promotion

DG TipSheet No. 1
June 2011
USDA is an equal opportunity provider and employer.

Go to www.ChooseMyPlate.gov for more information.

Figure 1-3 MyPlate food guidance system recommendations. (From the U.S. Department of Agriculture, Center for Nutrition Policy and Promotion. *Choose MyPlate mini-poster* (website): www.choosemyplate.gov. Accessed August 23, 2011.)

Key Recommendations

BALANCING CALORIES TO MANAGE WEIGHT

- Prevent and/or reduce overweight and obesity through improved eating and physical activity behaviors.
- Control total calorie intake to manage body weight. For people who are overweight or obese, this will mean consuming fewer calories from foods and beverages.
- Increase physical activity and reduce time spent in sedentary behaviors.
- Maintain appropriate calorie balance during each stage of life—childhood, adolescence, adulthood, pregnancy and breastfeeding, and older age.

FOODS AND FOOD COMPONENTS TO REDUCE

- Reduce daily sodium intake to less than 2,300 milligrams (mg) and further reduce intake to 1,500 mg among persons who are 51 and older and those of any age who are African American or have hypertension, diabetes, or chronic kidney disease. The 1,500 mg recommendation applies to about half of the U.S. population, including children, and the majority of adults.
- Consume less than 10 percent of calories from saturated fatty acids by replacing them with monounsaturated and polyunsaturated fatty acids.
- Consume less than 300 mg per day of dietary cholesterol.
- Keep trans fatty acid consumption as low as possible by limiting foods that contain synthetic sources of trans fats, such as partially hydrogenated oils, and by limiting other solid fats.
- Reduce the intake of calories from solid fats and added sugars.
- Limit the consumption of foods that contain refined grains, especially refined grain foods that contain solid fats, added sugars, and sodium.
- If alcohol is consumed, it should be consumed in moderation—up to one drink per day for women and two drinks per day for men—and only by adults of legal drinking age.[1]

FOODS AND NUTRIENTS TO INCREASE

Individuals should meet the following recommendations as part of a healthy eating pattern while staying within their calorie needs.

- Increase vegetable and fruit intake.
- Eat a variety of vegetables, especially dark-green and red and orange vegetables and beans and peas.
- Consume at least half of all grains as whole grains. Increase whole-grain intake by replacing refined grains with whole grains.
- Increase intake of fat-free or low-fat milk and milk products, such as milk, yogurt, cheese, or fortified soy beverages.[2]
- Choose a variety of protein foods, which include seafood, lean meat and poultry, eggs, beans and peas, soy products, and unsalted nuts and seeds.
- Increase the amount and variety of seafood consumed by choosing seafood in place of some meat and poultry.
- Replace protein foods that are higher in solid fats with choices that are lower in solid fats and calories and/or are sources of oils.
- Use oils to replace solid fats where possible.
- Choose foods that provide more potassium, dietary fiber, calcium, and vitamin D, which are nutrients of concern in American diets. These foods include vegetables, fruits, whole grains, and milk and milk products.

BUILDING HEALTHY EATING PATTERNS

- Select an eating pattern that meets nutrient needs over time at an appropriate calorie level.
- Account for all foods and beverages consumed and assess how they fit within a total healthy eating pattern.
- Follow food safety recommendations when preparing and eating foods to reduce the risk of foodborne illnesses.[5]

Recommendations for specific population groups

Women capable of becoming pregnant[3]

- Choose foods that supply heme iron, which is more readily absorbed by the body, additional iron sources, and enhancers of iron absorption such as vitamin C–rich foods.
- Consume 400 micrograms (mcg) per day of synthetic folic acid (from fortified foods and/or supplements) in addition to food forms of folate from a varied diet.[4]

Women who are pregnant or breastfeeding[3]

- Consume 8 to 12 ounces of seafood per week from a variety of seafood types.
- Due to their high methyl mercury content, limit white (albacore) tuna to 6 ounces per week and do not eat the following four types of fish: tilefish, shark, swordfish, and king mackerel.
- If pregnant, take an iron supplement, as recommended by an obstetrician or other health care provider.

Individuals ages 50 years and older

- Consume foods fortified with vitamin B_{12}, such as fortified cereals, or dietary supplements.

1. See Chapter 3, Foods and Food Components to Reduce, for additional recommendations on alcohol consumption and specific population groups. There are many circumstances when people should not drink alcohol.
DIETARY GUIDELINES FOR AMERICANS, 2010

2. Fortified soy beverages have been marketed as "soymilk," a product name consumers could see in supermarkets and consumer materials. However, FDA's regulations do not contain provisions for the use of the term soymilk. Therefore, in this document, the term "fortified soy beverage" includes products that may be marketed as soymilk.
3. Includes adolescent girls.
4. "Folic acid" is the synthetic form of the nutrient; whereas, "folate" is the form found naturally in foods.
5. Clean hands, food contact surfaces, and fruits and vegetables. Washing raw poultry, beef, pork, lamb, or veal before cooking it is not recommended. Bacteria in raw meat and poultry juices can be spread to other foods, utensils, and surfaces resulting in cross-contamination.
DIETARY GUIDELINES FOR AMERICANS, 2010

Figure 1-4 Summary of the *Dietary Guidelines for Americans, 2010.* (From the U.S. Department of Agriculture, U.S. Department of Health and Human Services. *Dietary Guidelines for Americans, 2010.* Washington, DC: U.S. Government Printing Office; 2010.)

Dietary Guidelines for Americans

The *Dietary Guidelines for Americans* were issued as a result of growing public concern that began in the 1960s and the subsequent Senate investigations studying hunger and nutrition in the United States. These guidelines are based on developing alarm about chronic health problems in an aging population and a changing food environment. An updated statement is issued every 5 years, but recent review by expert committees has led to minimal changes over the past decade. This publication encompasses a comprehensive evaluation of the scientific evidence regarding diet and health in a report jointly issued by the U.S. Department of Agriculture and the U.S. Department of Health and Human Services.[11]

Figure 1-4 shows the four key recommendations of the *Dietary Guidelines for Americans*. The current guidelines continue to serve as a useful general guide for promoting dietary and lifestyle choices that reduce the risk for chronic disease. Although no guidelines can guarantee health or well-being and although people differ widely with regard to their food needs and preferences, these general statements are meant to help evaluate food habits and move toward general improvements. Good food habits that are based on moderation and variety can help to build healthy bodies.

The current DRIs, MyPlate guidelines, and *Dietary Guidelines for Americans* are all in sync with one another and supported by scientific literature, and they reflect sound guidelines for a healthy diet.

Other Recommendations

Organizations such as the American Cancer Society and the American Heart Association also have their own independent dietary guidelines. In most cases, the guidelines set by various national organizations are modeled after the *Dietary Guidelines for Americans*. This may seem a bit repetitive, but the difference is the added emphasis on the prevention of specific chronic diseases, such as heart disease and cancer.

Individual Needs

Person-Centered Care

Regardless of the type of food guide or recommendations used, health care professionals must remember that food patterns vary with individual needs, tastes, habits, living situations, and energy demands. People who eat nutritionally balanced meals spread evenly throughout the day can usually work more efficiently and sustain a more even energy supply.

Changing Food Environment

Our food environment has been rapidly changing in recent years. American food habits may have deteriorated in some ways, with a heightened reliance on fast, processed, and prepackaged foods. Despite a plentiful food supply, surveys give evidence of malnutrition in all segments of the population. Nurses and other health care professionals have an important responsibility to observe patients' food intake carefully. However, in general, Americans are recognizing the relationship between food and health. Even fast-food restaurants are beginning to respond to their customers' desires for lower-fat, health-conscious alternatives to the traditional fare. Other chain, family, and university restaurants are developing and testing similar patterns in their new menu items. More than ever, Americans are being selective about what they eat. Guided by the U.S. Food and Drug Administration's nutrition labels, shoppers' choices indicate an increased awareness of nutritional values.

SUMMARY

- Good food and key nutrients are essential to life and health.
- In our changing world, an emphasis on health promotion and disease prevention by reducing health risks has become a primary health goal.
- The importance of a balanced diet for meeting this goal via the functioning of its component nutrients is fundamental. Functions of nutrients include providing energy, building tissue, and regulating metabolic processes.

- Malnutrition exists in the United States in both overnutrition and undernutrition states.
- Food guides that help with the planning of an individualized healthy diet include the DRIs, MyPlate, and the *Dietary Guidelines for Americans*.
- A person-centered approach is best when developing individual dietary recommendations that take personal factors into account.

CRITICAL THINKING QUESTIONS

1. What is the current U.S. national health goal? Define this goal in terms of health, wellness, and the differences between traditional and preventive approaches to health.
2. Why is a balanced diet important? List and describe some signs of good nutrition.
3. What are the three basic functions of foods and their nutrients? Describe the general roles of nutrients with regard to the following: (1) the main nutrients for each function and (2) other contributing nutrients.
4. With regard to both purpose and use, compare the DRIs with the MyPlate food guidelines.
5. Use the MyPlate guidelines to plan a day's food pattern for a selected person in accordance with the *Dietary Guidelines for Americans*.

CHAPTER CHALLENGE QUESTIONS

True-False

Write the correct statement for each statement that is false.

1. *True or False:* The diet-planning tool MyPlate is available only to health care professionals.
2. *True or False:* The focus of the DRIs is to promote health as opposed to exclusively centering on preventing disease.
3. *True or False:* Malnutrition is not a problem in the United States.

Multiple Choice

1. Nutrients are
   a. chemical elements or compounds in foods that have specific metabolic functions within the body.
   b. whole foods that are necessary for good health.
   c. exclusively energy-yielding compounds.
   d. nourishing foods that are used to cure certain illnesses.

2. All nutrients needed by the body
   a. must be obtained by specific food combinations.
   b. must be obtained by vitamin or mineral supplements.
   c. have only one function and use in the body.
   d. are supplied by a variety of foods in many different combinations.

3. All people throughout life, as indicated by the DRIs, need
   a. the same nutrients in varying amounts.
   b. the same amount of nutrients in any state of health.
   c. the same nutrients at any age in the same amounts.
   d. different nutrients in varying amounts.

⊖volve **Please refer to the Students' Resource section of this text's Evolve Web site for additional study resources.**

REFERENCES

1. U.S. Department of Health and Human Services. *Healthy people 2020*. Washington, DC: U.S. Government Printing Office; 2010.
2. Xu J, Kochanek KD, Murphy SL, Tejada-Vera B, Division of Vital Statistics. *Deaths: final data for 2007*. Hyattsville, Md: National Center for Health Statistics; 2010.
3. Hughes S, Kelly P. Interactions of malnutrition and immune impairment, with specific reference to immunity against parasites. *Parasite Immunol*. 2006;28(11):577-588.
4. Food and Nutrition Board, Institute of Medicine. *Dietary reference intakes for calcium, phosphorous, magnesium, vitamin D, and fluoride*. Washington, DC: National Academies Press; 1997.
5. Food and Nutrition Board, Institute of Medicine. *Dietary reference intakes for thiamin, riboflavin, niacin, vitamin B6, folate, vitamin B12, pantothenic acid, biotin, and choline*. Washington, DC: National Academies Press; 2000.
6. Food and Nutrition Board, Institute of Medicine. *Dietary reference intakes for water, potassium, sodium, chloride, and sulfate*. Washington, DC: National Academies Press; 2004.
7. Food and Nutrition Board, Institute of Medicine. *Dietary reference intakes for vitamin C, vitamin E, selenium, and carotenoids*. Washington, DC: National Academies Press; 2000.
8. Food and Nutrition Board, Institute of Medicine. *Dietary reference intakes for vitamin A, vitamin K, arsenic, boron, chromium, copper, iodine, iron, manganese, molybdenum, nickel, silicon, vanadium, and zinc*. Washington, DC: National Academies Press; 2001.
9. Food and Nutrition Board, Institute of Medicine. *Dietary reference intakes for energy, carbohydrate, fiber, fat, fatty acids, cholesterol, protein, and amino acids*. Washington, DC: National Academies Press; 2002.
10. U.S. Department of Agriculture, Center for Nutrition Policy and Promotion. *USDA's myplate home page* (website): www.choosemyplate.gov. Accessed August 23, 2011.
11. U.S. Department of Agriculture, U.S. Department of Health and Human Services. *Dietary guidelines for Americans, 2010*. Washington, DC: U.S. Government Printing Office; 2010.

FURTHER READING AND RESOURCES

The following organizations are key sources of up-to-date information and research regarding nutrition. Each site has a unique focus and may be helpful for keeping abreast of current topics.

Academy of Nutrition and Dietetics. www.eatright.org

American Society for Nutrition. www.nutrition.org

Dietary Guidelines for Americans. www.health.gov/dietaryguidelines

Food and Agriculture Organization of the United Nations. www.fao.org

Healthy People 2020. http://healthypeople.gov/2020/

National Research Council (National Academies of Science). http://sites.nationalacademies.org/NRC/index.htm

Society for Nutrition Education and Behavior. www.sne.org

USDA Choose My Plate. www.choosemyplate.gov

World Health Organization. www.who.int

Bachman JL, Reedy J, Subar AF, Krebs-Smith SM. Sources of food group intakes among the US population, 2001-2002. *J Am Diet Assoc.* 2008;108(5):804-814.
Despite substantial research and efforts to make recommendations known, Americans do not eat appropriate ratios of food from the recommended food groups. Instead, the average person consumes excess fat and sugar throughout the day.

Reedy J, Krebs-Smith SM. A comparison of food-based recommendations and nutrient values of three food guides: USDA's mypyramid, NHLBI's dietary approaches to stop hypertension eating plan, and Harvard's healthy eating pyramid. *J Am Diet Assoc.* 2008;108(3):522-528.
The authors compare three food guide systems that are regularly referred to in the United States. Although the research used for the basis of each of the three guides varied, the general recommendations are the same.

CHAPTER 2

Carbohydrates

KEY CONCEPTS

- Carbohydrate foods provide practical energy sources because of their wide availability, relatively low cost, and excellent storage capabilities.

- Carbohydrate structures vary from simple to complex, thus providing both quick and extended energy for the body.
- Dietary fiber, which is an indigestible carbohydrate, serves separately as a regulatory agent within the gastrointestinal tract.

As discussed in Chapter 1, key nutrients in food sustain life and promote health. The unique use of nutrients provides the body with three essential elements for life: (1) energy to do its work; (2) building materials to maintain its form and functions; and (3) control agents to regulate these processes efficiently. These three basic life and health functions of nutrients are closely related, and it is important to remember that no nutrient ever works alone.

This chapter looks specifically at the body's primary fuel source: carbohydrates. Carbohydrates are plentiful in the food supply, and they are an important contribution to a well-balanced diet. Recent controversy surrounding the use, abuse, and misunderstanding of this critical macronutrient should be better interpreted after evaluating its functions within the body.

NATURE OF CARBOHYDRATES

Relation to Energy

Basic Fuel Source

Energy is necessary for life. It is the power that an organism requires to do work. Any energy system must first have a basic fuel supply. In the Earth's energy system, vast energy resources from the sun enable plants, through photosynthesis, to transform solar energy into carbohydrate, which is the stored fuel form in plants. The human body can rapidly break down carbohydrates (i.e., sugars and starches), and they provide the major source of energy that is measured in calories.

Throughout this text, the term *energy* is used interchangeably with the terms *calorie, kilocalorie,* and *kcal* (see the definition of *kilocalorie* in Chapter 1). Our bodies need energy to survive. Both involuntary (e.g., heart, lung function) and voluntary actions (e.g., walking, talking) require energy, and that energy is derived from the digestion and metabolism of food.

Energy-Production System

A successful energy system, whether a living organism or a machine, must be able to do the following three things to produce energy from a fuel source:

1. Change the basic fuel to a refined fuel that the machine is designed to use
2. Carry this refined fuel to the places that need it
3. Burn this refined fuel in the special equipment set up at these places

The body easily does these three things more efficiently than any manmade machine. It digests its basic fuel, carbohydrate, thereby releasing glucose. The body then absorbs and, through blood circulation, carries this refined fuel to cells that need it. Glucose is burned in the specific and intricate equipment in these cells, and energy in the form of adenosine triphosphate is released through the process of cell metabolism. Because the human body can rapidly digest the starches and sugars that are eaten to yield energy, carbohydrates are considered quick-energy foods.

Dietary Importance

Practical reasons also exist for the large quantities of carbohydrates found in diets all over the world. First, carbohydrates are widely available and easily grown (e.g., grains, legumes, vegetables, fruits). In some countries, carbohydrate foods make up almost the entire diet. Second, carbohydrates are relatively low in cost as compared with many other food items. Third, carbohydrate foods are easily stored. They can be kept in dry storage for relatively long periods without spoilage, and modern processing and packaging can extend the shelf life of carbohydrate products for years.

The U.S. Department of Agriculture regularly surveys food intake. These reports indicate that approximately half (49.3%) of the total kilocalories in the typical American diet comes from carbohydrates. The daily intake of grain products by Americans accounts for 39.8% of total carbohydrate kilocalories, and almost as many carbohydrate kilocalories (37.3%) come from added sugars and sweeteners, with the remainder coming from dairy, fruit, and vegetable products.[1] It is worth noting that the consumption of whole grains has increased and the intake of refined sugar has decreased slightly since 1970; this is an overall positive change.

Classes of Carbohydrates

The word *carbohydrate* is derived from the chemical nature of the substance. A carbohydrate is composed of carbon (C), hydrogen (H), and oxygen (O). Its abbreviated name, *CHO,* is the combination of the chemical symbols of its three components. The term *saccharide* is used as a carbohydrate class name, and it comes from the Latin word *saccharum,* which means "sugar." Carbohydrates are classified according to the number of sugar (or saccharide) units that make up their structure: *mono*saccharides have one sugar unit; *di*saccharides have two sugar units; and *poly*saccharides have many sugar units. Monosaccharides and disaccharides are small, simple structures of only one- and two-sugar units; thus, they are referred to as *simple carbohydrates*. However, polysaccharides are large, complex compounds of many saccharide units in long chains; thus, they are called *complex carbohydrates*. For example, starch, which is the most significant polysaccharide in human nutrition, is composed of many coiled and branching chains in a treelike structure. Each of the multiple branching chains is composed of 24 to 30 units

of glucose, which gradually split off during digestion to supply a steady source of energy over time. Table 2-1 summarizes these classes of carbohydrates.

Monosaccharides

The three single sugars in nutrition are glucose, fructose, and galactose. Monosaccharides, which are the building blocks for all carbohydrates, require no digestion. They are quickly absorbed from the intestine into the bloodstream and transported to the liver. Energy demands will determine if the monosaccharides are then used for immediate energy or stored as glycogen for later use.

Glucose. The basic single sugar in human metabolism is glucose, which is the form of sugar circulating in the blood. It is the primary fuel for cells. Glucose, a moderately sweet sugar, usually is not found as such in the diet, except in corn syrup or processed food items. The body supply of glucose mainly comes from the digestion of starch. Glucose is also called *dextrose* to denote the structure of the molecule (i.e., six carbons).

Fructose. Fructose is primarily found in fruits (from which it gets its name) and in honey. Although honey is sometimes thought of as a sugar substitute, it is a sugar itself; therefore, it cannot be considered a substitute. The amount of fructose found in fruits depends on the degree of ripeness. As a fruit ripens, some of its stored starch turns to sugar. Fructose is the sweetest of the simple sugars.

---

photosynthesis the process by which plants that contain chlorophyll are able to manufacture carbohydrate by combining carbon dioxide and water; sunlight is used as energy, and chlorophyll is a catalyst.

saccharide the chemical name for sugar molecules; may occur as single molecules in monosaccharides (glucose, fructose, galactose), two molecules in disaccharides (sucrose, lactose, maltose), or multiple molecules in polysaccharides (starch, dietary fiber, glycogen).

simple carbohydrates sugars with a simple structure of one or two single-sugar (saccharide) units; a monosaccharide is composed of one sugar unit, and a disaccharide is composed of two sugar units.

complex carbohydrates large complex molecules of carbohydrates composed of many sugar units (polysaccharides); the complex forms of dietary carbohydrates are starch, which is digestible and provides a major energy source, and dietary fiber, which is indigestible (humans lack the necessary enzymes) and thus provides important bulk in the diet.

glycogen a complex carbohydrate found in animal tissue that is composed of many glucose units.

TABLE 2-1 **SUMMARY OF CARBOHYDRATE CLASSES**

Chemical Class Name	Class Members	Sources
Monosaccharides (single sugars, simple carbohydrates)	Glucose (dextrose)	Corn syrup (commonly used in processed foods)
	Fructose	Fruits, honey
	Galactose	Lactose (milk)
Disaccharides (double sugars, simple carbohydrates)	Sucrose	Table sugar (sugar cane, sugar beets)
	Lactose	Milk
	Maltose	Molasses
		Starch digestion, intermediate
		Sweetener in food products
Polysaccharides (multiple sugars, complex carbohydrates)	Starch	Grains and grain products (cereal, bread, crackers, baked goods)
		Rice, corn, bulgur
		Legumes
		Potatoes and other vegetables
	Glycogen	Storage form of carbohydrate in animal tissue (not a dietary source)

High-fructose corn syrups, which are manufactured by changing the glucose in cornstarch into fructose, are heavily used in processed food products, canned and frozen fruits, and soft drinks. These syrups are inexpensive sweeteners, and contribute to increased sugar intake in the United States. The per-capita consumption of high-fructose corn syrup increased from 0.12 tsp daily in 1970 to 11.18 tsp daily in 2008[2] (Figure 2-1).

Galactose. Galactose is not usually found as a free monosaccharide in the diet; rather, it is a product of lactose (milk sugar) digestion.

Disaccharides

Disaccharides are simple double sugars that are composed of two single-sugar units linked together. The three disaccharides that are important in human nutrition are sucrose, lactose, and maltose.

Sucrose = Glucose + Fructose

Lactose = Glucose + Galactose

. Maltose = Glucose + Glucose

Sucrose. Sucrose is common table sugar. Its two single-sugar units are glucose and fructose. Sucrose is used in the form of granulated, powdered, or brown sugar, and it is made from sugar cane or sugar beets. Molasses, which is a by-product of sugar production, is also a form of

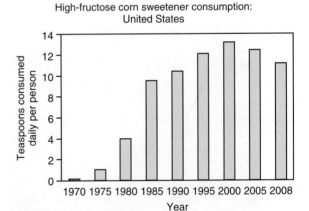

High-fructose corn sweetener consumption: United States

Figure 2-1 High-fructose corn sweetener: per capita consumption adjusted for loss. (Data from the U.S. Department of Agriculture, Economic Research Service. *High fructose corn sweetener [HFCS]: per capita consumption adjusted for loss* (website): www.ers.usda.gov/Data/FoodConsumption/FoodGuideSpreadsheets.htm#sugar. Accessed March 17, 2010.)

sucrose. When people speak of sugar in the diet, they usually mean sucrose.

Lactose. The sugar in milk, which is formed in mammary glands, is lactose. Its two single-sugar units are glucose and galactose. Lactose is the only common sugar that is not found in plants. It is less soluble and less sweet than sucrose. Lactose remains in the intestine longer than other sugars, and it encourages the growth of certain useful bacteria. Cow's milk contains 4.8% lactose, and human milk contains 7% lactose. Because lactose promotes the absorption of calcium and phosphorus, the presence of all three nutrients in milk is a fortunate circumstance.

Maltose. Maltose is not usually found as such in the diet. It is derived within the body from the intermediate digestive breakdown of starch. Because starch is made up entirely of many single-glucose units, the two single-sugar units that compose maltose are both glucose. Synthetically derived maltose is used as a sweetener in various processed foods.

Polysaccharides

Polysaccharides are complex carbohydrates that are composed of many single-sugar units. The important polysaccharides in nutrition include starch, glycogen, and dietary fiber.

Starch. Starches are by far the most significant polysaccharides in the diet. They are found in grains, legumes, and other vegetables and in some fruits in minute amounts. Starches are more complex in structure than simple sugars, so they break down more slowly and supply energy over a longer period of time. For starch to be used more promptly by the body, the outer membrane can be broken down by grinding or cooking. Cooking starch improves its flavor and also softens and ruptures the starch cells, thereby making digestion easier. Starch mixtures thicken when cooked, because the portion that encases the starch granules has a gel-like quality that thickens the starch mixture in the same way that pectin causes jelly to set.

Starch is the most important dietary carbohydrate worldwide. The Dietary Reference Intakes (DRIs; see Chapter 1) recommend that 45% to 65% of total kilocalories consumed come from carbohydrates, with a greater portion of that intake coming from complex carbohydrates.[3] For countries in which starch is the staple food, carbohydrates make up an even higher proportion of the diet. The major food sources of starch (Figure 2-2) include grains in the form of cereal, pasta, crackers, bread, and other baked goods; legumes in the form of beans and peas; potatoes, rice, corn, and bulgur; and other vegetables, especially of the root variety.

The term *whole grain* is used for food products such as flours, breads, or cereals that are produced from unrefined grain. Unrefined grains retain the outer bran layers, the inner germ, and the endosperm (Figure 2-3) and thus their nutrients (i.e., dietary fiber, vitamins, and minerals). *Enriched grains* are refined grain products to which some

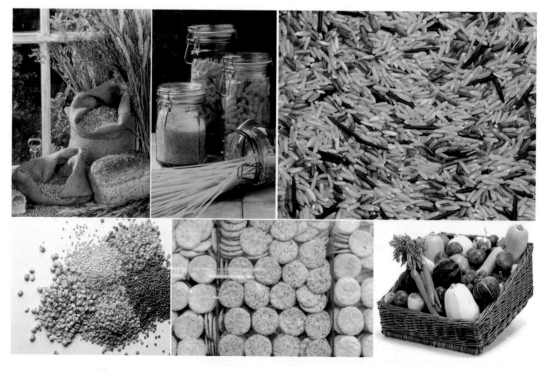

Figure 2-2 Complex carbohydrate foods. (Copyright JupiterImages Corp.)

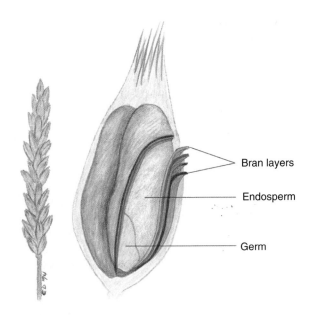

Figure 2-3 Kernel of wheat showing bran layers, endosperm, and germ. (Courtesy Eileen Draper.)

nutrients that were removed during the refining process—usually minerals (e.g., iron) and vitamins (e.g., A, C, D, thiamin, riboflavin, niacin)—have been added back. Ready-to-eat breakfast cereals usually contain additional nutrients such as vitamins D, E, B_6, and folic acid as well as the minerals phosphorus, magnesium, and zinc. These cereals, which are a favorite breakfast item for children, have become a major source of vitamin and mineral intake in the United States.

Glycogen. Glycogen is not a significant source of carbohydrate in the diet. Rather, it is a carbohydrate that is formed within the body's tissues, and it is crucial to the body's metabolism and energy balance. Glycogen is found in the liver and muscles, where it is constantly recycled (i.e., broken down to form glucose for immediate energy needs and synthesized for storage). These small stores of glycogen help to sustain normal blood glucose during short-term fasting periods (e.g., sleep), and they provide immediate fuel for muscle action. These reserves also protect cells from depressed metabolic function and injury. The process of blood glucose regulation with regard to glycogen breakdown is discussed in greater detail in Chapter 20.

Dietary Fiber. Human beings lack the necessary enzymes to digest dietary fiber; therefore, these polysaccharides do not have a direct energy value like other carbohydrates. However, their inability to be digested makes them important dietary assets. Increasing attention has focused on the beneficial relationship between fiber and disease prevention (especially cardiovascular disease and

---

BOX 2-1 **SUMMARY OF SOLUBLE AND INSOLUBLE FIBERS**

Insoluble
Cellulose
Most hemicelluloses
Lignin

Soluble
Gums
Mucilages
Algal polysaccharides
Most pectins

---

gastrointestinal problems) as well as the management of diabetes.[4-7]

As a means of simplification, dietary fiber is usually divided into two groups on the basis of solubility. Cellulose, lignin, and most hemicelluloses are not soluble in water. The rest of the dietary fibers (i.e., most pectins and other polysaccharides [e.g., gums, mucilages]) are water soluble. These two classes of dietary fiber are listed in Box 2-1. The looser physical structure and greater water-holding capacity of gums, mucilages, pectins, and algal polysaccharides (i.e., those derived from seaweed) partly account for their greater water solubility. Recommendations for specific types of fiber to consume often are based on the water-solubility distinction. Soluble fiber is noted for its ability to bind bile acids and ultimately lower blood cholesterol levels. Alternatively, insoluble fiber is recommended for relief from constipation. The types of dietary fiber that are important in human nutrition are described later in this chapter.

Cellulose. Cellulose is the chief component of cell walls in plants. It remains undigested in the gastrointestinal tract, and it adds important bulk to the diet. This bulk helps to move the food mass along, it stimulates normal muscle action in the intestine, and it forms feces for the elimination of waste products. The main sources of cellulose are the stems and leaves of vegetables and the coverings of seeds and grains. Within the same area of the plant, phosphorus is stored in the form of phytic acid; this compound is undigested in humans because of the lack of a necessary enzyme (phytase). Phytic acid is a strong chelator of important minerals (see the Drug-Nutrient Interaction box, "Phytic Acid and Mineral Absorption").

Lignin. Lignin, which is the only noncarbohydrate type of dietary fiber, is a large compound that forms the

---

chelator a ligand that binds to a metal to form a metal complex.

DRUG-NUTRIENT INTERACTION

PHYTIC ACID AND MINERAL ABSORPTION

Some compounds that are naturally found in food bind minerals, thereby making them unavailable for absorption. Phytic acid is one such compound, and it is found in legumes, wheat bran, and seeds. Iron also is naturally found in these foods, but, because of the phytic acid interference, as little as 2% of the available iron is absorbed.

A diet that consists of high-fiber foods that contain phytic acid and a low intake of iron-rich foods (e.g., meat, poultry) may exacerbate iron deficiency. This can especially be a problem in the developing world.[1]

In the United States and other developed nations, iron deficiency is rarely caused by this alone. However, iron deficiency is still common among pregnant and premenopausal women. If the anemia is severe enough, a physician may prescribe an iron supplement. The intake of foods that contain high amounts of phytic acid with the supplement would inhibit iron absorption just as it would if the iron were part of the food.

Phytic acid binds to other minerals that have a similar charge as iron, including calcium, magnesium, and zinc. Calcium supplements are often prescribed for those who may be losing bone mass (e.g., postmenopausal women) or for those who do not get enough calcium in the diet (e.g., teens, the elderly). Food sources of phytic acid that are eaten with calcium supplements may inhibit absorption. When recommending that patients take an iron or calcium supplement, also advise them to take the supplement with foods that do not contain phytate.

Sara Harcourt

1. World Health Organization; Centers for Disease Control and Prevention; de Benoist B, McLean E, Egli I, Cogswell M, editors. *Worldwide prevalence of anaemia 1993-2005: WHO Global Database on Anaemia* (website): http://whqlibdoc.who.int/publications/2008/9789241596657_eng.pdf. Accessed August 29, 2011.

TABLE 2-2 **SUMMARY OF DIETARY FIBER CLASSES**

Dietary Fiber Class	Source	Function
Cellulose	Main cell wall constituent of plants (stalks and leaves of vegetables; outer coverings of seeds, such as are found in whole grains)	Holds water; reduces elevated colonic intraluminal pressure
Noncellulose polysaccharides		Slow gastric emptying; provide fermentable material for colonic bacteria with the production of gas and volatile fatty acids; bind bile acids and cholesterol
Gums and mucilages	Secretions of plants and seeds (oats, legumes, barley)	
Algal polysaccharides	Algae, seaweeds	
Pectin substances	Intercellular plant material (fruit)	
Hemicellulose	Cell-wall plant material (bran, whole grains)	Holds water and increases stool bulk; reduces elevated colonic pressure; binds bile acids
Lignin	Woody part of plants (broccoli stems; fruits with edible seeds, such as strawberries and flaxseeds)	Antioxidant; binds bile acids, cholesterol, and metals

woody part of certain plants. It binds the cellulose fibers in plants, thereby giving added strength and stiffness to plant cell walls. Although it is an insoluble fiber, it also combines with bile acids and cholesterol in the human intestine to prevent their absorption.

Noncellulose Polysaccharides. Hemicellulose, pectins, gums, mucilages, and algal substances are noncellulose polysaccharides. They absorb water and swell to a larger bulk, thus slowing the emptying of the food mass from the stomach, binding bile acids (including cholesterol)[8] in the intestine, and preventing spastic colon pressure by providing bulk for normal muscle action. Noncellulose polysaccharides also provide fermentation material on which colon bacteria can work.

Table 2-2 provides a summary of these dietary fiber classes along with the sources and functions of each.

In general, the food groups that provide needed dietary fiber include whole grains, legumes, vegetables, and fruits with as much of their skin remaining as possible. Whole grains provide a special natural "package" of both the complex carbohydrate starch and the fiber in its coating. In addition, whole grains contain an abundance of vitamins and minerals (see the Clinical Applications box, "Case Study: Identifying Carbohydrates and Fiber").

Many health organizations have recommended increasing the intake of complex carbohydrates in general and dietary fiber in particular (see the For Further Focus box, "Fiber: What's All the Fuss About?").[3,9] The Food and Nutrition Board of the Institute of Medicine has always indicated that a desirable fiber intake should not be exclusively achieved by adding concentrated fiber supplements to the diet. Instead, the recommendations are to eat a high-fiber diet that is rich in whole grains, fruits, vegetables, and legumes, which also provide essential vitamins and minerals. The recommended daily intake of fiber for men and women who are 50 years old or younger is 38 and 25 g/day, respectively. The DRIs are reduced to 30 and 21 g/day for men and women who are older than 50 years of age.[3] This intake requires the consistent use of whole grains, legumes, vegetables, fruits, seeds, and nuts. Unfortunately, the average American does not consume the recommended servings of whole grains, vegetables, and fruit on a daily basis. In fact, results from the National Health and Nutrition Examination Survey (NHANES) revealed that only 40% of Americans meet the recommended servings of fruits and vegetables per day.[10] Another study found that only 8% of the U.S. population consumes the recommended three servings per day of whole grains.[11] The dietary fiber content of some commonly used foods is provided in Table 2-3 and Appendix B.

As with many things in nutrition, too much of a good thing also can be problematic. Sudden increases in fiber intake can result in uncomfortable gas, bloating, and constipation. Fiber intake should be gradually increased (along with water intake) to an appropriate amount for the individual. In addition, excessive amounts of dietary fiber can trap (by chelation) small amounts of minerals and prevent their absorption in the gastrointestinal tract. This function of fiber is beneficial when trapping or binding bile acids, but it may compromise nutritional status if fiber intake greatly exceeds the recommendations to the point of reducing mineral absorption.

CLINICAL APPLICATIONS

CASE STUDY: IDENTIFYING CARBOHYDRATES AND FIBER

A patient comes to you for dietary analysis. He is trying to eat a diet that is consistent with the dietary guidelines of 45% to 65% carbohydrate and 38 g of dietary fiber per day. On the basis of the 1-day diet record that he provides you, answer the questions that follow regarding his dietary analysis.

Breakfast:
- 2 cups Cheerios
- 1.25 cups skim milk
- 1 medium banana
- 16 oz coffee with 1 Tbsp sugar and 2 Tbsp whole-milk creamer

Lunch:
- Turkey sandwich (2 slices whole-wheat bread, 3 oz lean turkey, 1 oz cheddar cheese, 1 slice tomato, 2 lettuce leaves, 2 tsp yellow mustard, and ½ Tbsp mayonnaise)
- 1 oz pretzels
- 1½ cups mixed green salad with 2 Tbsp crushed pecans and 2 Tbsp fat-free Italian dressing
- 20 oz water

Snack:
- 1 medium apple
- 1 package peanut-butter crackers (6 crackers)

Dinner:
- 4 oz grilled chicken breast
- ½ cup green beans
- ¾ cup mashed potatoes made with skim milk and butter
- ½ cup roasted red peppers
- 1 whole-wheat roll
- 16 oz sweet tea

Questions for Analysis
1. Identify all of the foods that contain carbohydrates.
2. With the use of the dietary analysis CD-ROM included with this book or the Choose MyPlate Food Tracker available at www.choosemyplate.gov, analyze this 1-day diet to determine the following:
   a. How many total grams of carbohydrate did this individual consume?
   b. How many grams of sugar did he consume?
   c. How many grams of soluble and total fiber did he consume?
   d. What was the percentage of total calories from carbohydrates?
3. Did this individual meet the dietary guidelines for the percentage of calories from carbohydrates and grams of fiber on this day?
4. What additional recommendations would you make for improvement?

℮volve   Please refer to this text's Evolve Web site for answers to Case Study.

FOR FURTHER FOCUS

FIBER: WHAT'S ALL THE FUSS ABOUT?

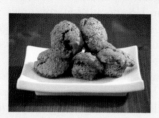

The National Institutes of Health and the World Health Organization—along with almost all other health-related agencies in the world—have been promoting the intake of fiber for years. The benefits have been defined in several clinical trials related to a variety of chronic illnesses.[1-4]

However, the average fiber intake in a typical American diet remains substantially lower than the current recommendations. Scientists are confident that consuming adequate amounts of fiber imparts the following health benefits:

- It lowers blood cholesterol levels.
- It promotes normal bowel function and prevents constipation.

- It increases satiety, which helps with the prevention of obesity.
- It protects against colon cancer.
- It slows glucose absorption, thereby reducing blood glucose spikes and insulin secretion.
- It prevents and helps to manage diverticulosis.

Health professionals can assist members of the public with evaluating their fiber intake by educating and encouraging the use of food labels. Food labels list the total dietary fiber found in each serving of food. Manufacturers may also voluntarily list the specific type of fiber (i.e., soluble or insoluble). Increases in dietary fiber intake should be made gradually, with extra attention paid to fluid intake. A sudden boost in dietary fiber can lead to uncomfortable bloating, gas, and cramping; this can be avoided by making small changes over time and by including an appropriate fluid intake of 8 glasses of water per day.

1. Behall KM, Scholfield DJ, Hallfrisch J. Whole-grain diets reduce blood pressure in mildly hypercholesterolemic men and women. *J Am Diet Assoc.* 2006;106(9):1445-1449.
2. Bijkerk CJ, de Wit NJ, Muris JW, et al. Soluble or insoluble fibre in irritable bowel syndrome in primary care? Randomised placebo controlled trial. *BMJ.* 2009;339:b3154.
3. Van Horn L, McCoin M, Kris-Etherton PM, et al. The evidence for dietary prevention and treatment of cardiovascular disease. *J Am Diet Assoc.* 2008;108(2):287-331.
4. Ventura E, Davis J, Byrd-Williams C, et al. Reduction in risk factors for type 2 diabetes mellitus in response to a low-sugar, high-fiber dietary intervention in overweight Latino adolescents. *Arch Pediatr Adolesc Med.* 2009;163(4):320-327.
(Copyright JupiterImages Corp.)

Other Sweeteners

Sugar alcohols and alternative sweeteners often are used as a sugar replacements. Sweeteners that contribute to total calorie intake (e.g., sugar alcohols) are considered *nutritive* sweeteners. *Nonnutritive sweeteners* or *alternative sweeteners* are sugar substitutes that do not have any caloric value.

Nutritive Sweeteners. The sugar alcohols sorbitol, mannitol, and xylitol are the alcohol forms of sucrose, mannose, and xylose, respectively. Sugar alcohols provide 2 to 3 kcal/g as compared with other carbohydrates, which provide 4 kcal/g. The most well-known sugar alcohol is sorbitol, which has been widely used as a sucrose substitute in various foods, candies, chewing gum, and beverages. Both glucose and sugar alcohols are absorbed in the small intestine. However, the sugar alcohols are absorbed more slowly and do not increase the blood sugar as rapidly as glucose. Therefore, sugar alcohols are often used in products that are intended for individuals who cannot tolerate a high blood sugar level (e.g., those with diabetes). The downside of using excessive

amounts of sugar alcohols in food products is that the slowed digestion may result in osmotic diarrhea. The advantage of using a sugar alcohol to replace sugar is a lowered risk of dental caries, because oral bacteria cannot use the alcohol for fuel.

Nonnutritive Sweeteners. Nonnutritive sweeteners are specifically manufactured to be used as alternative or artificial sweeteners in food products. Because

sugar alcohols nutritive sweeteners that provide 2 to 3 kcal/g; examples include sorbitol, mannitol, and xylitol; these are produced in food-industry laboratories for use as sweeteners in candies, chewing gum, beverages, and other foods.

sorbitol a sugar alcohol that is often used as a nutritive sugar substitute; it is named for where it was discovered in nature, in ripe berries of the *Sorbus aucuparia* tree; it also occurs in small quantities in various other berries, cherries, plums, and pears.

TABLE 2-3 **DIETARY FIBER AND CALORIC VALUE FOR SELECTED FOODS**

Food	Serving Size	Dietary Fiber (g)	Kilocalories	Food	Serving Size	Dietary Fiber (g)	Kilocalories
Breads and Cereals				Prunes, dried	1	0.6	20
All-Bran	⅓ cup	13	75	Raisins, seedless	½ cup (not packed)	3	217
Complete Oat Bran	¾ cup	4	105	Strawberries	½ cup sliced	1.9	25
Complete Wheat Bran	¾ cup	5	92	**Legumes**			
Cracklin' Oat Bran	¾ cup	6.4	225	Black beans	½ cup	7.5	113
Fiber One	½ cup	14.4	60	Garbanzo beans	½ cup	6.2	134
Oatmeal	1 cup	4	138	Kidney beans	½ cup	5.6	112
Popcorn, air popped	1 cup	1.2	30	Lima beans	½ cup	6.5	108
Raisin Bran	½ cup	3.5	94	**Vegetables**			
100% Bran	⅓ cup	8.3	83	Asparagus, cooked	½ cup	1.4	21
Shredded Wheat'N Bran	⅔ cup	4	98	Black-eyed peas	½ cup	4.1	80
Whole-wheat bread	1 slice	2	69	Broccoli, cooked	½ cup	2.3	22
Fruit				Carrots, raw strips	½ cup	1.8	26
Apple, raw, with skin	1 medium (2¾ inches in diameter)	3.7	81	Cauliflower, cooked	½ cup	1.7	14
Apricot	1 medium	0.7	17	Corn	½ cup	2.2	88
Banana	1 medium (7 to 8 inches long)	2.8	108	Green beans (snap beans), cooked	½ cup	2	22
Blueberries	½ cup	2	40	Green peas	½ cup	4.4	67
Cherries	½ cup	0.8	26	Potato, baked, with skin	1 medium (2¼ to 3¼ inches in diameter)	3.8	160
Dates, dried	1	0.6	23				
Grapefruit	½ cup of pieces	1.25	38				
Orange	1 medium (2½ inches in diameter)	3.1	61	Sweet potato, baked, with skin	1 medium (2 × 5 inches)	3.4	117
Peach	1 medium (2½ inches in diameter)	2	42	Tomato, raw, chopped	½ cup	1	19

Data from the U.S. Department of Agriculture, Agricultural Research Service, Nutrient Data Laboratory. *USDA national nutrient database for standard reference* (website): www.nal.usda.gov/fnic/foodcomp/search/. Accessed August 10 2010.

nonnutritive sweeteners do not provide any kilocalories, they present the sweet taste without contributing to an individual's total energy intake. People typically associate these sweeteners with diet foods. The alternative sweeteners that are most commonly used in the United States are acesulfame-K, aspartame, neotame, saccharin, and sucralose. Nonnutritive sweeteners are much sweeter than sucrose; therefore, extremely small quantities can be used to produce the same sweet taste. Table 2-4 provides a summary of artificial sweeteners and their relative sweetness value as compared with table sugar.

FUNCTIONS OF CARBOHYDRATES

Primary Energy Function

Basic Fuel Supply

The main function of carbohydrates is to provide fuel for the body. Carbohydrates burn in the body at the rate of 4 kcal/g; thus, the fuel factor of carbohydrates is 4. Carbohydrates furnish readily available energy that is needed for physical activities as well as for the work of body cells. Fat also serves as a source of fuel for the body, but the

TABLE 2-4 SWEETNESS OF SUGARS AND ARTIFICIAL SWEETENERS

Substance	Sweetness Value
Sugar or Sugar Product	
Levulose, fructose	173
Invert sugar*	130
Sucrose	100
Glucose	74
Sorbitol	60
Mannitol	50
Galactose	32
Maltose	32
Lactose	16
Artificial Sweeteners	
Cyclamate (banned in the United States)	30
Aspartame (NutraSweet and Equal)†	180
Acesulfame-K (Sunette and Sweet One)	200
Stevia (Enliten, Stevia, Truvia)	250 to 300
Saccharin (Sweet'N Low and Sugar Twin)	300
Sucralose (Splenda)	600
Neotame	7000 to 13,000

*Inverted sugar is sucrose (table sugar) that has been broken down into equal parts fructose and glucose.
†Nutritive (i.e., has calories).
Revised from Mahan LK, Escott-Stump S. *Krause's food & nutrition therapy*. 12th ed. Philadelphia: Saunders; 2008.

body only needs a small amount of dietary fat to supply the essential fatty acids (see Chapter 3).

Reserve Fuel Supply

The total amount of carbohydrate in the body, including both stored glycogen and blood sugar, is relatively small. Healthy, well-nourished adults store approximately 100 g of glycogen in the liver, which is about 8% of the liver mass weight. On average, 300 to 400 g of glycogen can be stored in the muscle, which is about 1% to 2% of the muscle mass weight. Glycogen in the liver is primarily reserved to maintain blood glucose levels and to ensure brain function. Without refueling, the total amount of available glucose in the muscle only provides enough energy for 1 to 2 hours of aerobic activity at 66% maximum capacity. Therefore, to maintain a normal blood glucose level and to prevent a breakdown of fat and protein in tissue, individuals must eat carbohydrate foods regularly to meet energy demands.

Special Tissue Functions

Carbohydrates also serve special functions in many body tissues and organs.

Liver. Glycogen reserves in the liver provide a constant exchange with the body's overall energy balance system. These reserves protect cells from depressed metabolic function and resulting injury.

Protein and Fat. Carbohydrates help to regulate both protein and fat metabolism. If dietary carbohydrate is sufficient to meet general body energy needs, protein does not have to be broken down to supply energy. This protein-sparing action of carbohydrate protects protein for its major roles in tissue growth and maintenance; these are crucial functions for which other macronutrients cannot serve as a substitute. Likewise, with sufficient carbohydrate for energy, fat is not needed to supply large amounts of energy. This is significant, because a rapid breakdown of fat may result in the production of ketones, which are products of incomplete fat oxidation in the cells. Ketones are strong acids. The condition of acidosis or ketosis upsets the normal acid–base balance of the body and may result in cellular damage in severe cases. This protective action of carbohydrate is called its *antiketogenic effect*.

Central Nervous System. Constant carbohydrate intake and reserves are necessary for the proper functioning of the central nervous system. The master center of the central nervous system, the brain, has no stored supply of glucose; therefore, it is especially dependent on a minute-to-minute supply of glucose from the blood. Sustained and profound shock from low blood sugar may cause brain damage and can result in coma or death.

FOOD SOURCES OF CARBOHYDRATES

Starches

Starch is the most important carbohydrate in a balanced diet. Whole grain starches such as rice, wheat, corn, and potatoes provide important sources of fiber and other nutrients. Table 2-5 outlines the carbohydrate content of commonly consumed foods.

Sugars

Sugar per se is not necessarily a villain. After all, the form of carbohydrate that is found in fruit is a disaccharide or simple sugar. The difference between this type of sugar and the sugar in candy is that fruit also provides fiber, water, and vitamins. The health problem with regard to added sugar (e.g., sweets, desserts, candy, soda) lies in the large quantities of "empty calories" that many people consume, often to the exclusion of other important foods. The average American consumes approximately 28.7 tsp of added sugar per day (460 kcal).[12] As with most things, moderation is the key.

TABLE 2-5 **CARBOHYDRATE CONTENT OF SELECT FOODS**

Food Source	Serving Size	Carbohydrate (g)	Total Kilocalories
Concentrated Sweets			
Sugar:			
Granulated	1 tsp	4.2	16
Powdered	1 tsp	2.49	10
Brown	1 tsp, packed	4.48	17
Maple	1 tsp	2.73	11
Honey	1 Tbsp	17.3	64
Syrup:			
High-fructose corn	1 Tbsp	14.44	53
Maple	1 Tbsp	13.42	52
Jam and preserves	1 Tbsp	13.77	56
Carbonated beverage, cola	12 oz	35.18	136
Candy:			
Skittles	1 package (2.17 oz)	56.28	251
Starburst fruit chews	1 package (2.07 oz)	48.72	241
Twizzlers	4 pieces from an 8 oz package	35.88	158
Baked goods:			
Brownie	1 square (1 oz)	18.12	115
Butter cookie	1 medium (1 oz)	19.53	132
Doughnut, glazed	1 medium (3-inch diameter)	22.86	192
Fruit			
Apple, with skin	1 medium (2¾-inch diameter)	19.06	72
Banana	1 medium (7.5 inches long)	26.95	105
Cherries, sweet, raw	15 cherries	16.33	64
Orange	1 medium (2½-inch diameter)	15.39	62
Pineapple	1 slice (3½-inch diameter × ¾-inch thick)	10.6	40
Strawberries	10 medium (1¼-inch diameter)	9.22	38
Dried fruit, mixed (prune, apricot, pear)	1 package (5.5 oz)	93.85	356
Vegetables			
Beans, kidney, cooked	½ cup	19.34	109
Carrots, raw	½ cup chopped, raw	6.13	26
Corn, sweet, yellow, cooked	½ cup, drained	20.59	89
Lettuce, green leaf, raw	1 cup shredded	1	5
Potato, with skin, baked	1 medium (2¼- to 3¼-inch diameter)	36.59	161
Squash, summer	½ cup cooked slices	3.88	18
Tomatoes, red, raw	½ medium (2¾-inch diameter)	2.4	11
Dairy Products			
Milk:			
Skim	1 cup	12.15	88
2%	1 cup	13.5	138
Whole	1 cup	11.03	146

Continued

TABLE 2-5 **CARBOHYDRATE CONTENT OF SELECT FOODS—cont'd**

Food Source	Serving Size	Carbohydrate (g)	Total Kilocalories
Cheese:			
Cheddar	½ cup, shredded	0.72	228
Cottage, 2% milk fat	½ cup	4.1	102
Grain Products			
Bread:			
Wheat	1 slice	11.8	65
White	1 slice	12.6	66
Rye	1 slice	15.46	83
Cereal (dry):			
Corn flakes	1 cup	24.28	101
Rice, puffed	1 cup	12.57	56
Wheat, shredded, presweetened	1 cup	43.58	183
Cereal (cooked):			
Grits, corn, cooked with water	1 cup	31.15	143
Oatmeal, cooked with water	1 cup	25.27	147
Wheat, cooked with water	1 cup	32.96	160
Crackers, saltines	5	10.72	65
Pasta, cooked	1 cup	39.07	176
Rice:			
Brown	½ cup, cooked	22.92	109
White	½ cup, cooked	26.59	121

Data from the U.S. Department of Agriculture, Agricultural Research Service, Nutrient Data Laboratory. *USDA national nutrient database for standard reference* (website): www.nal.usda.gov/fnic/foodcomp/search/. Accessed August 10 2010.

See the For Further Focus box, "Carbohydrate Complication," for a brief discussion of two controversial hot topics in mass-media coverage of nutrition, the glycemic index and "net carbs."

DIGESTION OF CARBOHYDRATES

Mouth

The digestion of carbohydrate foods, starches, and sugars begins in the mouth and progresses through the successive parts of the gastrointestinal tract, and it is accomplished by two types of actions: (1) mechanical or muscle functions that break the food mass into smaller particles; and (2) chemical processes in which specific enzymes break down the food nutrients into still smaller usable metabolic products. The chewing of food, which is called *mastication,* breaks food into fine particles and mixes it with saliva. During this process, the salivary enzyme salivary amylase (also called *ptyalin*) is secreted by the parotid glands, which lie under each ear at the back of the jaw. Salivary amylase acts on starch to begin its breakdown into dextrins (i.e., intermediate starch breakdown products) and disaccharides (primarily maltose). Carbohydrates eaten in the form of monosaccharides travel to the stomach and small intestines for absorption without further digestion.

Stomach

Wavelike contractions of the stomach muscles continue the mechanical digestive process. This action, called *peristalsis,* further mixes food particles with gastric secretions to facilitate chemical digestion. The gastric secretions contain no specific enzymes for the breakdown of carbohydrates. Gastric secretions do include hydrochloric acid, which inhibits the action of salivary amylase. However,

enzymes the proteins produced in the body that digest or change nutrients in specific chemical reactions without being changed themselves during the process, so their action is that of a catalyst; digestive enzymes in gastrointestinal secretions act on food substances to break them down into simpler compounds. (An enzyme usually is named after the substance [i.e., substrate] on which it acts, with the common word ending of *-ase;* for example, sucrase is the specific enzyme for sucrose, which it breaks down into glucose and fructose.)

FOR FURTHER FOCUS

CARBOHYDRATE COMPLICATION

Glycemic Index

The glycemic index (GI), which was developed by researchers at the University of Toronto in 1987, was thought to be an ideal tool for controlling blood glucose levels, specifically for individuals with diabetes. However, the use of this tool has been controversial throughout the past decade.

How it Works

The GI ranks foods according to how fast blood glucose levels rise after consuming a specific amount (50 g) as compared with a reference food such as white bread or pure glucose. Foods that produce a higher peak in blood sugar within 2 hours of eating them are given a higher GI ranking. Thus, low GI foods do not produce high blood glucose spikes and are favorable. In addition, low GI foods are generally high in fiber.

Complications of Use

The primary reason why this tool is controversial is because of its high variability. The GI of a food can vary significantly in the following ways:
- From person to person
- With the quantity of food eaten
- From one time of day to another
- When a food is eaten alone versus when it is eaten with other foods
- Depending on the ripeness, variety, cooking method used, degree of processing, and site of origin

The GI of a food also does not indicate the nutritious quality of the food. For example, ice cream has a lower GI value than pineapple.

Benefits of Consistent Use

Despite the limitations, a recent meta-analysis of 45 peer-reviewed publications concluded that individuals who were consuming a low-GI diet had favorable health markers for conditions including obesity, diabetes mellitus, and risk factors for coronary heart disease.[1] In a separate publication, authors supported the use of low-GI diets over high-protein diets for long-term weight loss as a result of the associated overall health benefits and disease prevention.[2] The Academy of Nutrition and Dietetics continues to recommend that people with diabetes monitor their total grams of carbohydrates and use the GI to fine-tune their food choices.

Net Carbs

Food manufacturers invented a category of carbohydrates called "net carbs" as a marketing tactic to capitalize on the low-carbohydrate diet craze. The U.S. Food and Drug Administration regulates all information provided in the Nutrition Facts label, including total carbohydrates, dietary fiber, and sugars, and it does not acknowledge or approve of the "net carb" category.

The concept was developed during the height of carbohydrate-phobic diets. Food manufacturers reasoned that, because dietary fiber and sugar alcohols have lower GI values, these carbohydrates can simply be subtracted from the total carbohydrates in a food serving. For example, a food may have 30 g of total carbohydrates with 18 g of sugar alcohols and 3 g of fiber, thereby leaving 9 "net carbs"; these are sometimes also referred to as "impact carbs" or "active carbs."

Problems With the "Net Carb" Theory

- Sugar alcohols do have calories and can raise blood sugar.
- The excessive use of sugar alcohols in foods has not been studied, but this type of labeling encourages manufacturers to increase the use of products such as sorbitol to lower their "net carb" claim.
- Excess intake of sugar alcohols can cause diarrhea.
- The idea of zero "net carbs" does not explain the fact that the food still has calories.

The bottom line is that the U.S. Food and Drug Administration maintains that, for weight management, no substitute exists for the formula of "calories in must equal calories out." Total calories count more than the quantity—or lack thereof—of high-GI carbohydrates, low-GI carbohydrates, or "net carbs."

1. Livesey G, Taylor R, Hulshof T, Howlett J. Glycemic response and health—a systematic review and meta-analysis: the database, study characteristics, and macronutrient intakes. *Am J Clin Nutr*. 2008;87(1):223S-236S.
2. Brand-Miller J, McMillan-Price J, Steinbeck K, Caterson I. Dietary glycemic index: health implications. *J Am Coll Nutr*. 2009;28(Suppl):446S-449S.

before the food completely mixes with the acidic stomach secretions, up to 20% to 30% of the starch may have been changed to maltose. Muscle action continues to mix the food mass and then moves the food to the lower part of the stomach. Here, the food mass is a thick and creamy chyme, ready for its controlled emptying through the pyloric valve and into the duodenum, which is the first portion of the small intestine.

Small Intestine

Peristalsis continues to help with digestion in the small intestine by mixing and moving chyme along the length of the organ. The chemical digestion of carbohydrate is completed in the small intestine by specific enzymes from both the pancreas and the intestine.

CULTURAL CONSIDERATIONS

ETHNICITY AND LACTOSE INTOLERANCE

Lactose intolerance or malabsorption results when the enzyme that is necessary for lactose digestion is absent or deficient from the brush border cells of the small intestine. This condition is known as *hypolactasia*. If the disaccharide lactose cannot be hydrolyzed into its respective monosaccharides (i.e., glucose and galactose), then the unabsorbed sugar attracts excess fluid into the gut. Lactose then entering the large intestine can be partially metabolized by normal bacteria found in the colon, thereby producing large amounts of gas and discomfort.

About 10% of the American population experiences lactose intolerance. However, within the United States, several ethnic groups—African Americans, Native Americans, Hispanic Americans, and Asian Americans—have significantly higher rates of lactose intolerance as compared with Americans of Northern European descent.[1] Some subgroups, such as Native Americans, report a prevalence of up to 100% lactose intolerance, and the prevalence of this condition among African Americans is approximately 75%.

Individuals with lactose intolerance can usually tolerate some low-lactose milk products, such as cheese. Lactose intolerance is not an allergy, and most affected individuals can handle varying levels of lactose in their diet. The amount tolerated varies and should be explored by gradually introducing small amounts of lactose-containing foods into the diet while keeping note of any side effects. Generally, in most people, the equivalent of 8 oz of milk is tolerated before symptoms arise. The strong genetic link to lactose intolerance indicates that it is not likely a drastic change will occur in response to dietary lactose over a lifetime. However, many individuals do experience slight changes. Most people become more intolerant with age, whereas others are able to gradually accept more.

1. National Institutes of Health, National Institute of Diabetes and Digestive and Kidney Diseases, National Digestive Diseases Clearinghouse. *Lactose intolerance* (website): http://digestive.niddk.nih.gov/ddiseases/pubs/lactoseintolerance. Accessed August 29, 2011.

Pancreatic Secretions

Secretions from the pancreas enter the duodenum through the common bile duct. These secretions contain the starch enzyme pancreatic amylase for the continued breakdown of starch into disaccharides and monosaccharides.

Intestinal Secretions

Enzymes from the brush border (i.e., microvilli) of the intestinal tract contain three disaccharidases: sucrase, lactase, and maltase. These specific enzymes act on their respective disaccharides to render the monosaccharides—glucose, galactose, and fructose—ready for absorption directly into the portal blood circulation.

Lactose intolerance, which is the inability to break lactose down into its monosaccharide units, results from a deficiency of lactase. Symptoms include bloating, gas, abdominal pain, and diarrhea. Lactose intolerance affects approximately 75% of adults worldwide, with a much higher prevalence in certain countries and ethnic groups (see the Cultural Considerations box, "Ethnicity and Lactose Intolerance").

A summary of the major aspects of carbohydrate digestion through the successive parts of the gastrointestinal tract is shown in Figure 2-4. The overall process of the absorption and metabolism of all energy-yielding nutrients (i.e., carbohydrate, fat, and protein) is discussed in Chapter 5.

RECOMMENDATIONS FOR DIETARY CARBOHYDRATE

Dietary Reference Intakes

Energy needs are listed as total kilocalories, and these amounts include caloric intake from fat and protein as well as carbohydrate. According to the most recent DRIs, 45% to 65% of an adult's total caloric intake should come from carbohydrate foods.[3] This translates to 225 to 325 g of carbohydrates for a 2000-kcal/day diet. The recommended fiber intake can be achieved by choosing carbohydrate foods such as whole-grain cereals, legumes, vegetables, and fruits, which also provide vitamins and minerals. In addition, the DRIs recommend limiting added sugar to no

brush border the cells that are located on the microvilli within the lining of the intestinal tract; the microvilli are tiny hair-like projections that protrude from the mucosal cells that help to increase surface area for the digestion and absorption of nutrients.

portal an entrance or gateway; for example, the portal blood circulation designates the entry of blood vessels from the intestines into the liver; it carries nutrients for liver metabolism, and it then drains into the body's main systemic circulation to deliver metabolic products to body cells.

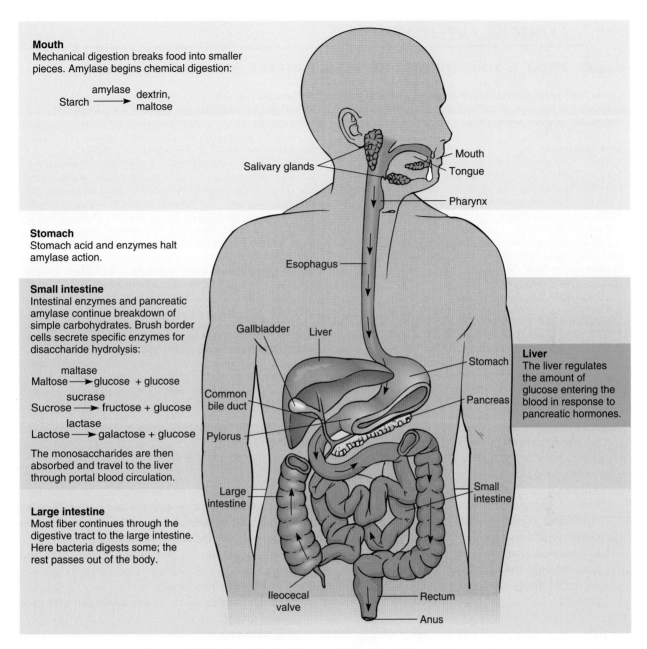

Mouth
Mechanical digestion breaks food into smaller pieces. Amylase begins chemical digestion:

$$Starch \xrightarrow{amylase} dextrin, maltose$$

Stomach
Stomach acid and enzymes halt amylase action.

Small intestine
Intestinal enzymes and pancreatic amylase continue breakdown of simple carbohydrates. Brush border cells secrete specific enzymes for disaccharide hydrolysis:

$$Maltose \xrightarrow{maltase} glucose + glucose$$

$$Sucrose \xrightarrow{sucrase} fructose + glucose$$

$$Lactose \xrightarrow{lactase} galactose + glucose$$

The monosaccharides are then absorbed and travel to the liver through portal blood circulation.

Large intestine
Most fiber continues through the digestive tract to the large intestine. Here bacteria digests some; the rest passes out of the body.

Liver
The liver regulates the amount of glucose entering the blood in response to pancreatic hormones.

Salivary glands
Mouth
Tongue
Pharynx
Esophagus
Gallbladder
Liver
Stomach
Common bile duct
Pancreas
Pylorus
Large intestine
Small intestine
Ileocecal valve
Rectum
Anus

Figure 2-4 Summary of carbohydrate digestion. (Courtesy Rolin Graphics.)

more than 25% of the total calories consumed. See the Clinical Applications box entitled "What Is Your Dietary Reference Intake for Carbohydrates?" to calculate specific carbohydrate recommendations.

Dietary Guidelines for Americans

The *Dietary Guidelines for Americans* are general guidelines for the promotion of health; therefore, they do not specifically outline calorie consumption or where those kilocalories should come from (refer to Figure 1-4). Instead, the *Guidelines* advise individuals to do the following with regard to carbohydrate-rich foods[9]:

- Reduce the intake of calories from added sugars.
- Limit the consumption of foods that contain refined grains, especially refined grain foods that contain solid fats, added sugars, and sodium.
- Consume at least half of all grains as whole grains. Increase whole-grain intake by replacing refined grains with whole grains.

CLINICAL APPLICATIONS

WHAT IS YOUR DIETARY REFERENCE INTAKE FOR CARBOHYDRATES?

On the basis of the current Dietary Reference Intakes (DRIs), calculate the amount of calories and grams of carbohydrates that you are recommended to consume daily. This requires you to know how many total calories you consume on a daily basis.

Step 1: Keep track of everything you eat for 1 day. You can use the CD-ROM that is included with this book to calculate your daily food intake. This is your *total energy intake.* (Chapter 6 discusses the evaluation of total energy intake relative to weight and activity needs.)

Total energy intake = _____ kcal.

Step 2: Multiply your total energy intake by 45% (0.45) and 65% (0.65) to get the recommended number of *kilocalories from carbohydrates (CHO).*

_____ total kcal × 0.45 = _____ kcal
_____ total kcal × 0.65 = _____ kcal

Example:
2200 total kcal × 0.45 = 990 kcal
2200 total kcal × 0.65 = 1430 kcal

Thus, the recommended range of total kilocalories from CHO for this example is 990 to 1430 kcal/day

Step 3: Determine how many *grams of CHO* you need on the basis of these recommendations.

Each gram of CHO has 4 kcal; therefore, divide your recommended range of kilocalories from CHO (as determined previously) by 4.

_____ kcal/day from CHO ÷ 4 = _____ g of CHO/day

Example:
990 to 1430 kcal/day from CHO ÷ 4 = 247.5 to 357.5 g of CHO/day

Thus, the recommended range of total grams of CHO for this example is 247.5 to 357.5 g of CHO/day.

Step 4: What is the maximum amount of total kilocalorie consumption that can come from *added sugars,* according to the DRIs? Added sugars are added to food and beverages during production. The majority of added sugars in American diets come from candy, soft drinks, fruit drinks, pastries, and other sweets. The DRIs recommend limiting added sugar intake to no more than 25% of the total kilocalories consumed.

Multiply your total energy intake by 25% (0.25) to get the maximum number of *kilocalories from added sugars.*

_____ total kcal × 0.25 = _____ kcal

Example:
2200 total kcal × 0.25 = 550 kcal

Thus, the maximum amount of total kilocalories from added sugar for this example is 550 kcal/day.

Step 5: Determine the number of grams of added sugar by dividing the maximum kcal/day of added sugar by 4.

_____ kcal/day from added sugar ÷ 4 = _____ g of added sugar/day

Example:
550 kcal/day from added sugar ÷ 4 = 137.5 g of added sugar/day

Therefore, the 137.5 g of added sugar is the recommended *limit* per day for this example.

- Increase vegetable and fruit intake. Eat a variety of vegetables, especially dark-green and red and orange vegetables as well as beans and peas.
- Choose foods that provide more potassium, dietary fiber, calcium, and vitamin D. These foods include vegetables, fruits, whole grains, and milk and milk products.

MyPlate

The MyPlate food guidance system provides recommendations that are specific to age, gender, height, weight, and physical activity when reported as part of the MyPlate plan (see Figure 1-3), which is available online at www.choosemyplate.gov. After this basic information is entered, the system will produce a plan with recommendations for appropriate intake from each of the food groups. Other helpful information can be found on the plan's Web site, including the following[13]:

- Tips for consuming more whole grains, fruits, and vegetables
- Serving size information
- Health benefits and nutrients associated with each food group
- Sample menus

In addition, the MyPlate Tracker is an assessment tool that allows the user to enter his or her own menu for an evaluation of diet quality. This is a great resource for feedback about dietary sources of carbohydrate, including the consumption of fiber, whole grains, fruits, vegetables, and added sugars.

SUMMARY

- The primary source of energy for most of the world's population is carbohydrate foods. These foods are from widely distributed plant sources, such as grains, legumes, vegetables, and fruits. For the most part, these food products can be stored easily and are relatively low in cost.

SUMMARY—cont'd

- Two basic types of carbohydrates supply energy: simple and complex. Simple carbohydrates are single- and double-sugar units (i.e., monosaccharides and disaccharides, respectively). Because simple carbohydrates are easy to digest and absorb, they provide quick energy. Complex carbohydrates (i.e., polysaccharides) are composed of many sugar units. They break down more slowly and thus provide sustained energy over a longer period.
- Dietary fiber is a complex carbohydrate that is not digestible by humans. It mainly occurs as the structural parts of plants, and it provides important bulk in the diet, affects nutrient absorption, and benefits health.

- Carbohydrate digestion starts briefly in the mouth with the initial action of salivary amylase to begin digesting starch into smaller units. No enzyme for starch digestion is present in the stomach, but muscle action continues to mix the food mass and move it to the small intestine, where pancreatic amylase continues the chemical digestion. Final starch and disaccharide digestion occurs in the small intestine with the action of sucrase, lactase, and maltase to produce single-sugar units of glucose, fructose, and galactose. These monosaccharides are then absorbed into the portal blood circulation to the liver.

CRITICAL THINKING QUESTIONS

1. Why are carbohydrates the predominant type of food in the world's diets? Give some basic examples of these carbohydrate foods.
2. How would you describe each of the main classes of carbohydrates in terms of general nature, functions, and main food sources to an individual who comes to you for advice about a no- or low-carbohydrate diet?
3. Compare starches and sugars as basic fuel. Why are complex carbohydrates a significant part of a healthy diet? What are the recommendations regarding the use of sugars in such a diet? Why?
4. Describe the types and functions of dietary fiber. What are the main food sources? How would you recommend increasing dietary fiber consumption, and how much per day would you recommend for an adult?
5. What is glycogen? Why is it a vital tissue carbohydrate?

CHAPTER CHALLENGE QUESTIONS

True-False
Write the correct statement for each statement that is false.
1. *True or False:* Carbohydrates are composed of carbon, hydrogen, oxygen, and nitrogen.
2. *True or False:* Starch is the main source of carbohydrate in the diet.
3. *True or False:* Lactose is a very sweet simple monosaccharide that is found in a number of foods.
4. *True or False:* Glucose is the form of sugar that circulates in the blood.
5. *True or False:* Modern food processing and refinement have reduced dietary fiber.
6. *True or False:* Glycogen is an important long-term storage form of energy, because large amounts are stored in the liver and muscles.

Multiple Choice
1. Which of the following carbohydrate foods provides energy the quickest?
   a. Slice of bread
   b. Oat-bran muffin
   c. Milk
   d. Orange juice
2. A quickly available but limited form of energy is stored in the liver by conversion of glucose to
   a. glycerol.
   b. glycogen.
   c. protein.
   d. fat.
3. The current DRIs recommend that _____ of a person's total daily caloric intake come from carbohydrate sources.
   a. 5% to 15%
   b. 20% to 35%
   c. 35% to 50%
   d. 45% to 65%

4. Which of the following is not a monosaccharide?
- **a.** Lactose
- **b.** Glucose
- **c.** Galactose
- **d.** Fructose

5. The disaccharide sucrose is hydrolyzed to the monosaccharides glucose and
- **a.** galactose.
- **b.** glucose.

- **c.** fructose.
- **d.** starch.

6. Which type of fiber would be specifically beneficial for someone with elevated blood cholesterol levels?
- **a.** Soluble
- **b.** Insoluble

⊖volve **Please refer to the Students' Resource section of this text's Evolve Web site for additional study resources.**

REFERENCES

1. U.S. Department of Agriculture, Economic Research Service. *U.S. food supply: nutrients and other food components, per capita per day, 1909 to 2004* (website): www.ers. usda.gov/Data/FoodConsumption/NutrientAvailIndex. htm. Accessed February 16, 2010.
2. U.S. Department of Agriculture, Economic Research Service. *High fructose corn sweetener (HFCS): per capita consumption adjusted for loss* (website): www.ers.usda.gov/ Data/FoodConsumption/FoodGuideSpreadsheets. htm#sugar. Accessed March 17, 2010.
3. Institute of Medicine, Food and Nutrition Board. *Dietary reference intakes for energy, carbohydrate, fiber, fat, fatty acids, cholesterol, protein, and amino acids*. Washington, DC: National Academies Press; 2002.
4. Behall KM, Scholfield DJ, Hallfrisch J. Whole-grain diets reduce blood pressure in mildly hypercholesterolemic men and women. *J Am Diet Assoc*. 2006;106(9):1445-1449.
5. Bijkerk CJ, de Wit NJ, Muris JW, et al. Soluble or insoluble fibre in irritable bowel syndrome in primary care? Randomised placebo controlled trial. *BMJ*. 2009;339:b3154.
6. Ventura E, Davis J, Byrd-Williams C, et al. Reduction in risk factors for type 2 diabetes mellitus in response to a low-sugar, high-fiber dietary intervention in overweight Latino adolescents. *Arch Pediatr Adolesc Med*. 2009;163(4):320-327.
7. Van Horn L, McCoin M, Kris-Etherton PM, et al. The evidence for dietary prevention and treatment of cardiovascular disease. *J Am Diet Assoc*. 2008;108(2):287-331.
8. Queenan KM, Stewart ML, Smith KN, et al. Concentrated oat beta-glucan, a fermentable fiber, lowers serum cholesterol in hypercholesterolemic adults in a randomized controlled trial. *Nutr J*. 2007;6:6.
9. U.S. Department of Agriculture, U.S. Department of Health and Human Services. *Dietary guidelines for Americans, 2010*. Washington, DC: U.S. Government Printing Office; 2010.
10. Guenther PM, Dodd KW, Reedy J, Krebs-Smith SM. Most Americans eat much less than recommended amounts of fruits and vegetables. *J Am Diet Assoc*. 2006;106(9): 1371-1379.
11. Cleveland LE, Moshfegh AJ, Albertson AM, Goldman JD. Dietary intake of whole grains. *J Am Coll Nutr*. 2000;19(3 Suppl):331S-338S.
12. U.S. Department of Agriculture, Economic Research Service. *Average daily per capita servings from the U.S. food supply, adjusted for spoilage and other waste* (website): www. ers.usda.gov/Data/FoodConsumption/FoodGuideSpreadsheets.htm. Accessed March 17, 2010.
13. U.S. Department of Agriculture, Center for Nutrition Policy and Promotion. *USDA's myplate home page* (website): www.choosemyplate.gov. Accessed August 29, 2011.

FURTHER READING AND RESOURCES

The following organizations are valuable resources for nutrition and health-related information.

Centers for Disease Control and Prevention. www.cdc.gov

Continuum Health Partners. Fiber content chart: www.slrhc. org/healthinfo/dietaryfiber/fibercontentchart.html

International Food Information Council Foundation. www.ific. org

U.S. Department of Health and Human Services. www.dhhs.gov

Whole Grains Council. www.wholegrainscouncil.org

Livesey G, Taylor R, Hulshof T, Howlett J. Glycemic response and health—a systematic review and meta-analysis: relations between dietary glycemic properties and health outcomes. *Am J Clin Nutr*. 2008;87(1):258S-268S.
The authors discuss the collective findings of 45 publications regarding the usefulness of adhering to a low glycemic index diet.

Brinkworth GD, Noakes M, Buckley JD, et al. Long-term effects of a very-low-carbohydrate weight loss diet compared with an isocaloric low-fat diet after 12 mo. *Am J Clin Nutr*. 2009;90(1):23-32.

Wycherley TP, Brinkworth GD, Keogh JB, et al. Long-term effects of weight loss with a very low carbohydrate and low fat diet on vascular function in overweight and obese patients. *J Intern Med*. 2010;267(5):452-461.
Carbohydrates are the topic of much debate in weight loss programs. Traditional weight loss programs focus on low-fat diets. However, more recent diets are centered on low levels of carbohydrate consumption. These studies examine the long-term effects of a low-carbohydrate diet as compared with a traditional low-fat diet with regard to cardiovascular risk factors.

CHAPTER 3

Fats

KEY CONCEPTS

- Dietary fat supplies essential body tissue needs as both an energy fuel and a structural material.
- Foods from animal and plant sources supply distinct forms of fat that affect health in different ways.
- Excess dietary fat, especially from animal food sources, is a risk factor for poor health.

General awareness regarding health concerns and the risk of chronic disease from excess saturated fat in the diet has influenced overall dietary choices. More knowledge of "heart-healthy" fats is helpful for the public to distinguish beneficial sources of dietary fat from unfavorable sources.

This chapter examines the various aspects of fat as an essential nutrient, a concentrated storage fuel, and a savory food component. In addition, the types of fat and the health implications when dietary fat or body fat goes unchecked are reviewed.

THE NATURE OF FATS

Dietary Importance

Fats are a concentrated fuel source for the human energy system. A large amount of energy can be stored in a relatively small space within adipose tissue as compared with carbohydrates that are stored as glycogen. As such, fats supplement carbohydrates (the primary fuel) as an additional energy source. In food, fats may be in the form of either solid fat or liquid oil. Fats are not soluble in water, and they have a greasy texture.

Structure and Classes of Fats

The overall name of the chemical group of fats and fat-related compounds is *lipids*, which comes from the Greek word *lipos*, meaning "fat." The word *lipid* appears in combination words that are used for fat-related health conditions. For example, an elevated level of blood fat is called *hyperlipidemia*.

All lipids are composed of the same basic chemical elements as carbohydrates: carbon, hydrogen, and oxygen. The majority of dietary fats are glycerides, which are composed of fatty acids attached to glycerol. Most natural fats, whether in animal or plant sources, have three fatty acids attached to their glycerol base, thus the chemical name of *triglyceride* (Figure 3-1).

Classification of Fatty Acids

Fatty acids, which are the building blocks of triglycerides, can be classified by their length as short-, medium-, or long-chain fatty acids. The chains contain carbon atoms with a methyl group (CH_3) on one end (also known as the *omega end*) and an acid carboxyl group (COOH) on the other end. Short-chain fatty acids have two to four carbons, whereas medium and long chains have 6 to 10 and more than 12 carbons, respectively. Fatty acids can also be classified according to their saturation or essentiality, both of which are significant characteristics.

Saturated Fatty Acid

When a substance is described as *saturated*, it contains all of the material that it is capable of holding (Figure 3-2, *A*). For example, a sponge is saturated with water when it holds all of the water that it can contain. Similarly, fatty

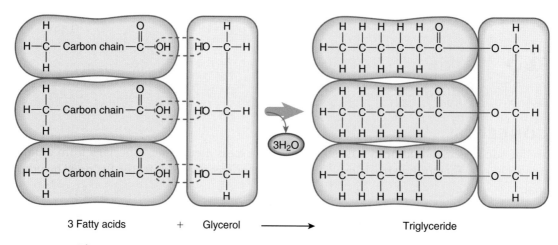

3 Fatty acids   +   Glycerol   ⟶   Triglyceride

Figure 3-1 A triglyceride contains three fatty acids bound to a glycerol molecule.

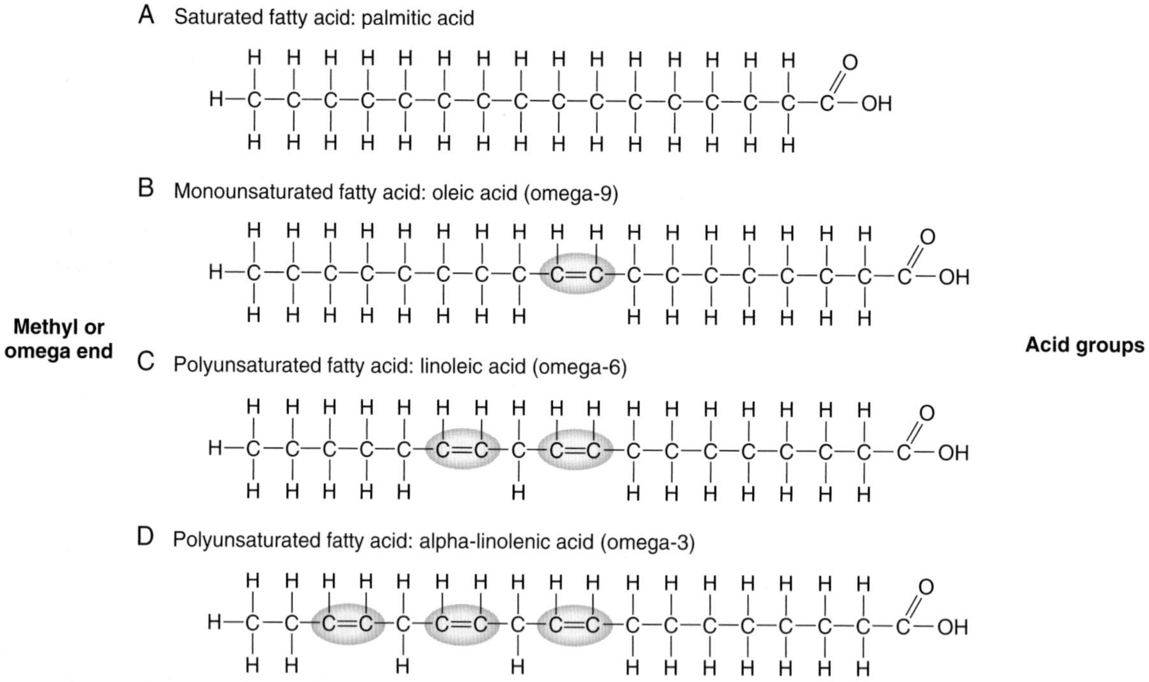

A Saturated fatty acid: palmitic acid

B Monounsaturated fatty acid: oleic acid (omega-9)

Methyl or omega end

Acid groups

C Polyunsaturated fatty acid: linoleic acid (omega-6)

D Polyunsaturated fatty acid: alpha-linolenic acid (omega-3)

Figure 3-2 Types of fatty acids. **A,** Saturated palmitic acid. **B,** Monounsaturated oleic acid (omega-9). **C,** Polyunsaturated linoleic acid (omega-6). **D,** Polyunsaturated alpha-linolenic acid (omega-3). (Modified from Grodner M, Long Roth S, Walkingshaw BC. *Foundations and clinical applications of nutrition.* 5th ed. St. Louis: Mosby; 2012.)

acids are saturated or unsaturated according to whether each carbon is filled with hydrogen. Thus, a saturated fatty acid is heavy and dense (i.e., solid at room temperature). If most of the fatty acids in a triglyceride are saturated, that fat is said to be a *saturated fat.* Most saturated fats are of animal origin. Figure 3-3 shows a variety of foods with saturated fat, including meat, dairy, and eggs.

Unsaturated Fatty Acid

A fatty acid that is not completely filled with all of the hydrogen that it can hold is unsaturated; as a result, it is less heavy and less dense (i.e., liquid at room temperature). If most of the fatty acids in a triglyceride are unsaturated, that fat is said to be an *unsaturated fat.* If the fatty acids have one unfilled spot (i.e., one double bond

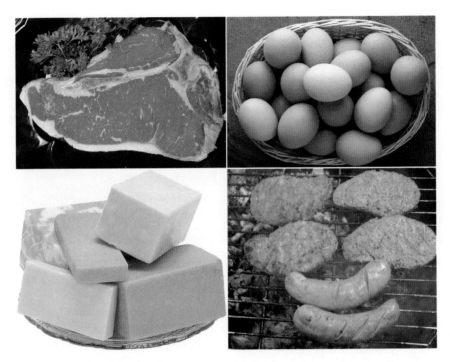

Figure 3-3 Dietary sources of saturated fats. (Copyright JupiterImages Corp.)

between the carbon atoms), the fat is called a *monoun-saturated fat* (see Figure 3-2, *B*). Examples of foods that contain some monounsaturated fats include olive oil, peanut oil, canola (rapeseed) oil, almonds, pecans, and avocados. If the fatty acids have two or more unfilled spots (i.e., more than one double bond between the carbon atoms), the fat is called a *polyunsaturated fat* (see Figure 3-2, *C* and *D*). Examples of foods that contain some polyunsaturated fats are the vegetable oils: saf-flower, corn, cottonseed, and soybean. Fats from plant and fish sources are mostly unsaturated (Figure 3-4). However, notable exceptions are the tropical oils, which are saturated. Although the world production of satu-rated tropical oils (e.g., palm, palm kernel, coconut) has increased rapidly since the 1970s, the use of these oils in the United States has not followed suit.

Trans-Fatty Acids. Naturally occurring unsaturated fatty acid molecules have a bend in the chain of atoms at the point of the carbon double bond. This form is called *cis,* meaning "same side," because both of the hydrogen atoms around the carbon double bond are on the same side of the bond. When vegetable oils are partially hydro-genated to produce a more solid, shelf-stable fat, the normal bend is changed so that the hydrogen atoms around the carbon double bond are on opposite sides. This form is called *trans,* meaning "opposite side," and the process is called *hydrogenation.* The illustration on page 34 shows the cis form and the trans form of a mol-ecule of oleic acid, which is a common monounsaturated fatty acid with a chain of 18 carbon atoms.

Commercially hydrogenated fats in margarine, snack items, fast food, and many other food products are typi-cally high in trans fat. Trans fats are unnecessary in

---

lipids the chemical group name for organic substances of a fatty nature; the lipids include fats, oils, waxes, and other fat-related compounds such as cholesterol.

glycerides the chemical group name for fats; fats are formed from a glycerol base with one, two, or three fatty acids attached to make monoglycerides, diglyc-erides, and triglycerides, respectively; glycerides are the principal constituents of adipose tissue, and they are found in animal and vegetable fats and oils.

fatty acids the major structural components of fats.

triglycerides the chemical name for fats in the body or in food; three fatty acids attached to a glycerol base.

saturated the state of being filled; the state of fatty acid components being filled in all their available carbon bonds with hydrogen, thus making the fat harder and more solid; such solid food fats are generally from animal sources.

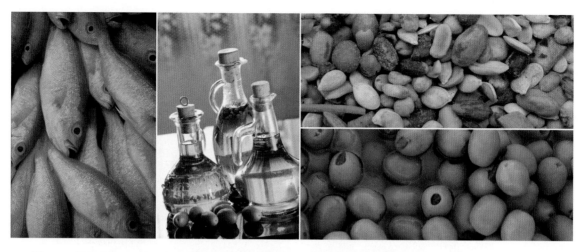

Figure 3-4 Dietary sources of monounsaturated and polyunsaturated fats. (Copyright JupiterImages Corp.)

Cis form   *Trans* form

human nutrition and pose a great number of negative health consequences related to cardiovascular disease.[1] The current dietary recommendations by the American Heart Association, the Academy of Nutrition and Dietetics, the Institute of Medicine, and the *Dietary Guidelines for Americans* are to avoid all trans fat in the diet.

Omega-3 and Omega-6 Fatty Acids. Unsaturated fatty acids can be distinguished by the occurrence of the first carbon involved in the double bond from the omega end (i.e., the methyl group end). When the first carbon double bond starts on the third carbon from the omega end, it is known as an *omega-3 fatty acid* (see Figure 3-2, *D*). When the first carbon double bond starts on the sixth carbon from the omega end, it is known as an *omega-6 fatty acid* (see Figure 3-2, *C*).

Essentiality of Fatty Acids. The term *essential* or *non-essential* is applied to a nutrient according to its necessity in the diet. A nutrient is essential if either of the following is true: (1) its absence will create a specific deficiency disease; or (2) the body cannot manufacture it in sufficient amounts and must obtain it from the diet. A diet with 10% or less of its total kilocalories from fat cannot supply adequate amounts of essential fatty acids. The only fatty acids known to be essential for complete human nutrition are the polyunsaturated fatty acids linoleic acid (an omega-6 fatty acid), and alpha-linolenic acid (an omega-3 fatty acid). Both essential fatty acids serve important functions related to tissue strength, cholesterol metabolism, muscle

---

linoleic acid an essential fatty acid that consists of 18 carbon atoms and two double bonds; found in vegetable oils.

alpha-linolenic acid an essential fatty acid with 18 carbon atoms and three double bonds; found in soybean, canola, and flaxseed oil.

cholesterol a fat-related compound called a *sterol* that is synthesized only in animal tissues; a normal constituent of bile and a principal constituent of gallstones; in the body, cholesterol is primarily synthesized in the liver; in the diet, cholesterol is found in animal food sources.

lipoproteins chemical complexes of fat and protein that serve as the major carriers of lipids in the plasma; they vary in density according to the size of the fat load being carried (i.e., the lower the density, the higher the fat load); the combination package with water-soluble protein makes possible the transport of non–water-soluble fatty substances in the water-based blood circulation.

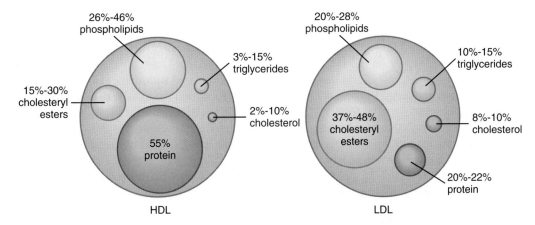

Figure 3-5 Composition of high-density lipoproteins (HDL) and low-density lipoproteins (LDL).

tone, blood clotting, and heart action. Essential fatty acids must come from the foods we eat. The body is capable of producing saturated fatty acids, monounsaturated fatty acids, and cholesterol. Therefore, no set recommendations of daily intake exist for these.

Lipoproteins

Lipoproteins, which are the major vehicles for lipid transport in the blood stream, are combinations of triglycerides, protein (apoprotein), phospholipids, cholesterol, and other fat-soluble substances (e.g., fat-soluble vitamins). Because fat is insoluble in water and because blood is predominately water, fat cannot freely travel in the bloodstream; it needs a water-soluble carrier. The body solves this problem by wrapping small particles of fat in a covering of protein, which is hydrophilic (i.e., "water loving"). The blood then carries these packages of fat to and from the cells to supply needed nutrients. A lipoprotein's relative load of fat and protein determines its density. The higher the protein load, the higher the lipoprotein's density. The higher the fat load, the lower the lipoprotein's density. Low-density lipoproteins carry fat and cholesterol to cells. High-density lipoproteins carry free cholesterol from body tissues to the liver for breakdown and excretion (Figure 3-5). All lipoproteins are closely associated with lipid disorders and with the underlying blood-vessel disease atherosclerosis. These relationships are discussed in greater detail in Chapter 19.

Phospholipids

Phospholipids are triglyceride derivatives in which the one fatty acid has been replaced with a phosphate group. The result is a molecule that is partially hydrophobic (i.e., "water fearing") and partially hydrophilic (because of the

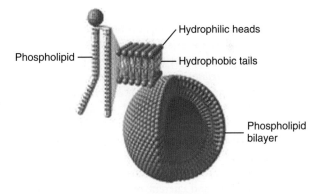

Figure 3-6 Phospholipid bilayer. (Reprinted from the NASA Astrobiology Institute. *Project 4. Prebiotic Molecular Selection and Organization (website):* http://nai.nasa.gov. Accessed July 6, 2007.)

phosphate group). This combination results in what is called an *amphiphilic molecule,* in which the hydrophilic heads face outward to the aqueous environment and the hydrophobic heads bind fats and oils and face each other (Figure 3-6). Phospholipids are major constituents in cell membranes and allow for the transport of fats through the bloodstream.

Lecithin. Lecithin, which is a lipid substance produced by the liver, is a key building block of the cell membranes. It is a combination of glycolipids, triglycerides, and phospholipids. The amphiphilic quality in lecithin makes it ideal for transporting fats and cholesterol.

Eicosanoids. Eicosanoids are signaling hormones that exert control over multiple functions in the body (e.g., the inflammatory response, immunity), and they are messengers for the central nervous system. Eicosanoids are divided into four classes: (1) prostaglandins; (2) prostacyclins; (3) thromboxanes; and (4) leukotrienes. Eicosanoids are derived from the essential fatty acids.

Sterols

Sterols are a subgroup of steroids, and they are amphipathic in nature. Sterols made by plants are called *phytosterols,* and sterols produced by animals are called *zoosterols.* Sterols play a variety of important roles, including membrane fluidity and cellular signaling. Cholesterol is the most significant zoosterol.

Cholesterol. Cholesterol is vital to membranes; it is a precursor for some hormones, and it plays other important roles in human metabolism. It occurs naturally in animal foods, and it is not present in plant products. The main food sources of cholesterol are egg yolks, organ meats (e.g., liver, kidney), and other meats (see Appendix A). To ensure that it always has the relatively small amount of cholesterol necessary for sustaining life, the human body synthesizes endogenous cholesterol in many body tissues, particularly in the liver as well as in small amounts in the adrenal cortex, the skin, the intestines, the testes, and the ovaries. Consequently, no biologic requirement for dietary cholesterol exists, and no Dietary Reference Intake (DRI) has been set for cholesterol consumption. The *Dietary Guidelines for Americans* and the DRIs recommend consuming a diet that is low in cholesterol.[2,3] Epidemiologic studies have found strong correlations between the dietary intake of saturated fats and trans fats with coronary heart disease. The association with such risk factors and dietary cholesterol is less well defined; however, research shows that a diet that is low in cholesterol is beneficial, and current recommendations are to limit cholesterol intake.[4]

FUNCTIONS OF FAT

Fat in Foods

Energy

In addition to carbohydrates, fats serve as a fuel for energy production. Fat is also an important storage form of body fuel. Excess caloric intake from any macronutrient source is converted into stored fat. Fat is a much more concentrated form of fuel, yielding 9 kcal/g when burned by the body as compared with carbohydrate's yield of 4 kcal/g.

Essential Nutrients

Dietary triglycerides supply the body with essential fatty acids. As long as an adequate amount of essential fatty acids are consumed, the body is capable of endogenously producing other fats and cholesterol as needed. Food fats are also a source of fat-soluble vitamins (see Chapter 7), and they aid in the absorption of those vitamins.

Flavor and Satisfaction

Some fat in the diet adds flavor to foods and contributes to a feeling of satiety and satisfaction after a meal. These effects are partly caused by the slower rate of digestion of fats as compared with that of carbohydrates. This satiety also results from the fuller texture and body that fat gives to food mixtures and the slower emptying time of the stomach that it necessitates. The absence of this satiation while on a low-fat diet may contribute to dissatisfaction and problems with necessary changes in food habits to establish a lowered fat and cholesterol intake for the long term.

Fat Substitutes

Several fat substitutes, which are compounds that are not absorbed and thus contribute little or no kilocalories, are available to provide improved flavor and physical texture to low-fat foods and to help reduce total dietary fat intake. Fat substitutes that are currently on the market are considered safe by the U.S. Food and Drug Administration (FDA); however, the safety of long-term use is not well established. Two examples of these fat substitutes are Simplesse (CP Kelco, Atlanta, Ga), which is made by reshaping the protein of milk whey or egg whites, and Olean (Olestra) (Procter & Gamble, Cincinnati, Ohio), which is an indigestible form of sucrose.

Fat in the Body

Adipose Tissue

Fat that is stored in various parts of the body is called *adipose tissue,* from the Latin word *adiposus,* meaning "fatty." A web-like padding of fat tissue supports and protects vital organs, and a layer of fat directly under the skin is important for the regulation of body temperature. In addition, the protective myelin sheath that surrounds neurons is largely composed of fat.

Cell Membrane Structure

Fat forms the fatty center of cell membranes, thereby creating the selectively permeable lipid bilayer. Proteins are embedded within this layer and allow for the transport of various nutrients in and out of the cells.

---

glycolipid a lipid with a carbohydrate attached.

adipose fat stored in the cells of adipose (fatty) tissue.

FOOD SOURCES OF FAT

Variety of Sources

Animal Fats

The predominant supply of saturated fats comes from animal sources, the most concentrated of which include meat fats (e.g., bacon, sausage), dairy fats (e.g., cream, ice cream, butter, cheese), and egg yolks. Because these are animal sources, they also contain considerable amounts of cholesterol. The exceptions are coconut and palm oils, which also contain saturated fatty acids. The American diet has traditionally featured meats and other foods of animal origin. The U.S. Department of Agriculture reports that animal products in particular (e.g., meat, poultry, fish, eggs, dairy products) contribute 32.7% of the total fat to U.S. diets as well as 45.3% of the saturated fat and 95% of the cholesterol.[5]

Although animal products supply saturated fat and cholesterol to the diet, all types of animal protein are not created equal. One study found that, regardless of the protein source, when consuming lean beef, lean fish, and poultry without skin in a well-balanced diet that also includes a high ratio of polyunsaturated fat to saturated fat and ample fiber, similar benefits for blood cholesterol levels are found.[6] In other words, although animal products can have a hefty dose of cholesterol and saturated fat, lean portions do not have the same hypercholesterolemic effects as their full-fat counterparts when they are consumed with diets that are high in fiber. However, even greater cholesterol-lowering effects can be achieved from a diet that is low in trans-fatty acids and that involves the regular moderate use of polyunsaturated oils in the place of saturated fat.[7]

Some animal fats contain small amounts of unsaturated fats. Specifically, fish oils are a good source of the polyunsaturated omega-3 fatty acids (i.e., docosahexaenoic acid and eicosapentaenoic acid).

Plant Fats

Plant foods supply mostly monounsaturated and polyunsaturated fats, including the essential fatty acids. Food sources for unsaturated fats include vegetable oils (e.g., safflower, corn, cottonseed, soybean, peanut, olive; see Figure 3-4). However, as indicated previously, coconut and palm oils are exceptions; these saturated fats are used mainly in commercially processed food items.

Characteristics of Food Fat Sources

For practical purposes, food fats can be classified as visible or invisible fats.

Visible Fat

The obvious fats are easy to see and include butter, margarine, separate cream, salad oils and dressings, lard, shortening, fatty meats (e.g., bacon, sausage, salt pork), and the visible fat of any meat. Visible fats are easier to control in the diet than those that are less apparent.

Invisible Fat

Some dietary fats are less visible, so individuals who want to control dietary fat must be aware of these food sources. Invisible fats include cheese, the cream portion of homogenized milk, nuts, seeds, olives, avocados, and lean meat. Basically, invisible fats are those that you cannot cut out of the food. Even when all of the visible fat has been removed from meat (e.g., the skin on poultry and the obvious fat on the lean portions), approximately 6% of the total fat surrounding the muscle fibers remains.

Table 3-1 provides a list of commonly eaten foods and their fat content.

FOOD LABEL INFORMATION

The FDA food-labeling regulations for nutrition facts panel content provide the following mandatory and voluntary (italicized below) information relating to dietary fat in food products[8] (Figure 3-7):

- Calories from fat
- *Calories from saturated fat*
- Total fat
- Saturated fat
- Trans fat
- *Polyunsaturated fat*
- *Monounsaturated fat*
- Cholesterol

The nature and amount of dietary fat and cholesterol contribute to disease risk for some forms of cancer, coronary heart disease, diabetes, and obesity (see the Cultural Considerations box, "Ethnic Differences in Lipid Metabolism"). The FDA has approved a series of health claims that link one or more dietary components to the reduced risk of a specific disease.[9] Approved and well-supported health claims that involve dietary fat include the following:

- A diet that is low in total fat may reduce the risk of some cancers.
- Diets that are low in saturated fat and cholesterol may reduce the risk of coronary heart disease.

The following are claims pending approval:

- The consumption of eicosapentaenoic acid and docosahexaenoic omega-3 fatty acids may reduce the risk of coronary heart disease.

TABLE 3-1 **FAT IN FOOD SERVINGS**

Food	Serving Size	Fat Content (g)	Food	Serving Size	Fat Content (g)
Fats			**Dairy**		
Butter or margarine	1 Tbsp	11	American cheese	2 oz	18
Cream cheese	1 Tbsp	10	Cheddar cheese	1½ oz	14
Mayonnaise	1 Tbsp	11	Frozen yogurt	½ cup	2
Salad dressing	1 Tbsp	7	Ice cream	⅓ cup	7
Vegetables			Low-fat milk	1 cup	5
Broccoli	½ cup	Trace	Skim milk	1 cup	Trace
Carrots	½ cup	Trace	Whole milk	1 cup	8
Potato, baked	1	Trace	**Eggs, Fish, Meat,**		
Fruit			**and Nuts**		
Apple	1	Trace	Bologna (2 slices)	1 oz	16
Banana	1	Trace	Egg	1	5
Fruit juice	1 cup	Trace	Fish	3 oz	6
Orange	1	Trace	Ground beef	3 oz	16
Bread and Grains			Lean beef	3 oz	6
Bagel	1	Trace	Poultry	3 oz	6
Muffin	1 medium	6	Nuts (⅓ cup)	1 oz	22
Rice or pasta	½ cup	Trace	**Other**		
			Danish pastry	1 medium	13
			French fries	1 cup	8

Adapted from Grodner M, Long Roth S, Walkingshaw BC. *Foundations and clinical applications of nutrition.* 5th ed. St. Louis: Mosby; 2012.

CULTURAL CONSIDERATIONS

ETHNIC DIFFERENCES IN LIPID METABOLISM

Dietary patterns and habits form at an early age as a result of both family influence and environmental factors. The dietary fat intake of some individuals is much lower than that of others simply because of how the individuals were raised. However, since the unveiling of the human genome, we are learning that biologic differences also exist that may affect dietary patterns and determine the ways in which our bodies handle the nutrients we eat. The prevalence of obesity has long been known to differ among ethnic and racial populations, but the exact cause remains uncertain.

Women are often the subjects of study in obesity research. A significant difference in ethnicity exists with regard to the incidence of women 20 years old or older who are overweight in the United States[1]:

- 79.8% of African-American women
- 73.9% of Mexican women
- 57.9% of white women

Evidence is accumulating to suggest that biologic differences in lipid metabolism among ethnic groups may be the cause. Bower and colleagues found that African-American women have an increased capacity to synthesize fat from glucose in adipose tissue as compared with white women[2]; thus they are more efficient at converting excess kilocalories into stored fat. Another group found that obese African-American women have an inhibition of lipolysis (i.e., the metabolic breakdown of fat) that contributes to the difficulty that they have losing weight as compared with white women.[3]

These types of differences continue to unfold with ongoing genetic studies. Differences such as these will also guide individuals in their dietary choices with regard to how their bodies will respond to specific nutrients. The path from fat in our food to fat on our bodies continues to provide many questions for inspection and evaluation. The science of lipid digestion, metabolism, and use will remain a hot topic for debate and research for years to come.

1. National Center for Health Statistics. *Heath, United States, 2009,* with special feature on medical terminology. Hyattsville, Md: U.S. Government Printing Office; 2010.
2. Bower JF, Vadlamudi S, Barakat HA. Ethnic differences in in vitro glyceride synthesis in subcutaneous and omental adipose tissue. *Am J Physiol Endocrinol Metab.* 2002;283(5):E988-E993.
3. Barakat H, Davis J, Lang D, et al. Differences in the expression of the adenosine A1 receptor in adipose tissue of obese black and white women. *J Clin Endocrinol Metab.* 2006;91(5):1882-1886.

Nutrition Facts

Serving Size 1 cup (228g)
Servings Per Container 2

Amount Per Serving

Calories 260	Calories from Fat 120

	% Daily Value*
Total Fat 13g	**20%**
Saturated Fat 5g	**25%**
Trans Fat 2g	
Cholesterol 30 mg	**10%**
Sodium 660 mg	**28%**
Total Carbohydrate 31g	**10%**
Dietary Fiber 0g	**0%**
Sugars 5g	
Protein 5g	

Vitamin A 4%	•	Vitamin C 2%
Calcium 15%	•	Iron 4%

* Percent Daily Values are based on a 2,000 calorie diet,
Your Daily Values may be higher or lower depending on
your calorie needs:

	Calories:	2,000	2,500
Total Fat	Less than	65g	80g
Sat Fat	Less than	20g	25g
Cholesterol	Less than	300mg	300mg
Sodium	Less than	2,400mg	2,400mg
Total Carbohydrate		300g	375g
Dietary Fiber		25g	30g

Calories per gram:
Fat 9 • Carbohydrate 4 • Protein 4

Figure 3-7 Example of nutrition facts panel listing the trans fat content. (From the U.S. Food and Drug Administration, U.S. Department of Health and Human Services. *Examples of revised nutrition facts panel listing trans fat* (website): www.fda.gov/Food/GuidanceCompliance RegulatoryInformation/GuidanceDocuments/FoodLabelingNutrition/ucm173838.htm. Accessed August 17, 2009.)

- Eating 2 tablespoons of olive oil (monounsaturated fat) daily may reduce the risk of coronary heart disease.
- Consuming about 1½ tablespoons of canola oil (unsaturated fat) daily may reduce the risk of coronary heart disease.

See the label claim information published by the FDA at www.fda.gov/Food/LabelingNutrition/LabelClaims/default.htm for more information about FDA-approved health claims. This Web site provides updates regarding approved health claims, pending claims, and the appropriate use of the claims on food products. Food labels and health claims are discussed further in Chapter 13.

DIGESTION OF FATS

Mouth

As with other macronutrients (i.e., carbohydrates and proteins), fats are broken down into their basic building blocks, fatty acids, through the process of digestion (Figure 3-8). When foods are eaten, some initial fat breakdown may begin in the mouth by action of lingual lipase, an enzyme that is secreted by Ebner's glands at the back of the tongue. Of note is that lingual lipase is only important for digestion during infancy. For adults, the primary digestive action that occurs in the mouth is mechanical. Foods are broken into smaller particles through chewing and moistened for passage into the stomach.

Stomach

Little if any chemical digestion of fat occurs in the stomach. General muscle action continues to mix the fat with the stomach contents. No significant amounts of fat enzymes are present in the gastric secretions except gastric lipase (tributyrinase), which acts on emulsified butterfat. While the primary gastric enzymes act on other macronutrients in the food mix, fat is separated out and prepared for its major, enzyme-specific breakdown in the small intestine.

Small Intestine

Fat digestion largely occurs in the small intestine, where the major enzymes that are necessary for the chemical changes are present. These digestive agents come from three major sources: an emulsification agent from the gallbladder and two specific enzymes from the pancreas and the small intestine itself.

Bile From the Gallbladder

The bile is first produced in large dilute amounts in the liver, and the liver then sends the bile to the gallbladder for concentration and storage so that it is ready for use during fat digestion as needed. The fat that comes into the duodenum, which is the first section of the small intestine, stimulates the secretion of cholecystokinin, a hormone that is released from glands in the intestinal walls. In turn, cholecystokinin causes the gallbladder to contract, relax its opening, and subsequently secrete bile into the intestine by way of the common bile duct. Bile is not an enzyme that acts in the chemical digestive process; rather, it functions as an emulsifier. This preparation process accomplishes two important tasks: (1) it breaks the fat into small particles, thereby greatly increasing the total surface area

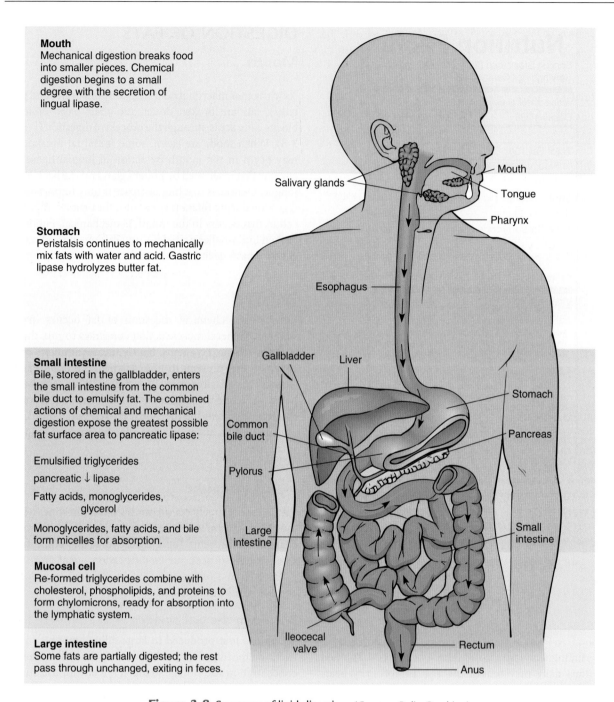

Mouth
Mechanical digestion breaks food into smaller pieces. Chemical digestion begins to a small degree with the secretion of lingual lipase.

Stomach
Peristalsis continues to mechanically mix fats with water and acid. Gastric lipase hydrolyzes butter fat.

Small intestine
Bile, stored in the gallbladder, enters the small intestine from the common bile duct to emulsify fat. The combined actions of chemical and mechanical digestion expose the greatest possible fat surface area to pancreatic lipase:

Emulsified triglycerides

pancreatic ↓ lipase

Fatty acids, monoglycerides, glycerol

Monoglycerides, fatty acids, and bile form micelles for absorption.

Mucosal cell
Re-formed triglycerides combine with cholesterol, phospholipids, and proteins to form chylomicrons, ready for absorption into the lymphatic system.

Large intestine
Some fats are partially digested; the rest pass through unchanged, exiting in feces.

Mouth · Salivary glands · Tongue · Pharynx · Esophagus · Gallbladder · Liver · Stomach · Common bile duct · Pancreas · Pylorus · Large intestine · Small intestine · Ileocecal valve · Rectum · Anus

Figure 3-8 Summary of lipid digestion. (Courtesy Rolin Graphics.)

available for enzymatic action; and (2) it lowers the surface tension of the finely dispersed and suspended fat particles, thus allowing the enzymes to penetrate more easily. This process is similar to the emulsification action of detergents. The bile also provides an alkaline medium that is necessary for the action of pancreatic lipase, which is the chief lipid enzyme.

Enzymes From the Pancreas

Pancreatic juice flowing into the small intestine contains one enzyme for triglycerides and another for cholesterol. First, pancreatic lipase breaks off one fatty acid at a time from the glycerol base of triglycerides. One fatty acid plus a diglyceride and then another fatty acid plus a monoglyceride are produced in turn. Each succeeding step of this breakdown occurs with increasing difficulty. In fact, the separation of the final fatty acid from the remaining monoglyceride is such a slow process that less than one third of the total fat present reaches complete breakdown. The final products of fat digestion to be absorbed are fatty acids, monoglycerides, and glycerol. Some remaining fat may pass into the large intestine for fecal elimination. The enzyme cholesterol esterase acts on cholesterol esters (not free cholesterol) to form a combination of free cholesterol and fatty acids in preparation for absorption into the lacteal (lymph vessel) and finally into the bloodstream (see Chapter 5).

Enzyme From the Small Intestine

The small intestine secretes an enzyme in the intestinal juice called *lecithinase,* which breaks down lecithin for absorption. Figure 3-8 summarizes fat digestion in the successive parts of the gastrointestinal tract.

Absorption

Fat absorption into the gastrointestinal cells and bloodstream is more involved than the absorption of other macronutrients (i.e., the products of digestion of carbohydrate and protein). Triglycerides are not soluble in water and thus cannot directly enter the bloodstream, which is mostly water. Within the small intestines, bile salts surround the monoglycerides and fatty acids to form micelles. The non–water-soluble fat particles (e.g., fatty acids, monoglycerides) are found in the middle of the packaged micelle, whereas the water-soluble part faces outward. This structure allows the products of lipid digestion to travel to the brush border membrane. Once there, fats are absorbed into the epithelial cells of the intestine, and bile is absorbed and transported by the portal vein to the liver for reprocessing; this process is called *enterohepatic circulation.* Inside the intestinal cells, monoglycerides and fatty acids again form triglycerides, which are then packaged into a chylomicron. Chylomicrons are made of triglycerides, cholesterol, phospholipids, and proteins (Figure 3-9). This structure also forms within the intestinal cell and allows the products of fat digestion to enter the circulation. Chylomicrons first enter the lacteals, then the lymphatic circulatory system, and then eventually the bloodstream. A summary of fat absorption through the process of micelle production and the formation of chylomicrons is provided in Figure 3-10.

Digestibility of Food Fats

The digestibility of fats varies somewhat according to the food source and the cooking method used. Butter digests

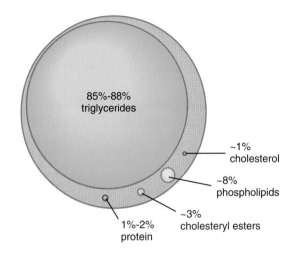

85%-88% triglycerides

~1% cholesterol

~8% phospholipids

~3% cholesteryl esters

1%-2% protein

Figure 3-9 Composition of a chylomicron.

more completely than meat fat. Fried foods, especially those that are saturated with fat during the frying process, are digested more slowly than baked or broiled foods. When fried foods are cooked at too high of a temperature, they are more difficult to digest, and substances in the fat break down into carcinogenic materials. Fried foods should be consumed sparingly, and the temperature of the fat should be carefully controlled during frying, grilling,

bile an emulsifying agent produced by the liver and transported to the gallbladder for concentration and storage; it is released into the duodenum with the entry of fat to facilitate enzymatic fat digestion by acting as an emulsifier.

emulsifier an agent that breaks down large fat globules into smaller, uniformly distributed particles; the action is chiefly accomplished in the intestine by bile acids, which lower the surface tension of the fat particles, thereby breaking the fat into many smaller droplets and thus greatly increasing the surface area of fat and facilitating contact with the fat-digesting enzymes.

micelles packages of free fatty acids, monoglycerides, and bile salts; the non–water-soluble fat particles are found in the middle of the package, whereas the water-soluble part faces outward and allows for the absorption of fat into intestinal mucosal cells.

chylomicron a lipoprotein formed in the intestinal cell that is composed of triglycerides, cholesterol, phospholipids, and protein; chylomicrons allow for the absorption of fat into the lymphatic circulatory system before entering the blood circulation.

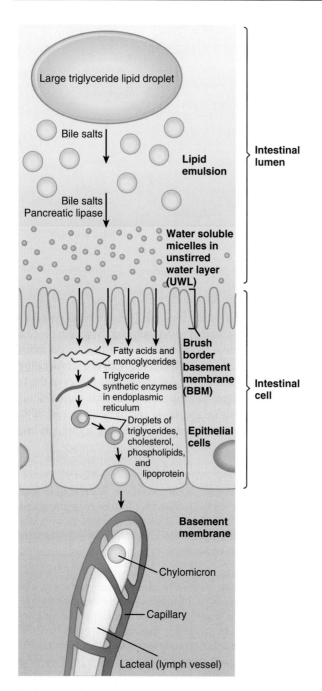

Figure 3-10 Summary of fat absorption. (From Mahan LK, Escott-Stump S. *Krause's food & nutrition therapy*. 12th ed. St. Louis: Saunders; 2008.)

and broiling. Although lower-fat food products are now generally more available in food markets, many high-fat products still compete for the customer's attention. Fat is an essential part of a healthy, well-balanced diet. However, one of the overall health goals is to reduce the amount of excessive fat used in the diet.

RECOMMENDATIONS· FOR DIETARY FAT

Dietary Fat and Health

American Diet

Fats in the diet supply flavor to food, thereby providing a sense of satisfaction and an enhancement of eating pleasure. The American diet has traditionally been high in fat. The U.S. Department of Agriculture nutrient intake records show that 31% of the total kilocalories came from fat in 1909, with an increase to 33% in 2008. However, Americans have succeeded in reducing the amount of fat coming from decidedly unhealthy saturated fat from 13% of total kcals to 11% over the same time frame.[5,10] Still, the average amount of saturated fat consumed per person in the United States for all individuals 2 years old and older exceeds the recommendations of the DRIs. Total kilocalories coming from fat should not exceed 20% to 35%, with a maximum of 10% of total kilocalories from saturated and trans fats combined.[3] Many individuals with health problems are encouraged to adjust to lower amounts of fat, with goals such as 15% to 25% of the total kilocalories and no more than 7% of total kilocalories from saturated and trans fats combined. This amount could easily provide an adequate amount of the essential fatty acids (i.e., linolenic acid and linoleic acid) to meet the physiologic needs of the body.

Health Problems

If fat is vital to human health, what is the concern about fat in the diet? Research continues to indicate that health problems from fat are related to too much dietary fat and specifically to saturated fat.

Amount of Fat. Too many kilocalories in the diet, regardless of the source—fat, carbohydrates, or protein—will exceed the requirement of immediate energy needs. The surplus is stored as body fat. Excess body fat is associated with risk factors for chronic diseases such as diabetes, hypertension, and heart disease. How much fat is in your own daily diet? See the Clinical Applications box entitled "How Much Fat Are You Eating?" to assess your fat intake.

Type of Fat. An excess of cholesterol and saturated fat in the diet, which comes from animal food sources, has been identified as a specific risk factor for atherosclerosis, the underlying blood vessel disease that contributes to heart attacks and strokes (see Chapter 19). A decrease in dietary saturated fats (e.g., using polyunsaturated and monounsaturated fats instead) has been shown to produce favorable lipid profiles.[7,11] When substituted for saturated fat in the diet, monounsaturated fats reduce low-density lipoprotein cholesterol levels and

CLINICAL APPLICATIONS

HOW MUCH FAT ARE YOU EATING?

Keep an accurate record of everything that you eat and drink for one day. Be sure to include all fat or other nutrient seasonings used with your foods (e.g., salad dressing, sugar, mayonnaise). If you want a more representative picture, use the nutrient analysis program that came with this text or another program to which you have access, and keep a 3- to 7-day record.

Step 1: Calculate the total kilocalories and grams for each of the energy-yielding nutrients (i.e., carbohydrates, fat, and protein) in everything that you eat. Multiply the total grams of each energy nutrient by its respective fuel value:

Fat: _____ g × 9 = _____ kcal
Protein: _____ g × 4 = _____ kcal
Carbohydrate: _____ g × 4 = _____ kcal

Step 2: Add the kcals from each macronutrient to determine the total kcals consumed.

Step 3: Calculate the percentage of each energy nutrient in your total diet:

Example: (Fat kcal/Total kcal) × 100 = % fat kcal in diet

Step 4: Compare the amount of fat in your diet with the amount of fat in a typical American diet (31% to 35% fat) and with the U.S. dietary goal (20% to 35% fat).

---

increase high-density lipoprotein levels, thereby improving overall cardiovascular health risk.

Essential Fatty Acid Deficiency. Fat-free diets may lead to essential fatty acid deficiency with clinical manifestations. Because essential fatty acids play an important role in maintaining the integrity of biologic membranes, one indication of essential fatty acid deficiency is dermatitis. Omega-3 fatty acids are especially required for normal function of the brain, the central nervous system, and the cell membranes. Low levels of omega-3 and omega-6 fatty acids are linked to hair loss, low blood platelet levels, impaired vision, compromised brain function, and growth retardation in children.

Trans-Fatty Acids. Observed effects of diets that are high in trans-fatty acids include an elevation of total cholesterol and low-density lipoprotein cholesterol levels, reduced high-density lipoprotein cholesterol levels, endothelial dysfunction, and the increased production of atherosclerotic inflammatory cytokines.[12] In response to these growing health concerns, the FDA now requires that all food products identify the amount of trans fats on the nutrition facts label, thereby making the identification of these products much easier (see Figure 3-7). This has motivated the food industry to develop alternative fats and oils to avoid the use of trans fats and to improve the fatty acid composition with regard to cardiovascular health risk.

Health Promotion

The ongoing movement in American health care is toward health promotion and disease prevention through the reduction of risk factors related to chronic disease. Heart disease continues to be a leading cause of death, and much attention is given to reducing the various risk factors that lead to this disease. Excess dietary fat—particularly saturated fat, trans fat, and cholesterol—contributes to these risk factors, which include obesity,

diabetes, elevated triglycerides, and elevated blood pressure. Such risk factors have previously been thought of as only affecting adults, but they are becoming increasingly apparent among obese children and adolescents. The Centers for Disease Control and Prevention reported that 20.3% of all youth between the ages of 12 and 19 years have abnormal lipid levels. Overweight children have a significantly higher prevalence of cardiovascular health risk than normal-weight children.[13] Healthier eating habits are especially important for children in high-risk families (e.g., families with identified lipid disorders and heart disease at young ages).

Additional lifestyle risk factors include smoking, increased stress, and physical inactivity, especially among middle-aged and older individuals. Emphasis is placed on the importance of keeping the body's total daily energy use in balance with the total daily caloric intake to maintain an ideal body weight. Low-fat diets, fad diets, and other issues that affect weight loss are discussed in more detail in Chapter 15.

In addition, changes are gradually being made in the fast-food industry to reduce the traditional high-fat content of menu items. For example, most of the fast-food chains are shifting to leaner meat for hamburgers; more variety in food choices (e.g., grilled chicken and fish sandwiches; breakfast items such as fruit, waffles, pancakes, and hot and cold cereals; baked potatoes; fresh and packaged salads and fruit); and using vegetable oil for frying.

Dietary Reference Intakes

Healthy diet guidelines stress the benefits of a diet that is low in fat, saturated fat, trans-fatty acids, and cholesterol. All guidelines recommend that the fat content of the diet not exceed 20% to 35% of the total kilocalories, that less than 10% of the kilocalories should come from saturated fats, and that dietary cholesterol be limited to a maximum of 300 mg/day (see Chapter 1). No DRI or Tolerable Upper Intake Level is set for trans-fatty acids. The National Academy of Sciences recommends limiting trans-fat intake to as low as possible while maintaining a nutritionally adequate diet.[3] As mentioned previously, fat is an essential part of the diet; therefore, diets that are completely devoid of fat are equally unhealthy and can result in a deficiency of essential fatty acids.

The DRI for linoleic acid, which is found in polyunsaturated vegetable oils, is set at 17 g/day for men and 12 g/day for women. Linolenic acid is primarily found in fish, soybeans, and flaxseed oil, and it is generally consumed in much lesser quantities than linoleic acid. The recommendation for linolenic acid intake is 1.6 and 1.1 g/day for men and women, respectively.[3] The average American diet contains significantly more omega-6 fatty acids than omega-3 fatty acids at a ratio of approximately 15-20:1 and 1-4:1. However, consuming more omega-3 fatty acids from vegetables and fish would help to achieve a preferred omega-6 to omega-3 ratio of 1-4:1 and thus reduce the risk for several chronic diseases.[14]

Dietary Guidelines for Americans

In line with the current national health goal of health promotion through disease prevention by reducing identified risks of chronic disease, the *Dietary Guidelines for Americans* recommends the general control of fat in the diet, especially saturated fat and cholesterol. The following guidelines address dietary fat intake[2]:

- Consume less than 10% of calories from saturated fatty acids by replacing them with monounsaturated and polyunsaturated fatty acids.
- Consume less than 300 mg/day of cholesterol.
- Keep trans-fatty acid consumption as low as possible by limiting foods that contain synthetic sources of trans fats (e.g., partially hydrogenated oils) and by limiting other solid fats.
- Reduce the intake of calories from solid fats.
- Choose fat-free or low-fat milk and milk products.
- Replace protein foods that are higher in solid fats with choices that are lower in solid fats and calories and/or are sources of oils.
- Use oils to replace solid fats where possible.

MyPlate

The MyPlate food guidance system provides recommendations for designing a diet that reflects the DRI and *Dietary Guidelines for Americans* recommendations for fat intake within a well-balanced diet. After an individual plan is determined on the basis of age, gender, height, weight, and physical activity level, other helpful tips and resources are available through the free Web site, www.choosemyplate.gov/, such as information about how to choose lean meats, where to find essential fatty acids, how to avoid saturated fat intake, tips for eating out, and sample menus.[15]

SUMMARY

- Fat is an essential body nutrient that serves important body needs as a backup storage fuel (secondary to carbohydrate) for energy. Fat also supplies important tissue needs as a structural material for cell membranes, a protective padding for vital organs, an insulation to maintain body temperature, and a covering for nerve fibers.
- Food fats have different forms and health implications. Saturated fats primarily come from animal food sources and carry health risks for the body. Plant food sources are the richest source of unsaturated fats and may reduce health risks when used in place of saturated and trans fats.
- Cholesterol is a sterol that is synthesized only by animals. When it is consumed in excessive amounts,

cholesterol also contributes to health risks for the development of cardiovascular disease.
- When various foods that contain triglycerides and cholesterol are eaten, specific digestive agents, including bile and pancreatic lipase, prepare and break down fats. Fatty acids and monoglycerides are incorporated into chylomicrons and absorbed through the lymphatic system into the bloodstream.
- Americans generally consume more saturated fat than recommended. Reducing saturated and trans-fat intake and maintaining a low-cholesterol diet are ideal for health promotion and disease prevention.

CRITICAL THINKING QUESTIONS

1. Compare fat and carbohydrate as fuel sources in the body's energy system. Name several other important functions of fat in human nutrition and health.
2. Differentiate the components of lipids, triglycerides, fatty acids, cholesterol, and lipoproteins.
3. Compare the structure of a saturated fat, a monounsaturated fat, a polyunsaturated fat, and a trans fat. Give food sources for each.
4. Why is a controlled amount of dietary fat recommended for health promotion? How much fat should a healthy diet contain?

CHAPTER CHALLENGE QUESTIONS

True-False

Write the correct statement for each statement that is false.

1. *True or False:* Fat has the same energy value as carbohydrate.
2. *True or False:* Fat is composed of the same basic chemical elements as carbohydrate.
3. *True or False:* Corn oil is a saturated fat.
4. *True or False:* Polyunsaturated fats predominantly come from animal food sources.
5. *True or False:* Lipoproteins, which are produced mainly in the liver, carry fat in the blood.

Multiple Choice

1. The fuel form of fat found in food sources is
   a. triglyceride.
   b. fatty acid.
   c. glycerol.
   d. lipoprotein.

2. Which of the following statements about the saturation of fats is correct?
   a. The degree of saturation does not depend on the amount of hydrogen in the fatty acids that make up the fat.
   b. Unsaturated fats come from animal food sources.
   c. The more saturated the fat, the softer it tends to be.
   d. Fats that are composed of fatty acids with two or more double bonds in their structure are called *polyunsaturated*.

3. If an individual implemented a diet that was low in saturated fat to lower the risk for heart disease, which of the following foods would be consumed more frequently than the others?
   a. Whole milk
   b. Olive oil and vinegar salad dressing
   c. Butter
   d. Cheddar cheese

4. Once absorbed into the enterocyte, monoglycerides and fatty acids again form triglycerides, which are then packaged into lipoproteins called _____ for absorption into the lymphatic structure.
   a. low-density lipoprotein cholesterol
   b. high-density lipoprotein cholesterol
   c. micelles
   d. chylomicrons

⊖volve **Please refer to the Students' Resource section of this text's Evolve Web site for additional study resources.**

REFERENCES

1. Remig V, Franklin B, Margolis S, et al. Trans fats in America: a review of their use, consumption, health implications, and regulation. *J Am Diet Assoc.* 2010;110(4):585-592.
2. U.S. Department of Agriculture, U.S. Department of Health and Human Services. *Dietary guidelines for Americans, 2010.* Washington, DC: U.S. Government Printing Office; 2010.
3. Food and Nutrition Board, Institute of Medicine. *Dietary reference intakes for energy, carbohydrate, fiber, fat, fatty acids, cholesterol, protein, and amino acids.* Washington, DC: National Academies Press; 2002.
4. Djousse L, Gaziano JM. Dietary cholesterol and coronary artery disease: a systematic review. *Curr Atheroscler Rep.* 2009;11(6):418-422.
5. U.S. Department of Agriculture, Economic Research Service. *U.S. food supply: nutrients and other food components, per capita per day, 1909 to 2004* (website): www.ers.usda.gov/Data/FoodConsumption/NutrientAvailIndex.htm. Accessed February 16, 2010.
6. Beauchesne-Rondeau E, Gascon A, Bergeron J, Jaques H. Plasma lipids and lipoproteins in hypercholesterolemic men fed a lipid-lowering diet containing lean beef, lean fish, or poultry. *Am J Clin Nutr.* 2003;77(3):587-593.
7. Binkoski AE, Kris-Etherton PM, Wilson TA, et al. Balance of unsaturated fatty acids is important to a cholesterol-lowering diet: comparison of mid-oleic sunflower oil and olive oil on cardiovascular disease risk factors. *J Am Diet Assoc.* 2005;105(7):1080-1086.
8. U.S. Food and Drug Administration, U.S. Department of Health and Human Services. *Examples of revised nutrition*

facts panel listing trans fat (website): www.fda.gov/Food/GuidanceComplianceRegulatoryInformation/GuidanceDocuments/FoodLabelingNutrition/ucm173838.htm. Accessed August 17, 2009.

9. U.S. Food and Drug Administration. *Label claims* (website): www.fda.gov/Food/LabelingNutrition/LabelClaims/default.htm. Accessed August 21 2010.

10. U.S. Department of Agriculture, Agricultural Research Service. *Energy intakes: percentages of energy from protein, carbohydrate, fat, and alcohol, by gender and age, what we eat in America, NHANES 2007-2008.* (website): www.ars.usda.gov/SP2UserFiles/Place/12355000/pdf/0708/Table_5_EIN_GEN_07.pdf. Accessed October 5 2011.

11. Allman-Farinelli MA, Gomes K, Favaloro EJ, Petocz P. A diet rich in high-oleic-acid sunflower oil favorably alters low-density lipoprotein cholesterol, triglycerides, and factor VII coagulant activity. *J Am Diet Assoc.* 2005;105(7):1071-1079.

12. Mozaffarian D, Aro A, Willett WC. Health effects of trans-fatty acids: experimental and observational evidence. *Eur J Clin Nutr.* 2009;63(Suppl 2):S5-S21.

13. Centers for Disease Control and Prevention. Prevalence of abnormal lipid levels among youths — United States, 1999-2006, *MMWR Morb Mortal Wkly Rep.* 2010;59(2):29-33.

14. Simopoulos AP. The importance of the omega-6/omega-3 fatty acid ratio in cardiovascular disease and other chronic diseases. *Exp Biol Med (Maywood).* 2008;233(6):674-688.

15. U.S. Department of Agriculture, Center for Nutrition Policy and Promotion. *USDA's myplate home page* (website): www.choosemyplate.gov. Accessed September 6, 2011.

FURTHER READING AND RESOURCES

Lipids in Health and Disease. www.lipidworld.com
An online journal of peer-reviewed articles about all aspects of lipids that is open access and free to the public

Mayo Clinic. www.mayoclinic.com
A site search for "dietary fat" results in several informative articles.

USDA Nutrient Data Laboratory. www.nal.usda.gov/fnic/foodcomp/search
A useful Web site for finding the nutrient content of the foods that you most enjoy, including their trans fat content

Lin CT, Yen ST. Knowledge of dietary fats among US consumers. *J Am Diet Assoc.* 2010;110(4):613-618.

Misra A, Singhal N, Khurana L. Obesity, the metabolic syndrome, and type 2 diabetes in developing countries: role of dietary fats and oils. *J Am Coll Nutr.* 2010;29(3 Suppl):289S-301S.

CHAPTER 4

Proteins

KEY CONCEPTS

- Protein in food provides the amino acids that are necessary for building and maintaining body tissue.
- Protein balance—both within the body and in the diet—is essential to life and health.

- The quality of a protein food and its ability to meet the body's needs are determined by the composition of amino acids.

Many different proteins in the body make human life possible. Each of these thousands of specific body proteins has a unique structure that is designed to perform an assigned task. Amino acids are the building blocks of all proteins. People obtain amino acids from a variety of foods. This chapter looks at the specific nature of proteins, both in food and in human bodies; it explains why protein balance is essential to life and health, and it discusses how that balance is maintained.

THE NATURE OF PROTEINS

Amino Acids: Basic Building Matter

Role as Building Units

All protein, whether in our bodies or in the food we eat, is composed of building blocks known as amino acids. Amino acids are joined in unique chain sequences to form specific proteins. Each amino acid is joined by a peptide bond (Figure 4-1). Two amino acids joined together are called a *dipeptide*. Polypeptides are chains of up to 100 amino acids. Hundreds of amino acids are linked together to form a single protein. When foods rich in protein are eaten, the protein is broken down into amino acids during the digestive process. The specific types of protein found in different foods are unique. For example, casein is the protein that is found in milk and cheese; albumin is in egg whites, and gluten is in wheat products. After they are absorbed into the body, amino acids are then reassembled in a specific order to form a variety of important body proteins. To maintain its solvency, each protein chain adopts a folded form, which can fold and unfold in accordance with metabolic need.

Because proteins are relatively large, complex molecules, they are occasionally subject to mutations or malformations in structure. For example, protein-folding mistakes are involved in Alzheimer's disease, which robs many older adults of their mental capacity.

Dietary Importance

Amino acids are named for their chemical nature. The word *amino* refers to compounds that contain nitrogen. Like carbohydrates and fats, proteins have a basic structure of carbon, hydrogen, and oxygen. However, unlike carbohydrates and fats, protein is approximately 16% nitrogen. As such, protein is the primary source of nitrogen in the diet. In addition, some proteins contain small but valuable amounts of the minerals sulfur, phosphorus, iron, and iodine.

Classes of Amino Acids

Twenty common amino acids have been identified, all of which are vital to life and health. These amino acids are classified as *indispensable*, *dispensable*, or *conditionally indispensable* in the diet according to whether the body

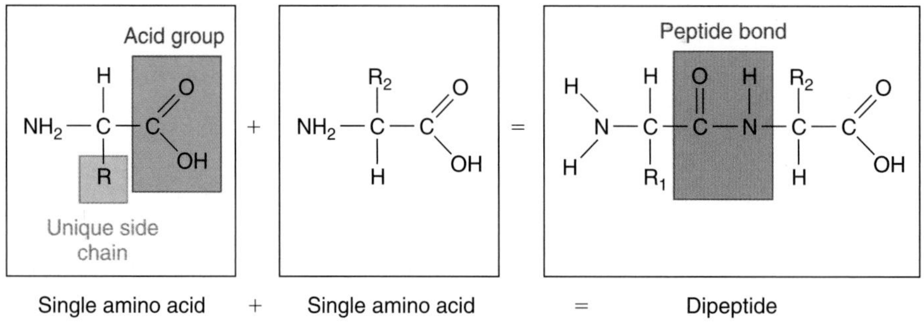

Figure 4-1 **Amino acid structure.** (Modified from Mahan LK, Escott-Stump S. *Krause's food & nutrition therapy.* 12th ed. Philadelphia: Saunders; 2008.)

can make them (Box 4-1).[1] These classifications were formerly known as *essential, nonessential,* or *conditionally essential,* respectively.

Indispensable Amino Acids

Nine amino acids are classified as indispensable because the body cannot manufacture them in sufficient quantity or at all (see Box 4-1). As the word *indispensable* implies, these amino acids are necessary in the diet and cannot be left out. Under normal circumstances, the remaining 11 amino acids are synthesized by the body to meet continuous metabolic demands throughout the life cycle.

Dispensable Amino Acids

The word *dispensable* can be confusing; all amino acids have essential tissue-building and metabolic functions in the body. However, the term refers to five amino acids that the body can synthesize from other amino acids, provided that the necessary building blocks and enzymes

---

BOX 4-1	**INDISPENSABLE, DISPENSABLE, AND CONDITIONALLY INDISPENSABLE AMINO ACIDS**

INDISPENSABLE	DISPENSABLE	CONDITIONALLY INDISPENSABLE
Histidine	Alanine	Arginine
Isoleucine	Aspartic acid	Cysteine
Leucine	Asparagine	Glutamine
Lysine	Glutamic acid	Glycine
Methionine	Serine	Proline
Phenylalanine		Tyrosine
Threonine		
Tryptophan		
Valine		

---

are present (see Box 4-1). These amino acids are needed by the body for a healthy life, but they are dispensable (i.e., not necessary) in the diet.

---

indispensable amino acids the nine amino acids that must be obtained from the diet because the body does not make adequate amounts to support body needs.

dispensable amino acids the five amino acids that the body can synthesize from other amino acids that are supplied through the diet and thus do not have to be consumed on a daily basis.

conditionally indispensable amino acids the six amino acids that are normally considered dispensable amino acids because the body can make them; however, under certain circumstances (e.g., illness), the body cannot make them in high enough quantities, and they become indispensable to the diet.

Conditionally Indispensable Amino Acids

The remaining six amino acids are classified as *conditionally indispensable* (see Box 4-1). Under certain physiologic conditions, these amino acids, which are normally synthesized in the body (along with the dispensable amino acids), must be consumed in the diet. Arginine, cysteine, glutamine, glycine, proline, and tyrosine are indispensable when endogenous sources cannot meet the metabolic demands. For example, the human body can make cysteine from the essential amino acid methionine. However, when the diet is deficient in methionine, cysteine must be consumed in the diet, thereby making it an indispensable amino acid during that time. Severe physiologic stress, illness, and genetic disorders also may render an amino acid conditionally indispensable. Phenylketonuria is a genetic disorder in which the affected

DRUG-NUTRIENT INTERACTION

ASPARTAME AND PHENYLKETONURIA

Aspartame is a nonnutritive sweetener (i.e., it does not provide any nutrients or calories) that is composed of two amino acids: aspartic acid and phenylalanine. It is made synthetically, and its structure more closely resembles a protein than a carbohydrate. However, by adding a methanol group, the resulting product provides a sweet taste. It is used in foods and beverages as a high-potency sweetener, and it is approximately 200 times sweeter than table sugar or sucrose. Therefore, much less is needed to sweeten a food to the same degree.

As mentioned previously, phenylketonuria (PKU) is a disease in which an individual lacks the enzyme phenylalanine hydroxylase. Without this enzyme, phenylalanine cannot be metabolized and thus accumulates in the blood. High levels in the blood are toxic to brain tissue, and this can result in mental degradation and possibly death. Individuals with PKU must follow a strict diet with careful intake of phenylalanine that supports growth but that does not exceed tolerance. Those with PKU should avoid all foods that contain aspartame because of its concentrated phenylalanine content.

Foods that contain phenylalanine, such as aspartame—which is also known by the trade names *NutraSweet* and *Equal*—have warnings on their packages for PKU patients.

Following is a list of common foods that contain aspartame:

- Chewing gum
- Diet sodas
- Frozen desserts
- Gelatins
- Puddings
- Sugar-free candies
- Yogurt

Sara Harcourt

---

individual lacks the enzyme that is needed to convert phenylalanine to tyrosine. Because the conversion of phenylalanine cannot take place, amounts in the blood may rise to toxic levels. A specific phenylketonuria diet must be followed and certain foods avoided (see the Drug-Nutrient Interaction box, "Aspartame and Phenylketonuria"). With this condition, tyrosine must be supplied by the diet, and thus it is conditionally indispensable.

Balance

In terms of nutrition, the term *balance* refers to the relative intake and output of substances in the body to maintain the equilibrium that is necessary for health in various circumstances throughout the lifespan. This concept of balance can be applied to life-sustaining protein and the nitrogen that it supplies.

Protein Balance

The body's tissue proteins are constantly being broken down into amino acids through a process called *catabolism,* and they are then resynthesized into tissue proteins as needed through a process called *anabolism.* To maintain nitrogen balance, the part of the amino acid that contains nitrogen may be removed by a process called *deamination,* converted into ammonia, and then excreted as urea in the urine. The remaining nonnitrogen residue will be used to make carbohydrate or fat, or it may be reattached to make another amino acid, if necessary. The rate of this protein and nitrogen turnover varies in different tissues in accordance with the degree of metabolic activity and the available supply of amino acids.

Tissue turnover is a continuous process of reshaping, building, and adjusting to maintain overall protein balance within the body. The body maintains a delicate balance among tissue protein, plasma protein, and dietary protein. With this finely balanced system, healthy individuals have a small pool of amino acids from both tissue protein and dietary protein that is available to meet metabolic needs (Figure 4-2).

Nitrogen Balance

The body's nitrogen balance indicates how well its tissues are being maintained. The intake and use of dietary protein are measured by the amount of nitrogen intake in food protein and the amount of nitrogen excreted in the urine. For example, 1 g of urinary nitrogen results from the digestion and metabolism of 6.25 g of protein. Thus, if 1 g of nitrogen is excreted in the urine for every 6.25 g of protein consumed, then the body is said to be in nitrogen balance. This balance is the normal pattern in adult health. However, at different times of life or in states of malnutrition or illness, the balance may shift to be either positive or negative.

Positive Nitrogen Balance. A positive nitrogen balance exists when the body holds on to more nitrogen than it excretes, thus storing more nitrogen (by building tissue) than it is losing (by breaking down

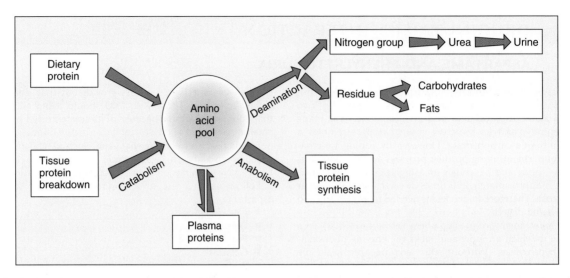

Figure 4-2 The balance between protein compartments and the amino acid pool.

tissue). This situation occurs normally during periods of rapid growth, such as infancy, childhood, adolescence, pregnancy, and lactation. A positive nitrogen balance also occurs in individuals who have been ill or malnourished and who are being "built back up" with increased nourishment. In such cases, protein is used to meet increased needs for tissue building and its associated metabolic activity.

Negative Nitrogen Balance. A negative nitrogen balance occurs when the body holds on to less nitrogen than it excretes. This means that the body has an inadequate protein intake and is losing nitrogen by breaking down more tissue than it is building up. This situation arises in states of malnutrition and illness. For example, negative nitrogen balance is seen in individuals when protein deficiency—even when kilocalories from carbohydrate and fat are adequate—causes the classic protein deficiency disease kwashiorkor. The failure to maintain the nitrogen balance may not become apparent for some time, but it eventually causes the loss of muscle tissue, the impairment of body organs and functions, and an increased susceptibility to infection. In children, negative nitrogen balance for an extended period causes growth retardation and may be fatal.

FUNCTIONS OF PROTEIN

Primary Tissue Building

Protein is the fundamental structural material of every cell in the body. In fact, the largest dry-weight portion of the body is protein. Body protein (e.g., the lean mass of muscles) accounts for approximately three fourths of the dry matter in most tissues, excluding bone and adipose tissue. Protein makes up the bulk of the muscles, internal organs, brain, nerves, skin, hair, and nails, and it is also a vital part of regulatory substances such as enzymes, hormones, and blood plasma. All such tissues must be constantly repaired and replaced. The primary functions of protein are to repair worn-out, wasted, or damaged tissue and to build new tissue. Thus, protein meets growth needs and maintains tissue health during the adult years. In fact, protein is central to the biochemical machinery that makes cells work.

Additional Body Functions

In addition to its basic tissue-building function, protein has other body functions related to energy, water balance, metabolism, and the body's defense system. Box 4-2 lists the major functions of protein.

Water and pH Balance

Fluids within the body are divided into three compartments: intravascular, intracellular, and interstitial (see Chapter 9). The body compartments are separated with cell membranes that are not freely permeable to protein. Because water is attracted to protein, plasma proteins such as albumin help to control water balance throughout the body by exerting osmotic pressure. This pressure maintains the normal circulation of tissue fluids within the appropriate compartments.

The normal pH of blood is between 7.35 and 7.45. However, constantly occurring bodily functions release acidic and alkaline substances, thereby affecting the overall acidity and alkalinity of blood. The unique structure of proteins—a combination of a carboxyl acid group and a base group—allows them to act as buffering agents by releasing or taking up excess acid within the body. If blood reaches a pH in either extreme (i.e., too acidic or too alkaline), plasma proteins denature and can result in death.

Metabolism and Transportation

Protein aids metabolic functions through enzymes, transport agents, and hormones. Digestive and cell enzymes are proteins that control metabolic processes. Enzymes that are necessary for the digestion of carbohydrates (amylase), fats (lipase), and proteins (proteases) are all proteins in structure. Protein also acts as the vehicle in which nutrients are carried throughout the body. Lipoproteins are necessary to transport fats in the water-soluble blood supply. Other examples are hemoglobin, which is the vital oxygen carrier in the red blood cells, and transferrin, which is the iron transport protein in blood. Peptide hormones (e.g., insulin, glucagon) are also proteins that play a major function in the metabolism of glucose (see Chapter 20).

Body Defense System

Protein is used to build special white blood cells (i.e., lymphocytes) and antibodies as part of the body's immune system to help defend against disease and infection.

Energy System

As described in previous chapters, carbohydrates are the primary fuel source for the body's energy system, and they are assisted by fat as a stored fuel. In times of need, protein may furnish additional fuel to sustain body heat and energy, but this is a less-efficient backup source for use only when the supply of carbohydrate and fat is insufficient. The available fuel factor of protein is 4 kcal/g.

FOOD SOURCES OF PROTEIN

Types of Food Proteins

Fortunately most foods contain a mixture of proteins that complement one another. In a mixed diet, animal and plant foods provide a wide variety of many nutrients, including protein. Thus, the key to a balanced diet is variety. Food proteins are classified as complete or incomplete proteins, depending on their amino acid composition.

Complete Proteins

Protein foods that contain all nine indispensable amino acids in sufficient quantity and ratio to meet the body's needs are called *complete proteins*. These proteins are primarily of animal origin (e.g., egg, milk, cheese, meat, poultry, fish; Figure 4-3). However, soybeans and soy products are the exception. Soy products are the only plant sources of complete proteins. Another exception is gelatin, which is an incomplete animal protein. Although gelatin is a protein of animal origin, it is a relatively insignificant protein, because it lacks the three essential amino acids tryptophan, valine, and isoleucine, and it has only small amounts of leucine.

Incomplete Proteins

Protein foods that are deficient in one or more of the nine indispensable amino acids are called *incomplete proteins*. These proteins are generally of plant origin (e.g., grains, legumes, nuts, seeds), but they are found in foods that make valuable contributions to the total amount of dietary protein.

Vegetarian Diets

Complementary Protein

Current knowledge of protein metabolism and the pooling of amino acid reserves (see Figure 4-2) indicates that a mixture of plant proteins can provide adequate amounts of amino acids when the basic use of various grains is expanded to include soy protein and other dried legume proteins (i.e., beans and peas). Because most plant proteins are incomplete and thereby lacking one or more of the indispensable (or essential) amino acids, vegetarians can mix plant foods so that the amino acids missing in one food are supplied by another. This is the art of combining plant protein foods so that they complement one another and supply all nine indispensable amino acids.

A normal eating pattern throughout the day, together with the body's small reserve of amino acids, usually ensures an overall amino acid balance. The underlying

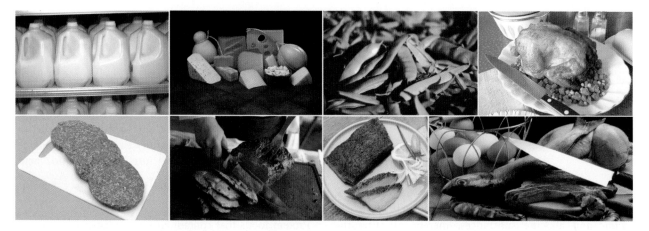

Figure 4-3 Sources of complete proteins. (Copyright JupiterImages Corp.)

CULTURAL CONSIDERATIONS

INDISPENSABLE AMINO ACIDS AND THEIR COMPLEMENTARY FOOD PROTEINS

A large percentage of the worldwide population follows various forms of vegetarian diets for religious, traditional, or economic reasons. Seventh-Day Adventists follow a lacto-ovo-vegetarian diet, whereas individuals of the Hindu and Buddhist faith generally are lacto-vegetarian. The Mediterranean diet has such a strong emphasis on grains, pastas, vegetables, and cheese that few other animal products (i.e., beef, chicken, and fish) are consumed. In other areas of the world, the economic burden of animal products does not allow for the consumption of such foods. Any form of a vegetarian diet can be healthy; however, a good understanding of how to achieve complete protein balance is necessary.

All nine indispensable (or essential) amino acids must be supplied by the diet. Protein from both animal and plant sources can meet protein requirements. One concern related to a vegetarian diet is getting a balanced amount of the indispensable amino acids to complement each other and to make complete protein combinations.

When making complementary food combinations to balance the needed amino acids, families of foods (e.g.,

grains, legumes, dairy) must be mixed. For example, grains are low in threonine and high in methionine, whereas legumes are the opposite and as such are low in methionine and high in threonine. Therefore, grains and legumes help to balance one another with regard to the accumulation of all indispensable amino acids. The addition of milk products and eggs enhances the amino acid adequacy of lacto-ovo-vegetarians. Following are sample food combinations to illustrate complementary protein combinations:

- *Grains and peas, beans, or lentils:* brown rice and beans; whole-grain bread with pea or lentil soup; wheat or corn tortilla with beans; peanut butter on whole wheat bread; Indian dishes of rice and dal (a legume); Chinese dishes of tofu and rice
- *Legumes and seeds:* falafel; soybeans and pumpkin or sesame seeds; Middle Eastern hummus (garbanzo beans and sesame seeds) or tahini
- *Grains and dairy:* whole-wheat pasta and cheese; yogurt and a multigrain muffin; cereal and milk; a cheese sandwich made with whole-grain bread

requirement for vegetarians—as for all people—is to eat a sufficient amount of varied foods to meet normal nutrient and energy needs (see the Cultural Considerations box, "Indispensable Amino Acids and Their Complementary Food Proteins").

Types of Vegetarian Diets

Vegetarian diets differ according to the beliefs or needs of the individuals who are following such food patterns. Approximately 2.3% of the U.S. adult population (roughly

4.9 million people) consistently followed a vegetarian diet in 2006.[2] A variety of reasons lead people to choose a vegetarian diet, including environmental and animal cruelty concerns, health incentives, religious adherence (e.g., Buddhists, Hindus, Seventh-Day Adventists), and aversion to the consumption of animal products. Alternatively, a diet that is void of animal products is not always a choice. In some areas in the world, vegetarianism is simply a result of the lack of resources and availability of animal products.

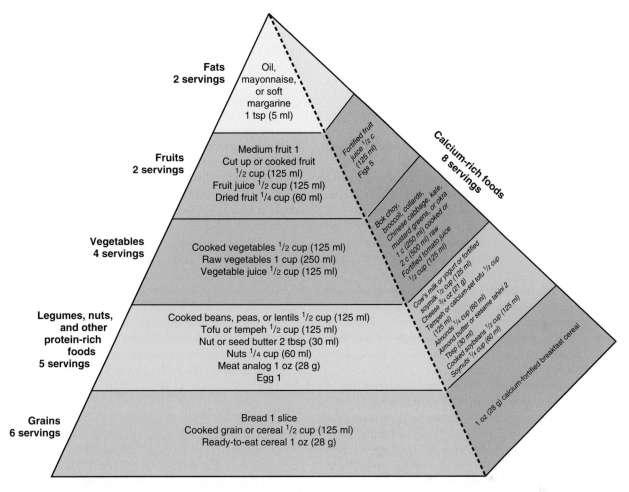

Figure 4-4 The lacto-ovo-vegetarian diet pyramid. (Reprinted from Messina V, Melina V, Mangels AR. A new food guide for North American vegetarians. *J Am Diet Assoc.* 2003; 103(6):771-775.)

In general, vegetarians can be described as one of the following four basic types:

1. *Lacto-ovo-vegetarians:* These are vegetarians who follow a food pattern that allows for the consumption of dairy products and eggs (Figure 4-4). Their mixed diet of plant and animal food sources that excludes meat, poultry, pork, and fish poses no nutritional concerns.

2. *Lacto-vegetarians:* These vegetarians accept only dairy products from animal sources to complement their basic diet of plant foods. The use of milk and milk products (e.g., cheese) with a varied mixed diet of whole or enriched grains, legumes, nuts, seeds, fruits, and vegetables in sufficient quantities to meet energy needs provides a balanced diet.

3. *Ovo-vegetarians:* The only animal foods included in the ovo-vegetarian diet are eggs. Because eggs are an excellent source of complete proteins,

individuals who are following this diet do not have to be overly concerned with complementary proteins if eggs are consumed consistently.

4. *Vegans:* Vegans follow a strict vegetarian diet and consume no animal foods. Their food pattern consists entirely of plant foods (e.g., whole or enriched grains, legumes, nuts, seeds, fruits, vegetables). The use of soybeans, soy milk, soybean curd (tofu), and processed soy protein products enhances the nutritional value of the diet. Careful planning and sufficient food intake ensure adequate nutrition.

The most recent position paper from the Academy of Nutrition and Dietetics (formerly known as the American Dietetic Association) and Dietitians of Canada states that a vegetarian diet (including the vegan option) can meet the current recommendations for all essential nutrients, including protein.[3] The experts also indicate that the former mindful combination of complementary plant proteins within every given meal is unnecessary; achieving a balance throughout the day is more important. In addition, vegetarian diets are appropriate throughout all stages of life, including pregnancy, infancy, childhood, adolescence, and older age as well as for those with an athletic lifestyle.

Health Benefits and Risk

Some of the most notable benefits of vegetarianism include the following[3,4]:

- Lower levels of dietary saturated fat and cholesterol
- Higher intake of fruits, vegetables, whole grains, nuts, soy products, fiber, and phytochemicals
- Lower body mass index and prevalence of obesity
- Better lipid profiles and lower rates of death from cardiovascular disease, including ischemic heart disease and hypertension
- Lowered risk of renal disease from high glomerular filtration rates as compared with long-term high protein intake
- Effective management of type 2 diabetes[5] and lowering of the risk of type 2 diabetes and some forms of cancer (e.g., prostate, colon)
- Other possible benefits include a lowered risk of dementia, diverticulitis, and gallstones

After an extensive review of the effects of vegetarian diets with regard to various medical conditions, some researchers have concluded that "dietary intervention with a vegetarian diet seems to be a cheap, physiologic, and safe approach for the prevention and possible management of modern lifestyle diseases."[6] The preventive mechanism at work in the vegetarian diet is the rich supply of monounsaturated and polyunsaturated fatty acids, fiber, complex carbohydrates, and antioxidants and a restriction of saturated fat. To reap the benefits of a vegetarian diet, a well-balanced diet from a variety of foods is necessary. It should be noted that not all vegetarians follow an ideal well-balanced diet and therefore do not obtain the possible health benefits.

Key nutrients of concern for practicing vegetarians are protein, iron, zinc, calcium, vitamin D, vitamin B_{12}, and omega-3 fatty acids.[3,7] Reasons for concern and effective ways to overcome these barriers are outlined in Table 4-1.

DIGESTION OF PROTEINS

Mouth

After a food that contains protein is consumed, the protein must be broken down into the necessary ready-to-use building blocks: amino acids. This is done through the successive parts of the gastrointestinal tract by mechanical and chemical digestion. The mechanical breaking down of protein begins with chewing in the mouth. The food particles are mixed with saliva and passed on to the stomach as a semisolid mass.

Stomach

Because proteins are such large and complex structures, a series of enzymes is necessary for digestion and for the release of individual amino acids, which is the primary form needed for absorption. Unlike the enzymes that are needed for carbohydrate and fat digestion, all enzymes involved in protein digestion (i.e., proteases) are stored as inactive proenzymes called zymogens. Zymogens are then activated according to need. The enzymes that are needed for protein digestion cannot be stored in an active form, because the cells and organs that produce and store them (which are made of structural proteins) would be digested as well.

The chemical digestion of protein begins in the stomach. In fact, the stomach's chief digestive function is the first stage of the enzymatic breakdown of protein. The following three agents in the gastric secretions help with this task.

Hydrochloric Acid

Hydrochloric acid begins the unfolding and denaturing of the complex protein chains. This unfolding makes the individual peptide bonds more available for enzymatic action. Hydrochloric acid also provides the acid medium that is necessary to convert pepsinogen into active pepsin, which is the gastric enzyme that is specific to proteins.

Pepsin

Pepsin is first produced as an inactive proenzyme called *pepsinogen* by a single layer of chief cells in the stomach wall. The hydrochloric acid within gastric juices then changes pepsinogen to the active enzyme pepsin.

---

proenzyme an inactive precursor (i.e., a forerunner substance from which another substance is made) that is converted to the active enzyme by the action of an acid, another enzyme, or other means.

zymogen an inactive enzyme precursor.

pepsin the main gastric enzyme specific for proteins; pepsin begins breaking large protein molecules into shorter chain polypeptides, and it is activated by gastric hydrochloric acid.

TABLE 4-1 **NUTRIENT CONSIDERATIONS FOR VEGETARIANS**

Nutrient	Problem	Solution
Protein	Plant protein quality varies; lower bioavailability than animal protein	Consume a variety of plant foods throughout the day, including soy products
Iron	Plant foods contain nonheme iron, which is less bioavailable than the heme iron found in animal foods and which is sensitive to inhibitors such as phytate, calcium, tea, coffee, and fiber	Iron intake recommendations are 1.8 times higher than for nonvegetarians; consume high-iron plant foods with dietary sources of vitamin C, which is an enhancer of iron absorption
Zinc	Plant foods high in phytates bind zinc	Regularly consume foods such as nuts, soy products, zinc-fortified cereals, and soaked and sprouted beans, grains, and seeds
Calcium	Oxalates reduce the absorption of calcium found in spinach, beet greens, and Swiss chard	Regularly consume plant foods that are high in calcium and low in oxalates, such as Chinese cabbage, broccoli, Napa cabbage, collards, kale, okra, and turnip greens in addition to calcium-fortified foods such as orange juice
Vitamin D	Other than endogenously produced vitamin D from sunlight exposure, the primary source of this vitamin is fortified cow's milk	Sun exposure to the face, hands, and forearms for 5 to 15 minutes per day during the summer provides enough sunlight for light-skinned people to produce adequate amounts of vitamin D, and dark-skinned people require more sun exposure; otherwise, choose foods or dietary supplements that are fortified with vitamin D, such as soy milk, rice milk, orange juice, and breakfast cereal
Vitamin B_{12}	No plant food contains active vitamin B_{12}	Choose foods that are fortified with B_{12}, such as soy milk, breakfast cereal, nutritional yeast, or use dietary supplements
Omega-3 fatty acid (alpha-linolenic)	Few plant foods are good sources of alpha-linolenic acid	Regularly include sources of alpha-linolenic acid in the diet, such as flaxseeds, walnuts, canola oil, soy products, and breakfast bars fortified with DHA, or take DHA supplements that are derived from microalgae

Adapted from Craig WJ. Health effects of vegan diets. *Am J Clin Nutr*. 2009; 89(5):1627S-1633S; and Craig WJ, Mangels AR. Position of the American Dietetic Association: vegetarian diets. *J Am Diet Assoc*. 2009; 109(7):1266-1282.

Pepsin begins splitting the bonds between the protein's amino acids, which changes the large protein into short chains called *polypeptides*. If the protein were held in the stomach longer, pepsin could continue this breakdown until only the individual amino acids of the protein remained. However, with the normal gastric emptying time, pepsin only completes the first stage of breakdown.

Rennin

The gastric enzyme rennin is only present during infancy and childhood, and it is especially important for the infant's digestion of milk. Rennin and calcium act on the casein of milk to produce a curd. By coagulating milk into a more solid curd, rennin prevents the food from passing too rapidly from the infant's stomach to the small intestine.

Small Intestine

Protein digestion begins in the acidic medium of the stomach, and it is completed in the alkaline medium of the small intestine. Enzymes from the secretions of both the pancreas and the intestine take part in this process.

Pancreatic Secretions

The following three enzymes produced by the pancreas continue breaking down proteins into more and more simple substances:

1. **Trypsin,** which is secreted first as inactive trypsinogen, is activated by the enzyme enterokinase. Enterokinase is secreted from the intestinal cells on contact with food entering the duodenum, which is the first section of the small intestine. The active trypsin then works on proteins and large polypeptide fragments that are carried from the stomach. This enzymatic action produces small polypeptides and dipeptides.

2. **Chymotrypsin,** which is secreted first as the inactive chymotrypsinogen, is activated by trypsin that is already present in the gut. The active enzyme then continues the same protein-splitting action of trypsin.

3. **Carboxypeptidase** attacks the acid (i.e., carboxyl) end of the peptide chains, thereby producing small peptides and some free amino acids. Carboxypeptidase is also first released as an inactive proenzyme (procarboxypeptidase), and it is activated by trypsin.

Intestinal Secretions

Glands in the intestinal wall produce the following two protein-splitting enzymes to complete the breakdown and free the remaining amino acids:

1. **Aminopeptidase** attacks the nitrogen-containing (i.e., amino) end of the peptide chain and releases amino acids one at a time, thereby producing peptides and free amino acids.
2. **Dipeptidase**, which is the final enzyme in the protein-splitting system, completes the job by breaking the remaining dipeptides into two free amino acids.

This finely coordinated system of protein-splitting enzymes breaks down the large, complex proteins into progressively smaller peptide chains and frees each individual amino acid. This is a tremendous overall task. The free amino acids are now ready to be absorbed directly into the portal blood circulation for use in the building of body tissues. This remarkable system of protein digestion is summarized in Figure 4-5.

RECOMMENDATIONS FOR DIETARY PROTEIN

Influential Factors of Protein Needs

The following three factors influence the body's requirement for protein: (1) tissue growth; (2) the quality of the dietary protein; and (3) the additional needs that result from illness or disease.

Tissue Growth

During rapid growth periods of the human life cycle, more protein per unit of body weight is necessary to build new tissue and to maintain present tissue. Human growth is most rapid during fetal growth, infant growth during the first year of life, and adolescent growth. Childhood is a sustained time of continued growth, but this occurs at a somewhat slower rate. For adults, protein requirements level off to meet tissue-maintenance needs, but individual needs may vary.

Dietary Protein Quality

The nature of a protein and its pattern of amino acids significantly influence its dietary quality.[8] Sufficient

energy intake—especially from nonprotein foods—is necessary to conserve protein for tissue structure. In addition, the digestion and absorption of the protein consumed are affected by the complexity of its structure as well as its preparation and cooking. The comparative quality of protein foods has been determined by the following methods:

1. *Chemical score,* which is derived from the amino acid pattern of the food; a high-quality protein food, such as an egg (with a value of 100), is compared with other foods according to their amino acid ratios
2. *Biological value,* which is based on nitrogen balance
3. *Net protein utilization,* which is based on the biologic value and the degree of the food protein's digestibility

---

rennin the milk-curdling enzyme of the gastric juice of human infants and young animals (e.g., calves); rennin should not be confused with renin, which is an important enzyme produced by the kidneys that plays a vital role in the activation of angiotensin.

trypsin a protein-splitting enzyme secreted as the inactive proenzyme trypsinogen by the pancreas and that is activated and works in the small intestine to reduce proteins to shorter-chain polypeptides and dipeptides.

enterokinase an enzyme produced and secreted in the duodenum in response to food entering the small intestine; it activates trypsinogen to its active form of trypsin.

chymotrypsin a protein-splitting enzyme secreted as the inactive zymogen chymotrypsinogen by the pancreas; after it has been activated by trypsin, it acts in the small intestine to continue breaking down proteins into shorter-chain polypeptides and dipeptides.

carboxypeptidase a specific protein-splitting enzyme secreted as the inactive zymogen procarboxypeptidase by the pancreas; after it has been activated by trypsin, it acts in the small intestine to break off the acid (i.e., carboxyl) end of the peptide chain, thereby producing smaller-chained peptides and free amino acids.

aminopeptidase a specific protein-splitting enzyme secreted by glands in the walls of the small intestine that breaks off the nitrogen-containing amino end (i.e., NH_2) of the peptide chain, thereby producing smaller-chained peptides and free amino acids.

dipeptidase the final enzyme in the protein-splitting system that produces the last two free amino acids.

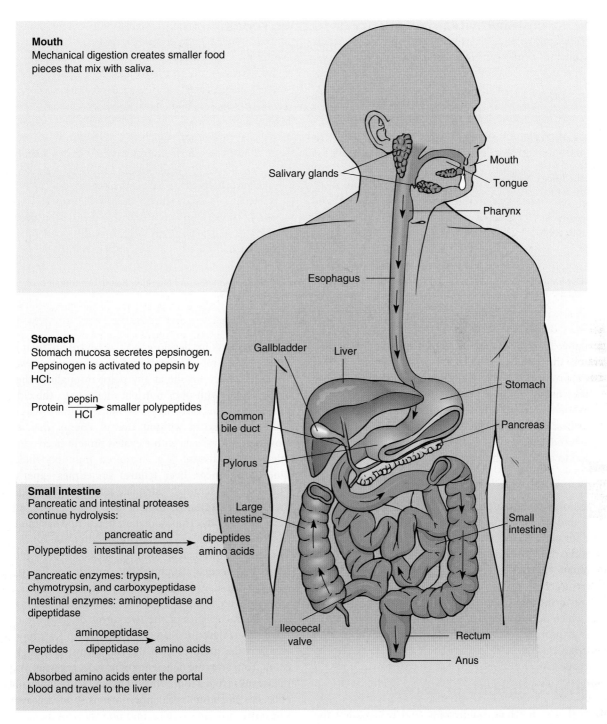

Mouth
Mechanical digestion creates smaller food pieces that mix with saliva.

Stomach
Stomach mucosa secretes pepsinogen. Pepsinogen is activated to pepsin by HCl:

Protein $\xrightarrow[\text{HCl}]{\text{pepsin}}$ smaller polypeptides

Small intestine
Pancreatic and intestinal proteases continue hydrolysis:

Polypeptides $\xrightarrow[\text{intestinal proteases}]{\text{pancreatic and}}$ dipeptides amino acids

Pancreatic enzymes: trypsin, chymotrypsin, and carboxypeptidase
Intestinal enzymes: aminopeptidase and dipeptidase

Peptides $\xrightarrow[\text{dipeptidase}]{\text{aminopeptidase}}$ amino acids

Absorbed amino acids enter the portal blood and travel to the liver

Salivary glands — Mouth — Tongue — Pharynx — Esophagus — Gallbladder — Liver — Stomach — Common bile duct — Pancreas — Pylorus — Large intestine — Small intestine — Ileocecal valve — Rectum — Anus

Figure 4-5 Summary of protein digestion. (Courtesy Rolin Graphics.)

4. *Protein efficiency ratio,* which is based on the weight gain of a growing test animal in relation to its protein intake

Table 4-2 compares various protein food scores on the basis of protein quality. As seen in the table, egg and cow's milk proteins have the highest protein quality score. The quality and digestibility of most plant proteins are significantly lower than those of animal proteins. Therefore, the dietary protein needs of vegans who rely solely on plant foods of lower protein quality (e.g., cereal, legumes) may

TABLE 4-2 COMPARATIVE PROTEIN QUALITY OF SELECTED FOODS

Food	Chemical Score*	Biologic Value	Net Protein Utilization	Protein Efficiency Ratio
Egg	100	100	94	3.92
Cow's milk	95	93	82	3.09
Fish	71	76	—	3.55
Beef	69	74	67	2.30
Unpolished rice	67	86	59	—
Peanuts	65	55	55	1.65
Oats	57	65	—	2.19
Polished rice	57	64	57	2.18
Whole wheat	53	65	49	1.53
Corn	49	72	36	—
Soybeans	47	73	61	2.32
Sesame seeds	42	62	53	1.77
Peas	37	64	55	1.57

*Amino acid.

Modified from Guthrie H. *Introductory nutrition.* 6th ed. New York: McGraw-Hill; 1986; and Food and Nutrition Board, Institute of Medicine. *Recommended dietary allowances.* 10th ed. Washington, DC: National Academies Press; 1989.

be higher than those of nonvegetarians.[3] In other words, because the protein provided by whole-wheat products is only approximately half as bioavailable as the protein that comes from eggs, more protein from whole-wheat products should be eaten to obtain equivalent useable protein. Regardless of dietary preferences for protein foods, a varied and balanced diet is the best way for a healthy person to obtain quality protein.

Illness or Disease

Illness or disease, especially when it is accompanied by fever and catabolic tissue breakdown, raises the body's need for protein and kilocalories for rebuilding tissue and meeting the demands of an increased metabolic rate. Traumatic injury requires extensive tissue rebuilding. After surgery, extra protein is needed for wound healing and restoring losses. Extensive tissue destruction, such as that which occurs with burns and pressure sores, requires a large protein increase for the healing and grafting processes.

Dietary Deficiency or Excess

As with any nutrient, moderation and balance are the keys to health. Too much or too little dietary protein can be problematic for overall body function.

Protein-Energy Malnutrition

Protein-energy malnutrition (PEM) may occur in a variety of situations. The most severe cases are found in less-industrialized countries where all foods—not just protein-rich foods—are in short supply. Children are at

the highest risk for developing PEM because of their high needs during rapid growth and development. However, PEM can affect anyone at any point throughout the life cycle. People with poor nutrient intake (e.g., the elderly, those with eating disorders) may suffer from PEM as well. PEM rarely exists without overall energy deficiency. However, individuals with elevated protein needs during infection or disease (e.g., acquired immunodeficiency syndrome, cancer, liver failure) sometimes experience PEM despite seemingly adequate total energy intake. As previously mentioned, protein has many critical functions in the body. Thus, a dietary deficiency has multiple consequences that are directly related to these functions. Without the amino acid building blocks, the body cannot synthesize needed structural (i.e., muscle) or functional (i.e., enzymes, antibodies, and hormones) proteins.

Two severe forms of PEM are kwashiorkor and marasmus. Characteristics of the two forms of PEM are quite different, as described later in this chapter. Kwashiorkor, which is the more fatal of the two forms, is thought to result from an acute deficiency of protein, whereas marasmus results from a more chronic deficiency of many nutrients. The end result with either form is stunted growth, a weakened immune system, and poor development.

Kwashiorkor. Kwashiorkor is more common among children who are between the ages of 18 and 24 months, who have been breastfed all their lives, and who are then are rapidly weaned, often because of the arrival of a younger sibling. These children are switched from nutritionally balanced breast milk to a dilute diet of mostly carbohydrates and little protein. The children may receive adequate total kilocalories, but they lack enough bioavailable protein sources. The term *kwashiorkor* is a Ghanaian word that refers to the disease that takes over the first child when the second child is born. Characteristics of kwashiorkor include generalized edema and fatty liver as a result of inadequate protein intake to maintain fluid balance and to transport fat from the liver (Figure 4-6).

To date, the exact pathogenesis of kwashiorkor is not well defined, and there may be additional factors involved in the development of the characteristic edema, such as oxidative stress and/or inappropriate antidiuretic hormone response.[9]

Marasmus. Individuals with marasmus have an emaciated appearance with little or no body fat. This is a chronic form of energy and protein deficiency; in other words, it is a result of basic starvation. Stunted growth and development are more severe with this form of PEM. Marasmus can affect individuals of all ages with inadequate food sources.

Excess Dietary Intake

Contrary to popular belief, one can ingest too much dietary protein. The body has a finite need for protein. When a person has met the dietary protein needs, additional protein is deaminated (i.e., the nitrogen is removed) and stored as fat or used as energy. Eating excess protein does not build muscle; only exercising with enough protein to support growth can do that. The following problems can occur with diets that are heavily laden with protein:

1. They are often high in saturated fat, which is a known risk for cardiovascular disease.
2. If a person fills up on protein foods, little room is left for fruits, vegetables, and other whole grains, which are packed with essential vitamins, minerals, and fiber (see the Further Focus box, "The High-Protein Diet").
3. The kidneys have the extra burden of getting rid of excess nitrogen.

Although most protein and amino acid supplements are not harmful in small doses, they are unnecessary in a balanced diet. However, taking excessive single amino acid dietary supplements can be harmful if it is to the exclusion of other essential amino acids, thereby creating an overall imbalance.

Dietary Guides

Dietary Reference Intakes

The Recommended Dietary Allowances (RDAs) continue to be the principal dietary guide for protein consumption, and they are part of the Dietary Reference Intake standards. Similar to carbohydrate and fat recommendations, the Dietary Reference Intakes for proteins have been set as a percentage of the total kilocalorie consumption by the National Academy of Sciences. Children and adults should obtain 10% to 35% of their total caloric intake from protein. The RDA standards relate to the age, sex, and weight of the average person, and they are based on the analysis of available nitrogen-balance studies. The RDA for both men and women is set at 0.8 g of high-quality protein per kilogram of desirable body weight per day[1] (i.e., 0.8 g/kg per day; see the Clinical Applications box, "Calculating Dietary Reference Intake for Protein"). Dietary recommendations are higher for infants and for pregnant and breastfeeding women in order to meet metabolic needs.

The RDAs are set to meet the nutritional requirements of most healthy people. Severe physical stress (e.g., illness, disease, surgery) can increase a person's requirement for protein. Of note is that the U.S. Department of Agriculture's "What We Eat in America" report found that the average daily protein intake of men and women 20 years and older is 101.9 g and 70.1 g per day, respectively.[10] According to this report, men consume approximately 181% of their Dietary Reference Intakes for protein, and

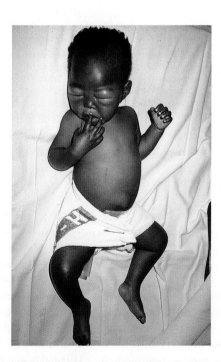

Figure 4-6 Kwashiorkor. The infant shows generalized edema, which is seen in the form of puffiness of the face, arms, and legs. (Reprinted from Kumar V, Abbas AK, Fausto N, Mitchell R. *Robbins basic pathology.* 8th ed. Philadelphia: Saunders; 2007.)

FOR FURTHER FOCUS

THE HIGH-PROTEIN DIET

The per-capita consumption of protein by Americans continues to rise, along with the total caloric intake. In the United States, the per-capita daily consumption of kilocalories and grams of protein rose from 3500 kcal and 101 g protein in 1909 to 3900 kcal and 111 g protein in 2006.[1] Not coincidentally, significant weight gains and the health risks associated with obesity (e.g., heart disease, diabetes, hypertension, some forms of cancer) have been noted. The Behavioral Risk Factor Surveillance System results indicate that 33% of men and 46% of women are actively trying to lose weight in the United States.[2]

Many health care professionals are concerned about the rising rate of obesity in this country as well as the methods by which people are trying to battle it. Current surveys report that, of those individuals who are trying to lose weight, only 19% of women and 22% of men reported using the recommended weight-loss strategy of fewer calories and more physical activity.[2] Some of the more popular diets are the high-protein, low-carbohydrate diets.

High-protein diets are generally higher in total fat, saturated fat, and cholesterol. Initial weight loss associated with a high-protein, high-fat diet is caused by the induction of metabolic ketosis and fluid loss from a lack of carbohydrates. Ketosis eventually suppresses the appetite, and this ultimately leads to reduced caloric intake and weight loss.

Clifton and colleagues[3] evaluated the long-term success of weight-loss maintenance among subjects after they followed either a high-protein (34% of total energy) or high-carbohydrate (64% of total energy) diet. Subjects were on the diet for 12 weeks and then assessed 52 weeks later to evaluate results. Authors concluded that sustained weight loss was not significantly different between groups but that the group with higher protein intake did experience some beneficial weight loss results, such as abdominal fat loss and total fat mass lost. Neither group reported long-term compliance with their assigned dietary regimen.

Krieger and associates[4] reviewed findings from 87 weight-loss studies of various macronutrient restrictions. Their conclusion was that weight-loss diets with low carbohydrate (35% to 41% total energy) and high protein intake resulted in a greater loss of fat mass. However, there was also a greater loss of lean tissue (i.e., a negative effect) in the low-carbohydrate, high-protein diet, unless protein intake exceeded 1.05 g/kg body weight.

Regardless of these findings, the American Heart Association has not changed its view regarding high-protein diets. In a statement for health care professionals from the Nutrition Committee of the Council on Nutrition, Physical Activity, and Metabolism of the American Heart Association, researchers concluded that "high-protein diets are not recommended because they restrict healthful foods that provide essential nutrients and do not provide the variety of foods needed to adequately meet nutritional needs."[5]

1. United States Department of Agriculture, Center for Nutrition Policy and Promotion. *U.S. food supply: nutrients and other food components, per capita per day, 1909 to 2006* (website): www.ers.usda.gov/Data/FoodConsumption/NutrientAvailIndex.htm. Accessed October 10 2011.
2. Bish CL, Blanck HM, Serdula MK, et al. Diet and physical activity behaviors among Americans trying to lose weight: 2000 Behavioral Risk Factor Surveillance System. *Obes Res*. 2005;13(3):596-607.
3. Clifton PM, Keogh JB, Noakes M. Long-term effects of a high-protein weight-loss diet. *Am J Clin Nutr*. 2008;87(1):23-29.
4. Krieger JW, Sitren HS, Daniels MJ, Langkamp-Henken B. Effects of variation in protein and carbohydrate intake on body mass and composition during energy restriction: a meta-regression 1. *Am J Clin Nutr*. 2006;83(2):260-274.
5. St Jeor ST, Howard BV, Prewitt TE, et al. Dietary protein and weight reduction: a statement for healthcare professionals from the Nutrition Committee of the Council on Nutrition, Physical Activity, and Metabolism of the American Heart Association. *Circulation*. 2001; 104(15):1869-1874.

women consume approximately 152% of their protein requirement daily.

Dietary Guidelines for Americans

Americans generally eat more protein than necessary, especially in the form of meat, which carries a considerable amount of saturated fat and cholesterol. There are no benefits from consuming a diet with a high animal protein content. However, some potential health risks do exist. These risks relate to certain cancers, coronary heart disease, kidney stones, and chronic renal failure (see Chapter 21) that are associated with excess protein and saturated fat.

The *Dietary Guidelines for Americans* recommend the following with regard to protein-rich foods[11]:

- Choose a variety of protein foods, including seafood, lean meat and poultry, eggs, beans and peas, soy products, and unsalted nuts and seeds.
- Increase the amount and variety of seafood consumed by choosing seafood in place of some meat and poultry.
- Replace protein foods that are higher in solid fats with choices that are lower in solid fats and calories and/or are sources of oils.

Table 4-3 provides a comparison of protein-rich food portions.

CLINICAL APPLICATIONS

CALCULATING DIETARY REFERENCE INTAKE FOR PROTEIN

There are two ways to calculate a person's dietary recommendation for protein.

1) *Dietary Reference Intakes of Acceptable Macronutrient Distribution Range:* To calculate the protein needs of an individual who is consuming 2200 kcal/day based on the Dietary Reference Intake recommendation of 10% to 35% of total kilocalories, complete the following calculations:

   (1) 2200 kcal × 0.10 = 220 kcal/day *and*
   (2) 2200 kcal × 0.35 = 770 kcal/day, thus giving a range of 220 to 770 kcal/day from protein
   (3) 220 kcal ÷ 4 kcal/g = 55 *and*
   (4) 770 kcal ÷ 4 kcal/g = 192.5 g of protein per day, thus giving a range of 55 to 192.5 g of protein per day

2) *Recommended Dietary Allowance relative to ideal body weight:* To calculate the protein needs of a woman who is 5 feet, 4 inches tall with an ideal body weight of 120 lb (see Chapter 15) based on the Recommended Dietary Allowance of 0.8 g protein/kg body weight per day, perform the following calculations:

   (1) Convert weight in pounds to weight in kg (2.2 lb = 1 kg) as follows: 120 lb ÷ 2.2 lb/kg = 54.5 kg
   (2) 54.5 kg × 0.8 g/kg = 43.6 g protein per day

Therefore, a woman who measures 5 feet, 4 inches tall and who is consuming 2200 kcal/day with a minimum of 10% of her calories coming from high-quality protein will safely obtain her Recommended Dietary Allowance for protein of 43.6 g per day.

TABLE 4-3 **FOODS THAT ARE HIGH IN PROTEIN***

Food	Approximate Amount	Protein (g)
Veal, leg, meat only, braised	3 oz cooked	31.2
Beef, top round, trimmed of fat	3 oz cooked	30.7
Chicken, breast, meat only, roasted	3 oz cooked	26.7
Tuna, fresh, bluefin, cooked with dry heat	3 oz cooked	25.4
Turkey, meat only, roasted	3 oz cooked	24.9
Goose, meat only, roasted	3 oz cooked	24.6
Pork, sirloin, boneless, roasted	3 oz cooked	24.5
Halibut, fresh, cooked with dry heat	3 oz cooked	22.7
Liver, chicken, pan fried	3 oz cooked	21.9
Lamb, shoulder, trimmed to $\frac{1}{4}$-inch of fat, broiled	3 oz cooked	21.7
Tuna, canned in water, drained	3 oz cooked	21.7
Beef, ground, 70% lean, 30% fat, pan browned	3 oz cooked	21.7
Haddock, cooked with dry heat	3 oz cooked	20.6
Duck, meat only, roasted	3 oz cooked	20
Scallops, steamed	3 oz cooked	19.7
Salmon, Atlantic, cooked with dry heat	3 oz cooked	18.8
Soy burger	3 oz cooked	16.1
Oysters, cooked with moist heat	3 oz cooked	16.1
Tofu, fried	3 oz	14.6
Ham, sliced, 11% fat	3 oz cooked	14.1
Cottage cheese, 2% milk fat	3 oz	11.7
Soy milk	1 cup	11
Milk, 1% fat	1 cup	9.7
Peanut butter, smooth	2 Tbsp	8
Lentils, boiled	3 oz cooked	7.7
Kidney beans, boiled	3 oz cooked	7.4
Cheddar cheese	1 oz	7
Egg, whole, scrambled	1 large	6.8
Yogurt, plain, skim milk	3 oz	4.9

*Listed in decreasing order of protein per serving.
Data from the U.S. Department of Agriculture, Agricultural Research Service, Nutrient Data Laboratory. *Nutrient Data Laboratory home page* (website): www.ars.usda.gov/ba/bhnrc/ndl. Accessed September 22, 2011.

MyPlate

As with the other macronutrient recommendations from the MyPlate, Americans are encouraged to consume a variety of foods to meet all of their nutrient needs (see Figure 1-3).[12] The MyPlate Web site (www.choosemyplate.gov/) includes tips for choosing lean sources of meat, poultry, and fish as well as protein alternatives such as beans, nuts, and seeds. A personalized plan can be obtained by entering an individual's age, sex, height, weight, and physical activity level. Sample menus for nonvegetarians and eating tips for vegetarian lifestyles are also available.

SUMMARY

- Protein provides the human body with amino acids, which are its primary tissue-building units. Of the 20 common amino acids, 9 are indispensable in the diet, because the body cannot manufacture them as it can the remaining 11.
- Foods that supply all of the indispensable amino acids are called *complete proteins;* these foods are mostly of animal origin. Plant protein foods are considered incomplete proteins, because they lack one or more of the indispensable amino acids. The exception is soy protein, which is of plant origin and provides complete proteins.
- Strict vegan diets involve only plant proteins, but other vegetarian diets may include dairy products, eggs, and sometimes fish. Without proper planning, only vegans risk protein imbalance and other nutritional deficiencies in iron, zinc, calcium, vitamin B_{12}, and omega-3 fatty acids.

- A constant turnover of tissue protein occurs between tissue anabolism and tissue catabolism. Adequate dietary protein and a reserve pool of amino acids help to maintain this overall protein balance. Nitrogen balance is a measure of overall protein balance.
- A mixed diet that includes a variety of foods, together with sufficient nonprotein kilocalories from the primary fuel foods (i.e., carbohydrates), supplies a balance of protein and other nutrients.
- After protein foods are eaten, a powerful digestive team of six protein-splitting enzymes frees individual amino acids for absorption.
- Protein requirements are principally influenced by growth needs and the nature of the diet in terms of protein quality and energy intake. Clinical influences on protein needs include fever, disease, surgery, and other trauma to body tissues.

CRITICAL THINKING QUESTIONS

1. What is the difference between indispensable and dispensable amino acids? Why is this difference important?
2. Compare complete and incomplete protein foods. Give examples of each.
3. Describe the different types of vegetarian diets. Compare each in terms of protein quality and risk for nutrient deficiencies. What recommendations would you offer to someone who is following a vegan diet?
4. Describe the factors that influence protein requirements.

CHAPTER CHALLENGE QUESTIONS

True-False

Write the correct statement for each statement that is false.

1. *True or False:* Complete proteins of high biologic value are found in whole grains, dried beans and peas, and nuts.
2. *True or False:* The primary function of dietary protein is to supply the necessary amino acids to build and repair body tissue.
3. *True or False:* Protein provides a main source of body heat and muscle energy.
4. *True or False:* The average American diet contains a relatively small amount of protein.
5. *True or False:* Because they are smaller, infants and young children need less protein per unit of body weight as compared with adults.
6. *True or False:* Healthy adults are in a state of nitrogen balance.
7. *True or False:* Positive nitrogen balance exists during periods of rapid growth (e.g., infancy, adolescence).
8. *True or False:* When negative nitrogen balance exists, an individual is less able to resist infection.
9. *True or False:* Egg protein has a higher biologic value than meat protein.

Multiple Choice

1. Nine of the 20 amino acids are indispensable, which means that
   a. the body cannot make them and must obtain them from the diet.
   b. they are required for body processes and the rest are not.
   c. the body makes them because they are essential to life.
   d. after making them, the body uses them for growth.

2. A complete protein food of high biologic value contains
   a. all 20 of the amino acids in sufficient amounts to meet human requirements.
   b. the nine indispensable amino acids in any proportion, because the body can always fill in the remaining differences.
   c. all of the 20 amino acids from which the body can make additional amounts of the nine indispensable ones as necessary.
   d. all nine of the indispensable amino acids in correct proportion to meet human requirements.

3. A state of negative nitrogen balance may occur during periods of
   a. pregnancy.
   b. adolescence.
   c. injury or surgery.
   d. infancy.

⊖volve Please refer to the Students' Resource section of this text's Evolve Web site for additional study resources.

REFERENCES

1. Food and Nutrition Board, Institute of Medicine. *Dietary reference intakes for energy, carbohydrate, fiber, fat, fatty acids, cholesterol, protein, and amino acids.* Washington, DC: National Academies Press; 2002.
2. Stahler C. How many adults are vegetarian? *Veg J.* 2006;25:14-15.
3. Craig WJ, Mangels AR. Position of the American dietetic association: vegetarian diets *J Am Diet Assoc.* 2009; 109(7):1266-1282.
4. Fraser GE. Vegetarian diets: what do we know of their effects on common chronic diseases? *Am J Clin Nutr.* 2009;89(5):1607S-1612S.
5. Barnard ND, Katcher HI, Jenkins DJ, et al. Vegetarian and vegan diets in type 2 diabetes management. *Nutr Rev.* 2009;67(5):255-263.
6. Segasothy M, Phillips PA. Vegetarian diet: panacea for modern lifestyle diseases? *QJM.* 1999;92(9):531-544.
7. Craig WJ. Health effects of vegan diets. *Am J Clin Nutr.* 2009;89(5):1627S-1633S.
8. Millward DJ, Layman DK, Tomé D, Schaafsma G. Protein quality assessment: impact of expanding understanding of protein and amino acid needs for optimal health. *Am J Clin Nutr.* 2008;87(5):1576S-1581S.
9. Ahmed T, Rahman S, Cravioto A. Oedematous malnutrition. *Indian J Med Res.* 2009;130(5):651-654.
10. U.S. Department of Agriculture, Agricultural Research Service. *What we eat in America* (website): www.ars.usda. gov/Services/docs.htm?docid=13793. Accessed September 22, 2011.
11. U.S. Department of Agriculture, U.S. Department of Health and Human Services. *Dietary guidelines for Americans, 2010.* Washington, DC: U.S. Government Printing Office; 2010.
12. U.S. Department of Agriculture, Center for Nutrition Policy and Promotion. *USDA's myplate home page* (website): www. choosemyplate.gov. Accessed August 23, 2011.

FURTHER READING AND RESOURCES

The following organizations are good sources of information about vegetarian diets.

Food and Nutrition Information Center. http://fnic.nal.usda.gov

Medline Plus (key search word: "vegetarianism"). www.nlm.nih.gov/medlineplus/vegetariandiet.html

North American Vegetarian Society. www.navs-online.org

Vegetarian Nutrition Dietetic Practice Group. www.vegetariannutrition.net

The Vegetarian Resource Group. www.vrg.org

Fuhrman J, Ferreri DM. Fueling the vegetarian (vegan) athlete. *Curr Sports Med Rep.* 2010;9(4):233-241.

CHAPTER 5

Digestion, Absorption, and Metabolism

KEY CONCEPTS

- Through a balanced system of mechanical and chemical digestion, food is broken down into smaller substances, and the nutrients are then released for biologic use.
- Special organ structures and functions accomplish these tasks through the successive parts of the overall system.

- Absorption, transport, and metabolism allow for the distribution, use, and storage of nutrients throughout the body.

As described in previous chapters, nutrients that the body requires do not come ready to use; rather, they are packaged as foods in a variety of forms. Therefore, whole food must be broken down into smaller substances for absorption and metabolism to meet the body's needs. Digestion of the macronutrients—carbohydrates, fat, and protein—has been discussed in preceding chapters.

This chapter views the overall process of food digestion and nutrient absorption as one continuous whole that involves a series of successive events. In addition, metabolism and the unique body structures and functions that make this process—as well as life—possible are reviewed.

DIGESTION

Basic Principles

Principle of Change

Body cells cannot use food as it is eaten. Food must be changed into simpler substances for absorption and then into even more simple substances that cells can use to sustain life. Preparing food for the body's use involves many steps, including digestion, absorption, transport, and metabolism.

Principle of Wholeness

The different parts of the gastrointestinal (GI) tract and accessory organs are shown in Figure 5-1. The individual parts of the GI system works systematically together as a

digestion the process by which food is broken down in the gastrointestinal tract to release nutrients in forms that the body can absorb.

absorption the process by which nutrients are taken into the cells that line the gastrointestinal tract.

transport the movement of nutrients through the circulatory system from one area of the body to another.

metabolism the sum of the vast number of chemical changes in the cell that ultimately produce the materials that are essential for energy, tissue building, and metabolic controls.

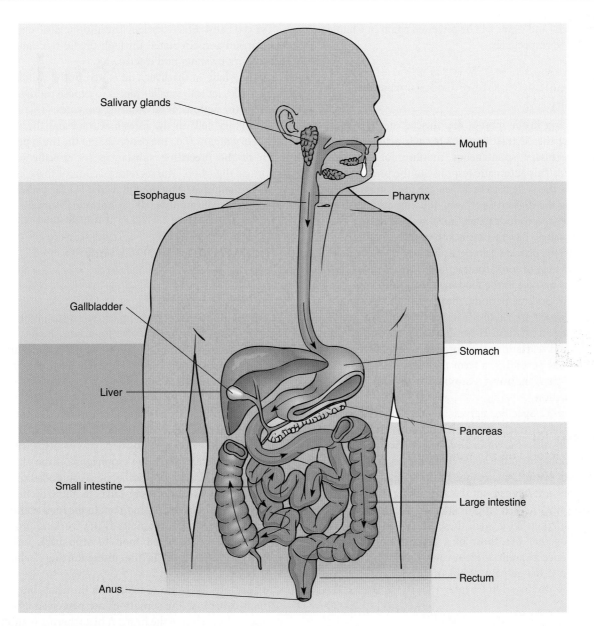

Figure 5-1 The gastrointestinal system. Through the successive parts of the system, multiple activities of digestion liberate food nutrients for use. (Courtesy Rolin Graphics.)

whole to complete the process of digestion and metabolism. Food components travel through this system until they ultimately are absorbed and delivered to the cells or excreted as waste.

Mechanical and Chemical Digestion

For nutrients to be absorbed, food must go through a series of mechanical and chemical changes. Together, these two actions encompass the overall process of digestion.

The specific mechanical and chemical actions that occur during the digestion of the macronutrients (i.e., carbohydrates, proteins, and fats) have previously been discussed. Of the micronutrients, most vitamins and minerals require little to no digestion. There are some exceptions (e.g., vitamins A and B_{12}, biotin) that require digestion before absorption can take place. Water does not require digestion, and it is easily absorbed into the general circulation. This chapter touches on those actions as a whole and as an interdependent process. Vitamins, minerals, and water will be reviewed again in Chapters 7, 8, and 9, respectively.

Mechanical Digestion: Gastrointestinal Motility

Beginning in the mouth, the muscles and nerves in the walls of the GI tract coordinate their actions to provide the necessary spontaneous motility for digestion to proceed. This automatic response to the presence of food enables the system to break up the food mass and move it along the digestive pathway. Muscles and nerves work together to produce steady motility.

Muscles. Layers of smooth muscle in the GI wall interact to provide two general types of movement: (1) muscle tone or tonic contraction, which ensures the continuous passage of the food mass and valve control along the way; and (2) periodic muscle contraction and relaxation, which are rhythmic waves that mix the food mass and move it forward. These alternating muscular contractions and relaxations that force the contents forward are known as *peristalsis,* a term that comes from the Greek words *peri,* meaning "around," and *stalsis,* meaning "contraction."

Nerves. Specific nerves regulate muscular action along the GI tract. A complex network of nerves in the GI wall called the *intramural nerve plexus* extends from the esophagus to the anus. These nerves do three things: (1) they control muscle tone in the wall; (2) they regulate the rate and intensity of the alternating muscle contractions; and (3) they coordinate all of the various movements. When all is well, these finely tuned movements flow together like those of a great symphony, without conscience awareness. However, when all is not well, the discord is felt as pain. Problems and diseases of the GI tract are discussed in Chapter 18.

Chemical Digestion: Gastrointestinal Secretions

A number of secretions work together to make chemical digestion possible. Five types of substances generally are involved.

Hydrochloric Acid and Buffer Ions. Hydrochloric acid and buffer ions are needed to produce the correct pH (i.e., the degree of acidity or alkalinity) that is necessary for enzymatic activity.

Enzymes. Digestive enzymes are proteins of a specific kind and quantity for breaking down nutrients.

Mucus. Secretions of mucus lubricate and protect the mucosal tissues that line the GI tract, and they help to mix the food mass.

Water and Electrolytes. The products of digestion are carried and circulated through the GI tract and into the tissues by water and electrolytes.

Bile. Made in the liver and stored in the gallbladder, bile divides fat into smaller pieces to expose more surface area for the actions of fat-splitting enzymes.

Secretory cells in the intestinal tract and the nearby accessory organs (i.e., the pancreas and the liver) produce each of the preceding substances for specific jobs in chemical digestion. The secretory action of these cells or glands is stimulated by the following: (1) the presence of food; (2) nerve impulses; or (3) hormonal stimuli.

Digestion in the Mouth and Esophagus

Mechanical Digestion

In the mouth, the process of mastication (i.e., biting and chewing) begins to break down food into smaller particles. The teeth and oral structures are particularly suited for this work. After the food is chewed, the mixed mass of food particles is swallowed, and it passes down the esophagus, largely as a result of peristaltic waves that are controlled by nerve reflexes. Muscles at the base of the tongue facilitate the swallowing process. Then, if the body is in the upright position, gravity helps with the movement of food down the esophagus. At the entrance to the stomach, the gastroesophageal sphincter muscle relaxes, much like a one-way valve, to allow the food to enter; it then constricts again to retain the food within the stomach cavity. If the sphincter is not working properly, it may allow acid-mixed food to seep back into the esophagus. The result is the discomforting feeling of heartburn.

Heartburn has nothing to do with the heart, but it was so named because the sensations are perceived as originating in the region of the heart. A hiatal hernia is another common cause of heartburn; this occurs when part of the stomach protrudes upward into the chest cavity (i.e., the thorax; see Chapter 18).

Chemical Digestion

The salivary glands secrete material that contains salivary amylase, which is also called *ptyalin. Amylase* is the general name for any starch-splitting enzyme. Small

---

salivary amylase a starch-splitting enzyme in the mouth that is secreted by the salivary glands and that is commonly called *ptyalin* (from the Greek word *ptyalon,* meaning "spittle").

glands at the back of the tongue (i.e., von Ebner's glands) secrete lingual lipase. *Lipase* is the general name for any fat-splitting enzyme. However, in this case, food does not remain in the mouth long enough for much chemical action to occur. During infancy, lingual lipase is a more relevant enzyme for the digestion of milk fat. The salivary glands also secrete a mucous material that lubricates and binds food particles to facilitate the swallowing of each food bolus (i.e., lump of food material). Mucous glands also line the esophagus, and their secretions help to move the food mass toward the stomach.

Digestion in the Stomach

Mechanical Digestion

Under sphincter-muscle control from the esophagus, which joins the stomach at the cardiac notch, the food enters the fundus (i.e., the upper portion of the stomach) in individual bolus lumps. Within the stomach, muscles gradually knead, store, mix, and propel the food mass forward in slow, controlled movements. By the time the food mass reaches the antrum (i.e., the lower portion of the stomach), it is now a semiliquid, acid–food mix called *chyme*. A constricting sphincter muscle at the end of the stomach called the *pyloric valve* controls the flow at this point. This valve slowly releases acidic chyme so that it can be quickly buffered by the alkaline intestinal secretions and not irritate the mucosal lining of the duodenum, which is the first section of the small intestine. The caloric density of a meal, which mainly results from its fat composition, influences the rate of stomach emptying at the pyloric valve. The major parts of the stomach are shown in Figure 5-2.

Chemical Digestion

The gastric secretions contain three types of materials that help with chemical digestion in the stomach.

Acid. The hormone gastrin stimulates parietal cells within the lining of the stomach to secrete hydrochloric acid. Hydrochloric acid creates the necessary degree of acidity for gastric enzymes to work, and it also activates the first protease, pepsinogen, in the stomach.

Mucus. Mucous secretions protect the stomach lining from the erosive effect of hydrochloric acid. Secretions also bind and mix the food mass and help to move it along.

Enzymes. The inactive enzyme pepsinogen is secreted by stomach cells, and it is activated by hydrochloric acid to become the protein-splitting enzyme pepsin. Other cells produce small amounts of a specific gastric lipase called *tributyrinase,* which works on tributyrin (i.e., butterfat); however, this is a relatively minor activity in the stomach.

Various sensations, emotions, and foods stimulate the nerve impulses that trigger these secretions. The concept that the stomach is said to "mirror the person within" is not without merit. For example, anger and hostility increase secretions, whereas fear and depression decrease secretions and inhibit blood flow and motility. Additional hormonal stimulus occurs in response to food entering the stomach.

Digestion in the Small Intestine

Up to this point, the digestion of food has largely been mechanical, and it has resulted in the delivery of a semifluid mixture of fine food particles and watery secretions to the small intestine. Chemical digestion has been minimal. Thus, the major task of digestion and the absorption that follows occurs in the small intestine. The structural parts, synchronized movements, and array of specific enzymes of the small intestine are highly developed for the final step of mechanical and chemical digestion.

chyme the semifluid food mass in the gastrointestinal tract that is present after gastric digestion.

gastrin a hormone that helps with gastric motility, that stimulates the secretion of gastric acid by the parietal cells of the stomach, and that stimulates the chief cells to secrete pepsinogen.

pepsin the main gastric enzyme specific to proteins; it begins breaking large protein molecules into shorter-chain polypeptides; gastric hydrochloric acid is necessary for its activation.

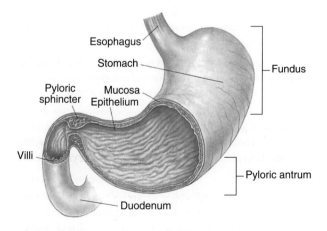

Esophagus
Stomach
Fundus
Pyloric sphincter
Mucosa
Epithelium
Villi
Pyloric antrum
Duodenum

Figure 5-2 Stomach. (Reprinted from Raven PH, Johnson GB. *Biology,* 3rd ed. New York: McGraw-Hill; 1992.)

Mechanical Digestion

Under the control of nerve impulses, the muscular walls of the small intestines stretch from the food mass or hormonal stimuli, and the intestinal muscles produce several types of movement that aid digestion, as follows:

- *Peristaltic waves* slowly push the food mass forward, sometimes with long, sweeping waves over the entire length of the intestine.
- *Pendular movements* from small, local muscles sweep back and forth, thereby stirring the chyme at the mucosal surface.
- *Segmentation rings* from the alternating contraction and relaxation of circular muscles progressively chop the food mass into successive soft lumps and then mix them with secretions.
- *Longitudinal rotation* by long muscles that run the length of the intestine rolls the slowly moving food mass in a spiral motion to mix it and expose new surfaces for absorption.
- *Surface villi motions* stir and mix the chyme at the intestinal wall, thereby exposing additional nutrients for absorption.

Chemical Digestion

The small intestines, together with the GI accessory organs (i.e., the pancreas, liver, and gallbladder), supply many secretory materials to accomplish the major chore of chemical digestion. The pancreas and intestines secrete enzymes that are specific for the digestion of each macronutrient.

Pancreatic Enzymes

1. *Carbohydrate:* Pancreatic amylase converts starch into the disaccharides maltose, and sucrose.
2. *Protein:* Trypsin and chymotrypsin split large protein molecules into smaller and smaller peptide fragments and finally into single amino acids. Carboxypeptidase removes end amino acids from peptide chains.
3. *Fat:* Pancreatic lipase converts fat into glycerides and fatty acids.

Intestinal Enzymes

1. *Carbohydrate:* Disaccharidases (i.e., maltase, lactase, and sucrase) convert their respective disaccharides (i.e., maltose, lactose, and sucrose) into monosaccharides (i.e., glucose, galactose, and fructose).
2. *Protein:* The intestinal enzyme enterokinase activates trypsinogen, which is released from the pancreas to become the protein-splitting enzyme trypsin. Amino peptidase removes end amino acids from polypeptides. Dipeptidase splits dipeptides into their two remaining amino acids.
3. *Fat:* Intestinal lipase splits fat into glycerides and fatty acids.

Mucus.   Large quantities of mucus, which are secreted by intestinal glands, protect the mucosal lining from the irritation and erosion caused by the highly acidic gastric contents that enter the duodenum.

Bile.   Bile is an emulsifying agent and an important part of fat digestion and absorption. It is produced by the liver and stored in the adjacent gallbladder, and it is ready for use when fat enters the intestine.

Hormones.   The hormone secretin, which is produced by the mucosal glands in the first part of the intestine, controls the acidity and secretion of enzymes from the pancreas. The resulting alkaline environment in the small intestine, with a pH greater than 8, is necessary for the activity of the pancreatic enzymes. The hormone cholecystokinin, which is secreted by intestinal mucosal glands when fat is present, triggers the release of bile from the gallbladder to emulsify fat.

The arrangement of accessory organs to the duodenum, which is the first section of the small intestine, is shown in Figure 5-3. These organs make up the biliary system. The liver is sometimes called the "metabolic capital" of the body, because it performs numerous functions for the metabolism of all converging nutrients (Box 5-1). The liver's many metabolic functions are reviewed in greater detail in Chapter 18.

The various nerve and hormone controls of digestion are illustrated in Figure 5-4. Although small individual summaries of digestion are given in each of the macronutrient chapters, a general summary of the entire digestive process is shown in Figure 5-5 so that the overall process can be viewed as it is: one continuous and integrated whole.

---

pancreatic amylase   a major starch-splitting enzyme that is secreted by the pancreas and that acts in the small intestine.

trypsin   a protein-splitting enzyme produced in the pancreas and released into the small intestine; the inactive precursor trypsinogen is activated by enterokinase.

chymotrypsin   one of the protein-splitting and milk-curdling pancreatic enzymes that is activated in the small intestine from the precursor chymotrypsinogen; it breaks specific amino acid peptide links of protein.

carboxypeptidase   a protein enzyme that splits off the carboxyl group (i.e., –COOH) at the end of peptide chains.

pancreatic lipase   a major fat-splitting enzyme produced by the pancreas and secreted into the small intestine to digest fat.

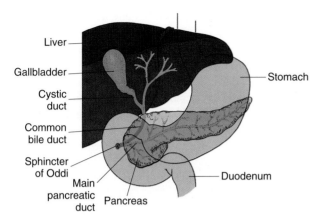

Figure 5-3 Organs of the biliary system and the pancreatic ducts.

ABSORPTION AND TRANSPORT

When digestion is complete, food has been changed into simple end products that are ready for cell use. Carbohydrate foods are reduced to the simple sugars glucose, fructose, and galactose, and fats are transformed into fatty acids and glycerides. Protein foods are changed into single amino acids, and vitamins and minerals are also liberated. With a water base for solution and transport in addition to the necessary electrolytes, the whole fluid food-derived mass is now prepared for absorption. For many nutrients, especially certain vitamins and minerals, the point of absorption becomes the vital gatekeeper that determines how much of a given nutrient is kept for body use. Although the GI tract is quite efficient, 100% of all

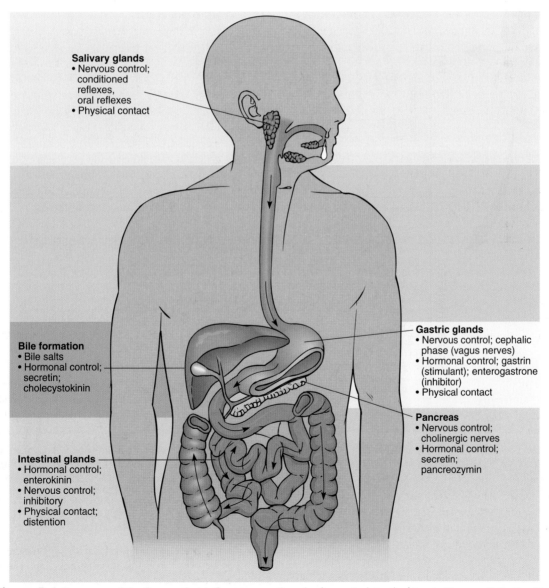

Figure 5-4 Summary of the factors that influence secretions in the gastrointestinal tract. (Courtesy Rolin Graphics.)

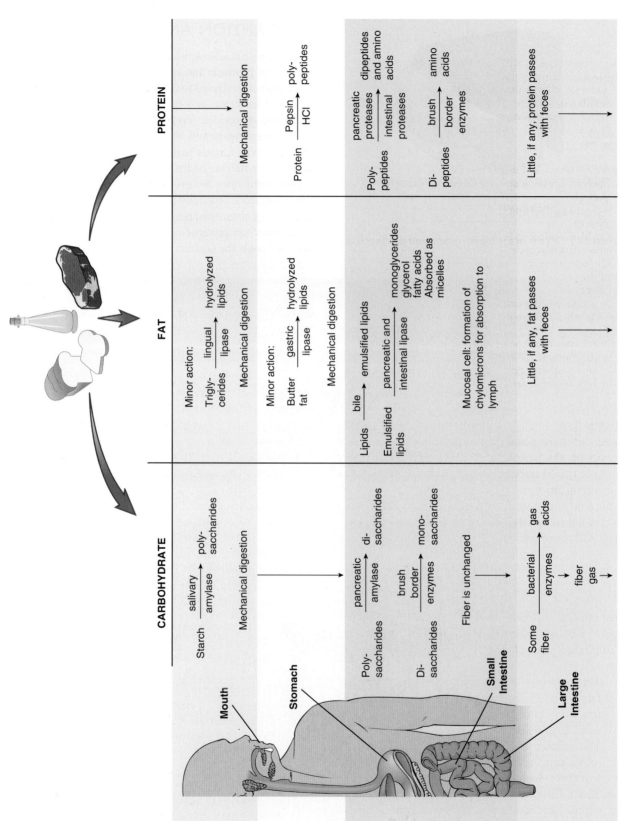

Figure 5-5 Summary of the digestive processes. (Courtesy Rolin Graphics.)

BOX 5-1   FUNCTIONS OF THE LIVER

Major Functions
- Bile production
- Synthesis of proteins and blood-clotting factors
- Metabolism of hormones and medications
- Regulation of blood glucose levels
- Urea production to remove the waste products of normal metabolism

Specific Metabolic Functions of the Macronutrients
- Lipolysis: breaking down lipids into fatty acids and glycerol
- Lipogenesis: building up lipids from fatty acids and glycerol
- Glycolysis: breaking down glucose into pyruvate to enter the Krebs cycle
- Gluconeogenesis: converting noncarbohydrate substances into glucose
- Glycogenolysis: breaking down glycogen into individual glucose units
- Glycogenesis: combining units of glucose to store as glycogen
- Protein degradation: breaking down proteins into single amino acids
- Protein synthesis: building complete proteins from individual amino acids

---

nutrients consumed is not absorbed as a result of varying degrees of bioavailability. A nutrient's bioavailability depends on the following: (1) the amount of nutrient present in the GI tract; (2) competition among nutrients for common absorptive sites; and (3) the form in which the nutrient is present. This degree of bioavailability is a factor in setting dietary intake standards for all macronutrients and micronutrients.[1-6]

Absorption in the Small Intestine

Absorbing Structures

Three important structures of the intestinal wall surface (Figure 5-6) are particularly adapted to ensure the maximal absorption of essential nutrients in the digestive process:

- *Mucosal folds:* Like the hills and valleys of a mountain range, the surface of the small intestine piles into many folds. Mucosal folds can easily be seen when such tissue is examined.
- *Villi:* Closer examination under a regular light microscope reveals small, finger-like projections that cover the piled-up folds of the mucosal lining. These little villi further increase the area of exposed surface. Each villus has an ample supply of blood vessels to receive protein and carbohydrate materials as well as a lymph vessel to receive

fat-soluble nutrients. This lymph vessel is called a *lacteal,* because the fatty chyme is creamy at this point and looks like milk.
- *Microvilli:* Even closer examination with an electron microscope reveals a covering of smaller projections on the surface of each tiny villus. The covering of microvilli on each villus is called the *brush border,* because it looks like bristles on a brush.

These three unique structures of the inner intestinal wall—folds, villi, and microvilli—combine to make the inner surface some 600 times greater than the area of the outer surface of the intestine. The length of the small intestine is approximately 660 cm (22 ft). This remarkable organ is well adapted to deliver nutrients into the circulation to the body's cells. If its entire surface were spread out on a flat plane, the total surface area is estimated to be as large as half of a basketball court. Far from being the lowly gut, the small intestine is one of the most highly developed, exquisitely fashioned, and specialized tissues in the body.

Absorption Processes

A number of absorbing processes complete the task of moving vital nutrients across the inner intestinal wall and into the body circulation (Figure 5-7). These processes include diffusion, energy-driven active transport, and pinocytosis:

- *Simple diffusion* is the force by which particles move outward in all directions from an area of greater concentration to an area of lesser concentration. Small materials that do not need the help of a specific protein channel to move across the mucosal cell wall use this method.
- *Facilitated diffusion* is similar to simple diffusion, but it makes use of a protein channel for the carrier-assisted movement of larger items across the mucosal cell membrane.

---

mucosal folds the large, visible folds of the mucous lining of the small intestine that increase the absorbing surface area.

villi small protrusions from the surface of a membrane; finger-like projections that cover the mucosal surfaces of the small intestine and that further increase the absorbing surface area; they are visible through a regular microscope.

microvilli extremely small, hair-like projections that cover all of the villi on the surface of the small intestine and that greatly extend the total absorbing surface area; they are visible through an electron microscope.

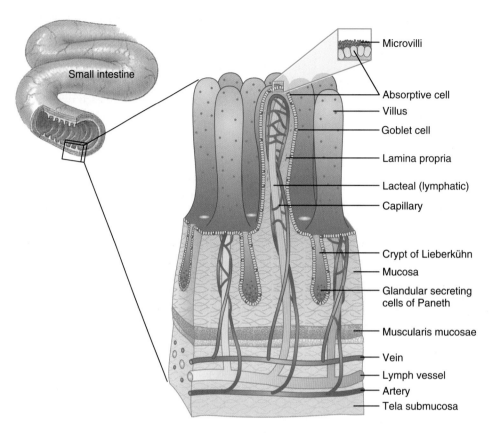

Figure 5-6 The intestinal wall. A diagram of the villi of the human intestine that shows its structure and the blood and lymph vessels. (Reprinted from Mahan LK, Escott-Stump S. *Krause's food & nutrition therapy*. 12th ed. Philadelphia: Saunders; 2008.)

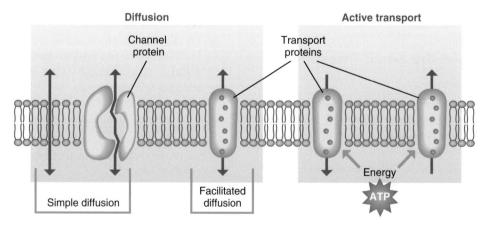

Figure 5-7 Transport pathways through the cell membrane. (Reprinted from Mahan LK, Escott-Stump S. *Krause's food & nutrition therapy*. 12th ed. Philadelphia: Saunders; 2008.)

- *Active transport* is the force by which particles move against their concentration gradient. Active transport mechanisms usually require some sort of carrier partner to help ferry the particles across the membrane. For example, glucose enters absorbing cells through an active transport mechanism that involves sodium as a partner.
- *Pinocytosis* is the penetration of larger materials by attaching to the thicker cell membrane and being engulfed by the cell.

Absorption in the Large Intestine

Water

The main absorptive task that remains for the large intestine is to absorb water. Most water in the chyme that enters the large intestine is absorbed in the first half of the colon. Only a small amount (approximately 100 mL) remains to form the feces and be eliminated.

Dietary Fiber

Food fiber is not digested, because humans lack the specific enzymes that are required to break the beta bonds between molecules. However, dietary fiber contributes important bulk to food mass and helps to form feces. The formation and passage of intestinal gas is a normal process of healthy digestion, but it can be problematic for some individuals (see the Clinical Applications box, "The Sometimes Embarrassing Effects of Digestion").

Macronutrients and Micronutrients

Table 5-1 summarizes the major features of intestinal nutrient absorption, including macronutrients and micronutrients. In addition, Figure 5-8 shows the location of absorption of each nutrient as well as the route through which it is absorbed (i.e., lymph or blood).

Transport

After being broken down from food and absorbed, nutrients must be transported to various cells throughout the body. This transportation requires the work of both the vascular and lymphatic systems (see Figure 5-6).

Vascular System

The vascular system is composed of veins and arteries, and it is responsible for supplying the entire body with nutrients, oxygen, and many other vital substances that are necessary for life via the blood. In addition, the vascular system transports waste (e.g., carbon dioxide, nitrogen) to the lungs and kidneys for removal.

Most of the products of digestion are water-soluble nutrients, which therefore can be absorbed into the vascular system (i.e., the blood circulatory system) directly from the intestinal cells. The nutrients travel first to the liver for immediate cell enzyme work before being dispersed to other cells throughout the body. The portion of circulation from the intestines to the liver is called the *portal circulation.*

Lymphatic System

Because fatty materials are not water soluble, another route must be provided. These fat molecules pass into the lymph vessels in the villi (e.g., the lacteals), flow into the larger lymph vessels of the body, and eventually enter the bloodstream through the thoracic duct.

Metabolism

At this point, the individual macronutrients in food have been broken down through digestion into the basic building blocks (i.e., monosaccharides, amino acids, and fatty acids) and absorbed into the bloodstream or the lymphatic system. Now these nutrients can be converted into needed energy or stored in the body for later use.

In addition, the micronutrients (i.e., vitamins and minerals) have been liberated from any bound proteins, and they are free for absorption. Once inside, the micronutrients are dispersed throughout the body for their many critical functions.

Energy for Fuel

Metabolism is the sum of the chemical reactions that occur within a living cell to maintain life. The mitochondrion of the cell is the work center in which all metabolic reactions take place. The two types of metabolism are catabolism and anabolism. Catabolism is the breaking down of large substances into smaller units. For example, breaking down stored glycogen into its smaller building blocks (i.e., glucose) is a catabolic reaction. Anabolism is the opposite; it is the process by which cells build large substances from smaller particles, such as building a complex protein from single amino acids.

catabolism the metabolic process of breaking down large substances to yield smaller building blocks.

anabolism the metabolic process of building large substances from smaller parts; the opposite of catabolism.

CLINICAL APPLICATIONS

THE SOMETIMES EMBARRASSING EFFECTS OF DIGESTION

After eating certain foods, some people complain of the discomfort or embarrassment of gas. Gas is a normal by-product of digestion, but when it becomes painful or apparent to others, it may become a physical and social dilemma.

The gastrointestinal tract normally holds approximately 3 oz of gas that moves along with the food mass and is silently absorbed into the bloodstream. Sometimes extra gas collects in the stomach or intestine, thereby creating an embarrassing—although usually harmless—situation.

Stomach Gas

Gas in the stomach results from trapped air bubbles. It occurs when a person eats too fast, drinks through a straw, or otherwise takes in extra air while eating. Burping releases some gas, but the following tips may help to avoid uncomfortable situations:

- Avoid carbonated beverages.
- Do not gulp.
- Chew with the mouth closed.
- Do not drink from a can or through a straw.
- Do not eat while overly nervous.

Intestinal Gas

The passing of gas from the intestine can be a social embarrassment. This gas forms in the colon, where bacteria attack undigested items and cause them to decompose and produce gas. Carbohydrates release hydrogen, carbon dioxide, and—in some people with certain types of bacteria in the gut—methane. All three products are odorless (although noisy) gases. Protein produces hydrogen sulfide and volatile compounds such as indole and skatole, which add a distinctive aroma to the expelled air. The following suggestions may help to control flatulence:

- Cut down on simple carbohydrates (e.g., sugars). Especially observe milk's effect, because lactose intolerance may be the culprit. Substitute cultured forms, such as yogurt or milk treated with a lactase product such as Lactaid (McNeil Nutritionals, Fort Washington, Pa).
- Use a prior leaching process before cooking dry beans to remove indigestible saccharides such as raffinose and stachyose. Although humans cannot digest these substances, they provide a feast for bacteria in the intestines. This simple procedure eliminates a major portion of these gas-forming saccharides. First, put washed, dry beans into a large pot, add 4 cups of water for each pound of beans (approximately 2 cups), and boil the beans uncovered for 2 minutes. Remove the pot from the heat, cover it, and let it stand for 1 hour. Finally, drain and rinse the beans, add 8 cups of fresh water, bring the water to a boil, reduce the heat, and simmer the beans in a covered pot for 1 to 2 hours or until beans are tender. Season as desired.
- Eliminate known food offenders. These vary from person to person, but some of the most common offenders are beans (if they are not prepared for cooking as described), onions, cabbage, and high-fiber wheat products.

When relief has been achieved, slowly add more complex carbohydrates and high-fiber foods back into the diet. After small amounts are tolerated, try moderate increases. If no relief occurs, medical help may be needed to rule out or treat an overactive gastrointestinal tract.

The Krebs cycle, which is also known as the *citric acid cycle* or the *TCA cycle,* is the hub of energy production that occurs in the mitochondria of the cell. The combined processes of metabolism (i.e., catabolic and anabolic reactions) ensure that the body has much needed energy in the form of adenosine triphosphate (ATP). The rate of ATP production fluctuates, and it speeds up or slows down depending on energy needs at a given time. Energy needs are minimal during sleep, but they increase dramatically during strenuous physical activity. Energy supply and demand are discussed further in Chapter 6. Figure 5-9 (on page 77) illustrates a brief breakdown of the macronutrients and how they enter the final step of energy production to ultimately supply cells with ATP.

Because carbohydrates have 4 kcal/g and fat has 9 kcal/g, the metabolism of glucose yields less energy (i.e., ATP) than the metabolism of fat, gram for gram. However, the body prefers to use glucose as its primary source of energy. Protein can be used as a source of energy as well, but this is a relatively inefficient method of producing energy, and it results in extra nitrogen waste. The body only breaks down protein for energy when glucose and fatty acids are in short supply.

Stored Energy

If the amount of food consumed yields more energy than is needed to maintain voluntary and involuntary actions,

TABLE 5-1 **INTESTINAL ABSORPTION OF SOME MAJOR NUTRIENTS**

Nutrient	Form	Means of Absorption	Control Agent or Required Cofactor	Route
Carbohydrate	Monosaccharides (glucose or galactose)	Competitive	—	Blood
		Selective	—	
		Active transport by sodium pump	Sodium	
	Fructose	Facilitated diffusion	Protein carrier	Blood
Protein	Amino acids	Selective	—	Blood
	Some dipeptides	Facilitated diffusion	Pyridoxine (pyridoxal phosphate)	Blood
	Whole protein (rare)	Pinocytosis	Protein carrier	Blood
Fat	Fatty acids	Fatty acid–bile complex (micelles)	Bile	Lymph
	Glycerides (monoglycerides and diglycerides)			
	Few triglycerides (neutral fat)	Pinocytosis	—	Lymph
Vitamins	B$_{12}$	Facilitated diffusion	Intrinsic factor	Blood
	A, D, E, and K	Bile complex (micelles)	Bile	Blood
	K from bacterial synthesis			From the large intestine to the blood
Minerals	Sodium	Active transport by sodium pump	—	Blood
	Calcium	Active transport	Vitamin D	Blood
	Iron	Active transport	Ferritin mechanism	Blood (as transferrin)
Water	Water	Osmosis	—	Blood, lymph, and interstitial fluid

the remaining energy is stored for later use in the body. The human body is a highly efficient organism. Energy or kilocalories in excess of needs are not wasted. Excess glucose can easily be stored as glycogen in the liver and muscles for quick energy at a later time. The anabolic process of converting extra glucose into glycogen is called *glycogenesis*.

When the glycogen reserves are full, additional excess energy from carbohydrates, fat, or protein are stored as fat in adipose tissue. **Lipogenesis** is the building up of triglycerides for storage in the **adipose tissue** of the body. Both glycogen and stored fat are available for use when energy demands require it. Energy balance and the factors that influence it are discussed further in Chapter 6.

Excess protein intake is not stored as muscle. The body uses amino acids to build functional and structural proteins as needed, and the liver stores some free amino acids to meet rapid needs of the body. However, protein intake above and beyond the body's requirements is broken down further so that the nitrogen unit is removed, and the remaining carbon chain can be converted to glucose or fat for storage. The conversion of amino acids to glucose is referred to as *gluconeogenesis*.

Although alcohol is not a nutrient, it does provide 7 kcal/g. Therefore, alcohol intake adds to the overall supply of energy (see the For Further Focus box, "What About Alcohol?").

ERRORS IN DIGESTION AND METABOLISM

The Genetic Defect

Certain food intolerances stem from underlying genetic disease. For each genetic disease, the necessary enzyme that controls the cell's metabolism of a specific nutrient

---

glycogenesis the anabolic process of creating stored glycogen from glucose.

lipogenesis the anabolic process of forming fat.

adipose tissue the storage site for excess fat.

gluconeogenesis the formation of glucose from non-carbohydrate substances such as amino acids.

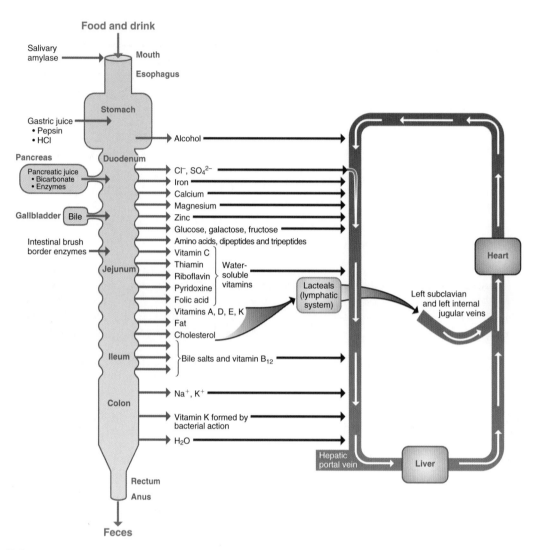

Figure 5-8 Sites of secretion and absorption in the gastrointestinal tract. (Mahan LK, Escott-Stump S. *Krause's food & nutrition therapy.* 12th ed. Philadelphia: Saunders; 2008.)

is missing, thereby preventing the normal nutrient metabolism. Three examples of genetic defects are phenylketonuria (PKU), galactosemia, and glycogen storage disease.

Phenylketonuria

PKU is an autosomal recessive genetic disorder that results when phenylalanine hydroxylase, which is the enzyme that is responsible for metabolizing the essential amino acid phenylalanine, is not produced by the body. If left untreated, this condition causes permanent mental retardation and central nervous system damage. Other possible symptoms and side effects include irritability, hyperactivity, convulsive seizures, and psychiatric disorders. PKU affects approximately 1 in every 10,000 to 15,000 live births in the United States. Screening tests

began during the 1960s, and they are now mandatory at birth in all areas of the United States. A simple blood test can identify affected infants, and thus, treatment can start immediately. With proper treatment, children with PKU grow normally and have healthy lives. The treatment is a low-phenylalanine diet of special formulas and low-protein food products for life. Unfortunately, the prescribed diet is somewhat unpalatable, and lifelong adherence is low. Intensive family counseling by a metabolic team is needed. Research into cell-directed therapy and more permanent treatments is ongoing.[7]

Galactosemia

Galactosemia is a genetic disease that affects carbohydrate metabolism and that also results from a missing enzyme. Similar to PKU, galactosemia is an autosomal recessive

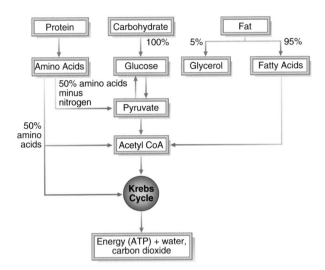

Figure 5-9 **Metabolic pathways.** (Reprinted from Peckenpaugh NJ. *Nutrition essentials and diet therapy.* 10th ed. Philadelphia: Saunders; 2007.)

disorder; it affects 1 in every 10,000 to 30,000 live births. The missing enzyme, galactose-1-phosphate uridyltransferase, is one that converts galactose to glucose. Because galactose comes from the breakdown of lactose (milk sugar), all sources of lactose in the diet must be eliminated. When it is not treated, galactosemia causes brain and liver damage. Newborn screening programs, which are required in all states, identify affected infants.[8] If treatment begins immediately, life-threatening damage may be avoided and thus, enable the child to grow normally. Treatment is a galactose-free diet, with special formulas for infants and lactose-free food guides. The treatment diet must be followed for life.

Glycogen Storage Diseases

Glycogen storage diseases (GSDs) are a group of rare genetic defects that inhibit the normal metabolic pathways of glycogen. This disease occurs in 1 of every 20,000 to 40,000 live births in the United States.[9] Twelve distinct forms of GSD result from the absence of the enzymes that are required for the synthesis or breakdown of glycogen. The specific form of GSD is distinguished by the enzyme

FOR FURTHER FOCUS

WHAT ABOUT ALCOHOL?

Does Alcohol Provide Energy?
Yes. Alcohol contributes to the overall energy intake in the form of calories. Alcohol yields 7 kcal/g consumed. This is more than both carbohydrates and protein, which yield 4 kcal/g each.

Is Alcohol a Nutrient?
No. Unlike carbohydrates, fats, proteins, vitamins, minerals, and water, alcohol performs no essential function in the body. Alcohol is not stored in the body, but the by-products of metabolism can accumulate to toxic amounts when alcohol is consumed in large quantities.

How Is Alcohol Digested?
The majority (i.e., 85% to 95%) of alcohol is absorbed without any chemical digestion. Alcohol is one of the few substances that can be absorbed directly into the circulation from the stomach. Small amounts of alcohol can enter the blood circulation from the mouth and the esophagus. What is not absorbed in the stomach is absorbed in the small intestine and sent directly to the liver for metabolism.

How Is Alcohol Metabolized?
Alcohol metabolism takes precedence over the metabolism of any other nutrient in the body because it is a toxin. The primary by-product of alcohol metabolism is acetaldehyde, which is the culprit for the destruction of healthy tissue that

is associated with alcoholism. After detoxifying the alcohol, the liver uses remaining by-products to produce fatty acids. Fatty acids are combined with glycerol through lipogenesis to form triglycerides, and they are stored in the liver. A single drinking binge can result in an accumulation of fat in the liver. Repeated episodes over time can lead to fatty liver disease, which is the first stage of alcoholic liver disease.

Alcohol metabolism is a priority for the liver. Blood alcohol concentrations peak at approximately 30 to 45 minutes after one drink, which is defined as 12 oz of beer, 5 oz of wine, or 1.5 oz of 80-proof distilled spirits. The liver can only work so fast to metabolize and rid the body of alcohol, regardless of how much has been consumed. When consumption exceeds the rate of metabolism, alcohol and its metabolites begin to accumulate in the blood.

Several factors influence an individual's ability to metabolize alcohol, including gender, food intake, body weight, sex hormones, and medications.

More Information
To find out more about alcohol and its dangers, benefits, and associated diseases, refer to the following Web sites:
- Alcoholics Anonymous: www.aa.org
- The National Council on Alcoholism and Drug Dependence: www.ncadd.org
- National Institute on Alcohol Abuse and Alcoholism: www.niaaa.nih.gov

that is missing and the tissue affected. The liver is the primary site of glycogen metabolism; therefore, hepatic forms of GSD (e.g., von Gierke's disease or type I glycogenosis) affect the glucose availability of the whole body. Myopathic forms of GSD inhibit normal glycogen metabolism in the striated muscles, and they are less severe than hepatic forms. An example of a myopathic form is McArdle's disease (i.e., type V glycogenosis).

Other Intolerances or Allergies

Not all intolerances are genetic inborn errors of metabolism. Some problems with digestion and metabolism are the result of food intolerances or allergies. An example of a food intolerance that is caused by the inability to complete digestion is lactose intolerance.

Lactose Intolerance

A deficiency of any one of the disaccharidases (i.e., lactase, sucrase, or maltase) in the small intestine may produce a wide range of GI problems and abdominal pain because the specific sugar involved cannot be digested (see Chapter 2). Lactose intolerance is the most common, and it presents as varying degrees of intolerance. With this condition, there is insufficient lactase to break down the milk sugar lactose; thus, lactose accumulates in the intestine, causing abdominal cramping and diarrhea. Milk and all products containing lactose are carefully avoided. Milk that is treated with a commercial lactase product and soymilk products are safe substitutes.

Allergies

This chapter is limited to digestion, metabolism, transport, and absorption; therefore, allergic reactions (e.g., celiac disease) are not covered here. Allergies are inappropriate immune responses to substances that are not otherwise harmful and not necessarily problems with digestion or metabolism. Issues that are specific to GI disorders and allergies are covered in more detail in Chapter 18.

SUMMARY

- Necessary nutrients as they occur in food are not usable by the human body; they must be changed, released, regrouped, and rerouted into forms that body cells can use. The closely related activities of digestion, absorption, and transport ensure that key food nutrients are delivered to the cells so that the multiple metabolic tasks that sustain life can be completed.
- Mechanical digestion consists of spontaneous muscular activity that is responsible for the initial mechanical breakdown by mastication and the movement of the food mass along the GI tract by motions such as peristalsis.
- Chemical digestion involves enzymatic action that breaks food down into progressively smaller components and then releases its nutrients for absorption.
- Absorption involves the passage of nutrients from the intestines into the mucosal lining of the intestinal wall. It primarily occurs in the small intestine as a result of the work of highly efficient intestinal wall structures that, together with a number of effective absorbing mechanisms, increase the absorbent surface area. Nutrients that are absorbed are then transported throughout the body by the blood circulation.
- The nutrients that we eat are converted into ATP through the cycles of metabolism. Metabolism is the sum of the body processes that change food energy from the macronutrients into various forms of energy. Metabolism is a balance of both anabolic and catabolic reactions.
- Genetic diseases of metabolism result from missing enzymes that control the metabolism of specific nutrients. Special diets in each case limit or eliminate the particular nutrient involved.

CRITICAL THINKING QUESTIONS

1. Describe the types of muscle movement that are involved in mechanical digestion. What does the word *motility* mean?
2. Identify the digestive enzymes and any related substances secreted by the salivary and mucosal glands, the pancreas, and the liver. What activities do they perform on carbohydrates, proteins, and fats? What stimulates the release of these enzymes?
3. Describe four mechanisms of nutrient absorption from the small intestine. Describe the routes taken by the breakdown products of carbohydrates, proteins, and fats after absorption. Why must an alternate route to the bloodstream be provided for fat?
4. What functions does the large intestine perform?

CHAPTER CHALLENGE QUESTIONS

True-False

Write the correct statement for each statement that is false.

1. *True or False:* The digestive products of a large meal are difficult to absorb because the absorbent surface of the intestines is relatively small.
2. *True or False:* Before they can work, some enzymes must be activated by hydrochloric acid or another enzyme.
3. *True or False:* Bile is an enzyme that is specifically used for the chemical breakdown of fat.
4. *True or False:* The GI circulation provides a constant supply of water and electrolytes to carry digestive secretions and other substances.
5. *True or False:* Secretions from the GI accessory organs (i.e., the gallbladder and the pancreas) mix with gastric secretions in the stomach to help with digestion.
6. *True or False:* One enzyme may work on both carbohydrate and fat breakdown.
7. *True or False:* Bile is released from the gallbladder in response to a hormonal stimulus.

Multiple Choice

1. During digestion, the major muscle action that moves the food mass forward in regular rhythmic waves is called
   a. valve contraction.
   b. segmentation ring motion.
   c. muscle tone.
   d. peristalsis.
2. Mucus is an important GI secretion because it
   a. causes chemical changes in substances to prepare for enzyme action.
   b. helps to create the proper degree of acidity for enzymes to act.
   c. lubricates and protects the GI lining.
   d. helps to emulsify fats for enzyme action.
3. Pepsin is
   a. produced in the small intestine to act on protein.
   b. a gastric enzyme that acts on protein.
   c. produced in the pancreas to act on fat.
   d. produced in the small intestine to act on fat.
4. Bile is an important secretion that is
   a. produced by the gallbladder.
   b. stored in the liver.
   c. an aid to protein digestion.
   d. a fat-emulsifying agent.
5. The route of fat absorption is
   a. the lymphatic system by way of the villi lacteals.
   b. directly into the portal blood circulation.
   c. with the aid of bile directly into the villi blood capillaries.
   d. with the help of protein directly into the portal blood circulation.

⊖volve Please refer to the Students' Resource section of this text's Evolve Web site for additional study resources.

REFERENCES

1. Food and Nutrition Board, Institute of Medicine. *Dietary reference intakes for calcium, phosphorous, magnesium, vitamin D, and fluoride.* Washington, DC: National Academies Press; 1997.
2. Food and Nutrition Board, Institute of Medicine. *Dietary reference intakes for thiamin, riboflavin, niacin, vitamin B6, folate, vitamin B12, pantothenic acid, biotin, and choline.* Washington, DC: National Academies Press; 2000.
3. Food and Nutrition Board, Institute of Medicine. *Dietary reference intakes for vitamin C, vitamin E, selenium, and carotenoids.* Washington, DC: National Academies Press; 2000.
4. Food and Nutrition Board, Institute of Medicine. *Dietary reference intakes for vitamin A, vitamin K, arsenic, boron, chromium, copper, iodine, iron, manganese, molybdenum, nickel, silicon, vanadium, and zinc.* Washington, DC: National Academies Press; 2001.
5. Food and Nutrition Board, Institute of Medicine. *Dietary reference intakes for energy, carbohydrate, fiber, fat, fatty acids, cholesterol, protein, and amino acids.* Washington, DC: National Academies Press; 2002.
6. Food and Nutrition Board, Institute of Medicine. *Dietary reference intakes for water, potassium, sodium, chloride, and sulfate,* Washington, DC: National Academies Press; 2004.
7. Harding C. Progress toward cell-directed therapy for phenylketonuria. *Clin Genet.* 2008;74(2):97-104.
8. Kaye CI, Committee on Genetics, Accurso F, et al. Introduction to the newborn screening fact sheets. *Pediatrics.* 2006; 118(3):1304-1312.
9. Mayatepek E, Hoffmann B, Meissner T. Inborn errors of carbohydrate metabolism. *Best Pract Res Clin Gastroenterol* 2010;24(5):607-618.

FURTHER READING AND RESOURCES

The following organizations provide up-to-date research and reliable information about matters of the GI tract and metabolism.

The American College of Gastroenterology. www.acg.gi.org

The American Gastroenterological Association. www.gastro.org

The American Journal of Gastroenterology. www.amjgastro.com

Metabolism. www.metabolism.com

Nutrition & Metabolism. www.nutritionandmetabolism.com

Duggan S, O'Sullivan M, Feehan S, et al. Nutrition treatment of deficiency and malnutrition in chronic pancreatitis: a review. *Nutr Clin Pract*. 2010;25(4):362-370.

This article will give the reader insight into the complex issues that result when one accessory organ fails to provide the necessary enzymes for normal digestion.

CHAPTER **6**

Energy Balance

KEY CONCEPTS

- Food energy is changed into body energy to do work.
- The body uses most of its energy supply for basal metabolic needs.

- A balance between the intake of food energy and the output of body work maintains life and health.
- States of being underweight and overweight reflect degrees of energy imbalance.

Efficient human bodies constantly convert energy from food into the energy that is used for work and activity. Fuel is used and stored as necessary according to intake and output demands. This chapter looks at the big picture of energy balance among all of the energy-yielding nutrients and shows how energy intake is measured, cycled, and used to meet all of the body's energy demands.

HUMAN ENERGY SYSTEM

Basic Energy Needs

The body needs constant energy to do the work that is necessary for maintenance of life and health. Both voluntary and involuntary actions require energy.

Voluntary Work and Exercise

Voluntary work includes all of the actions related to a person's conscious activities of daily living and physical exercise. Although these intentional actions seem to use most of the energy output, that usually is not the case.

Involuntary Body Work

The greatest energy output is the result of involuntary work, which includes all of the activities in the body that are not consciously performed. These activities include such vital processes as circulation, respiration, digestion, and absorption (this is referred to as the *thermic effect of food*) as well as many other internal activities that maintain life. Involuntary body functions require energy in various forms, such as chemical energy (in many metabolic products), electrical energy (in brain and nerve activities), mechanical energy (in muscle contraction), and thermal (i.e., heat) energy to maintain body temperature.

Sources of Fuel

Energy that is needed for voluntary and involuntary body work requires fuel, which is provided in the form of adenosine triphosphate. As explained earlier in this book, the only three energy-yielding nutrients are the macronutrients carbohydrate, fat, and protein. Carbohydrates are the body's primary fuel, with fat assisting as a storage fuel. Protein is used for energy only when other fuel sources are not available. The body must have an adequate supply of fuel to balance energy demands for healthy weight maintenance.

Measurement of Energy

Unit of Measure: Kilocalorie

In common usage, the word *calorie* refers to the amount of energy in food or the amount that is expended in physical actions. However, in human nutrition, the term kilocalorie (i.e., 1000 calories) is used to designate the large calorie unit that is used in nutrition science to avoid dealing with such large numbers. A kilocalorie, which is abbreviated as *kcalorie* or *kcal,* is the amount of heat that is necessary to raise 1 kg of water 1° C. The international unit of measure for energy is the joule (J). To convert kilocalories (kcal) into kilojoules (kJ), multiply the number of kilocalories by 4.184 (e.g., 200 kcal × 4.184 = 836.8 kJ).

Food Energy: Fuel Factors

As discussed previously, the macronutrients have basic fuel factors. Ethanol (i.e., beverage alcohol from fermented grains and fruits) also supplies fuel. These factors reflect their relative fuel densities: carbohydrate, 4 kcal/g; fat, 9 kcal/g; protein, 4 kcal/g; and alcohol, 7 kcal/g.

Caloric and Nutrient Density

The term *density* refers to the degree of concentrated material in a given substance. More material in a smaller amount of substance increases the density. Thus, the concept of *caloric density* refers to a high concentration of energy (i.e., kilocalories) in a small amount of food. Of the three energy nutrients, fat or foods that are high in fat have the highest caloric density. Similarly, foods may be evaluated in terms of their relative nutrient density. A food with a high nutrient density has a relatively high concentration of all nutrients, including vitamins and minerals, in smaller amounts of a given food. Food guides such as MyPlate (www.choosemyplate.gov/guidelines; see Figure 1-3) recommend foods that are nutrient dense as opposed to only calorie dense. Some foods are both calorie and nutrient dense, which means that they provide a lot of both kilocalories and nutrients.

ENERGY BALANCE

Energy—like matter—is neither created nor destroyed. When energy is referred to as "being produced," it really means that it is transformed (i.e., changed in form and cycled through a system). Consider the human energy system as part of the total energy system on Earth. In this sense, two energy systems support human life—one within the body and the much larger one surrounding us—as follows:

1. *External energy cycle:* In the environment, the ultimate source of energy is the sun and its vast nuclear reactions. With the use of water and carbon dioxide as raw materials, plants transform the sun's radiation into stored chemical energy that is mainly carbohydrate with some fat and protein. The food chain continues as animals, including humans, eat plants and the products of other animals (e.g., meat, milk, eggs).
2. *Internal energy cycle:* When people eat plant and animal foods, the stored energy changes into body fuels (i.e., glucose and fatty acids) and cycles into various other energy forms to serve body needs. These forms include the involuntary actions mentioned previously: chemical, electrical, mechanical, and thermal energy. As this internal energy cycle continues, water is excreted, carbon dioxide is exhaled, and heat is radiated, thereby returning these end products to the external environment. The overall energy cycle continually repeats itself to sustain life.

Energy Intake

The total overall energy balance within the body depends on the energy intake in relation to the energy output. The main source of energy for all body work is food, and this is supplemented with stored energy in the body tissues.

Sources of Food Energy

The three energy-yielding nutrients in food keep human bodies supplied with fuel. Personal energy intake can easily be estimated by recording a day's actual food consumption and calculating its energy value. Nutritrac, which is the nutrition analysis program that is available on the Evolve Web site for this book (see the front matter for instructions and details on page 000), is an excellent tool for evaluating energy intake as well as several other components of an individual's diet (e.g., vitamins, minerals, fat, carbohydrates, sugar, protein). The MyPlate Tracker (www.choosemyplate.gov) is another free software tool that is available through the Internet and that can be used to assess total energy intake.

Sources of Stored Energy

When food is not available, such as during sleep, longer periods of fasting, or the extreme stress of starvation, the body draws from its stored energy.

---

thermic effect of food an increase in energy expenditure caused by the activities of digestion, absorption, transport, and storage of ingested food; a meal that consists of a usual mixture of carbohydrates, protein, and fat increases the energy expenditure equivalent to approximately 10% of the food's energy content (e.g., a 300-kcal piece of pizza would elicit an energy expenditure of 30 kcal to digest the food).

calorie a measure of heat; the energy necessary to do work is measured as the amount of heat produced by the body's work; the energy value of a food is expressed as the number of kilocalories that a specified portion of the food will yield when it is oxidized in the body.

Glycogen. A 12- to 48-hour reserve of glycogen exists in the liver and in the body's muscles, and it is quickly depleted if it is not replenished by daily food intake. For example, glycogen stores maintain normal blood glucose levels for body functions during the hours of sleep. The first meal, breakfast (which is so named because it "breaks the fast"), has a significant function for energy intake.

Adipose Tissue. Although the amount of fat storage is larger than that of glycogen storage, the supply varies from person to person. As an additional energy resource, stored fat provides more kilocalories per gram than any other fuel source.

Muscle Mass. Energy in the form of protein may be elicited from muscle mass. However, this lean tissue serves important structural functions, and it is ideally not sacrificed for energy use. Only during longer periods of fasting or starvation does the body turn to this tissue for energy.

Energy Output

The necessary activities to sustain life—normal body functions, the regulation of body temperature, and the processes of tissue growth and repair—use energy from food and body reserves. The sum of the total chemical changes that occur during all of these activities is called *metabolism.* The following three demands for energy determine the body's total energy requirements: (1) resting energy expenditure; (2) physical activity; and (3) the thermic effect of food.

Resting Energy Expenditure and Basal Energy Expenditure

The term *resting energy expenditure (REE)* or *resting metabolic rate (RMR)* refers to the sum of all internal working activities of the body at rest; it is expressed in kilocalories per day. For example, if an individual's REE is 1500 kcal, that would represent the amount of energy that this particular person would need to consume, on average, over a 24-hour period to maintain his or her current weight while at complete rest. In general use, the terms *REE, RMR,* and *basal energy expenditure* (BEE) are used interchangeably to describe a vast amount of physiologic work. However, a technical difference exists between BEE and REE. BEE must be measured when an individual is at complete digestive, physical, mental, thermal, and emotional rest. Maintaining the stringent conditions required to measure a true BEE is rather difficult; therefore, measurements are most often expressed as REE. The REE is slightly higher than a true BEE measurement.[1]

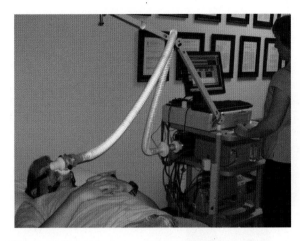

Figure 6-1 Measuring resting metabolic rate with a metabolic cart.

Most of the body's total energy expenditure (i.e., 60% to 75%) is spent maintaining necessary bodily functions in the form of REE. The majority of that energy is used by small but highly active tissues (e.g., liver, brain, heart, kidney) that only amount to 5% to 6% of the total body weight. A recent study of healthy adults found that the relative size of skeletal muscle mass and liver mass accounted for 81% of individual variability with regard to REE.[2]

Measuring Basal Metabolic Rate or Resting Metabolic Rate. A measure of basal metabolic rate (BMR) or RMR is sometimes made in clinical practice (e.g., on metabolic wards or in research laboratories) with the use of indirect calorimetry. This method measures the amount of energy that a person uses while at rest. A portable metabolic cart allows the person to breathe into an attached mouthpiece or ventilated hood system while lying down, and the normal exchange of oxygen and carbon dioxide is measured (Figure 6-1). The metabolic rate can be calculated with a high degree of accuracy from the rate of oxygen use.

resting energy expenditure (REE) the amount of energy (in kcal) needed by the body for the maintenance of life at rest over a 24-hour period; this is often used interchangeably with the term *basal energy expenditure,* but in actuality it is slightly higher.

basal energy expenditure (BEE) the amount of energy (in kcal) needed by the body for the maintenance of life when a person is at complete digestive, physical, mental, thermal, and emotional rest (i.e., 10 to 12 hours after eating and 12 to 18 hours after physical activity; measured immediately upon waking).

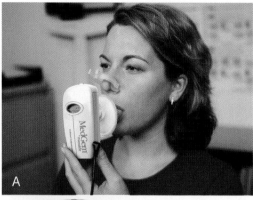

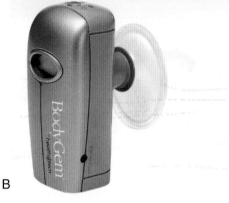

Figure 6-2 A, MedGem and **B,** BodyGem devices, which are used to determine the resting metabolic rate. (Courtesy Microlife USA, Dunedin, Fla.)

The MedGem and BodyGem (Microlife USA, Dunedin, Fla) are alternative methods for determining RMR with fast and portable devices (Figure 6-2). Both devices are handheld and come with disposable mouthpieces and nose clips. The individual being tested holds the device while breathing exclusively into the mouthpiece. The MedGem and BodyGem measure oxygen consumption to determine an individual's RMR by using a modified Weir equation with a constant respiratory quotient of 0.85 (RMR = 6.931 × Maximal oxygen consumption [i.e., VO_2max]).

Predicting Basal Metabolic Rate or Resting Metabolic Rate. A general formula for calculating basal energy needs is to multiply 0.9 or 1 kcal/kg body weight by the number of hours in a day. Thus, the daily basal metabolic needs (in kilocalories) are calculated as follows:

For a 154-lb man:

1 kcal × kg body weight × 24 hours

(1) Convert pounds to kilograms: 154 lb ÷ 2.2 = 70 kg

(2) 1 kcal × 70 kg × 24 hr = 1680 kcal/24 hr

For a 121-lb woman:

0.9 kcal × kg body weight × 24 hours

(1) Convert pounds to kilograms: 121 lb ÷ 2.2 = 55 kg

(2) 0.9 kcal × 55 kg × 24 hr = 1188 kcal/24 hr

The Mifflin-St. Jeor equations, the Harris-Benedict equations, and the equations that were used for the 2002 Dietary Reference Intake values provide an alternate method of estimating the BMR or RMR that is more specific to the individual (Box 6-1). Of these equations, studies found the Mifflin-St. Jeor equation to give the most reliable RMR measures.[3]

In addition, thyroid function tests may be used as an indicator of BMR, because the thyroid hormone regulates metabolism. Thyroid function tests measure the activity of the thyroid, the serum thyroxin levels, and the serum protein-bound iodine and radioactive iodine uptake levels. Iodine's basic function is in the synthesis of the prohormone thyroxine. Such tests are not associated with a kilocalorie amount in terms of total energy needs. However, they can be used as a gauge of normal metabolic function. Abnormal results require the attention of a physician for treatment.

Factors That Influence Basal Metabolic Rate. Several factors influence the BMR and should be kept in mind when related test results are interpreted. The major factors that affect BMR relate to lean body mass, growth periods, body temperature, and hormonal status, as follows:

- *Lean body mass:* One of the largest contributors to overall metabolic rate is the relative percent of lean body mass. This is caused by the greater metabolic activity that occurs in lean tissues (i.e., muscles and organs) as compared with fat and bones. Overall metabolic rates are higher in lean bodies, thereby requiring more energy.[4] Other factors (e.g., gender) only influence the metabolic rate as they relate to the lean body mass.[5,6] Although lean body mass is lost with advanced age, lowered metabolic rate in the elderly population is not exclusively caused by changes in body composition.[7,8]

- *Growth periods:* During rapid growth periods, human growth hormone stimulates cell regeneration and raises BMR to support anabolic metabolism. Thus, growth spurts during childhood and adolescence reflect periods of elevated BMR and energy needs per kilogram of body weight. As growth and the rate of cellular regeneration decline into old age, so does BMR. BMR rises significantly

thyroxine   (T₄) thyroid prohormone; the active hormone form is T₃; it is the major controller of basal metabolic rate.

BOX 6-1 EQUATIONS FOR ESTIMATING RESTING ENERGY NEEDS

Mifflin-St. Jeor
Men:
TEE (kcal/day) = (Weight [kg] × 10 + Height [cm] × 6.25 − Age × 5 + 5) × PA

Women:
TEE (kcal/day) = (Weight [kg] × 10 + Height [cm] × 6.25 − Age × 5 − 161) × PA

PA coefficient:
1.200 = Sedentary (little or no exercise)
1.375 = Lightly active (light exercise/sports 1 to 3 days/wk)
1.550 = Moderately active (moderate exercise/sports 3 to 5 days/wk)
1.725 = Very active (hard exercise/sports 6 to 7 days/wk)
1.900 = Extra active (very hard exercise/sports and physical job)

Harris-Benedict
Men:
TEE (kcal/day) = 66.5 + 13.75 × Weight (kg) + 5 × Height (cm) − 6.76 × Age × PA

Women:
TEE (kcal/day) = 655 + 9.56 × Weight (kg) + 1.7 × Height (cm) − 4.7 × Age × PA

PA coefficient:
1.200 = Sedentary (little or no exercise; desk job)
1.375 = Lightly active (light exercise/sports 1 to 3 days/wk)
1.550 = Moderately active (moderate exercise/sports 3 to 5 days/wk)
1.725 = Heavy exercise (hard exercise/sports 6 to 7 day/wk)

2002 Dietary Reference Intake Energy Calculation
EER = TEE + Energy deposition

Children 0 to 36 Months Old:
0 to 3 months: (89 × Weight [kg] − 100) + 175 kcal
4 to 6 months: (89 × Weight [kg] − 100) + 56 kcal
7 to 12 months: (89 × Weight [kg] − 100) + 22 kcal
13 to 36 months: (89 × Weight [kg] − 100) + 20 kcal

Boys 3 to 8 Years Old:
EER = 88.5 − (61.9 × Age [yr]) + PA × (26.7 × Weight [kg] + 903 × Height [m]) + 20 kcal

PA coefficient:
1.00 if PAL is estimated to be ≥1.0 but <1.4 (sedentary)
1.13 if PAL is estimated to be ≥1.4 but <1.6 (low active)
1.26 if PAL is estimated to be ≥1.6 but <1.9 (active)

1.42 if PAL is estimated to be ≥1.9 but <2.5 (very active)

Girls 3 to 8 Years Old:
EER = 135.3 − (30.8 × Age [yr]) + PA × (10.0 × Weight [kg] + 934 × Height [m]) + 20 kcal

PA coefficient:
1.00 if PAL is estimated to be ≥1.0 but <1.4 (sedentary)
1.16 if PAL is estimated to be ≥1.4 but <1.6 (low active)
1.31 if PAL is estimated to be ≥1.6 but <1.9 (active)
1.56 if PAL is estimated to be ≥1.9 but <2.5 (very active)

Boys 9 to 18 Years Old:
EER = 88.5 − (61.9 × Age [yr]) + PA × (26.7 × Weight [kg] + 903 × Height [m]) + 25 kcal

PA coefficient:
1.00 if PAL is estimated to be ≥1.0 but <1.4 (sedentary)
1.13 if PAL is estimated to be ≥1.4 but <1.6 (low active)
1.26 if PAL is estimated to be ≥1.6 but <1.9 (active)
1.42 if PAL is estimated to be ≥1.9 but <2.5 (very active)

Girls 9 to 18 Years Old:
EER = 135.3 − (30.8 × Age [yr]) + PA × (10.0 × Weight [kg] + 934 × Height [m]) + 25 kcal

PA coefficient:
1.00 if PAL is estimated to be ≥1.0 but <1.4 (sedentary)
1.16 if PAL is estimated to be ≥1.4 but <1.6 (low active)
1.31 if PAL is estimated to be ≥1.6 but <1.9 (active)
1.56 if PAL is estimated to be ≥1.9 but <2.5 (very active)

Men 19 Years Old and Older:
EER = 662 − (9.53 × Age [yr]) + PA × (15.91 × Weight [kg] + 539.6 × Height [m])

PA coefficient:
1.00 if PAL is estimated to be ≥1.0 but <1.4 (sedentary)
1.11 if PAL is estimated to be ≥1.4 but <1.6 (low active)
1.25 if PAL is estimated to be ≥1.6 but <1.9 (active)
1.48 if PAL is estimated to be ≥1.9 but <2.5 (very active)

Women 19 Years Old and Older:
EER = 354 − (6.91 × Age [yr]) + PA × (9.36 × Weight [kg] + 726 × Height [m])

PA coefficient:
1.00 if PAL is estimated to be ≥1.0 but <1.4 (sedentary)
1.12 if PAL is estimated to be ≥1.4 but <1.6 (low active)
1.27 if PAL is estimated to be ≥1.6 but <1.9 (active)
1.45 if PAL is estimated to be ≥1.9 but <2.5 (very active)

EER, Estimated energy requirement; *PA,* physical activity; *PAL,* physical activity level; *TEE,* total energy expenditure.

DRUG-NUTRIENT INTERACTION

ABSORPTION OF LEVOTHYROXINE

Levothyroxine (Synthroid) is a synthetic hormone that is prescribed to treat hypothyroidism and to regulate energy balance. It is absorbed primarily in the jejunum and ileum of the small intestine. Many nutritional factors affect the absorption of the drug[1,2]:

- Levothyroxine absorption is maximized in an empty stomach, which suggests the importance of gastric acid. Food also tends to delay the drug's absorption.
- Dietary fiber reduces the bioavailability of levothyroxine by binding the drug and causing it to be eliminated.
- Calcium and iron supplements or soy products interfere with the drug's absorption and reduce its bioavailability.
- Gastrointestinal disorders: Celiac disease, lactose intolerance, *Helicobacter pylori* infection, and chronic gastritis all affect the absorptive ability of the

digestive system and consequently interfere with the absorption of the drug.

Levothyroxine should be taken at least 1 hour before or 2 hours after a meal, especially a meal that is high in fiber. If an appropriate meal and drug regimen cannot be implemented, higher doses of the drug may be required. Therefore, a consistent schedule is key.[1] Levothyroxine should be taken at least 4 hours before consuming soy products or before taking calcium or iron supplements (however, normal amounts of these minerals in foods do not seem to pose a problem).[1]

The prevalence of celiac disease is higher among patients with autoimmune thyroid disorders.[3] When a patient has celiac disease or lactose intolerance, drug absorption does not improve sufficiently with higher doses of the drug until dietary restrictions for the disorder are followed.[2]

Kelli Boi

1. American Thyroid Association. *ATA hypothyroidism booklet.* Falls Church, Va: American Thyroid Association; 2003.
2. Liwanpo L, Hershman JM. Conditions and drugs interfering with thyroxine absorption. *Best Pract Res Clin Endocrinol Metab.* 2009; 23(6):781-792.
3. Sattar N, Lazare F, Kacer M, et al. Celiac disease in children, adolescents, and young adults with autoimmune thyroid disease. *J Pediatr.* 2011;158(2):272-275, e1.

during pregnancy, which is a period of rapid growth that requires an additional 340 to 450 kcal/day on average. However, this value is highly variable among women, and it is correlated with total weight gain and prepregnancy percentage of body fat. BMR increases above prepregnancy rates with the progression of pregnancy; average increases with each trimester are 4.5%, 10.8%, and 24%, respectively.[9] During the period of lactation, the breast-feeding mother's BMR remains elevated to cover the added metabolic cost of producing milk.

- *Body temperature:* Fever increases BMR by approximately 7% for each 1° F rise above normal body temperature. In states of starvation and malnutrition, the process of adaptive thermogenesis results in lowered heat production (i.e., body temperature) to conserve energy and thus BMR decreases.[10] It has also been speculated that a lower core body temperature may be a contributing factor to the efficiency of storing fat in obese individuals.[11] In cold weather, especially in freezing temperatures, BMR rises in response to the generation of more body heat to maintain normal core temperature.
- *Hormonal status:* Energy expenditure is also influenced by hormonal secretions. As previously mentioned, the thyroid function test is a means of measuring metabolism. Individuals with an underactive thyroid gland may develop hypothyroidism,

which results in a decreased metabolic rate. Hypothyroidism is easily treated with medication (see the Drug-Nutrient Interaction box, "Absorption of Levothyroxine," for more information about hypothyroidism medication interactions). Conversely, hyperthyroidism occurs when the thyroid gland is overactive (see the Cultural Considerations box, "Hypermetabolism and Hypometabolism: What Are They, and Who Is at Risk?"). The fight-or-flight reflexes increase metabolic rate in response to the hormone epinephrine. Growth hormone increases metabolism; alternately, a deficiency of normal growth hormone secretions attenuates the metabolic rate and has recently been linked to obesity as a causative factor.[12] Other hormones (e.g., insulin, cortisol) also increase metabolism, and they may fluctuate daily.

Physical Activity

The exercise that is involved in work or recreation (Figure 6-3) accounts for wide individual variations in energy output (see Chapter 16). In addition to increasing energy

---

adaptive thermogenesis **an adjustment to heat production in response to changing environmental influences (e.g., external temperature, diet).**

CULTURAL CONSIDERATIONS

HYPERMETABOLISM AND HYPOMETABOLISM: WHAT ARE THEY AND WHO IS AT RISK?

Hypermetabolism and hypometabolism are conditions in which the metabolic rate is either significantly higher (hyper) or lower (hypo) than normal. Because the thyroid gland is responsible for producing the hormone thyroxine, which controls the metabolic rate, such conditions usually result from malfunctions of the thyroid gland. Clinically, hypermetabolism and hypometabolism are referred to as *hyperthyroidism* and *hypothyroidism*, respectively.

An individual with hyperthyroidism has a significantly higher metabolic rate and higher energy needs than normal. Such increases in energy needs are not explained by lean tissue, age, or gender. This individual has an overactive thyroid gland, which means that he or she produces too much thyroxine. As a result, the normal energy intake recommendations do not meet this individual's needs. For example, a woman who is 25 years old, 5 feet and 5 inches tall, and weighs 125 lb normally needs approximately 2200 kcal/day to maintain her weight if she engages in a moderate level of activity. However, the same woman with hyperthyroidism may need 1.5 to 2.5 times as many kilocalories per day to maintain her current weight.

Hypothyroidism is the opposite of hyperthyroidism. Individuals with hypothyroidism do not produce enough thyroxine and therefore require less energy than normal to maintain their current body weight. The Dietary Reference Intakes for energy intake for an individual with hypothyroidism are too high and thus, result in weight gain. However, effective medications are available for hypothyroidism. Typically, both hyperthyroidism and hypothyroidism are discovered during young adulthood.

Congenital hypothyroidism (CH), which occurs in 4 out of every 10,000 live births in the United States, is a type of hypothyroidism that is present at birth and that can result in mental retardation if it is not treated. Newborn screening for CH began during the 1970s and is now standard. Studies have found that the risk of CH is linked to birth weight, gender, and ethnicity. Both male and female infants who weigh less than 4.5 lb or more than 10 lb have a significantly higher risk of developing CH, and females of any weight have 50% more risk than males. A recent report in the United States noted that the incidence rate of CH was 100% higher in Hispanic newborns and 44% higher in Asian and Native Hawaiian or other Pacific Islander newborns as compared with Caucasian newborns; it was 30% lower in African-American newborns as compared with Caucasian newborns.[1]

Another risk factor for the development of abnormal thyroid function and thus, abnormal metabolism is iodine intake. The mineral iodine is an important part of the thyroid hormone thyroxine. The incidence of hyperthyroidism and hypothyroidism has been linked to iodine, with both high and low iodine intakes being associated with thyroid disease.[2]

The close monitoring of basal metabolism and total energy expenditure is an important aspect of the treatment of thyroid disease. Medications and energy intake are then modified to control weight and prevent complications.

1. Hinton CF, Harris KB, Borgfeld L, et al. Trends in incidence rates of congenital hypothyroidism related to select demographic factors: data from the United States, California, Massachusetts, New York, and Texas. *Pediatrics.* 2010;125 (Suppl 2):S37-S47.
2. Laurberg P, Jørgensen T, Perrild H, et al. The Danish investigation on iodine intake and thyroid disease, DanThyr: status and perspectives. *Eur J Endocrinol.* 2006;155(2):219-228.

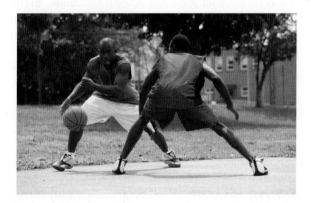

Figure 6-3 Energy output increases during exercise. (Copyright PhotoDisc.)

expenditure and reducing the risk of chronic diseases such as heart disease, diabetes, and certain types of cancer, exercise has positive effects on both physical and mental quality of life.[13] Table 6-1 gives some representative kilocalorie expenditures of different types of work and recreation. Although mental work or study does not require additional kilocalories, muscle tension, restlessness, and agitated movements may increase energy needs for some individuals.

The energy expenditure that is used for physical activity goes above and beyond the RMR. Keeping track of all energy that is used explicitly for physical activity to calculate total energy requirements is somewhat difficult. Instead, the energy that is used for physical activity can be estimated as a factor of RMR by categorizing the physical activity (PA) level in accordance with standard values (1.0 to 2.5, depending on lifestyle). This factor is then multiplied by the RMR. For example, an individual who

TABLE 6-1   ENERGY EXPENDITURE PER POUND PER HOUR DURING VARIOUS ACTIVITIES

Activity	kcal/lb/hr*
Aerobics, moderate	2.95
Bicycling	
Light: 10 to 11.9 mph	2.72
Moderate: 12 to 13.9 mph	3.63
Fast: 14 to 15.9 mph	4.54
Mountain biking	3.85
Daily Activities	
Cleaning	1.36
Cooking	0.91
Driving a car	0.91
Eating, sitting	0.68
Gardening, general	1.81
Office work	0.82
Reading, writing while sitting	0.70
Sleeping	0.41
Shoveling snow	2.72
Running	
5 mph (12 min/mile)	3.63
7 mph (8.5 min/mile)	5.22
9 mph (6.5 min/mile)	6.80
10 mph (6 min/mile)	7.26
Sports	
Boxing, in ring	5.44
Field hockey	3.63
Golf	2.04
Rollerblading	4.42
Skiing, cross country, moderate	3.63
Skiing, downhill, moderate	2.72
Soccer	3.85
Swimming, moderate	3.14
Tennis, doubles	2.27
Tennis, singles	3.63
Ultimate Frisbee	3.63
Volleyball	1.81
Walking	
Moderate: ≈3 mph (20 min/mile), level	1.50
Moderate: ≈3 mph (20 min/mile), uphill	2.73
Brisk: ≈3.5 mph (17.14 min/mile), level	1.72
Fast: ≈4.5 mph (13.33 min/mile), level	2.86
Weight Training	
Light or moderate	1.36
Heavy or vigorous	2.72

*Multiply the activity factor by the weight in pounds by the fraction of hour spent performing the activity.

Example: A 150-lb person plays soccer for 45 minutes. Therefore, the equation would be as follows: 3.85 (i.e., the factor from the table) × 150 (lb) × 0.75 (hr) = 433.13 calories burned.

Energy expenditure depends on the physical fitness of the individual and the continuity of exercise.

Modified from Nieman DC. *Exercise testing and prescription: a health-related approach.* 5th ed. New York: McGraw-Hill; 2003.

works at a desk job and who has little or no leisure activity would have a PA of approximately 1.2 according to the Mifflin-St. Jeor equation. To get a range of total energy expenditure, multiply the person's RMR by 1.2 (see the Clinical Applications box, "Evaluate Your Daily Energy Requirements," for physical activity factors).

Thermic Effect of Food

After eating, food stimulates the metabolism and requires extra energy for the digestion, absorption, and transportation of nutrients to the cells. This overall stimulating effect is called the *thermic effect of food.* Approximately 5% to 10% of the body's total energy needs for metabolism relates to the digestion and storing of nutrients from food.

Total Energy Requirement

The RMR, physical activities, and the thermic effect of food make up a person's overall total energy requirements (Figure 6-4). To maintain a daily energy balance, food energy intake must match body energy output. An energy imbalance (i.e., when energy intake exceeds energy output) can lead to weight gain (Table 6-2). Treatment should include a decrease in food kilocalories and an increase in physical activity. Extreme and unhealthy weight loss (i.e., anorexia nervosa or starvation) results when food energy intake does not meet body energy requirements for extended periods. Treatment should include a gradual increase in food kilocalories along with moderate activity and rest (see Chapter 15).

The Clinical Applications box entitled "Evaluate Your Daily Energy Requirements" provides a step-by-step example for evaluating your energy needs. You may also wish to record your food and activities for a day and to calculate your energy intake (i.e., kilocalories) and output (i.e., kilocalorie expenditure in activities). Total your

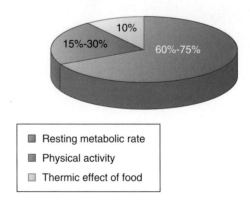

Figure 6-4 The contributions of resting metabolic rate, physical activity, and the thermic effect of food to total energy expenditure.

CLINICAL APPLICATIONS

EVALUATE YOUR DAILY ENERGY REQUIREMENTS

Your estimated energy requirement (in kcal) per day is the sum of your body's three uses of energy, which are as follows:

1. Resting metabolic rate
2. Thermic effect of food
3. Physical activity

Estimated Energy Requirement (EER) as Calculated by the 2002 Dietary Reference Intakes

Men 19 years old and older = 662 − (9.53 × Age [yr]) + Physical activity (PA) × (15.91 × Weight [kg] + 539.6 × Height [m])

Women 19 years old and older = 354 − (6.91 × Age [yr]) + PA × (9.36 × Weight [kg] + 726 × Height [m])

Physical Activity

Estimate your average level of PA. The PA level is the ratio of the total energy expenditure to the basal energy expenditure.

Lifestyle	PA Factor for Men	PA Factor for Women
Sedentary: Mostly resting with little or no planned strenuous activity and only performing those tasks that are required for independent living	1.0	1.0
Low Active: In addition to the activities of a sedentary lifestyle, the added equivalent of a 1.5- to 3-mile walk at a speed of 3 to 4 mph for the average-weight person*	1.11	1.12
Active: In addition to the activities identified for a sedentary lifestyle, an average of 60 minutes of daily moderate-intensity physical activity (e.g., walking at 3 to 4 mph for 3 to 6 miles/day) or shorter periods of more vigorous exertion (e.g., jogging for 30 minutes at 5.5 mph)	1.25	1.27

Lifestyle	PA Factor for Men	PA Factor for Women
Very Active: In addition to the activities of a sedentary lifestyle, an activity level equivalent to walking at 3 to 4 mph for 12 to 22 miles/day (approximately 5 to 7 hours per day) or shorter periods of more vigorous exertion (e.g., running 7 mph for approximately 2.5 hours/day)	1.48	1.45

Example 1

A 32-year-old woman weighs 130 lb (59 kg), is 5 feet and 4 inches tall, and has started and is maintaining a regular physical exercise program. She is currently consuming approximately 2600 kcal/day:

Conversions: 1 pound = 2.2 kg; 39.37 in = 1 m. Thus, 130 ÷ 2.2 = 59 kg; 5 feet 4 inches = 64 inches ÷ 39.37 = 1.626 m.

EER = 354 − (6.91 × 32) + 1.27 [PA] × (9.36 × 59 + 726 × 1.626)

EER = 354 − 221.12 + 1.27 × (552.24 + 1180.5)

EER = 2333.5 kcal/day

Result: This woman will gain weight. Her energy intake is approximately 266 kcal/day more than her energy output. Because 1 lb of body weight equals approximately 3500 kcal, she will gain approximately 1 lb every 13 days with the preceding eating and exercise routine.

Example 2

A 41-year-old man weighs 180 lb (82 kg), is 6 feet tall, and eats an average of 3300 kcal/day while maintaining a very active lifestyle:

EER = 662 − (9.53 × 41) + 1.48 [PA] × (15.91 × 82 + 539.6 × 1.829 [m])

EER = 662 − 390.73 + 1.48 × (1304.62 + 986.93)

EER = 3663 kcal/day

Result: This man will tend to lose weight with his current exercise and meal plan, because he is consuming approximately 163 kcal less than he is expending. Approximately how many pounds will he lose per month?

*For example, a man who weighs 70 kg and is 1.77 m tall and a woman who weighs 57 kg and is 1.63 m tall, on the basis of the reference body weights for adults.

day's activity, and compare it with the general types of similar activities given in Table 6-1. Estimate the total time that you spent on a given activity by adding up the minutes that you spent on that activity at any time and then converting those minutes to hours (or decimal fractions of hours) for the day. For example, if you spent 10 minutes at one point and 5 minutes at another point doing the same thing, then your day's total for that activity is 15 minutes or 0.25 hr. Multiply this total time for a given type of activity by the average kilocalories per

TABLE 6-2   ENERGY BALANCE EXAMPLE: A 32-YEAR-OLD WOMAN WHO WEIGHS 120 LB AND WHO IS 5 FEET AND 4 INCHES TALL

Energy Intake	Energy Output	
Breakfast: 450 kcal	Resting metabolic rate: 1240.5 kcal (this includes the thermic effect of food)	Mifflin-St. Jeor equation
Midmorning snack: 175 kcal	Physical activity: an additional 899.4 kcal	Very active (RMR × 1.725)
Lunch: 500 kcal		
Afternoon snack: 250 kcal		
Dinner: 600 kcal		
Evening snack: 200 kcal		
Total intake: 2175 kcal	**Total output: 2140 kcal**	**Positive energy balance of an extra 35 kcal/day**

Although it is not much, an extra 35 kcal/day could lead to weight gain. Approximately 3500 kcal are in each pound of fat mass. Therefore, if the excess is maintained, this woman could gain 1 lb of fat in 100 days despite her very active lifestyle. By decreasing her energy intake by 35 kcal/day or by further increasing her energy expenditure by 35 kcal/day, she would then be in energy balance and weight stable.

TABLE 6-3   APPROXIMATE CALORIC ALLOWANCES FROM BIRTH TO THE AGE OF 18 YEARS

Age (yr)	kcal/lb
Infants	
0 to 0.5	33.4
0.6 to 1.0	35.6
Children	
1 to 2	36.2
Boys	
3 to 8	32
9 to 13	26.3
14-18	24
Girls	
3 to 8	29.7
9 to 13	23.8
14 to 18	19.3

Data from the Food and Nutrition Board, Institute of Medicine: *Dietary reference intakes for energy, carbohydrate, fiber, fat, fatty acids, cholesterol, protein, and amino acids.* Washington, DC: National Academies Press; 2005.

hour for that activity (see Table 6-1), and then add them up for the day's total kilocalories. Use the following basic steps to estimate your energy expenditure for a day's activities:

1. Total minutes of an activity ÷ 60 = Hours of that activity
2. Total time (hr) × kcal/hr = Total kcal/day for that activity
3. Total kcal/day of all activities = Total kcal energy expenditure for 1 day from activities

RECOMMENDATIONS FOR DIETARY ENERGY INTAKE

General Life Cycle

Growth Periods

During periods of rapid growth, extra energy per unit of body weight is necessary to build new tissue. During childhood, the most rapid growth occurs during infancy and adolescence, with continuous but slower growth taking place in between these periods (Table 6-3). The rapid growth of the fetus and the placenta as well as other maternal tissues make increased energy intake during pregnancy and lactation highly important.

Adulthood

With full adult growth achieved, energy needs level off to meet requirements for tissue maintenance and usual physical activities.

As the aging process continues, a gradual decline in BMR and physical activity decreases the total energy requirement. There is an average decline in BMR of 1% to 2% per decade (assuming that a constant weight is maintained). A more rapid decline occurs around 40 years of age in men and 50 years of age in women. The accelerated loss of fat-free mass during menopause among women is associated with a large drop in BMR.[1] Therefore, food choices should reflect a decline in caloric density and place greater emphasis on increased nutrient density.

Dietary Reference Intakes

To determine recommendations for energy intake, the Food and Nutrition Board of the Institute of Medicine considered the average energy intake of individuals who were healthy, free living, and maintaining a healthy body weight as determined by body mass index measurements.[1] Table 6-4 gives the average total energy expenditure

TABLE 6-4   MEDIAN HEIGHT, WEIGHT, AND RECOMMENDED ENERGY INTAKE

Age (yr)	Mean Weight (kg [lb])	Mean Height (m [in])	Mean Body Mass Index (kg/m²)	Basal Energy Expenditure (kcal/day)	Mean Physical Activity Level	Mean Total Energy Expenditure (kcal/day)
Infants						
0 to 0.5	6.9 (15)	0.64 (25)	16.86	—	—	501
0.6 to 1.0	9 (20)	0.72 (28)	17.20	—	—	713
Children						
1 to 2	11 (24)	0.82 (32)	16.19	—	—	869
Males						
3 to 8	20.4 (45)	1.15 (45)	15.42	1035	1.39	1441
9 to 13	35.8 (79)	1.44 (57)	17.20	1320	1.56	2079
14 to 18	58.8 (130)	1.70 (67)	20.37	1729	1.80	3116
19 to 30	71 (156)	1.80 (71)	22.02	1769	1.74	3081
31 to 50	71.4 (157)	1.78 (70)	22.55	1675	1.81	3021
51 to 70	70 (154)	1.74 (69)	22.95	1524	1.63	2469
71+	68.9 (152)	1.74 (69)	22.78	1480	1.52	2238
Females						
3 to 8	22.9 (50)	1.20 (47)	15.63	1004	1.48	1487
9 to 13	36.4 (80)	1.44 (57)	17.38	1186	1.60	1907
14 to 18	54.1 (119)	1.63 (64)	20.42	1361	1.69	2302
19 to 30	59.3 (131)	1.66 (65)	21.42	1361	1.80	2436
31 to 50	58.6 (129)	1.64 (65)	21.64	1322	1.83	2404
51 to 70	59.1 (130)	1.63 (63)	22.18	1226	1.70	2066
71+	54.8 (121)	1.58 (62)	21.75	1183	1.33	1564
Pregnant						
First trimester						+0
Second and third trimester						+300/day
Lactating						
First 12 months						+500/day

Data from Food and Nutrition Board, Institute of Medicine. *Dietary reference intakes for energy, carbohydrate, fiber, fat, fatty acids, cholesterol, protein, and amino acids.* Washington, DC: National Academies Press; 2005.

throughout life. Note the average height, weight, body mass index, and physical activity level within each age and gender group. Because a balance of energy intake and energy expenditure helps with the maintenance of a healthy weight, the Dietary Reference Intakes for energy intake are equal to the total energy expenditure in kilocalories.

Dietary Guidelines for Americans

The *Dietary Guidelines for Americans* address energy needs by making the following recommendations[14]:

- Prevent and/or reduce overweight and obesity through improved eating and physical activity behaviors.
- Control total calorie intake to manage body weight. For people who are overweight or obese, this will mean consuming fewer calories from foods and beverages.

- Increase physical activity and reduce the time spent in sedentary behaviors.
- Maintain appropriate calorie balance during each stage of life: childhood, adolescence, adulthood, pregnancy and breast-feeding, and older age.
- Select an eating pattern that meets nutrient needs over time at an appropriate calorie level.

MyPlate

The MyPlate Web site (www.choosemyplate.gov) can help you to determine an individualized calorie level and corresponding serving sizes from each of the food groups to meet nutrient and energy-density needs on the basis of age, gender, weight, height, and activity level.[15] The site also provides helpful information for maintaining a balance between food intake and energy output through physical activity.

SUMMARY

- Energy is the force or power to do work. In the human energy system, food provides energy. Energy is measured in kilocalories. Energy from food is cycled through the body's internal energy system in balance with the external environment's energy system, which is powered by the sun.
- The metabolism is the sum of the body processes that are involved in converting food into various forms of energy. These forms of energy include chemical, electrical, mechanical, and thermal energy.

When food is not available, the body draws on its stored energy, which is in the forms of glycogen, fat, and muscle protein.
- Total body energy requirements are based on the following: (1) basal metabolism needs, which make up the largest portion of energy needs; (2) energy for physical activities; and (3) the thermal effect of food (i.e., digesting food and absorbing and transporting nutrients).
- Energy requirements vary throughout life.

CRITICAL THINKING QUESTIONS

1. What are the fuel factors of the three energy nutrients? What is the fuel factor of alcohol? What do these figures mean? What is the primary energy nutrient? Give examples of foods that provide each of these nutrients.
2. Define *RMR*. What body tissues contribute most to resting metabolic needs? What factors influence basal energy requirements?
3. What factors influence nonbasal energy needs? Identify each as either voluntary or involuntary.

CHAPTER CHALLENGE QUESTIONS

True-False
Write the correct statement for each statement that is false.
1. *True or False:* Vitamins are energy-yielding nutrients in foods.
2. *True or False:* The RMR takes into account energy that is used for physical activity.
3. *True or False:* The thyroid hormone thyroxine is a controlling factor of body metabolism.
4. *True or False:* Because children are smaller, their energy requirements are less per kilogram (or pound) of body weight than those of adults.
5. *True or False:* The thermic effect of food refers to the energy that is necessary for the digestion of food.
6. *True or False:* Different people doing the same amount of physical activity require the same amount of energy in kilocalories.

Multiple Choice
1. In human nutrition, the kilocalorie is used to
   a. provide vitamins and water.
   b. measure energy input and output.
   c. control energy reactions.
   d. measure electrical energy.
2. In the following family of four, who has the highest energy needs per unit of body weight?
   a. The 32-year-old mother
   b. The 35-year-old father
   c. The 2-month-old son
   d. The 70-year-old grandmother
3. An overactive thyroid causes
   a. decreased energy needs.
   b. no effect on energy needs.
   c. increased energy needs.
   d. decreased protein needs.
4. Which one of the following people is using the most energy?
   a. A teenager who is playing basketball
   b. A woman who is walking uphill
   c. A student who is studying for her final examinations
   d. A man who is driving a car
5. Which of these foods has the highest energy value per unit of weight?
   a. Bread
   b. Meat
   c. Potato
   d. Butter
6. A slice of bread contains 2 g of protein, 1 g of fat, and 15 g of carbohydrate in the form of starch. What is its kilocalorie value?
   a. 17 kcal
   b. 68 kcal
   c. 77 kcal
   d. 92 kcal

⊖volve Please refer to the Students' Resource section of this text's Evolve Web site for additional study resources.

REFERENCES

1. Food and Nutrition Board, Institute of Medicine. *Dietary reference intakes for energy, carbohydrate, fiber, fat, fatty acids, cholesterol, protein, and amino acids.* Washington, DC: National Academies Press; 2002.
2. Bosy-Westphal A, Reinecke U, Schlörke T, et al. Effect of organ and tissue masses on resting energy expenditure in underweight, normal weight and obese adults. *Int J Obes Relat Metab Disord.* 2004;28(1):72-79.
3. Frankenfield D, Roth-Yousey L, Compher C. Comparison of predictive equations for resting metabolic rate in healthy nonobese and obese adults: a systematic review. *J Am Diet Assoc.* 2005;105(5):775-789.
4. Müller MJ, Bosy-Westphal A, Later W, et al. Functional body composition: insights into the regulation of energy metabolism and some clinical applications. *Eur J Clin Nutr.* 2009;63(9):1045-1056.
5. Johnstone AM, Murison SD, Duncan JS, et al. Factors influencing variation in basal metabolic rate include fat-free mass, fat mass, age, and circulating thyroxine but not sex, circulating leptin, or triiodothyronine, *Am J Clin Nutr.* 2005;82(5):941-948.
6. Geer EB, Shen W. Gender differences in insulin resistance, body composition, and energy balance. *Gend Med.* 2009;6 (Suppl 1):60-75.
7. Ahmed T, Haboubi N. Assessment and management of nutrition in older people and its importance to health. *Clin Interv Aging.* 2010;5:207-216.
8. St-Onge MP, Gallagher D. Body composition changes with aging: the cause or the result of alterations in metabolic rate and macronutrient oxidation? *Nutrition.* 2010;26 (2):152-155.
9. Butte NF, King JC. Energy requirements during pregnancy and lactation. *Public Health Nutr.* 2005;8(7A):1010-1027.
10. Hall KD. Computational model of in vivo human energy metabolism during semistarvation and refeeding. *Am J Physiol Endocrinol Metab.* 2006;291(1):E23-E37.
11. Landsberg L, Young JB, Leonard WR, et al. Do the obese have lower body temperatures? A new look at a forgotten variable in energy balance. *Trans Am Clin Climatol Assoc.* 2009;120:287-295.
12. Kreitschmann-Andermahr I, Suarez P, Jennings R, et al. GH/IGF-I regulation in obesity—mechanisms and practical consequences in children and adults. *Horm Res Paediatr.* 2010;73(3):153-160.
13. Martin CK, Church TS, Thompson AM, et al. Exercise dose and quality of life: a randomized controlled trial. *Arch Intern Med.* 2009;169(3):269-278.
14. U.S. Department of Agriculture, U.S. Department of Health and Human Services. *Dietary guidelines for Americans, 2010.* Washington, DC: U.S. Government Printing Office; 2010.
15. U.S. Department of Agriculture, Center for Nutrition Policy and Promotion. *USDA's MyPlate home page* (website): www.choosemyplate.gov. Accessed August 23, 2011.

FURTHER READING AND RESOURCES

The following Web sites provide methods for predicting total energy needs and for evaluating energy expenditure.

Adult energy needs and body mass index calculator. www.bcm.edu/cnrc/caloriesneed.cfm

Children's energy needs calculator. www.bcm.edu/cnrc/healthyeatingcalculator/eatingCal.html

Mayo Clinic. *Metabolism and weight loss: how you burn calories:* www.mayoclinic.com/health/metabolism/WT00006

Gardner DS, Rhodes P. Developmental origins of obesity: programming of food intake or physical activity? *Adv Exp Med Biol.* 2009;646:83-93.
This review article outlines theories regarding obesity. The authors briefly discuss the multifactorial elements that are involved in energy storage and energy expenditure.

CHAPTER 7

Vitamins

KEY CONCEPTS

- Vitamins are noncaloric, essential nutrients that are necessary for many metabolic tasks.
- Certain health problems are related to inadequate or excessive vitamin intake.
- Vitamins occur in a wide variety of foods and are packaged with the energy-yielding macronutrients (i.e., carbohydrate, fat, and protein).

- The body uses vitamins to make the coenzymes that are required for some enzymes to function.
- The need for particular vitamin supplements depends on a person's vitamin status.

More than any other group of nutrients, vitamins have captured public interest and concern. This chapter answers some of the questions about vitamins: What do they do? How much of each vitamin does the human body need? What foods do they come from? Do we need to take supplements? The scientific study of nutrition, on which the Dietary Reference Intake (DRI) guidelines are based, continues to expand the body of nutrition knowledge. Thus, the answers to these questions have evolved through years of research.

This chapter looks at the vitamins both as a group and as individual nutrients. It explores general and specific vitamin needs as well as reasonable and realistic supplement use.

DIETARY REFERENCE INTAKES

The study of vitamins and minerals and their many functions in human nutrition is a subject of intense scientific investigation. As discussed in Chapter 1, the DRIs are recommendations for nutrient intake by healthy population groups. The continuing development of DRIs under the direction of the National Academy of Sciences takes place over several years and involves numerous scientists from the United States and Canada. They include recommendations for each gender and age group, and they incorporate and expand upon the well-known Recommended Dietary Allowances (RDAs).

Within the DRIs are the following four interconnected categories of recommendations, which were also defined in Chapter 1:

1. *RDA:* The daily intake that meets the needs of almost all healthy individuals in a specified group
2. *Estimated Average Requirement (EAR):* The nutrient intake that meets the needs of half of the individuals in the reference population
3. *Adequate Intake (AI):* A guideline that is used when not enough scientific data is available to establish an RDA
4. *Tolerable Upper Intake Level (UL):* A guideline that sets the maximum nutrient intake that is unlikely to pose a risk of toxicity in healthy individuals

This chapter's discussion of vitamins and the following chapters that discuss minerals, fluids, and electrolytes refer to the various DRI recommendations (especially the RDAs) whenever possible.

THE NATURE OF VITAMINS

Discovery

Early Observations

Vitamins were largely discovered while searching for cures of classic diseases that were suspected to be associated with dietary deficiencies. As early as 1753, British naval surgeon Dr. James Lind observed that many sailors became ill and died on long voyages when they had to live on rations without fresh foods. When Lind provided the sailors with fresh lemons and limes, which were easily stored on a later voyage, no one became ill. Dr. Lind had discovered that scurvy, which had been the curse of sailors, was caused by a dietary deficiency and was prevented by adding lemons or limes to the diet. Because British sailors carried limes on these long voyages, they got the nickname *limeys.*

Early Animal Experiments

In 1906, Dr. Frederick Hopkins of Cambridge University performed an experiment in which he fed a group of rats a synthetic mixture of protein, fat, carbohydrate, mineral salts, and water. All of the rats became ill and died. In another experiment, he added milk to the purified ration, and all of the rats grew normally. This important discovery—that elements present in natural foods are essential to life—provided the necessary foundation for the individual vitamin discoveries that followed.

Era of Vitamin Discovery

Most of the vitamins that are known today were discovered during the first half of the 1900s. The nature of these vital molecules became more evident over time. A form of the name *vitamin* was first used in 1911, when Casimir Funk, a Polish chemist working at the Lister Institute in London, discovered a nitrogen-containing substance (in organic chemistry, known as an *amine*) that he speculated might be a common characteristic of all vital agents. He coined the word *vitamine,* meaning "vital amine." The final *e* was dropped later, when other vital substances turned out not to be amines, and the name *vitamin* was retained to designate compounds within this class of essential substances. At first scientists assigned letters of the alphabet to each vitamin in the order that they were discovered; however, as more vitamins were discovered, this practice was abandoned in favor of more specific names based on a vitamin's chemical structure or body function. Both letter designation and current name will be presented here.

Definition

As each vitamin was discovered during the first half of the 1900s, the following two characteristics that define a vitamin clearly emerged:

1. It must be a vital organic substance that is not a carbohydrate, fat, or protein, and it must be necessary to perform its specific metabolic function or to prevent its associated deficiency disease.
2. It cannot be manufactured by the body in sufficient quantities to sustain life, so it must be supplied by the diet.

Because the body only needs them in small amounts, vitamins are considered micronutrients. The total volume of vitamins that a healthy person normally requires each day would barely fill a teaspoon. Thus, the units of measure for vitamins—milligrams or micrograms—are exceedingly small and difficult to visualize (see the For Further Focus box, "Small Measures for Small Needs"). Nonetheless, all vitamins are essential to life.

Functions of Vitamins

Although each vitamin has its specific metabolic tasks, general functions of vitamins include the following: (1) as components of coenzymes; (2) as antioxidants; (3) as hormones that affect gene expression; (4) as components of cell membranes; and (5) as components of the light-sensitive rhodopsin molecule in the eyes (i.e., vitamin A).

Metabolism: Enzymes and Coenzymes

Coenzymes that are derived from vitamins are an integral part of some enzymes, without which these enzymes cannot catalyze their metabolic reactions. For example, several of the B vitamins (i.e., thiamin, niacin, and riboflavin) are part of coenzymes. These coenzymes are, in turn, integral parts of enzymes that metabolize glucose, fatty acids, and amino acids to extract energy. Enzymes act as catalysts; catalysts increase the rate at which their specific chemical reactions proceed, but they are not themselves consumed during the reactions.

---

scurvy a hemorrhagic disease caused by a lack of vitamin C that is characterized by diffuse tissue bleeding, painful limbs and joints, thickened bones, and skin discoloration from bleeding; bones fracture easily, wounds do not heal, gums swell and tend to bleed, and the teeth loosen.

FOR FURTHER FOCUS

SMALL MEASURES FOR SMALL NEEDS

By definition, vitamins are essential nutrients that are necessary in small amounts for human health. Just how small those amounts truly are is sometimes hard to imagine. Vitamins are measured in metric system terms such as *milligram* and *microgram*, but how much is that? Perhaps comparing these amounts with commonly used household measures will be helpful.

Early during the age of scientific development, scientists realized that they needed a common language of measures that could be understood by all nations to exchange rapidly developing scientific knowledge. Thus, the metric system was born. Like American money, it is a simple decimal system, but here it is applied to weights and measures. This system was developed in the mid-1800s by French scientists and named *Le Système International d'Unités,* which is abbreviated as *SI units.* The use of these more precise units is now widespread, especially because it is mandatory for all purposes in most countries besides the United States. The U.S. Congress passed the official Metric Conversion Act in 1975, but this country has been slower to apply the metric system to common use as compared with other countries (see

Appendix E). However, the use of this system in scientific work is worldwide.

Compare the two metric measures that are used for vitamins in the United States. Below are the Recommended Dietary Allowances equated with common measures to demonstrate just how small our needs really are:

- One *milligram* (mg) is equal to one thousandth of a gram (28 g = 1 oz; 1 g is equal to approximately ¼ tsp). Recommended Dietary Allowances are measured in milligrams for vitamins B_6, C, and E and for thiamin, riboflavin, niacin, pantothenic acid, and choline.
- A *microgram* (mcg or μg) is equal to one millionth of a gram. Recommended Dietary Allowances are measured in micrograms for vitamins A (retinol equivalents), B_{12}, D, and K and for folate and biotin.

It is a small wonder that the total amount of vitamins that we need each day would scarcely fill a teaspoon; however, that small amount makes the big difference between life and death.

Tissue Structure and Protection

Some vitamins are involved in tissue or bone building. For example, vitamin C is involved in the synthesis of collagen, which is a structural protein in the skin, ligaments, and bones. In fact, the word *collagen* comes from a Greek word meaning "glue." Collagen is like glue in its capacity to add tensile strength to body structures. Vitamins (e.g., A, C, and E) also act as antioxidants to protect cell structures and to prevent damage caused by free radicals.

Prevention of Deficiency Diseases

When a vitamin deficiency becomes severe, the nutritional deficiency disease associated with the specific function of that vitamin becomes apparent. For example, the classic vitamin deficiency disease scurvy is caused by insufficient dietary vitamin C. Scurvy is a hemorrhagic disease that is characterized by bleeding in the joints and other tissues and by the breakdown of fragile capillaries under normal blood pressure; these are all symptoms that are related to vitamin C's role in producing the collagen in strong capillary walls. Internal membranes disintegrate and death occurs, as previously mentioned regarding British sailors of earlier centuries. The name *ascorbic acid* comes from the Latin word *scorbutus,* meaning "scurvy," and the prefix *a-* means "without"; thus, the term *ascorbic* means "without scurvy." In developed countries today, we do not see frank scurvy often, but we do see vitamin C deficiency in combination with other forms and degrees

of malnutrition among low-income and poverty-stricken population groups.

Vitamin Metabolism

The way in which our bodies digest, absorb, and transport vitamins depends on the vitamin's solubility. Vitamins are traditionally classified as either fat soluble or water soluble. The fat-soluble vitamins are A, D, E, and K. The water-soluble vitamins are C and all of the B vitamins. This chapter is divided into the following sections: (1) Fat-Soluble Vitamins; (2) Water-Soluble Vitamins; (3) Phytochemicals; and (4) Vitamin Supplementation.

Fat-Soluble Vitamins

Intestinal cells absorb fat-soluble vitamins with fat as a micelle and then incorporate all fat-soluble nutrients into chylomicrons. From the intestinal cells, chylomicrons enter the lymphatic circulation and then the blood (see Chapter 3). The absorption of fat-soluble vitamins is enhanced by dietary fat. For instance, the vitamin A in a glass of vitamin–A-fortified milk is better absorbed from

---

antioxidant a molecule that prevents the oxidation of cellular structures by free radicals

whole or 2% milk than from skim milk, because skim milk contains no fat.

Unlike water-soluble vitamins, fat-soluble vitamins can be stored the liver and adipose tissue for long periods of time. The body uses this reserve in times of inadequate daily intake. Fat-soluble vitamin accumulation in the liver and in adipose tissue is the reason that excess intake can result in toxicity over time.

Water-Soluble Vitamins

Intestinal cells easily absorb water-soluble vitamins. From these cells, the vitamins move directly into the portal blood circulation. Because blood is mostly water, the transport of water-soluble vitamins does not require the assistance of carrier proteins.

With the exception of cobalamin (vitamin B_{12}) and pyridoxine (vitamin B_6), the body does not store water-soluble vitamins to any significant extent. Therefore, the body relies on the frequent intake of foods that are rich in water-soluble vitamins. The potential toxicity of each vitamin is determined by the body's capacity to store it and the capacity of the liver and kidneys to clear it.

Fat-soluble and water-soluble vitamins are absorbed throughout the small intestines. Refer to Figure 5-8 for the general absorptive sites of all nutrients in the gastrointestinal tract.

SECTION 1   **FAT-SOLUBLE VITAMINS**

VITAMIN A (RETINOL)

Functions

Vitamin A performs the functions of aiding vision, tissue strength and immunity, and growth.

Vision

The chemical name *retinol* was given to vitamin A because of its major function in the retina of the eye. The aldehyde form, retinal, is part of a light-sensitive pigment in retinal cells called *rhodopsin,* which is commonly known as *visual purple.* Rhodopsin enables the eye to adjust to different amounts of available light. A mild vitamin A deficiency may cause night blindness, slow adaptation to darkness, or glare blindness. Vitamin-A–related compounds (i.e., the carotenoids lutein and zeaxanthin) are specifically associated with the prevention of age-related macular degeneration.[1]

Tissue Strength and Immunity

The other retinoids (i.e., retinoic acid and retinol) help to maintain healthy epithelial tissue, which is the protective tissue that covers body surfaces (i.e., the skin and the inner mucous membranes in the nose, throat, eyes, gastrointestinal tract, and genitourinary tract). These tissues are the primary barrier to infection. Vitamin A is also important as an antioxidant and in the production of immune cells that are responsible for fighting bacterial, parasitic, and viral attacks.

Growth

Retinoic acid and retinol are involved in skeletal and soft-tissue growth through their roles in protein synthesis and the stabilization of cell membranes. The constant need to replace old cells in the bone matrix, the gastrointestinal tract, and other areas requires adequate vitamin A intake.

Requirements

Vitamin A requirements are based on its two basic forms in foods (i.e., preformed vitamin A and provitamin A) and its storage in the body. The established RDA for adults is 700 mcg retinol equivalents for women and 900 mcg retinol equivalents for men.[2]

retinol the chemical name of vitamin A; the name is derived from the vitamin's visual functions related to the retina of the eye, which is the back inner lining of the eyeball that catches the light refractions of the lens to form images that are interpreted by the optic nerve and the brain and that makes the necessary light–dark adaptations.

carotenoids organic pigments that are found in plants; known to have functions such as scavenging free radicals, reducing the risk of certain types of cancer, and helping to prevent age-related eye diseases; more than 600 carotenoids have been identified, with β-carotene being the most well-known.

Food Forms and Units of Measure

Vitamin A occurs in two forms, as follows:

1. Preformed vitamin A or retinol, which is the active vitamin A found in foods that are derived from animal products.
2. Provitamin A or β-carotene, which is a pigment in yellow, orange, and deep green fruits or vegetables that the human body can convert to retinol. Carotenoids are a family of compounds that are similar in structure; β-carotene and lutein are the most common in foods (Box 7-1).

In the typical American diet, a significant amount of vitamin A is in the *pro*vitamin A form (i.e., β-carotene). To account for all food forms, individual carotenoids and preformed vitamin A are measured, and the amounts are converted to retinol equivalents. For the body to make 1 mcg of retinol, 12 mcg of dietary β-carotene, 2 mcg of supplemental β-carotene, or 24 mcg of either of the carotenoids (α-carotene or β-cryptoxanthin) are necessary. An older measure that is sometimes used to quantify vitamin A is the International Unit (IU). One IU of vitamin A equals 0.3 mcg of retinol or 0.6 mcg of β-carotene.

Body Storage

The liver can store large amounts of retinol. In healthy individuals, the liver stores approximately 80% of the body's total vitamin A. Thus, the liver is particularly susceptible to toxicity as a result of excessive vitamin A supplementation. The remaining vitamin A may be stored in adipose tissue, the kidneys, and the lungs.

Deficiency Disease

Adequate vitamin A intake prevents two eye conditions: (1) xerosis, which involves itching, burning, and red, inflamed eyelids; and (2) xerophthalmia, which is blindness that is caused by severe deficiency. Dietary vitamin A deficiency is the leading cause of preventable blindness in children worldwide. A recent publication by the World Health Organization reports that vitamin A deficiency that results in night blindness currently affects 5.2 million preschool-aged children and 9.8 million pregnant women globally.[3]

Deficiency symptoms are directly related to vitamin A's functions. Therefore, a lack of dietary vitamin A may also result in epithelial and immune system disorders.

Toxicity Symptoms

The condition created by excessive vitamin A intake is called *hypervitaminosis A*. Symptoms include bone pain, dry skin, loss of hair, fatigue, and anorexia. Excessive vitamin A intake may cause liver injury with portal hypertension, which is elevated blood pressure in the portal vein, and ascites, which is fluid accumulation in the abdominal cavity. Because of the potential for toxicity, the UL of retinol for adults has been set at 3000 mcg/day.[2] Although vitamin A deficiency is more common worldwide than toxicity, children in the United States may consume excess vitamin A from fortified foods alone, without added vitamin A from dietary supplements.[4] Toxicity symptoms usually result from the overconsumption of preformed vitamin A rather than of carotenoids. The absorption of dietary carotenoids is dose dependent at high intake levels. However, the prolonged excessive intake of foods that are high in β-carotene will cause a harmless orange skin tint that disappears when the excessive intakes are discontinued. Alternatively, β-carotene supplements can reach concentrations in the body that promote oxidative damage, cell division, and the destruction of other forms of vitamin A.

Food Sources

Fish liver oils, liver, egg yolks, butter, and cream are sources of preformed natural vitamin A. Preformed vitamin A occurs naturally in milk fat. Low-fat and nonfat milks and margarine are significant sources of vitamin A, because they are fortified. Some good sources of β-carotene are dark green leafy vegetables such as Swiss

---

BOX 7-1   CAROTENOIDS

Carotenes: orange pigments that contain no oxygen
- α-Carotene
- β-Carotene
- γ-Carotene
- δ-Carotene
- Lycopene

Xanthophylls: yellow pigments that contain some oxygen
- Lutein
- Zeaxanthin
- Neoxanthin
- Violaxanthin
- α- and β-Cryptoxanthin

---

carotene a group name for three red and yellow pigments (α-, β-, and γ-carotene) that are found in dark green and yellow vegetables and fruits; β-carotene is most important to human nutrition because the body can convert it to vitamin A, thus making it a primary source of the vitamin.

chard, turnip greens, kale, and spinach as well as dark-orange vegetables and fruits such as carrots, sweet potatoes or yams, pumpkins, mangoes, and apricots. Table 7-1 provides some comparative food sources of vitamin A.

β-Carotene and preformed vitamin A require emulsification by bile salts to be absorbed by the intestine. Preformed vitamin A is efficiently absorbed at a rate of 70% to 90%, whereas provitamin A (carotenoids) are less bioavailable at an absorption rate of 20% to 50%. Inside the intestinal cells, both forms are incorporated into chylomicrons with fat, and the chylomicrons pass through the lymphatic system and into the bloodstream.

Stability

Retinol is unstable when it is exposed to heat and oxygen. Quick cooking methods that use little water help to preserve vitamin A in food.

TABLE 7-1   FOOD SOURCES OF VITAMIN A

Item	Quantity	Amount (mcg of Retinol Equivalents)
Vegetables		
Beet greens, boiled	½ cup	276
Bok choy, boiled	½ cup	180
Carrots, raw	½ cup	534
Collard greens, boiled	½ cup	386
Dandelion greens, boiled	½ cup	260
Kale, raw	½ cup	258
Mustard greens, boiled	½ cup	221
Pumpkin, boiled	½ cup	306
Spinach, boiled	½ cup	472
Sweet potato, baked, in skin	1 medium (114 g)	1096
Winter squash	½ cup	268
Fruits		
Cantaloupe	1 cup, diced	264
Meat, Poultry, Fish, Dry Beans, Eggs, and Nuts		
Beef liver, pan fried	3 oz	6582
Chicken liver, pan fried	3 oz	3652
Milk and Dairy Products		
Milk, low-fat 2%, fortified	8 oz	134
Milk, skim, fortified	8 oz	149
Ricotta cheese, whole milk	½ cup	149

Data from the U.S. Department of Agriculture, Agricultural Research Service: Nutrient Data Laboratory. *USDA nutrient database for standard reference* (website): www.ars.usda.gov/ba/bhnrc/ndl. Accessed October 12 2010.

VITAMIN D (CALCIFEROL)

Vitamin D was mistakenly classified as a vitamin in 1922 by its discoverers when they cured rickets with fish oil, which is a natural source of vitamin D. Today, we know that the compound produced by animals (i.e., cholecalciferol or vitamin D_3) and some organisms (i.e., ergocalciferol or vitamin D_2) is a prohormone rather than a vitamin. Vitamins D_2 and D_3 are both physiologically relevant to human nutrition, and they are collectively referred to as *calciferol*.

Upon exposure to ultraviolet light, humans are able to convert the precursor 7-dehydrocholesterol, a compound that is found in the epidermal layer of skin, into cholecalciferol. Similarly, organisms such as invertebrates and fungi are capable of converting the precursor ergosterol into ergocalciferol after they receive ultraviolet irradiation.

The activated and functional form of vitamin D is calcitriol (i.e., 1,25-dihydroxycholecalciferol). Vitamins D_2 and D_3 must be activated in two successive hydroxylation reactions to yield calcitriol. The first hydroxylation reaction occurs in the liver to produce 25-hydroxycholecalciferol. The enzyme 1-α-hydroxylase then catalyzes the second hydroxylation reaction in the kidneys to produce the most active form of vitamin D, calcitriol. Figure 7-1 illustrates the activation process of vitamin D in the body.

---

cholecalciferol the chemical name for vitamin D_3 in its inactive form; it is often shortened to *calciferol*.

ergocalciferol the chemical name for vitamin D_2 in its inactive form; it is produced by some organisms (not humans) upon ultraviolet irradiation from the precursor ergosterol.

prohormone a precursor substance that the body converts to a hormone; for example, a cholesterol compound in the skin is first irradiated by sunlight and then converted through successive enzyme actions in the liver and kidney into the active vitamin D hormone, which then regulates calcium absorption and bone development.

calcitriol the activated hormone form of vitamin D.

1-α-hydroxylase the enzyme in the kidneys that catalyzes the hydroxylation reaction of 25-hydroxycholecalciferol (i.e., calcidiol) to calcitriol, which is the active form of vitamin D; 1-α-hydroxylase activity is increased by parathyroid hormone when blood calcium levels are low.

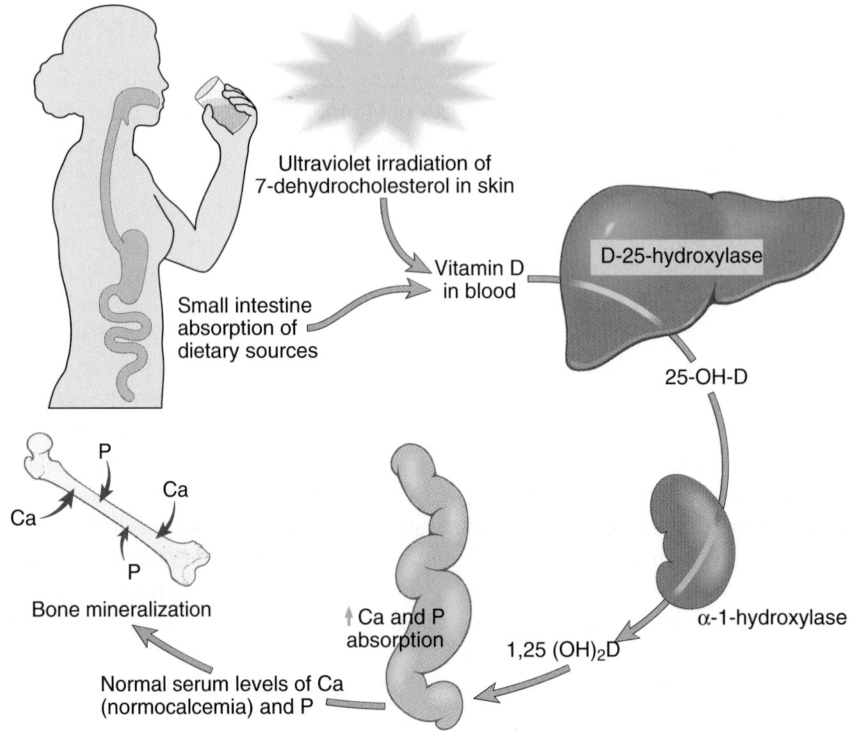

Figure 7-1 Vitamin D activation from skin synthesis and dietary sources. Normal vitamin D metabolism maintains blood calcium levels. (Reprinted from Kumar V, Abbas A, Fausto N, Mitchell R. *Robbins basic pathology*. 8th ed. Philadelphia: Saunders; 2007.)

Functions

Absorption of Calcium and Phosphorus and Bone Mineralization

Calcitriol acts physiologically with two other hormones—parathyroid hormone and the thyroid hormone calcitonin—to control calcium and phosphorus metabolism. Calcitriol stimulates the following: (1) the intestinal cell absorption of calcium and phosphorus; (2) the kidney reabsorption of calcium and phosphorus; and (3) the osteoclastic resorption of calcium and phosphorus from trabecular bone. All of these mechanisms maintain blood calcium and phosphorus homeostasis (see Figure 7-1).

Osteoporosis Treatment

Osteoporosis involves a loss of bone density that leads to brittle bones and spontaneous fractures. Because calcitriol regulates the rate of calcium and phosphorus resorption from bone, it has been clinically used to reduce the risk of osteoporosis.

Requirements

Establishing requirements for vitamin D is difficult because it is made in the skin by the sun's ultraviolet rays from 7-dehydrocholesterol and because the number of food sources are limited. Vitamin D requirement varies with individual exposure to sunlight, which is affected by season, the latitude at which a person resides, and even a person's skin color.

Recent research indicates that worldwide vitamin D deficiency is pandemic, with multifactorial health consequences.[5] The primary cause of inadequate circulating serum vitamin D is a lack of sun exposure. In the northern hemisphere, particularly above 40 degrees latitude, less sunlight is present during fall and winter than during spring and summer. Because the amount of vitamin D produced in the skin is relative to the intensity of the sun, significantly less vitamin D is produced during the winter and at higher latitudes. This also affects the vitamin D requirement of people with darker skin, because melanin absorbs ultraviolet B radiation in a way that is similar to that of sunscreen. Thus, less vitamin D is produced in darker-skinned people than in lighter-skinned people who receive the same sun exposure.

---

resorption the breaking down and releasing of minerals from bones.

A flurry of research over the past decade indicates that the dietary needs of vitamin D are higher than what was established at the time of publication of the previous DRIs in 1997. The current DRI for vitamin D is 600 IU/day for individuals who are between 1 and 70 years old and 800 IU/day for individuals who are older than 70 years of age.[6] The American Academy of Pediatrics recommends that infants receive a minimum of 400 IU of vitamin D beginning soon after birth to prevent rickets.[7]

Deficiency Disease

Calcitriol deficiency causes rickets, which is a condition seen in growing children that is characterized by the malformation of the bones. Children with rickets have soft long bones that bend under the child's weight (Figure 7-2). In addition to causing skeletal malformations, inadequate vitamin D intake prevents children from attaining their peak bone mass, thereby contributing to the development of osteoporosis or osteomalacia as adults. Many other chronic diseases have been linked with vitamin D deficiency, including muscle weakness, several types of cancer, coronary heart disease, hypertension, tuberculosis, and several autoimmune diseases (e.g., type 1 diabetes,

multiple sclerosis, Crohn's disease, rheumatoid arthritis).[5] It is currently estimated that 77% Americans have inadequate vitamin D stores, with a disproportionate prevalence occurring among non-Hispanic blacks (97%) and Mexican Americans (90%).[8]

Toxicity Symptoms

Excessive dietary intake of vitamin D can be toxic, especially for infants and children. Symptoms of toxicity or hypervitaminosis D include the calcification of the soft tissues (e.g., kidneys, heart, lungs), fragile bones, and kidney stones. The prolonged elevated intake of cholecalciferol may produce elevated blood calcium concentrations (i.e., hypercalcemia) and calcium deposits in the kidney nephrons, which interferes with overall kidney function. The UL for vitamin D among people who are older than 9 years of age is 4000 IU/day.[9] Vitamin D intoxication cannot occur as a result of the cutaneous production of vitamin D. For most people, vitamin D intake from food and dietary supplements is not likely to exceed the UL. However, individuals who consume diets that are high in fatty fish and fortified milk in addition to dietary supplements that contain vitamin D may be at risk for toxicity.

Food Sources

Fatty fish are one of the only good natural sources of vitamin D. Therefore, a large portion of daily vitamin D intake comes from fortified foods (Table 7-2). Because it is a common food that also contains calcium and phosphorus, milk is a practical food to fortify with vitamin D. The standard commercial practice is to add 400 IU per quart. Butter substitutes such as margarines also are fortified with vitamin D. Children who are consuming vitamin-D–deficient diets (e.g., a rigid macrobiotic diet with no vitamin-D–fortified food products) are especially vulnerable to stunted bone development and rickets.

Stability

Vitamin D is relatively stable under most conditions that involve heat, aging, and storage.

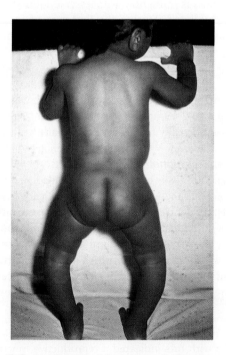

Figure 7-2 A child with rickets; note the bowlegs.
(Reprinted from Kumar V, Abbas A, Fausto N, Mitchell R. *Robbins basic pathology.* 8th ed. Philadelphia: Saunders; 2007.)

rickets a disease of childhood that is characterized by the softening of the bones from an inadequate intake of vitamin D and insufficient exposure to sunlight; it is also associated with impaired calcium and phosphorus metabolism.

TABLE 7-2 FOOD SOURCES OF VITAMIN D

Item	Quantity	Amount (International Units)
Bread, Cereal, Rice, and Pasta		
All Bran, Kellogg's cereal	½ cup	50
Total Whole Grain, General Mills cereal	1 cup	53
Meat, Poultry, Fish, Dry Beans, Eggs, and Nuts		
Herring or trout, cooked	3 oz	177
Salmon, Atlantic, cooked	3 oz	255
Salmon, canned (includes Chinook, coho, pink, and sockeye)	3 oz	689
Sardines, Pacific, canned	3 oz	408
Tuna, canned, albacore or ahi	3 oz	119
Tuna, bluefin, cooked	3 oz	782
Milk and Dairy Products		
Milk, vitamin-D fortified	1 cup (8 fl oz)	100
Soy or rice milk, vitamin-D fortified	1 cup (8 fl oz)	80
Fats, Oils, and Sugars		
Fish oil, cod liver	1 Tbsp	1360

Data from the U.S. Department of Agriculture, Agricultural Research Service: Nutrient Data Laboratory. *USDA nutrient database for standard reference* (website): www.ars.usda.gov/ba/bhnrc/ndl. Accessed October 2010; and the British Columbia Ministry of Health. *Food sources of calcium and vitamin D* (website): www.bchealthguide.org/healthfiles/hfile68e.stm#hf004. Accessed August 2007.

VITAMIN E (TOCOPHEROL)

Early vitamin studies identified a substance that was necessary for animal reproduction. This substance was named *tocopherol* from two Greek words: *tophos,* meaning "childbirth," and *phero,* meaning "to bring," with the *-ol* ending used to indicate its alcohol functional group. Tocopherol became known as the antisterility vitamin, but it was soon demonstrated to have this effect only in rats and a few other animals and not in people. A number of related compounds have since been discovered. Tocopherol is the generic name for this entire group of homologous fat-soluble nutrients, which are designated as α-, β-, γ-, and δ-tocopherol or tocotrienol. Of these eight, α-tocopherol is the only one that is significant in human nutrition and thus, used to calculate dietary needs.[10]

Functions

The most vital function of α-tocopherol is its antioxidant action in tissues. In addition to the potent antioxidant activity of vitamin E, it has been associated with antipro-

liferative effects in the eye that are seemingly protective against conditions such as cataracts and glaucoma.[11]

Antioxidant Function

α-Tocopherol is the body's most abundant fat-soluble antioxidant. The polyunsaturated fatty acids (see Chapter 3) in the phospholipids of cell and organelle membranes are particularly susceptible to free radical oxidation. α-Tocopherol intercepts this oxidation process and protects the polyunsaturated fatty acids from damage.

Relation to Selenium Metabolism

Selenium is a trace mineral that, as part of the selenium-containing enzyme glutathione peroxidase, works with α-tocopherol as an antioxidant. Glutathione peroxidase is the second line of defense for preventing free radical damage to membranes. Glutathione peroxidase spares α-tocopherol from oxidation, thereby reducing the dietary requirement for α-tocopherol. Similarly, α-tocopherol spares glutathione peroxidase from oxidation, thus reducing the dietary requirement for selenium.

Requirements

α-Tocopherol requirements are expressed in milligrams per day. The RDA for men and women who are 14 years old and older is 15 mg/day, with lesser amounts necessary during childhood. During the first year of infancy, no RDA has been determined, but the AI is 4 to 6 mg/day.[10]

Deficiency Disease

Young infants—especially premature infants who missed the final 1 to 2 months of gestation, when α-tocopherol stores are normally filled—are particularly vulnerable to hemolytic anemia. With hemolytic anemia, red blood cell membrane phospholipids and proteins are left unprotected and are easily oxidized and degraded, and the continued loss of functioning red blood cells leads to anemia.

A dietary deficiency of vitamin E is rare; the only cases occur in individuals who cannot absorb or metabolize fat. In such cases, the α-tocopherol deficiency disrupts the normal synthesis of myelin, which is the protective phospholipid-rich membrane that covers the nerve cells. The

tocopherol the chemical name for vitamin E, which was named by early investigators because their initial work with rats indicated a reproductive function; in people, vitamin E functions as a strong antioxidant that preserves structural membranes such as cell walls.

major nerves that are affected are the spinal cord fibers that affect physical activity and the retina of the eye, which affects vision.

Toxicity Symptoms

α-Tocopherol from food sources has no known toxic effects in people. Supplemental α-tocopherol intakes that exceed the UL of 1000 mg/day may interfere with vitamin K activity and blood clotting. Although the exact mechanism is unknown, this may be particularly problematic for individuals who are deficient in vitamin K or for patients who are receiving anticoagulation therapy.[12]

Food Sources

The richest sources of α-tocopherol are vegetable oils (e.g., wheat germ, soybean, safflower). Note that vegetable oils are also the richest sources of polyunsaturated fatty acids, which α-tocopherol protects. Other food sources of α-tocopherol include nuts, fortified cereals, and avocados. Table 7-3 provides a list of food sources of vitamin E.

TABLE 7-3 **FOOD SOURCES OF VITAMIN E AS α-TOCOPHEROL**

Item	Quantity	Amount (mg of α-tocopherol)
Bread, Cereal, Rice, and Pasta		
Total Whole Grain, General Mills cereal	1 cup	18.0
Wheat germ, toasted, plain	1 oz	4.53
Fruits		
Avocado	¼ medium	1.04
Mango, raw	½ medium	1.16
Meat, Poultry, Fish, Dry Beans, Eggs, and Nuts		
Almonds, dried	1 oz	7.33
Hazelnuts, dried	1 oz	4.26
Sunflower seeds	2 Tbsp	6.21
Fats, Oils, and Sugars		
Corn oil	1 Tbsp	2.83
Cottonseed oil	1 Tbsp	4.80
Palm oil	1 Tbsp	2.17
Peanut oil	1 Tbsp	2.12
Safflower oil	1 Tbsp	4.64
Sunflower oil	1 Tbsp	5.59

Data from the U.S. Department of Agriculture, Agricultural Research Service: Nutrient Data Laboratory. *USDA nutrient database for standard reference* (website): www.ars.usda.gov/ba/bhnrc/ndl. Accessed October 2010.

Stability

α-Tocopherol is unstable to heat and alkalis.

VITAMIN K

In 1929, Henrik Dam, a biochemist at the University of Copenhagen, discovered a hemorrhagic disease in chicks that were fed a diet from which all lipids had been removed. Dam hypothesized that an unidentified lipid factor had been removed from the chicks' feed. Dam called it *koagulations vitamin* or *vitamin K,* and the letter that he assigned it is still used today. Dam later succeeded in isolating the agent from alfalfa and identifying it, for which he received the Nobel Prize for physiology and medicine. As with many of the vitamins, not just one but several homologous forms of vitamin K make up the group. The major form in plants that was initially isolated from alfalfa by Dam is phylloquinone, which is the dietary form of vitamin K. Menaquinone, a second form, is synthesized by intestinal bacteria. Menaquinone contributes approximately half of our daily supply of vitamin K. Menadione is a synthetic precursor of vitamin K, but it has not been used as a dietary supplement since the U.S. Food and Drug Administration banned it because of its toxicity effects.

Functions

Vitamin K has two well-established functions in the body: blood clotting and bone development.

Blood Clotting

The most well-known and the earliest discovered function of vitamin K is in the blood-clotting process. Vitamin K is essential for maintaining the normal blood concentrations of four blood-clotting factors. The first of these vitamin–K–dependent blood factors to be identified and characterized was prothrombin (i.e., clotting factor II). Prothrombin, which is synthesized in the liver, is converted to thrombin, which then initiates the conversion of fibrinogen to fibrin to form the blood clot (Figure 7-3).

Phylloquinone is an antidote for the effects of excessive anticoagulant drug doses, and it is often used to control and prevent certain types of hemorrhages. Fat-soluble vitamins are more completely absorbed when bile is

phylloquinone a fat-soluble vitamin of the K group that is found primarily in green plants.

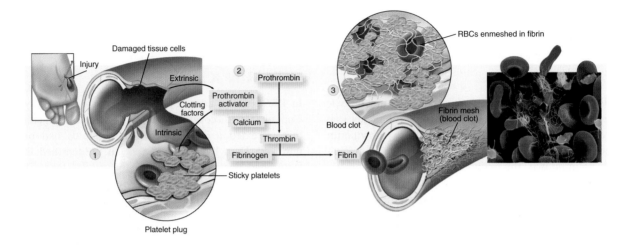

Figure 7-3 The blood-clotting mechanism. The complex clotting mechanism can be distilled into three steps: (1) the release of clotting factors from both injured tissue cells and sticky platelets at the injury site, which form a temporary platelet plug; (2) a series of chemical reactions that eventually result in the formation of thrombin; and 3) the formation of fibrin and the trapping of blood cells to form a clot. (Modified from Thibodeau GA, Patton KT. *Anatomy & physiology.* 6th ed. St. Louis: Mosby; 2007.)

DRUG-NUTRIENT INTERACTION

VITAMIN K CONSIDERATIONS WITH ANTICOAGULANT AND ANTIBIOTIC MEDICATIONS

Anticoagulation medications such as warfarin act to reduce the overall production of blood-clotting factors. Because the primary action of vitamin K is the manufacturing of these same proteins, the amount of vitamin-K–rich foods that a patient eats can affect the medication level that is needed for optimal anticoagulation. Many patients believe that they should avoid foods that are rich in vitamin K while they are taking warfarin, but this can lead to unstable anticoagulation and the restriction of the other nutrients that are found in these foods. Patients should strive to eat a consistent diet rather than limiting vitamin-K–rich foods like dark leafy greens. A dietitian can educate the patient about foods that are rich in vitamin K and help them to achieve a balance between their medication level and their desired vitamin K intake.

One form of vitamin K, menaquinone, is synthesized by healthy bacteria in the gut. This source is significant for meeting overall vitamin K needs. Therefore, the long-term use of medications that destroy gastrointestinal bacteria (e.g., antibiotics) also obliterates a valuable source of vitamin K. Patients should be advised to maintain their daily intakes of food sources of vitamin K (Table 7-4).

present. Thus, conditions that hinder the release of bile into the small intestine decrease the absorption of vitamin K and ultimately increase the length of time that is required for blood to clot. When bile salts are given with vitamin K concentrate, the blood-clotting time returns to normal. See the Drug-Nutrient Interaction box entitled "Vitamin K Considerations With Anticoagulant and Antibiotic Medications" for additional information about special medication-related considerations with vitamin K.

Bone Development

Five proteins in bone and cartilage require vitamin–K-dependent modifications to function.[13] The most abundant noncollagenous protein in bone matrix, osteocalcin, is one of the vitamin–K-dependent proteins. Vitamin K is involved in the modification of the glutamic acid residues of osteocalcin to form calcium-binding γ-carboxyglutamic acid residues. Like the blood-clotting proteins, osteocalcin binds calcium; unlike the blood-clotting proteins, it forms bone crystals.

Requirements

Because intestinal bacteria synthesize a form of vitamin K (menaquinone), a constant supply is normally available to support body needs. Currently not enough scientific evidence is available to establish an RDA. Therefore, the DRIs for vitamin K are AIs. Values gradually increase from birth to adulthood. The AI for men is 120 mcg/day; for women, it is 90 mcg/day.[2]

Deficiency Disease

Deficiency diseases related to vitamin K are not common. A deficiency (i.e., hypoprothrombinemia) may present as a secondary result of another clinical condition as opposed to a dietary deficiency. Patients who have severe malabsorption disorders (e.g., Crohn's disease) or who are treated chronically with antibiotics that kill intestinal bacteria are susceptible to blood loss induced by vitamin K deficiency.

Vitamin K is routinely given at birth to prevent hemorrhaging, because vitamin K does not efficiently transfer through the placenta during gestation, and the intestinal tract of a newborn does not yet have vitamin-K–producing gut flora. Thus, infants are deficient in vitamin K at birth.

Toxicity Symptoms

Toxicity from vitamin K—even when large amounts are taken over extended periods—has not been observed. Therefore, no UL has been established.

TABLE 7-4 FOOD SOURCES OF VITAMIN K

Item	Quantity	Amount (mcg)
Vegetables		
Broccoli, raw	½ cup, chopped	45
Brussels sprouts, cooked, drained	½ cup	109
Kale, raw	½ cup, chopped	273
Mustard greens, raw	½ cup, chopped	139
Spinach, raw	½ cup	72
Turnip greens, raw	½ cup	69

Data from the U.S. Department of Agriculture, Agricultural Research Service: Nutrient Data Laboratory. *USDA nutrient database for standard reference* (website): www.ars.usda.gov/ba/bhnrc/ndl. Accessed October 2010.

Food Sources

Green leafy vegetables such as spinach, turnip greens, and broccoli are the best dietary sources of vitamin K, providing 40 to 80 mcg of phylloquinone per half cup of raw food. Small amounts of phylloquinone are contributed by milk, dairy products, meats, fortified cereals, fruits, and vegetables (see Table 7-4).

Stability

Phylloquinone is fairly stable, although it is sensitive to light and irradiation. Therefore, clinical preparations are kept in dark bottles.

Table 7-5 provides a summary of the fat-soluble vitamins.

SECTION 2 **WATER-SOLUBLE VITAMINS**

VITAMIN C (ASCORBIC ACID)

Functions

Vitamin C has several critical functions in the body. It acts as an antioxidant and a cofactor of enzymes, and it plays a role in many metabolic and immunologic activities.

Connective Tissue

Ascorbic acid is necessary to build and maintain strong tissues through its involvement in collagen synthesis. Collagen is especially important in tissues of mesodermal origin, including connective tissues (e.g., ligaments, tendons, bone matrix, other binding lattices that hold together and give tensile strength to tissues) and other tissues that contain connective tissue (e.g., cartilage, tooth dentin, capillary walls).

Each time that the amino acids proline or lysine are added during collagen synthesis, they are hydroxylated (i.e., OH is added) to form hydroxyproline and hydroxylysine by the ascorbic–acid-dependent enzymes prolyl hydroxylase and lysyl hydroxylase. Iron is a cofactor for

ascorbic acid the chemical name for vitamin C; the vitamin was named after its ability to cure scurvy.

TABLE 7-5 **SUMMARY OF FAT-SOLUBLE VITAMINS**

Vitamin	Functions	Recommended Intake (Adults)	Deficiency	Tolerable Upper Intake Level (UL) and Toxicity	Sources
Vitamin A (retinol, retinal, and retinoic acid) Provitamin A (carotene)	Vision cycle: adaptation to light and dark; tissue growth, especially skin and mucous membranes; reproduction; immune function	Men, 900 mcg/day; women, 700 mcg/day	Night blindness; xerosis; xerophthalmia; susceptibility to epithelial infection; dry skin; impaired immunity, growth, and reproduction	UL: 3000 mcg/day Hair loss; irritated skin; bone pain, liver damage; birth defects	Retinol (animal foods): liver, egg yolk, cream, butter or fortified margarine, fortified milk Provitamin A (plant foods): dark green and deep orange vegetables (e.g., spinach, collard greens, broccoli, pumpkin, sweet potatoes, carrots)
Vitamin D (cholecalciferol, ergocalciferol)	Absorption of calcium and phosphorus; calcification of bones and teeth; growth	Between the ages of 1 and 70 years, 600 IU/day; 70 years of age or older, 800 IU/day	Rickets and growth retardation in children; osteomalacia (soft bones) in adults	UL: 1000 to 4000 IU/day Calcification of soft tissue; kidney damage; growth retardation	Synthesized in the skin with exposure to sunlight, fortified milk, fish oils
Vitamin E (α-tocopherol)	Antioxidant (i.e., protection of materials that oxidize easily)	Adults, 15 mg/day	Breakdown of red blood cells; anemia; nerve damage; retinopathy	UL: 1000 mg/day (from supplements) Inhibition of vitamin K activity in blood clotting	Vegetable oils, vegetable greens, wheat germ, nuts, seeds
Vitamin K (phylloquinone, menaquinone)	Normal blood clotting and bone development	Men, 120 mcg/day; women, 90 mcg/day	Bleeding tendencies; hemorrhagic disease; poor bone growth	UL: Not set Interference with anticoagulation drugs	Synthesis by intestinal bacteria, dark green leafy vegetables, soybean oil

both enzymes, and ascorbic acid is required to maintain the iron atoms in these enzymes in their active ferrous (Fe^{2+}) form. Hydroxyproline and hydroxylysine form covalent bonds with other residues, which strengthen collagen's structure. When ascorbic acid is plentiful, collagen and the connective tissues in which it is integral quickly develop. Blood vessels are particularly dependent on ascorbic acid's role in collagen synthesis to help their walls resist stretching as blood is forced through them.

General Body Metabolism

The more metabolically active body tissues (e.g., adrenal glands, brain, kidney, liver, pancreas, thymus, spleen) contain greater concentrations of ascorbic acid. Ascorbic acid in the adrenal glands is drawn upon when the gland is stimulated. This use of ascorbic acid during adrenal stimulation suggests an increased need for ascorbic acid during stress. More ascorbic acid is present in a child's actively growing tissues than in adult tissues. Other enzymes that require ascorbic acid perform very diverse functions, including the following: (1) the conversion of the neurotransmitter dopamine to the neurotransmitter norepinephrine; (2) the synthesis of carnitine, a mitochondrial fatty acid transporter that is involved in extracting energy from fatty acids; (3) the oxidation of phenylalanine and tyrosine; (4) the metabolism of tryptophan and folate; and (5) the maturation of some bioactive neural and endocrine peptides. Furthermore, ascorbic acid helps the body to absorb nonheme iron by keeping it in its bioactive reduced ferrous form (Fe^{2+}), thereby making it available for hemoglobin production and helping to prevent iron-deficiency anemia.

CLINICAL APPLICATIONS

ASCORBIC ACID NEEDS IN SMOKERS

Free radicals are reactive molecules that can disrupt the normal structure of DNA, proteins, carbohydrates, and fatty acids. Such damage is linked to an increased risk of cancer and cardiovascular disease. Cigarette smoke is one environmental source of free radicals. The body fights these free radicals with antioxidants such as vitamins A, E, and C and minerals such as selenium and zinc. Antioxidants neutralize free radicals and work to protect the body from free radical damage.

As free radical production increases, antioxidant needs also increase. Cigarette smokers deplete their supply of ascorbic acid more rapidly than nonsmokers because of increased exposure to free radicals. The vitamin is needed to break down the toxic compounds found in cigarette smoke. Therefore, it is recommended that cigarette smokers consume an additional 35 mg of vitamin C per day to meet these increased needs; it is also recommended that they stop smoking.

Antioxidant Function

Similar to vitamin E in function, ascorbic acid is an antioxidant that works to protect the body from damage caused by free radicals. Free radicals lead to oxidative stress, which is associated with increased risks of inflammatory diseases, Alzheimer's disease, cancer, and heart disease.

Requirements

The DRI guidelines for ascorbic acid sets an RDA of 75 mg/day for women and 90 mg/day for men, with increases for women during pregnancy and lactation.[10] Because cigarette smoke increases oxidative stress and free radicals in body tissues, the DRI committee recommends an additional 35 mg/day for smokers (see the Clinical Applications box, "Ascorbic Acid Needs in Smokers").

Deficiency Disease

Signs of ascorbic acid deficiency include tissue bleeding (e.g., easy bruising, pinpoint skin hemorrhages), bone and joint bleeding, susceptibility to bone fracture, poor wound healing, and soft bleeding gums with loosened teeth. Extreme deficiency results in the disease scurvy.

Toxicity Symptoms

The UL for ascorbic acid is 2000 mg/day. Although most excessive intakes of water-soluble vitamins are efficiently excreted in the urine, levels of more than 2000 mg/day are cleared less efficiently and may result in gastrointestinal disturbances and osmotic diarrhea. The supplemental intake of vitamin C at 1000 mg/day is associated with increased oxalate stone (i.e., kidney stone) formation.[14] The Institute of Medicine states that further research into

the toxic effects of ascorbic acid is warranted because of the popularity of high intake of the vitamin in the United States.[10]

Food Sources

The best food sources of ascorbic acid include citrus fruits, red bell peppers, and kiwis (Figure 7-4). Additional good sources include tomatoes, cabbage, berries, melons, green peppers, broccoli, potatoes, and other green and yellow vegetables (Table 7-6).

Stability

Ascorbic acid is readily oxidized upon exposure to air and heat. Therefore, care must be taken when handling its food sources. Ascorbic acid is not stable in alkaline mediums; thus, baking soda, which often is added to foods to preserve color, destroys the ascorbic acid content. Acidic fruits and vegetables retain their ascorbic acid content better than nonacidic foods, and the vitamin is also highly soluble in water. The more water added for cooking, the more ascorbic acid leaches out of the fruit or vegetable into the cooking water.

THIAMIN (VITAMIN B$_1$)

The name of the vitamin *thiamin* comes from the presence of the thiazole ring in its structure.

---

thiamin the chemical name of vitamin B$_1$; this vitamin was discovered in relation to the classic deficiency disease beriberi, and it is important in body metabolism as a coenzyme factor in many cell reactions related to energy metabolism.

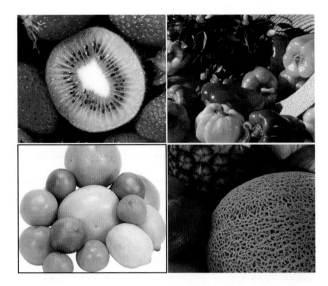

Figure 7-4 Foods that are high in Vitamin C. (Copyright JupiterImages Corp.)

TABLE 7-6 **FOOD SOURCES OF VITAMIN C**

Item	Quantity	Amount (mg)
Vegetables		
Green pepper, raw	½ cup, chopped	60
Peppers, hot chili, red, raw	½ cup, chopped	108
Red pepper, sweet, raw	½ cup, chopped	95
Fruits, Raw		
Kiwi	1 medium	70.5
Lemon juice, fresh	8 fl oz	112
Orange juice, fresh	8 fl oz	124
Orange, navel	1 medium	80
Papaya	½ medium	94
Strawberries	½ cup	49

Data from the U.S. Department of Agriculture, Agricultural Research Service: Nutrient Data Laboratory. *USDA nutrient database for standard reference* (website): www.ars.usda.gov/ba/bhnrc/ndl. Accessed October 2010.

Functions

Thiamin is a component of the coenzyme thiamin pyrophosphate, which is involved in several metabolic reactions that ultimately provide the body with energy in the form of adenosine triphosphate. Thiamin is especially necessary for the healthy function of systems that are in constant action and in need of energy, such as the gastrointestinal tract, the nervous system, and the cardiovascular system.

Requirements

The dietary requirement for thiamin is directly related to its function in energy and carbohydrate metabolism. For healthy people, the RDAs are based on average energy needs: 1.2 mg/day for men and 1.1 mg/day for women; children require less. For infants up to the age of 12 months, no RDA exists; the AI is 0.2 to 0.3 mg/day.[15] Increased thiamin intake is needed during pregnancy and lactation as well as during the treatment of infectious diseases and alcoholism.

Deficiency Disease

The gastrointestinal tract relies on glucose for muscular energy. Therefore, a lack of dietary thiamin may result in poor appetite, indigestion, and constipation. The central nervous system also depends on glucose for constant energy. Without sufficient thiamin, alertness and reflexes decrease, and apathy, fatigue, and irritability result. If the thiamin deficit continues, nerve irritation, pain, and prickly or numbing sensations may eventually progress to paralysis.

Chronic thiamin deficiency is known as beriberi; this paralyzing disease was especially prevalent in Asian countries that relied heavily on polished white rice as a food staple. The name describes the disease well; it is Singhalese for "I can't, I can't," because afflicted people were too ill to do anything. In industrialized societies, thiamin deficiency is largely associated with chronic alcoholism and poor diet. Alcohol inhibits the absorption of thiamin. Alcohol-induced thiamin deficiency causes a debilitating brain disorder known as *Wernicke's encephalopathy,* which affects mental alertness, short-term memory, and muscle coordination.

Toxicity Symptoms

The kidneys clear excess thiamin; therefore, there is no evidence of toxicity from oral intake, and no UL exists.

Food Sources

Although thiamin is widespread in most plant and animal tissues, the amount is usually small. Thus, thiamin deficiency is a distinct possibility when food

beriberi a disease of the peripheral nerves that is caused by a deficiency of thiamin (vitamin B₁) and is characterized by pain (neuritis) and paralysis of legs and arms, cardiovascular changes, and edema.

intake is markedly curtailed (e.g., with alcoholism or highly inadequate diets). Good food sources of thiamin include wheat germ, lean pork, beef, liver, whole or enriched grains (e.g., flour, bread, cereals), and legumes (Table 7-7). Eggs, fish, and a few vegetables are also fair sources. Some raw fish contain a thiamin-degrading enzyme (i.e., thiaminase) and consequently are not good sources.

Stability

Thiamin is a fairly stable vitamin, but it is destroyed by alkalis and prolonged exposure to high cooking temperatures. As with other water-soluble vitamins, prepared dishes retain more thiamin when their cooking water is used in the dish during preparation rather than discarded.

RIBOFLAVIN (VITAMIN B₂)

The name *riboflavin* comes from the vitamin's chemical nature. It is a yellow-green fluorescent pigment that contains ribose, which is a monosaccharide.

Functions

Riboflavin is active in its coenzyme forms: flavin adenine dinucleotide and flavin mononucleotide. These two flavin coenzymes are required for macronutrient metabolism

to produce adenosine triphosphate via the Krebs cycle and the electron transport chain. Flavoproteins are involved in a number of other metabolic reactions as well. Some examples of riboflavin-dependent reactions include converting tryptophan to niacin, converting retinal to retinoic acid, and synthesizing the active form of folate.

Requirements

Riboflavin needs are related to total energy requirements for age, level of exercise, body size, metabolic rate, and rate of growth. The RDA for adults who are 18 years old and older is 1.3 mg/day and 1.1 mg/day for men and women, respectively. The RDA is higher for women during pregnancy (1.4 mg/day) and lactation (1.6 mg/day). An AI of 0.3 to 0.4 mg/day has been established for infants who are up to 12 months old.[15]

Deficiency Disease

Areas of the body with rapid cell regeneration are most affected by riboflavin deficiency. Signs of riboflavin deficiency include cracked lips and mouth corners; a swollen, red tongue; burning, itching, or tearing eyes caused by extra blood vessels in the cornea; and a scaly, greasy dermatitis in the skin folds. Riboflavin deficiency usually occurs with other B vitamin and nutrient deficiencies (e.g., protein malnutrition) rather than by itself. No specific riboflavin deficiency disease is comparable to beriberi. A rare riboflavin deficiency condition has been given the general name *ariboflavinosis*. Its symptoms are tissue inflammation and breakdown and poor wound healing; even minor injuries become easily aggravated and do not heal well.

TABLE 7-7 FOOD SOURCES OF THIAMIN

Item	Quantity	Amount (mg)
Bread, Cereal, Rice, and Pasta		
Bran flakes cereal	1 cup	0.5
Complete, Kellogg's cereal	1 cup	2.08
Product 19, Kellogg's cereal	1 cup	1.5
Quaker Oat Life, Kellogg's cereal	1 cup	0.54
Total Whole Grain, General Mills cereal	1 cup	2.0
Wheaties, General Mills cereal	1 cup	0.75
Meat, Poultry, Fish, Dry Beans, Eggs, and Nuts		
Ham, sliced, regular (11% fat)	3 oz	0.53
Pork loin, lean, boneless, roasted	3 oz	0.75

Data from the U.S. Department of Agriculture, Agricultural Research Service: Nutrient Data Laboratory. *USDA nutrient database for standard reference* (website): www.ars.usda.gov/ba/bhnrc/ndl. Accessed October 2010.

enriched a word that is used to describe foods to which vitamins and minerals have been added back to a food after a refining process that caused a loss of some nutrients; for example, iron may be lost during the refining process of a grain, so the final product will be enriched with additional iron.

riboflavin the chemical name for vitamin B₂; this vitamin was discovered in relation to an early vitamin deficiency syndrome called *ariboflavinosis* that is mainly evidenced in the breakdown of skin tissues and resulting infections; it also has a role as a coenzyme factor in many cell reactions related to energy and protein metabolism.

Toxicity Symptoms

No adverse effects of riboflavin intake from food or supplements have been reported. Thus, there is no UL for riboflavin.

Food Sources

The most important food source of riboflavin is milk. Each serving of milk and milk products contains 0.3 to 0.5 mg of riboflavin. Other good sources include enriched grains and animal protein sources such as meats (especially beef liver), poultry, and fish. Vegetables such as mushrooms, spinach, and avocados are good natural sources. Table 7-8 provides a summary of riboflavin food sources.

Stability

Riboflavin is destroyed by light; therefore, milk is usually sold and stored in plastic or cardboard cartons instead of glass containers to preserve the vitamin.

NIACIN (VITAMIN B₃)

Functions

Niacin is part of two coenzymes. The role of one of the niacin-containing coenzymes (nicotinamide adenine dinucleotide) is the metabolism of the macronutrients (similar to the coenzymes that contain riboflavin and thiamin). The other niacin-containing coenzyme

TABLE 7-8 FOOD SOURCES OF RIBOFLAVIN

Item	Quantity	Amount (mg)
Bread, Cereal, Rice, and Pasta		
Bran flakes cereal	1 cup	0.57
Complete, Kellogg's cereal	1 cup	2.28
Product 19, Kellogg's cereal	1 cup	1.7
Total Whole Grain, General Mills cereal	1 cup	2.26
Wheaties, General Mills cereal	1 cup	0.85
Meat, Poultry, Fish, Dry Beans, Eggs, and Nuts		
Beef liver, fried	3 oz	2.9
Chicken liver, simmered	3 oz	1.7
Milk and Dairy Products		
Buttermilk, reduced fat	8 fl oz	0.51
Milk, skim or whole	8 fl oz	0.45
Yogurt, low fat	8 fl oz	0.52

Data from the U.S. Department of Agriculture, Agricultural Research Service: Nutrient Data Laboratory. *USDA nutrient database for standard reference* (website): www.ars.usda.gov/ba/bhnrc/ndl. Accessed October 2010.

(nicotinamide adenine dinucleotide phosphate) is involved in DNA repair and steroid hormone synthesis.

Requirements

Factors such as age, growth, pregnancy and lactation, illness, tissue trauma, body size, and physical activity—all of which affect energy needs—influence niacin requirements. Because the body can make some of its needed niacin from the essential amino acid tryptophan, the total niacin requirement is stated in terms of niacin equivalents (NE) to account for both sources. Approximately 60 mg of tryptophan can yield 1 mg of niacin; thus, 60 mg of tryptophan equals 1 NE. The DRI guidelines include an RDA for adults who are 14 years old and older of 16 mg NE/day for men and 14 mg NE/day for women. The RDA is higher during pregnancy (18 mg NE/day) and lactation (17 mg NE/day). No RDA has been determined for infants who are up to 12 months old, but the AI is 2 to 4 mg NE/day.[15]

Deficiency Disease

Symptoms of general niacin deficiency are weakness, poor appetite, indigestion, and various disorders of the skin and nervous system. Skin areas that are exposed to sunlight develop a dark, scaly dermatitis. Extended deficiency may result in central nervous system damage with resulting confusion, apathy, disorientation, and neuritis. Such signs of nervous system damage are seen in patients with chronic alcoholism. The deficiency disease that is associated with niacin is pellagra, which is characterized by the "four Ds": *d*ermatitis, *d*iarrhea, *d*ementia, and *d*eath (Figure 7-5). When therapeutic doses of niacin are given, pellagra symptoms improve. Pellagra was common in the United States and parts of Europe during the early twentieth century in regions where corn (which is low in niacin) was the staple food. Between 1900 and 1940 alone, more than 100,000 people living in the southern United States were estimated to have died as a result of pellagra.[16]

niacin the chemical name for vitamin B₃; this vitamin was discovered in relation to the deficiency disease pellagra, which is largely a skin disorder; it is important as a coenzyme factor in many cell reactions related to energy and protein metabolism.

pellagra the deficiency disease caused by a lack of dietary niacin and an inadequate amount of protein that contains the amino acid tryptophan, which is a precursor of niacin; pellagra is characterized by skin lesions that are aggravated by sunlight as well as by gastrointestinal, mucosal, neurologic, and mental symptoms.

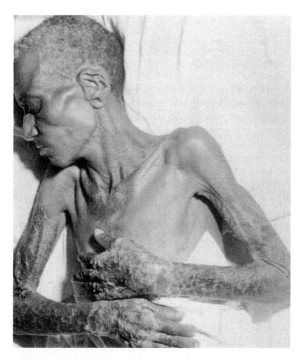

Figure 7-5 Pellagra, which results from a niacin deficiency. (Reprinted from McLaren DS. *A colour atlas and text of diet-related disorders.* 2nd ed. London: Mosby–Year Book; 1992.)

TABLE 7-9 FOOD SOURCES OF NIACIN

Item	Quantity	Amount (mg of Niacin Equivalents)
Bread, Cereal, Rice, and Pasta		
Bran flakes cereal	1 cup	6.7
Complete, Kellogg's cereal	1 cup	26.7
Mueslix Fine Grain, Kellogg's cereal	⅔ cup	5.5
Product 19, Kellogg's cereal	1 cup	20.0
Quaker Oat Life, Kellogg's cereal	1 cup	7.32
Total Whole Grain, General Mills cereal	1 cup	26.6
Wheaties, General Mills cereal	1 cup	9.9
Meat, Poultry, Fish, Dry Beans, Eggs, and Nuts*		
Beef liver, fried	3 oz	14.9
Chicken, white meat, boneless, roasted	3 oz	10.6
Chicken liver, simmered	3 oz	9.4
Mackerel, baked	3 oz	5.8
Salmon, cooked, dry heat	3 oz	7.25
Sirloin steak, lean, broiled	3 oz	6.64
Swordfish, cooked, dry heat	3 oz	10.0

*The amino acid tryptophan can be converted into niacin. Therefore, foods that are high in tryptophan also are significant sources of niacin.
Data from the U.S. Department of Agriculture, Agricultural Research Service: Nutrient Data Laboratory. *USDA nutrient database for standard reference* (website): www.ars.usda.gov/ba/bhnrc/ndl. Accessed October 2010.

Toxicity Symptoms

Excessive niacin intake can produce adverse physical effects, unlike high intakes of thiamin and riboflavin. The UL is 35 mg/day, which is based on the skin flushing that is caused by high supplemental intakes.[15] Although no evidence exists of adverse effects from consuming niacin that naturally occurs in foods, evidence does exist of excessive niacin consumption and adverse effects from nonprescription vitamin supplements and niacin-containing prescription medications. The primary reaction is a reddened flush on the skin of the face, arms, and chest that is accompanied by burning, tingling, and itching. This reaction also occurs in many patients who are therapeutically treated with niacin (see the Clinical Applications box, "Niacin as a Treatment for High Cholesterol").

Food Sources

Meat is a good source of niacin. Most dietary niacin in the United States comes from meat, poultry, fish, or enriched grain products. In addition, enriched and whole-grain breads and bread products and fortified ready-to-eat cereals have ample levels of niacin. Other good sources of niacin include legumes (e.g., peanuts, dried beans, peas). Table 7-9 gives the food sources of niacin.

Stability

Niacin is stable in acidic mediums and in heat, but it is lost in cooking water unless the water is retained and consumed (e.g., in soup).

VITAMIN B₆

The name *pyridoxine* comes from the pyridine ring in the structure of this vitamin. The term *vitamin B₆* collectively refers to a group of six related compounds: pyridoxine, pyridoxal, pyridoxamine, and their respective activated phosphate forms. Two of the phosphorylated compounds are the coenzymes pyridoxal 5′-phosphate and pyridoxamine 5′-phosphate.

---

pyridoxine the chemical name of vitamin B₆; in its activated phosphate form (i.e., B_2PO_4), pyridoxine functions as an important coenzyme factor in many reactions in cell metabolism that are related to amino acids, glucose, and fatty acids.

CLINICAL APPLICATIONS

NIACIN AS A TREATMENT FOR HIGH CHOLESTEROL

In addition to the many other important functions of niacin, improved blood lipid profiles are seen at supplemental doses of 1500 mg/day. At high doses, niacin decreases low-density lipoprotein cholesterol and triglyceride levels, both of which are linked with cardiovascular disease. In addition, pharmacologic doses of niacin improve high-density lipoprotein cholesterol levels; this is the "good" cholesterol. When niacin is used in this sense, it is functioning more as a drug than as a vitamin, and it should be used *only* under medical supervision. Niacin that is used in combination with other hypolipidemic agents is a common therapy regime, and it is more effective than medications that are used only to lower low-density lipoprotein cholesterol.[1]

To understand the potentially beneficial role of niacin at pharmacologic dosing, the potential side effects must also be understood. The Recommended Dietary Allowance for niacin in adult men and women is 16 mg/day and 14 mg/day, respectively. The Tolerable Upper Intake Level for niacin is 35 mg/day. Therefore, a long-term dose of 1500 mg/day has serious side effects. Adverse effects from pharmacologic dosing are the same as the toxicity effects: flushing of the skin, tingling sensation in the extremities, nausea, and vomiting. Some individuals may even experience liver damage if long-term use is continued unsupervised for months or years at a time.

1. Brooks EL, Kuvin JT, Karas RH. Niacin's role in the statin era. *Expert Opin Pharmacother* 2010;11(14):2291-3300.

Functions

Pyridoxal 5′-phosphate, which is the metabolically active form of vitamin B_6, has an essential role in protein metabolism and in many cell reactions that involve amino acids. It is involved in neurotransmitter synthesis and thus, in brain and central nervous system activity. Unlike most water-soluble vitamins, vitamin B_6 is stored in tissues throughout the body, particularly muscle. It participates in amino acid absorption, energy production, the synthesis of the heme portion of hemoglobin, and niacin formation from tryptophan. Enzymes that make use of vitamin B_6 coenzymes are also involved in carbohydrate and fat metabolism.

Requirements

Vitamin B_6 is involved in amino acid metabolism; therefore, needs vary directly in response to protein intake. The DRI guidelines set the RDA for healthy men and women up to the age of 50 years at 1.3 mg/day. For older adults, the RDA is slightly higher at 1.7 mg/day for men and 1.5 mg/day for women. The RDA is also higher for women during pregnancy (1.9 mg/day) and lactation (2.0 mg/day). The AI for infants up to 12 months old is 0.1 to 0.3 mg/day.[15]

Deficiency Disease

A vitamin B_6 deficiency is unlikely, because much more is available in a typical diet than is required. A vitamin B_6 deficiency causes abnormal central nervous system function with hyperirritability, neuritis, and possible convulsions. Vitamin B_6 deficiency is one cause of microcytic hypochromic anemia, because it is required for heme synthesis (part of the red blood cell protein hemoglobin).

Toxicity Symptoms

High vitamin B_6 intake from food does not result in adverse effects, but large supplemental doses can cause uncoordinated movement and nerve damage. Symptoms improve when supplemental overdosing is discontinued. The UL for adults is 100 mg/day on the basis of studies that related vitamin B_6 dosage to nerve damage.[15]

Food Sources

Vitamin B_6 is widespread in foods. Good sources include grains, enriched cereals, liver and kidney, and other meats. Limited amounts are in milk, eggs, and vegetables. Table 7-10 lists food sources of vitamin B_6.

Stability

Vitamin B_6 is stable to heat but sensitive to light and alkalis.

FOLATE

The given name *folate* comes from the Latin word *folium*, meaning "leaf," because it was originally discovered in dark green leafy vegetables. In nutrition, the term *folate* refers loosely to a large class of molecules that are derived from folic acid (i.e., pteroylglutamic acid) found in plants

TABLE 7-10 FOOD SOURCES OF VITAMIN B₆ (PYRIDOXINE)

Item	Quantity	Amount (mg)
Bread, Cereal, Rice, and Pasta		
Bran flakes cereal	1 cup	0.67
Complete, Kellogg's cereal	1 cup	2.71
Mueslix Fine Grain, Kellogg's cereal	⅔ cup	2.04
Quaker Oat Life, Kellogg's cereal	1 cup	0.73
Total Whole Grain, General Mills cereal	1 cup	2.66
Vegetables		
Potato, baked, with skin	1 medium (173 g)	0.54
Meat, Poultry, Fish, Dry Beans, Eggs, and Nuts		
Beef liver, fried	3 oz	0.87
Chicken, white meat, boneless, roasted	3 oz	0.51
Chicken liver, simmered	3 oz	0.64
Sirloin steak, lean, broiled	3 oz	0.52

Data from the U.S. Department of Agriculture, Agricultural Research Service: Nutrient Data Laboratory. *USDA nutrient database for standard reference* (website): www.ars.usda.gov/ba/bhnrc/ndl. Accessed October 2010.

and animals. The most stable form of folate is folic acid, which is rarely found in food but which is the form that is usually used in vitamin supplements and fortified food products. In the body, folate is converted to and used as the coenzyme tetrahydrofolic acid (TH₄).

Functions

TH₄ participates in DNA synthesis (with the enzyme thymidylate synthetase) as well as cell division. TH₄ is involved in the synthesis of the amino acid glycine, which in turn is required for heme synthesis and thus hemoglobin synthesis.

TH₄ also participates in the reduction of blood homocysteine concentration and indirectly in gene expression (with the enzyme methionine synthase). Blood homocysteine concentrations are high in patients with cardiovascular disease, although whether this contributes to or is merely an effect of cardiovascular disease has not been determined. Nonetheless, adequate dietary folate is one of the important factors for the prevention of hyperhomocysteinemia.

Requirements

The DRI standards give a general folate RDA for both men and women 14 years old and older of 400 mcg of dietary folate equivalent (DFE) per day. DFE is used because naturally occurring food folate has a lower bioavailability than synthetic folic acid.[17] One mcg of DFE equals 1 mcg of food folate, 0.5 mcg of folic acid taken on an empty stomach, or 0.6 mcg of folic acid taken with food. As a result of the role of folate in cell division during embryogenesis, adequate prepregnancy and pregnancy intake are linked to reduced neural tube defect occurrences. Thus, the DRIs include a special recommendation that all women who are capable of becoming pregnant take 400 mcg/day of synthetic folic acid from fortified foods or supplements in addition to natural folate from a varied diet. During pregnancy, the RDA is increased to 600 mcg DFE/day to meet the elevated needs for fetal growth. A lactating mother needs 500 mcg DFE/day. For infants, the observed AI is 65 mcg DFE/day during the first 6 months and 80 mcg DFE/day from the ages of 7 to 12 months. The DRI recommendations are aimed at providing adequate safety allowances that include specific population groups that are at risk for deficiency, such as pregnant women, adolescents, and older adults.[15]

Deficiency Disease

Folate deficiency impairs DNA and RNA synthesis. Thus, rapidly dividing cells are affected quickly by folate deficiency. When red blood cells cannot divide, the result is large and immature erythrocytes (i.e., megaloblastic macrocytic anemia). If the deficiency is not corrected, symptoms may progress to poor growth in children, weakness, depression, and neuropathy. Pregnant and lactating women are particularly susceptible to diminished blood folate concentrations and anemia as a result of their higher needs.

Neural tube defects such as spina bifida and anencephaly are some of the most common birth defects in the United States; they affect approximately 1 in every 1000 pregnancies (Figure 7-6). This defect occurs within the first 28 days after conception, often before a woman realizes that she is pregnant. Although the exact causes of neural tube defects are not known, studies show that, if women had adequate stores of folic acid before

hyperhomocysteinemia the presence of high levels of homocysteine in the blood; associated with cardiovascular disease.

spina bifida a neural tube defect in which the lower end of the neural tube does not close properly and the spinal cord may protrude through the spinal column.

anencephaly a neural tube defect in which the brain does not form.

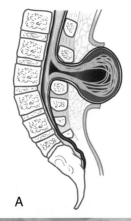

A

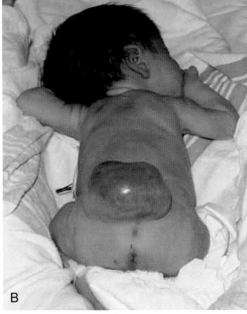

B

Figure 7-6 A, Myelomeningocele. **B,** Spina bifida in a child at birth with a cutaneous defect over the lumbar spine. (**B,** Courtesy Dr. Robert C. Dauser, Baylor College of Medicine, Houston, Texas.)

TABLE 7-11 **FOOD SOURCES OF FOLATE**

Item	Quantity	Amount (mcg DFE)
Bread, Cereal, Rice, and Pasta		
Bran flakes cereal	1 cup	221
Mueslix Fine Grain, Kellogg's cereal	⅔ cup	683
Product 19, Kellogg's cereal	1 cup	673
Quaker Oat Life, Kellogg's cereal	1 cup	553
Total Whole Grain, General Mills cereal	1 cup	901
Wheat Flakes, Kellogg's All-Bran Complete cereal	1 cup	901
Wheaties, General Mills cereal	1 cup	449
Vegetables		
Collard greens, boiled	½ cup	88
Spinach, boiled	½ cup	131
Fruits		
Orange juice, fresh	1 cup, 8 oz	74
Meat, Poultry, Fish, Dry Beans, Eggs, and Nuts		
Black beans, boiled	½ cup	128
Chicken liver, simmered	3 oz	491
Chickpeas (garbanzo beans)	½ cup	141
Kidney beans, boiled	½ cup	115

Data from the U.S. Department of Agriculture, Agricultural Research Service: Nutrient Data Laboratory. *USDA nutrient database for standard reference* (website): www.ars.usda.gov/ba/bhnrc/ndl. Accessed January 23 2012.

conception and during early gestation, approximately half of the neural tube defect cases could be prevented. Supplemental folic acid can significantly improve the folate status of women and improve pregnancy outcomes, including women with prior pregnancies that have been affected by neural tube defects.[18-20]

Toxicity Symptoms

No negative effects have been observed from the consumption of folate from foods. However, some evidence shows that excessive folic acid can mask biochemical indications of vitamin B_{12} deficiency. Prolonged B_{12} deficiency can result in permanent nerve damage; therefore, the UL for adults for supplemental folic acid (not DFE) has been set at 1000 mcg/day.[15]

Food Sources

Folate is widely distributed in foods (Table 7-11). Rich sources include green leafy vegetables, orange juice, dried beans, and chicken liver. Since January 1998, as part of an effort to reduce the occurrences of neural tube defects, the U.S. Food and Drug Administration has required all manufacturers of certain grain products (e.g., enriched white flour; white rice; corn grits; cornmeal; noodles; fortified breakfast cereals, bread, rolls, and buns) to fortify with folic acid. The fortification of the general food supply has successfully reduced the prevalence of neural tube defects in the United States by 22.9%.[21] The special DRI recommendation that women who are capable of becoming pregnant consume folic acid from supplements or fortified foods is one of only two current RDAs that specifically recommend consuming vitamin sources in addition to those available in a varied diet of natural foods. (The other supplementation recommendation concerns vitamin B_{12}.)

Stability

Folate is easily destroyed by heat, and it easily leaches into cooking water, especially when the food is submerged in the water. As much as 50% to 90% of food folate may be destroyed during food processing, storage, and preparation.

COBALAMIN (VITAMIN B_{12})

Vitamin B_{12} is the B vitamin designation for cobalamin. The name *cobalamin* was derived from cobalt, which is the trace mineral that is the single gray atom at the center of cobalamin's corrin ring. The term *vitamin B_{12}* originally referred to the synthetic pharmaceutical molecule cyanocobalamin. In nutrition, it has become a term for all cobalamin derivatives, including the two biologically active coenzyme derivatives methylcobalamin and deoxyadenosylcobalamin.

Functions

Methylcobalamin is a coenzyme that is required for the catalytic activity of two of the same enzymes as tetrahydrofolic acid: methionine synthase and serine hydroxymethyltransferase. Thus, like tetrahydrofolic acid, methylcobalamin participates in the reduction of blood homocysteine concentration and indirectly in gene expression as well as in the synthesis of the amino acid glycine, which in turn is required for heme synthesis and therefore hemoglobin synthesis. In addition, vitamin B_{12} is essential for DNA synthesis and cell division.

Deoxyadenosylcobalamin is a coenzyme for the mitochondrial enzyme methylmalonyl-coenzyme A mutase, which is involved in the metabolism of fatty acids that have an odd number of carbon atoms.

Requirements

The amount of dietary vitamin B_{12} needed for normal human metabolism is quite small, and it consists of only a few micrograms per day. A mixed diet that includes animal foods easily provides this much and more. The DRI guidelines list an RDA for men and women who are 19 years of age and older of 2.4 mcg/day. The RDA during pregnancy is 2.6 mcg/day and during lactation is 2.8 mcg/day. An observed AI during the first year is 0.4 to 0.5 mcg/

day. Evidence exists that approximately 20% of adults in industrialized countries may be deficient in cobalamin, and 60% to 70% of the cases in elderly adults are explained by poor absorption from food as opposed to inadequate intake.[22] Therefore, the DRIs include a special recommendation that both men and women who are 50 years old and older meet their RDA with vitamin-B_{12}–fortified foods or supplements.[15]

Deficiency Disease

Vitamin B_{12} deficiency usually results from malabsorption (most commonly) or inadequate intake (e.g., vegan diets). A component of the gastric digestive secretions called *intrinsic factor* is necessary for the absorption of vitamin B_{12} by intestinal cells (Figure 7-7). Gastrointestinal disorders that destroy the cells that line the stomach (e.g., atrophic gastritis) disrupt the secretion of intrinsic factor and hydrochloric acid, both of which are needed for vitamin B_{12} absorption. As mentioned previously, a significant contributor to vitamin B_{12} deficiency, especially in the elderly population, is the malabsorption of

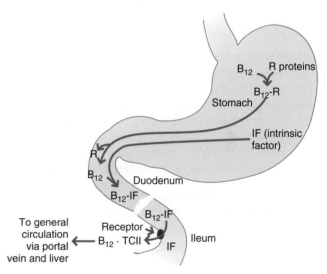

Figure 7-7 Digestion and absorption of vitamin B_{12}. (Reprinted from Mahan LK, Escott-Stump S. *Krause's food & nutrition therapy.* 12th ed. Philadelphia: Saunders; 2008.)

cobalamin the chemical name for vitamin B_{12}; this vitamin is found mainly in animal protein food sources; it is closely related to amino acid metabolism and the formation of the heme portion of hemoglobin; the absence of its necessary digestion and absorption agents in the gastric secretions, hydrochloric acid and intrinsic factor, leads to pernicious anemia and degenerative effects on the nervous system.

cobalamin in food. Other cases of vitamin B_{12} deficiency from inadequate intake have been reported in vegans (see Chapter 4); cobalamin supplements are recommended for vegans to prevent such deficiency, because their diets contain no animal foods, which are the only natural sources of vitamin B_{12}.[23]

The general symptoms of vitamin B_{12} deficiency include nonspecific symptoms such as fatigue, anorexia, and nausea. In the case of continued vitamin B_{12} deficiency, a multitude of conditions may develop, including hematologic (e.g., pernicious anemia), neurologic (e.g., myelosis funicularis), and digestive (e.g., glossitis) manifestations.[22] In such cases, vitamin B_{12} is most often administered via hypodermic injection to bypass the absorption defect.

Toxicity Symptoms

Vitamin B_{12} has not been shown to produce adverse effects in healthy individuals when intake from food or supplements exceeds body needs; therefore, no UL has been established.

Food Sources

Vitamin B_{12} is bound to protein in foods. All dietary vitamin B_{12} originates from bacteria that inhabit the gastrointestinal tracts of herbivorous animals. Thus, the only human food sources are of animal origin or come from bacteria found on unwashed plants. Human intestinal bacteria also synthesize vitamin B_{12}, but it is not bioavailable. The richest dietary sources are beef and chicken liver, lean meat, clams, oysters, herring, and crab (Table 7-12).

Stability

Vitamin B_{12} is stable throughout ordinary cooking processes.

PANTOTHENIC ACID

The name *pantothenic acid* refers to this substance's widespread functions in the body and its widespread availability in foods of all types. The name is based on the Greek word *pantothen,* meaning "from every side." Pantothenic acid is present in all living things, and it is essential to all forms of life.

Functions

Pantothenic acid is part of coenzyme A (CoA), which is a carrier of acetyl moieties or larger acyl moieties. It is involved in cellular metabolism as well as both protein acetylation and protein acylation.

Acetyl CoA is involved in energy extraction from the fuel molecules: glucose, fatty acids, and amino acids. CoA also is involved in the biosynthesis of the following: (1) sphingolipids, which are found in neural tissue; (2) some amino acids; (3) isoprenoid derivatives (e.g., cholesterol, steroid hormones, vitamins A and D); (4) δ-aminolevulinic acid, which is the precursor of the porphyrin rings in hemoglobin, the cytochromes of the electron transport chain, and the corrin ring of vitamin B_{12}; (5) the neurotransmitter acetylcholine; and (6) melatonin, which is a sleep inducer that is derived from the neurotransmitter serotonin.

Requirements

No specific RDA for pantothenic acid is given in the DRI guidelines. The usual intake range of the American diet is 4 to 7 mg/day. The DRI guidelines report an AI for people

TABLE 7-12 FOOD SOURCES OF VITAMIN B_{12} (COBALAMIN)

Item	Quantity	Amount (mcg)
Meat, Poultry, Fish, Dry Beans, Eggs, and Nuts*		
Beef liver, fried	3 oz	71
Clams, cooked, moist heat	3 oz	84
Mussels, steamed	3 oz	20
Oysters, cooked, moist heat	3 oz	25

*Several vegan-friendly meat and dairy substitute products (e.g., soy milk, tofu) are fortified with vitamin B_{12}.
Data from the U.S. Department of Agriculture, Agricultural Research Service: Nutrient Data Laboratory. *USDA nutrient database for standard reference* (website): www.ars.usda.gov/ba/bhnrc/ndl. Accessed October 2010.

pernicious anemia a form of megaloblastic anemia that is caused by destroyed gastric parietal cells that produce intrinsic factor; without intrinsic factor, vitamin B_{12} cannot be absorbed.

pantothenic acid a B-complex vitamin that is found widely distributed in nature and that occurs throughout the body tissues; it is an essential constituent of the body's main activating agent, coenzyme A; this special compound has extensive metabolic responsibility for activating a number of compounds in many tissues, and it is a key energy metabolism substance in every cell.

14 years of age and older of 5 mg/day. The AI is slightly higher during pregnancy (6 mg/day) and lactation (7 mg/day). For infants during the first year, the observed AI is 1.7 to 1.8 mg/day.[15]

Deficiency Disease

Given its widespread natural occurrence, pantothenic acid deficiencies are unlikely. The only cases of deficiency have been in individuals who are fed synthetic diets that contain virtually no pantothenic acid.

Toxicity Symptoms

No observed adverse effects have been associated with pantothenic acid intake in people or animals. Therefore, the DRI guidelines have not established an UL for this vitamin.

Food Sources

Pantothenic acid occurs as widely in foods as in body tissues. It is found in all animal and plant cells, and it is especially abundant in animal tissues, whole-grain cereals, and legumes (Table 7-13). Smaller amounts are found in milk, vegetables, and fruits.

Stability

Pantothenic acid is stable to acid and heat, but it is sensitive to alkalis.

BIOTIN

Functions

Biotin is a coenzyme for five carboxylase enzymes. Carboxylase enzymes transfer carbon dioxide moieties from one molecule to another in the following biotin enzymes:
1. *α-Acetyl-CoA carboxylase*, which is involved in fatty acid synthesis
2. *β-Acetyl-CoA carboxylase*, which is involved in inhibiting fatty acid breakdown during the hours after starch, sucrose, or fructose is consumed
3. *Pyruvate carboxylase*, which is involved in synthesizing glucose during fasting (gluconeogenesis) or during short bursts of energy (from lactic acid)
4. *Methylcrotonyl-CoA carboxylase*, which is involved in the degradation of the amino acid leucine
5. *Propionyl-CoA carboxylase*, which is involved in the breakdown of the three-carbon fatty acid propionic acid

TABLE 7-13 FOOD SOURCES OF PANTOTHENIC ACID

Item	Quantity	Amount (mg)
Bread, Cereal, Rice, and Pasta		
All-Bran cereal	1 cup	1.34
Mueslix Fine Grain, Kellogg's cereal	⅔ cup	2.53
Total Whole Grain, General Mills cereal	1 cup	13.3
Wheat Flakes, Kellogg's Complete cereal	1 cup	13.5
Vegetables		
Corn, yellow, boiled	½ cup	0.72
Portabella mushroom, grilled	1 medium (173 g)	0.65
Potato, baked, with skin	½ cup, pieces	0.97
Fruits		
Avocado, raw	¼ medium	0.70
Meat, Poultry, Fish, Dry Beans, Eggs, and Nuts		
Beef liver, fried	3 oz	5.90
Beef, ground, 70% fat, pan browned	3 oz	0.68
Chicken liver, simmered	3 oz	5.67
Egg, scrambled	1 large	0.61
Mackerel, baked	3 oz	0.84
Milk and Dairy Products		
Milk, skim	8 fl oz	0.88
Yogurt, low fat	8 fl oz	1.45

Data from the U.S. Department of Agriculture, Agricultural Research Service: Nutrient Data Laboratory. *USDA nutrient database for standard reference* (website): www.ars.usda.gov/ba/bhnrc/ndl. Accessed October 2010.

Requirements

The amount of biotin needed for metabolism is extremely small, and it is measured in micrograms. The DRI guidelines do not establish an RDA for biotin. An AI has been set on the basis of the intakes of healthy individuals. The AI for adults who are 18 years old and older is 30 mcg/day. For infants during the first 12 months, the observed AI is 5 to 6 mcg/day. The AI during pregnancy also is 30 mcg/day, and during lactation it is 35 mcg/day. The intestinal cells also absorb biotin, which is synthesized by the bacteria that normally inhabit the intestine.[15]

Deficiency Disease

Because the potency of biotin is great, despite the tiny microgram quantities present in the body, no known natural dietary deficiency occurs. Biotin is bound by avidin, a protein that is found in uncooked egg whites. Consequently, consuming raw eggs inhibits biotin absorption. Mice studies found that marginal biotin deficiency during gestation inhibited the availability of insulin-like growth factor (IGF-I), thereby resulting in malformations of the long bones.[24] Biotin deficiency may be teratogenic for humans as well. A rare inborn error of metabolism called *biotinidase deficiency* can result in neurologic disturbances if it is left untreated, but it is treatable with pharmacologic doses of biotin.[25]

Toxicity Symptoms

No toxicity or other adverse effects from the consumption of biotin by people or animals are known. No data currently support setting an UL for biotin.

Food Sources

Biotin is widely distributed in natural foods, but it is not equally absorbed from all of them. For example, the biotin in corn and soy meal is completely bioavailable (i.e., able to be digested and absorbed by the body). However, almost none of the biotin in wheat is bioavailable. The best food sources of biotin are liver, cooked egg yolk, soy flour, cereals (except bound forms in wheat), meats, tomatoes, and yeast.

Stability

Biotin is a stable vitamin, but it is water soluble. A summary of the water-soluble vitamins is given in Table 7-14.

CHOLINE

Choline is a water-soluble nutrient that is associated with the B-complex vitamins. The Institute of Medicine established choline as an essential nutrient for human nutrition in the 1998 DRIs.[15]

Functions

Choline is important for maintaining the structural integrity of cell membranes as a component of the phospholipid lecithin (i.e., phosphatidyl choline). Choline is also involved in lipid transport (i.e., lipoproteins), homocysteine reduction, and the neurotransmitter acetylcholine, which is involved in involuntary functions, voluntary movement, and long-term memory storage, among other things.

Requirements

The DRI guidelines provide an AI of 550 mg/day for men 14 years of age or older and of 425 mg/day for women 18 years of age or older. During pregnancy, the AI is 450 mg/day; during lactation, it is 550 mg/day, because an ample amount of choline is secreted into human milk. For infants, the observed AI is 125 to 150 mg/day during the first year of life.[15]

Deficiency Disease

Choline deficiency may cause liver and muscle damage. Other conditions associated with choline deficiency include neural tube defects, heart disease related to hyperhomocysteinemia, inflammation, and breast cancer. Some researchers conclude that suboptimal choline intake may be a public health concern and think that it warrants the attention of health professionals.[26]

Toxicity Symptoms

Very high doses of supplemental choline have caused lowered blood pressure, fishy body odor, sweating, excessive salivation, and reduced growth rate. The UL for adults is 3.5 g/day.[15]

Food Sources

Choline is found naturally in a wide variety of foods. Soybean products, milk, eggs, liver, and peanuts are especially rich sources of choline.

Stability

Choline is a relatively stable nutrient. It is water soluble, as are all of the B-complex vitamins.

SECTION 3 PHYTOCHEMICALS

In addition to the vitamins discussed so far in this chapter, there are other bioactive molecules called *phytochemicals* that have health benefits and that come from the plants that we eat. Phytochemicals are nonessential organic molecules. The term *phytochemical* comes from the Greek word *phyton*, meaning "plant." Scientists believe that

TABLE 7-14 SUMMARY OF VITAMIN C AND THE B-COMPLEX VITAMINS

Vitamin	Functions	Recommended Intake (Adults)	Deficiency	Tolerable Upper Intake Level (UL) and Toxicity	Sources
Vitamin C (ascorbic acid)	Antioxidant; collagen synthesis; helps prepare iron for absorption and release to tissues for red blood cell formation; metabolism	Men, 90 mg; women, 75 mg; smokers: an additional 35 mg/day	Scurvy (deficiency disease); sore gums; hemorrhages, especially around bones and joints; anemia; tendency to bruise easily; impaired wound healing and tissue formation; weakened bones	UL: 2000 mg Diarrhea	Citrus fruits, kiwi, tomatoes, melons, strawberries, dark leafy vegetables, chili peppers, cabbage, broccoli, chard, green and red peppers, potatoes
Thiamin (vitamin B₁)	Normal growth; coenzyme in carbohydrate metabolism; normal function of heart, nerves, and muscle	Men, 1.2 mg; women, 1.1 mg	Beriberi (deficiency disease); gastrointestinal: loss of appetite, gastric distress, indigestion, deficient hydrochloric acid; central nervous system: fatigue, nerve damage, paralysis; cardiovascular: heart failure, edema of the legs	UL not set; toxicity unknown	Pork, beef, liver, whole or enriched grains, legumes, wheat germ
Riboflavin	Normal growth and energy; coenzyme in protein and energy metabolism	Men, 1.3 mg; women, 1.1 mg	Ariboflavinosis; wound aggravation; cracks at the corners of the mouth; a swollen red tongue; eye irritation; skin eruptions	UL not set; toxicity unknown	Milk; meats, enriched cereals, green vegetables
Niacin (vitamin B₃, nicotinamide, nicotinic acid)	Coenzyme in energy production; normal growth; health of skin	Men, 16 mg of niacin equivalents; women: 14 mg of niacin equivalents	Pellagra (deficiency disease); weakness; loss of appetite; diarrhea; scaly dermatitis; neuritis; confusion	UL: 35 mg Skin flushing	Fortified cereals and grains
Vitamin B₆ (pyridoxine)	Coenzyme in amino acid metabolism: protein synthesis; heme formation; brain activity; carrier for amino acid absorption	Between the ages of 19 and 50 years, 1.3 mg; Men 50 years of age or older: 1.7 mg; women 50 years of age or older: 1.5 mg	Anemia; hyperirritability; convulsions; neuritis	UL: 100 mg Nerve damage	Wheat germ, legumes, meats, poultry, seafood
Folate (folic acid, folacin)	Coenzyme in DNA and RNA synthesis; amino acid metabolism; red blood cell maturation	400 mcg of dietary folate equivalents	Megaloblastic anemia (large immature red blood cells); poor growth; neural tube defects	UL: 1000 mcg Masks vitamin B₁₂ deficiency	Liver, green leafy vegetables, legumes, yeast, fortified orange juice
Cobalamin (vitamin B₁₂)	Coenzyme in synthesis of heme for hemoglobin; myelin sheath formation to protect nerves	2.4 mcg	Pernicious anemia; poor nerve function	UL not set; toxicity unknown	Liver; lean meats, fish, seafood
Pantothenic acid	Formation of coenzyme A; fat, cholesterol, protein, and heme formation	Adequate Intake 5 mg	Unlikely because of widespread distribution in most foods	UL not set; toxicity unknown	Meats, eggs, milk, whole grains, legumes, vegetables
Biotin	Coenzyme A partner; synthesis of fatty acids, amino acids, and purines	Adequate Intake 30 mcg	Natural deficiency unknown	UL not set; toxicity unknown	Liver, egg yolk, soy flour, nuts

Fortified cereals and grains

fruits, vegetables, beans, nuts, and whole grains provide thousands of phytochemicals, many of which have yet to be identified.

What prompted researchers to investigate phytochemicals were the health differences seen in people who were eating whole fruits and vegetables compared with people who were eating mostly refined foods and taking vitamin and mineral supplements. Those individuals who were obtaining their essential nutrients from a diet rich in plant foods benefited far more than those who did not.

FUNCTION

Phytochemicals have a wide variety of functions, some of which include antioxidant activity, hormonal actions, interactions with enzymes and DNA replication, and antibacterial effects. Studies show that diets that are high in phytochemicals protect against cardiovascular disease, counteract inflammatory compounds, help to prevent cancer, and increase antioxidant status.[27] The beneficial effects of phytochemicals are thought to result from the synergistic actions of multiple constituents as opposed to the actions of isolated compounds.[28]

RECOMMENDED INTAKE

There are no established DRIs for phytochemicals. Phytochemicals give fruits and vegetables their specific colors; thus, consuming a colorful variety of fruits, vegetables, whole grains, and nuts will provide a rich supply of phytochemicals. The Centers for Disease Control and Prevention (CDC) recommends consuming a combined total of five to nine servings of fruits and vegetables daily. At www.fruitsandveggiesmatter.gov, the CDC provides recommendations for the number of cups of fruits and vegetables that a person should consume daily on the basis of age, gender, and activity level. One cup of raw or cooked vegetables or vegetable juice or 2 cups of raw leafy greens are equivalent to 1 cup from the vegetable group. One cup of fruit or 100% fruit juice or half a cup of dried fruit is equivalent to 1 cup from the fruit group.[29]

This recommendation is based on the finding that consuming 400 to 600 g/day of fruits and vegetables reduces the risk of developing some forms of cancer. Current reports from the Economic Research Service of the U.S. Department of Agriculture show that the average American consumes much less than the recommendations: 0.8 servings of fruit per day and 1.7 servings of vegetables per day.[30]

FOOD SOURCES

Foods derived from animals and those that have been processed and refined are virtually devoid of phytochemicals. Phytochemicals are found in whole and unrefined foods such as vegetables, fruits, legumes, nuts, seeds, whole grains, and certain oils (e.g., olive oil).

The following is a list of seven typical fruit and vegetable colors along with the specific phytochemical (e.g., lycopene) or phytochemical class (e.g., flavonoids) that these fruits and vegetables may contain. The specified phytochemical or phytochemical class is present in fruits or vegetables of other colors, but color is one prominent indicator that a significant quantity of the specified phytochemical or phytochemical class may be present. One specific exception that is worth noting is flavonoids. Although orange-yellow foods are good sources of flavonoids, other significant sources include purple grapes, black tea, olives, onions, celery, green tea, oregano, and whole wheat, none of which have an orange-yellow color.

- *Red* foods provide lycopene.
- *Yellow-green* foods provide zeaxanthin.
- *Red-purple* foods provide anthocyanin.
- *Orange* foods provide β-carotene.
- *Orange-yellow* foods provide flavonoids.
- *Green* foods provide glucosinolate.
- *White-green* foods provide allyl sulfides.

By consuming one fruit or vegetable from each of these seven color categories daily, individuals get a variety of phytochemicals. Thousands of other phytochemicals are also widely distributed in fruits, vegetables, grains, soybeans, legumes, and nuts.

SECTION 4 **VITAMIN SUPPLEMENTATION**

The Dietary Supplement Health and Education Act (DSHEA) of 1994 officially defined supplements as a product (other than tobacco) that has the following characteristics:

- It is intended to supplement the diet.

- It contains one or more dietary ingredients (including vitamins, minerals, herbs or other botanicals, amino acids, and other substances) or their constituents.

- It is intended to be taken by mouth as a pill, capsule, tablet, or liquid.
- And it is labeled on the front panel as being a dietary supplement.

Dietary supplements are regulated in the United States by the U.S. Food and Drug Administration. The Office of Dietary Supplements (http://ods.od.nih.gov/), which is housed within the National Institutes of Health, has the following mission: "to strengthen knowledge and understanding of dietary supplements by evaluating scientific information, stimulating and supporting research, disseminating research results, and educating the public to foster an enhanced quality of life and health for the U.S. population."[31]

The use of dietary supplements is quite common in the United States. About half of the population regularly takes a dietary supplement. The most commonly used supplement is of the multivitamin or multimineral variety. It is the position of the Academy of Nutrition and Dietetics that "… the best nutrition-based strategy for promoting optimal health and reducing the risk of chronic disease is to wisely choose a wide variety of foods. Additional nutrients from supplements can help some people meet their nutritional needs …"[32] If people ate a healthy and varied diet in accordance with the *Dietary Guidelines for Americans* and the MyPlate guidelines, adequate nutrients should be provided by whole foods. However, since only about 3% to 4% of Americans currently eat in the ways that these guidelines recommend, inadequate nutrient consumption is quite possible.[32,33] Although dietary vitamin and mineral supplements may be beneficial for bridging this gap, it is also possible to exceed the UL for certain nutrients. Of interest is that the use of dietary supplements is most common among the healthiest people rather than among those who need it the most.

RECOMMENDATIONS FOR NUTRIENT SUPPLEMENTATION

Health care professionals should be aware that people often fail to notify their health care providers about the use of dietary supplements. Drug-nutrient interactions are more common with dietary supplements than with whole foods; thus, it is important to specifically ask patients about their use of supplements. Although dietary supplements may not be necessary for everyone, there are some instances in which supplemental forms of specific nutrients are recommended on the basis of age, lifestyle, or disease state.

Life Cycle Needs

Vitamin needs fluctuate with age and with situations that occur throughout the life cycle.

Pregnancy and Lactation

The DRI guidelines explicitly establish separate recommendations for women during pregnancy and lactation that take into account the increased nutrient demands that occur during this period. To reduce the risk of neural tube defects, the DRI committee recommends that pregnant women and women who are capable of becoming pregnant increase their intake of folic acid from fortified foods and/or dietary supplements in addition to the folate that is already present in their diets. Women may find meeting the increased nutrient needs of pregnancy difficult by diet alone as a result of nutrient bioavailability, tolerances, food preferences, or other factors that can marginalize their diet (i.e., effectively decrease the nutrients that their diet provides). Supplements may then become a viable way of ensuring adequate intake to meet increased nutrient demands.

Infants, Children, and Adolescents

The American Academy of Pediatrics recommends that all breast-fed infants receive 400 IU of supplemental vitamin D daily to help prevent rickets. Infants who are not breast fed, children, and adolescents who do not consume at least 1 qt/day of vitamin-D–fortified milk or otherwise have an intake of 400 IU of vitamin D should also receive 400 IU of supplemental vitamin D daily.[7]

Older Adults

The aging process may increase the need for some vitamins because of decreased food intake and less efficient nutrient absorption, storage, and usage (see Chapter 12). The Institute of Medicine recommends that people who are 50 years of age or older take 2.4 mcg/day of supplemental vitamin B_{12}. Advancing age also decreases the ability of the skin to produce vitamin D. Thus, older adults are encouraged to consume extra vitamin D from fortified foods or dietary supplements.[32]

Lifestyle

Personal lifestyle choices also influence individual needs for nutrient supplementation.

Restricted Diets

People who habitually follow fad diets may find meeting many of the nutrient intake standards difficult, particularly if their meals provide fewer than 1200 kcal/day. Very restrictive diets are not recommended, because they may cause multiple nutrient deficiencies. A wise weight-reduction program should meet all nutrient needs. People who are following strict vegan diets need supplemental vitamin B_{12} in fortified foods or dietary supplements, because the only natural food sources of this vitamin are of animal origin.

Smoking

Smoking cigarettes adversely affects health in many ways, including reducing the body's vitamin C pool. Research shows that smokers have significantly less serum vitamin C than nonsmokers.[34] The Institute of Medicine sets the RDA of vitamin C at 35 mg/day higher for smokers to compensate for the oxidative stress that is induced by smoking. The additional vitamin C does not necessarily need to come from a dietary supplement; however, if the person chooses to not quit smoking or to not consume additional vitamin-C–rich foods, a dietary supplement may be advisable.

Alcohol

The chronic or abusive use of alcohol can interfere with the absorption of B-complex vitamins, especially thiamin, folate, and vitamin B_6. Multivitamin supplements that are rich in B vitamins may partially mitigate the effects. However, decreased alcohol use must accompany this nutrition therapy to rectify the alcohol-induced deficiency.

Disease

Evidence does not support the use of multivitamin and multimineral dietary supplements to prevent chronic disease. However, for patients with certain diseases, dietary supplements may be warranted to help combat specific nutrient deficiencies. In states of disease, malnutrition, malabsorption, debilitation, or hypermetabolic demand, each patient requires careful nutrition assessment. Nutrition support, including therapeutic supplementation as indicated, is part of the total medical therapy. A dietitian plans dietary and supplemental therapy to meet the patient's clinical requirements.

MEGADOSES

At high pharmacologic concentrations, vitamins no longer operate strictly as nutritional agents. Nutrients and drugs can do the following: (1) participate in or improve physiologic conditions or illnesses; (2) prevent diseases; or (3) relieve symptoms. However, many people are ignorant of the similarities between drugs and vitamins. Most people realize that too much of any drug can be harmful or even fatal and take care to avoid overdosing. However, too many people do not apply this same logic to nutrients and only realize the dangers of vitamin megadoses when they experience toxic side effects.

The liver can store large amounts of fat-soluble vitamins, especially vitamin A. Therefore, the potential toxicity of fat-soluble vitamin megadoses, including liver and brain damage in extreme cases, is well known.[35-37] Megadoses of one vitamin can also produce toxic effects and lead to a secondary deficiency of another nutrient. Hyperphysiologic levels of one vitamin may increase the need for other nutrients with which it works in the body, thereby effectively inducing a deficiency. Deficiencies can also occur when a person suddenly stops overdosing, which is known as a *rebound effect*. For example, infants who are born to mothers who took ascorbic acid megadoses during pregnancy may develop rebound scurvy after birth, when their high doses of ascorbic acid are cut off.

SUPPLEMENTATION PRINCIPLES

The following basic principles may help to guide nutrient supplementation decisions:

- *Read the labels carefully.* The Nutrition Labeling and Education Act of 1990 standardized and defined label terminology on food products in an effort to ensure that health claims on food packaging are clear and truthful. Consumers can make better-informed decisions knowing that a product's ingredients, toxicity levels, potential side effects, and health claims are based on significant scientific evidence.
- *Vitamins, like drugs, can be harmful in large amounts.* The only time that larger vitamin doses may be helpful is when severe deficiency exists or when nutrient absorption or metabolism is inefficient.
- *Professionally determined individual needs govern specific supplement usage.* Each person's need should be the basis for supplementing nutrients. This prevents excessive intake, which may have a cumulative effect over time.
- *All nutrients work together to promote good health.* Consuming large amounts of one vitamin often induces deficiencies of other vitamins or nutrients.
- *Food is the best source of nutrients.* Most foods are the best "package deals" in nutrition. Foods provide a wide variety of nutrients in every bite as compared with the dozen or so that are found in a vitamin bottle. In addition, by itself, a vitamin can do nothing. It is catalytic, so it must have a substrate (i.e., carbohydrate, protein, fat, or their metabolites) on which to work. With the careful selection of a wide variety

of foods and with good storage techniques, meal planning, and preparation techniques, most people can obtain ample amounts of essential nutrients from their diets (see the Cultural Considerations box, "The American Diet"). Furthermore, the evidence still overwhelmingly supports whole foods as the superior vehicles for delivering nutrients to the body.

■ *Evaluate the information.* The Further Reading and Resources section at the end of the chapter provides a list of reliable organizations and resources related to dietary supplements.

CULTURAL CONSIDERATIONS

THE AMERICAN DIET

By consuming the recommended servings from each food group in accordance with the MyPlate guidelines, an individual's vitamin and mineral needs should be met. However, the average American does not consume the recommended servings per day of key vitamin-rich foods such as fruits and vegetables. Note that, in the map below, no state reported more than 20.1% of its adult population to be consuming the recommended minimum number of servings of fruits and vegetables per day.

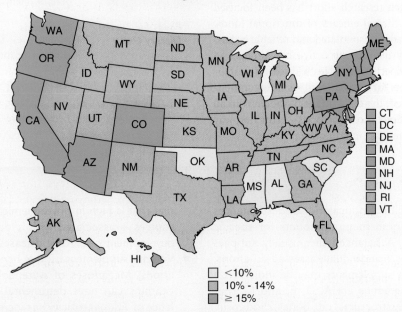

State Indicator Report on Fruits and Vegetables, 2009

Behavioral Indicators
Adult Fruit and Vegetable Consumption Maps

☐ <10%
☐ 10% - 14%
☐ ≥ 15%

Range (8.8% to 20.1%)

Instead, studies show that the average American overconsumes "nutrient-empty" foods such as fats and sugars. The average daily MyPlate equivalents consumed in the United States for each food group are as follows[1]:

■ Flour and cereal products   7.7 servings per day
■ Vegetables   1.7 servings per day
■ Fruit   0.8 servings per day
■ Dairy   1.7 servings per day
■ Meat, eggs, and nuts   6.6 servings per day
■ Added fats and oils   71.2 servings per day
■ Added sugars   28.7 servings per day

How do you measure up? What about your family and friends? The prevention of deficiency or any diseases associated with nutrient deficiency is always better than treatment.

(Data from Centers for Disease Control and Prevention. *State indicator report on fruits and vegetables,* 2009 (website): www. fruitsandveggiesmatter.gov/health_professionals/maps_adults.html. Accessed October 12 2010.)
1. U.S. Department of Agriculture Economic Research Service. *Average daily per capita MyPyramid equivalents from the U.S. food availability* (website): www.ers.usda.gov/Data/FoodConsumption/FoodGuideSpreadsheets.htm#servings. Accessed October 12 2010.

FUNCTIONAL FOODS

The term *functional food* technically has no legal definition or meaning. Generally, "functional foods" include any foods or food ingredients that may provide a health benefit beyond their basic nutritional value. Such foods are also referred to as *nutraceuticals* or *designer foods*. The position of the Academy of Nutrition and Dietetics is that such whole foods—having been fortified, enriched, or enhanced in some way—could be beneficial when regularly consumed as part of a varied diet.[38] The regulation of functional foods is complicated by the fact that they fall under different areas of federal jurisdiction, because they include conventional foods, food additives, dietary supplements, medical foods, and foods for special dietary use. Box 7-2 gives examples of functional food categories.

Recommendations for functional food intake have not been established, because scientific evidence on which to base such recommendations is insufficient. However, over the past decade, much research effort has been focused on determining the clinical efficacy of functional foods. When efficacy is clearly substantiated and reliable assessments for accurately quantifying active constituents in foods are in place, expert committees will work to establish recommendations for intake. Until such recommendations are established, the daily intake of foods from all food groups—including functional foods—is the best way to meet macronutrient and micronutrient needs.

BOX 7-2   FUNCTIONAL FOOD CATEGORIES ALONG WITH SELECTED FOOD EXAMPLES

Functional Food Category	Selected Functional Food Examples
Conventional Foods (whole foods)	Garlic Nuts Tomatoes
Modified Foods Fortified	Calcium-fortified orange juice Iodized salt
Enriched	Folate-enriched breads
Enhanced	Energy bars, snacks, yogurts, teas, bottled water, and other functional foods that are formulated with bioactive components such as lutein, fish oils, ginkgo biloba, St. John's wort, saw palmetto, or assorted amino acids
Medical Foods	Phenylketonuria formulas that are free of phenylalanine
Foods for Special Dietary Use	Infant foods Hypoallergenic foods such as gluten-free foods and lactose-free foods Weight-loss foods

Hasler CM, Brown AC. Position of the Academy of Nutrition and Dietetics: functional foods. *J Am Diet Assoc.* 2009; 109(4):735-746.

SUMMARY

- Vitamins are organic, noncaloric food substances that are necessary in minute amounts for specific metabolic tasks. A balanced diet usually supplies sufficient vitamins. In individually assessed situations, however, vitamin supplements may be indicated.
- The fat-soluble vitamins are A, D, E, and K. They mainly affect body structures (i.e., bones, rhodopsin, cell membrane phospholipids, and blood-clotting proteins).
- The water-soluble vitamins are vitamin C (ascorbic acid), the eight B-complex vitamins (i.e., thiamin, riboflavin, niacin, pyridoxine, folate, cobalamin, pantothenic acid, and biotin), and choline. Their major metabolic tasks relate to their roles in coenzyme factors, except for vitamin C, which is a biologic reducing agent that quenches free radicals and helps with collagen synthesis.
- Phytochemicals are compounds that are found in whole and unrefined foods derived from plants. A diet that is high in phytochemicals from a variety of sources is associated with a decreased risk of the development of chronic diseases.
- Vitamin supplementation is beneficial in some situations. Megadoses of water-soluble or fat-soluble vitamins can have detrimental effects. The prevalence of vitamin toxicity has increased along with the prevalence of taking dietary supplements.
- All water-soluble vitamins—especially vitamin C—are easily oxidized, so care must be taken to minimize the exposure of food surfaces to air or other oxidizers during storage and preparation. With few exceptions, all nutrients in foods are more bioavailable and beneficial to the body than nutrients in supplements.
- Functional foods are whole foods with added nutrients, such as vitamins, minerals, herbs, fiber, protein, or essential fatty acids that are thought to have beneficial health effects.

CRITICAL THINKING QUESTIONS

1. What are vitamins? Name them, and distinguish between fat-soluble and water-soluble vitamins.
2. Describe three general functions of vitamins, and give examples of each.
3. How would you advise a friend who was taking self-prescribed vitamin supplements? Give reasons and examples to support your answer.

4. Describe four situations in which vitamin supplements should be used. Give reasons and examples in each case.
5. What are phytochemicals? How can you incorporate them into your diet?

CHAPTER CHALLENGE QUESTIONS

True-False
Write the correct statement for each statement that is false.
1. *True or False:* A coenzyme acts alone to control a number of different types of reactions.
2. *True or False:* Carotene is preformed vitamin A that is found in animal food sources.
3. *True or False:* Exposure to sunlight produces vitamin D from a cholesterol precursor in the skin.
4. *True or False:* Extra vitamin C is stored in the liver to meet the demands of tissue infection.
5. *True or False:* Vitamin D and sufficient levels of calcium and phosphorus can prevent rickets.
6. *True or False:* Good sources of vitamin K are found in green leafy vegetables such as kale and spinach.
7. *True or False:* Dietary supplements are a necessary part of healthy living for all people.

Multiple Choice
1. Vitamin A is fat soluble and formed from carotene in plant foods, or it is consumed as a fully formed vitamin in animal foods. Which of the following supplies the greatest amount of this vitamin?
   a. Cantaloupe
   b. Collards
   c. Beef liver
   d. Carrots

2. If you wanted to increase the vitamin C content of your diet, which of the following foods would you choose in larger amounts?
   a. Liver, other organ meats, and seafood
   b. Potatoes, enriched cereals, and fortified margarine
   c. Green peppers, strawberries, and oranges
   d. Milk, cheese, and eggs

3. Which of the following statements is true about the sources of vitamin K?
   a. Vitamin K is found in a wide variety of foods, so no deficiency can occur.
   b. Vitamin K is easily absorbed without assistance, so we absorb all of the nutrient that we consume into our circulatory system.
   c. Vitamin K is rarely found in foods, so a natural deficiency can occur.
   d. A large portion of the amount of vitamin K that is required for metabolic purposes is produced by our own intestinal bacteria.

4. A food with nutrients that have been added through fortification or enrichment is considered a
   a. dietary supplement.
   b. functional food.
   c. phytochemical.
   d. None of the above

5. One of the primary functions of folate is as a(n)
   a. antioxidant.
   b. coenzyme in protein and energy metabolism.
   c. CoA partner.
   d. coenzyme in DNA and RNA synthesis.

6. Beriberi is the deficiency disorder that is associated with which vitamin?
   a. Thiamin
   b. Riboflavin
   c. Niacin
   d. Pantothenic acid

7. The formation of prothrombin for normal blood-clotting purposes is a primary function of which fat-soluble vitamin?
   a. Vitamin A
   b. Vitamin D
   c. Vitamin E
   d. Vitamin K

Ⓔvolve Please refer to the Students' Resource section of this text's Evolve Web site for additional study resources.

REFERENCES

1. Wang W, Connor SL, Johnson EJ, et al. Effect of dietary lutein and zeaxanthin on plasma carotenoids and their transport in lipoproteins in age-related macular degeneration. *Am J Clin Nutr.* 2007;85(3):762-769.
2. Food and Nutrition Board, Institute of Medicine. *Dietary reference intakes for vitamin A, vitamin K, arsenic, boron, chromium, copper, iodine, iron, manganese, molybdenum, nickel, silicon, vanadium, and zinc.* Washington, DC: National Academies Press; 2001.
3. World Health Organization. *Global prevalence of vitamin A deficiency in populations at risk 1995-2005,* Geneva: World Health Organization; 2009.
4. Briefel R, Hanson C, Fo MK, et al. Feeding Infants and Toddlers Study: do vitamin and mineral supplements contribute to nutrient adequacy or excess among US infants and toddlers? *J Am Diet Assoc.* 2006;106(1 Suppl 1): S52-S65.
5. Holick MF, Chen TC. Vitamin D deficiency: a worldwide problem with health consequences. *Am J Clin Nutr.* 2008;87(4):1080S-1086S.
6. Ross AC, Manson JE, Abrams SA, et al. The 2011 Dietary Reference Intakes for Calcium and Vitamin D: what dietetics practitioners need to know. *J Am Diet Assoc.* 2011; 111(4):524-527.
7. Wagner CL, Greer FR. Prevention of rickets and vitamin D deficiency in infants, children, and adolescents. *Pediatrics.* 2008;122(5):1142-1152.
8. Ginde AA, Liu MC, Camargo Jr CA. Demographic differences and trends of vitamin D insufficiency in the US population, 1988-2004. *Arch Intern Med.* 2009;169(6): 626-632.
9. Food and Nutrition Board, Institute of Medicine. *Dietary reference intakes for calcium and vitamin D.* Washington, DC: National Academy of Sciences; 2010.
10. Food and Nutrition Board, Institute of Medicine. *Dietary reference intakes for vitamin C, vitamin E, selenium, and carotenoids.* Washington, DC: National Academies Press; 2000.
11. Engin KN. Alpha-tocopherol: looking beyond an antioxidant. *Mol Vis.* 2009;15:855-860.
12. Traber MG. Vitamin E and K interactions—a 50-year-old problem. *Nutr Rev.* 2008;66(11):624-629.
13. Bonjour JP, Guéguen L, Palacios C, et al. Minerals and vitamins in bone health: the potential value of dietary enhancement. *Br J Nutr.* 2009;101(11):1581-1596.
14. Taylor EN, Curhan GC. Determinants of 24-hour urinary oxalate excretion. *Clin J Am Soc Nephrol.* 2008;3(5):1453-1460.
15. Food and Nutrition Board, Institute of Medicine. *Dietary reference intakes for thiamin, riboflavin, niacin, vitamin B6, folate, vitamin B12, pantothenic acid, biotin, and choline,* Washington, DC: National Academies Press; 2000.
16. Marks HM: Epidemiologists explain pellagra: gender, race, and political economy in the work of Edgar Sydenstricker. *J Hist Med Allied Sci.* 2003;58(1):34-55.

17. Winkels RM, Brouwer IA, Siebelink E, et al. Bioavailability of food folates is 80% of that of folic acid. *Am J Clin Nutr.* 2007;85(2):465-473.
18. Wilson RD, Johnson JA, Wyatt P, et al; Genetics Committee of the Society of Obstetricians and Gynaecologists of Canada and The Motherrisk Program. Pre-conceptional vitamin/folic acid supplementation 2007: the use of folic acid in combination with a multivitamin supplement for the prevention of neural tube defects and other congenital anomalies. *J Obstet Gynaecol Can.* 2007;29(12): 1003-1026.
19. Wolff T, Wiktop CT, Miller T, et al. Folic acid supplementation for the prevention of neural tube defects: an update of the evidence for the U.S. Preventive services task force. *Ann Intern Med.* 2009;150(9):632-639.
20. Grosse SD, Collins JS. Folic acid supplementation and neural tube defect recurrence prevention. *Birth Defects Res A Clin Mol Teratol.* 2007;79(11):737-742.
21. Centers for Disease Control and Prevention. Racial/ethnic differences in the birth prevalence of spina bifida—United States, 1995-2005. *MMWR Morb Mortal Wkly Rep.* 2009; 57(53):1409-1413.
22. Dali-Youcef N, Andres E. An update on cobalamin deficiency in adults. *QJM.* 2009;102(1):17-28.
23. Elmadfa I, Singer I. Vitamin B-12 and homocysteine status among vegetarians: a global perspective. *Am J Clin Nutr.* 2009;89(5):1693S-1698S.
24. Báez-Saldaña A, Gutiérrez-Ospina G, Chimal-Monroy J, et al. Biotin deficiency in mice is associated with decreased serum availability of insulin-like growth factor-I. *Eur J Nutr.* 2009;48(3):137-144.
25. Wolf B. Clinical issues and frequent questions about biotinidase deficiency. *Mol Genet Metab.* 2010;100(1):6-13.
26. Zeisel SH, da Costa KA. Choline: an essential nutrient for public health. *Nutr Rev.* 2009;67(11):615-623.
27. Heber D. Vegetables, fruits and phytoestrogens in the prevention of diseases. *J Postgrad Med.* 2004;50(2):145-149.
28. de Kok TM, van Breda SG, Manson MM. Mechanisms of combined action of different chemopreventive dietary compounds: a review. *Eur J Nutr.* 2008;47(Suppl 2):51-59.
29. Centers for Disease Control and Prevention. *What counts as a cup?* (website): www.fruitsandveggiesmatter.gov/what/index.html. Accessed October 12 2010.
30. U.S. Department of Agriculture Economic Research Service. *Average daily per capita MyPyramid equivalents from the U.S. food availability* (website): http://www.ers.usda.gov/Data/FoodConsumption/FoodGuide Spreadsheets.htm#servings. Accessed October 12 2010.
31. Office of Dietary Supplements. *Mission statement* (website): ods.od.nih.gov/About/about_ods.aspx. Accessed October 12 2010.
32. Marra MV, Boyar AP. Position of the academy of nutrition of dietetics: nutrient supplementation. *J Am Diet Assoc.* 2009;109(12):2073-2085.
33. King JC. An evidence-based approach for establishing dietary guidelines. *J Nutr.* 2007;137(2):480-483.
34. Schleicher RL, Carroll MD, Ford ES, Lacher DA. Serum vitamin C and the prevalence of vitamin C deficiency in the United States: 2003-2004 National Health and Nutrition Examination Survey (NHANES). *Am J Clin Nutr.* 2009; 90(5):1252-1263.

35. Ramanathan VS, Hensley G, French S, et al. Hypervitaminosis A inducing intra-hepatic cholestasis—a rare case report. *Exp Mol Pathol.* 2010;88(2):324-325.

36. Castano G, Etchart C, Sookoian S. Vitamin A toxicity in a physical culturist patient: a case report and review of the literature. *Ann Hepatol.* 2006;5(4):293-395.

37. Sheth A, Khurana R, Khurana V. Potential liver damage associated with over-the-counter vitamin supplements. *J Am Diet Assoc.* 2008;108(9):1536-1537.

38. Hasler CM, Brown AC. Position of the academy of nutrition of dietetics: functional foods. *J Am Diet Assoc.* 2009; 109(4):735-746.

FURTHER READING AND RESOURCES

For more information about the role of folic acid with regard to neural tube defects, see the following Web sites:

Centers for Disease Control and Prevention. www.cdc.gov/ncbddd/folicacid/index.html

Spina Bifida Association of America. www.sbaa.org

The following organizations and articles provide current information and guidelines regarding dietary recommendations for nutrient consumption:

Center for Science in the Public Interest. www.cspinet.org

Centers for Disease Control and Prevention, Fruit and Veggies Matter. www.fruitsandveggiesmatter.gov

Holick MF, Chen TC. Vitamin D deficiency: a worldwide problem with health consequences. *Am J Clin Nutr.* 2008;87(4):1080S-1086S.

Marra MV, Boyar AP. Position of the academy of nutrition of dietetics: nutrient supplementation. *J Am Diet Assoc.* 2009;109(12):2073-2085.

CHAPTER **8**

Minerals

KEY CONCEPTS

- The human body requires a variety of minerals to perform its numerous metabolic tasks.
- A mixed diet of varied foods and adequate energy value is the best source of the minerals that are necessary for health.
- Of the total amount of minerals that a person consumes, only a relatively limited amount is available to the body.

Over the course of Earth's history, shifting oceans and plate tectonics have deposited minerals throughout its crust. These minerals move from rocks to soil to plants to animals and people. Not surprisingly, the mineral content of the human body is quite similar to that of Earth's crust.

In nutrition, we focus only on mineral elements: single atoms that are simple compared with vitamins, which are large, complex, organic compounds. However, minerals perform a wide variety of metabolic tasks that are essential to human life.

This chapter looks at minerals and shows how they differ from vitamins with regard to the variety of their tasks and in the amounts, which range from relatively large to exceedingly small, that are necessary to do those tasks.

NATURE OF BODY MINERALS

Most living matter is composed of four elements: hydrogen, carbon, nitrogen, and oxygen, which are the building blocks of life. The minerals that are necessary to human nutrition are elements widely distributed in nature. Of the 118 elements on the periodic table, 25 are essential to human life. These 25 elements, in varying amounts, perform a variety of metabolic functions.

Classes of Body Minerals

Minerals occur in varying amounts in the body. For example, a relatively large amount (approximately 2%) of our total body weight is calcium, most of which is in the bones. An adult who weighs 150 lb has approximately 3 lb of calcium in the body. Iron, on the other hand, is found in much smaller quantities. The same adult who weighs 150 lb has only approximately 0.11 oz of iron in his or her body. In both cases, the amount of each mineral is specific to its task.

The varying amounts of individual minerals in the body are the basis for classification into two main groups.

Major Minerals

The term *major* describes the amount of a mineral in the body and not its relative importance to human nutrition. Major minerals have a recommended intake of more than 100 mg/day. The seven major minerals are calcium,

---

element a single type of atom; a total of 118 elements have been identified, of which 94 occur naturally on Earth; elements cannot be broken down into smaller substances.

major minerals the group of minerals that are required by the body in amounts of more than 100 mg/day.

BOX 8-1 MAJOR MINERALS AND TRACE MINERALS IN HUMAN NUTRITION

Major Minerals*
Calcium (Ca)
Phosphorus (P)
Sodium (Na)
Potassium (K)
Chloride (Cl)
Magnesium (Mg)
Sulfur (S)

Trace Minerals
Essential[†]
Iron (Fe)
Iodine (I)
Zinc (Zn)
Selenium (Se)
Fluoride (Fl)
Copper (Cu)
Manganese (Mn)
Chromium (Cr)
Molybdenum (Mo)
Cobalt (Co)
Boron (B)
Vanadium (V)
Nickel (Ni)

Essentiality Unclear
Silicon (Si)
Tin (Sn)
Cadmium (Cd)
Arsenic (As)
Aluminum (Al)

*Required intake of more than 100 mg/day.
†Required intake of less than 100 mg/day.

phosphorus, sodium, potassium, magnesium, chloride, and sulfur. Because the body cannot make any minerals, all minerals must be consumed in the foods that we eat.

Trace Minerals

The remaining 18 elements make up the group of trace minerals. These minerals are no less important to human nutrition than the major minerals; however, smaller amounts of them are in the body. Trace minerals have a recommended intake of less than 100 mg/day. Box 8-1 provides a list of all of the minerals that are essential to human nutrition.

Functions of Minerals

These simple single elements perform a wide variety of metabolic tasks in the body. They are involved in processes of building tissue as well as activating, regulating, transmitting, and controlling metabolic processes.

For example, sodium and potassium are key players in water balance. Calcium and phosphorus are required for osteoclasts to build bone. Iron is critical to the oxygen carrier hemoglobin. Cobalt is at the active site of vitamin B_{12}. Thyroid peroxidase in thyroid cells uses iodine to make thyroid hormone, which in turn regulates the overall rate of body metabolism. Minerals are essential, and they are involved in most of the body's metabolic processes.

Mineral Metabolism

Mineral metabolism is usually controlled either at the point of intestinal absorption or at the point of tissue uptake.

Digestion

Minerals are absorbed and used in the body in their ionic forms, which means that they are carrying either a positive or negative electric charge. Unlike carbohydrates, proteins, and fats, minerals do not require a great deal of mechanical or chemical digestion before absorption occurs.

Absorption

The following general factors influence how much of a mineral is absorbed into the body from the gastrointestinal tract: (1) food form—minerals from animal sources are usually more readily absorbed than those from plant sources; (2) body need—more is absorbed if the body is deficient than if the body has enough; and (3) tissue health—if the absorbing intestinal surface is affected by disease, its absorptive capacity is greatly diminished.

The absorptive method for each mineral depends on its physical properties. Some minerals require active transport to be absorbed, whereas others enter the intestinal cells by diffusion. Compounds found in foods may also affect the absorptive efficiency. For example, the presence of fiber, phytate, or oxalate—all of which are found in a variety of whole grains, fruits, and vegetables—can bind certain minerals in the gastrointestinal tract, thereby inhibiting or limiting their absorption.

Transport

Minerals enter the portal blood circulation and travel throughout the body bound to plasma proteins or mineral-specific transport proteins (e.g., iron is bound to transferrin in the circulation).

trace minerals the group of elements that are required by the body in amounts of less than 100 mg/day.

Tissue Uptake

The uptake of some minerals into their target tissue is controlled by hormones, and excess minerals are excreted into the urine. For example, thyroid-stimulating hormone (TSH) controls the uptake of iodine from the blood by the thyroid gland depending on the amount that the thyroid gland needs to make the hormone thyroxine. When more thyroxine is needed, TSH stimulates the thyroid gland to take up iodine and the kidneys to excrete less iodine into the urine. When the thyroxine concentration is normal, less TSH is released from the anterior pituitary gland, thereby resulting in less iodine uptake by the thyroid gland and more excretion of iodine into the urine by the kidneys.

Occurrence in the Body

Body minerals are found in several forms in body tissues. The two basic forms in which minerals occur in the body are as free ions in body fluids (e.g., sodium in tissue fluids, which influence water balance) and as covalently bound minerals that may be combined with other minerals (e.g., calcium and phosphorus in hydroxyapatite) or with organic substances (e.g., iron that is bound to heme and globin to form the organic compound hemoglobin).

MAJOR MINERALS

Calcium

The intestinal absorption of dietary calcium depends on the food form (e.g., plant forms are sometimes bound to oxalate or phytate and thus are not readily available) and the interaction of three hormones (i.e., vitamin D, parathyroid hormone, and calcitonin [from the thyroid gland]) that directly control calcium's intestinal absorption and use, along with indirect control by the estrogens (i.e., sex hormones produced primarily by the ovaries).

Functions

After it has been absorbed, calcium has four basic functions in the body.

Bone and Tooth Formation. More than 99% of the body's calcium is found in the bones and teeth. Approximately 1% to 2% of adult body weight is calcium. When hydroxyapatite is removed from bone, the remaining tissue is a collagen matrix. If dietary calcium is insufficient during critical periods (e.g., the initial formation of the fetal skeleton, childhood growth, or the rapid growth of long bones during adolescence), then the construction of healthy bones is hindered. Teeth are calcified before they erupt from the gums; thus, insufficient dietary

calcium later in life does not affect tooth structure as it does bone structure.

Blood Clotting. Calcium is essential for the formation of fibrin, which is the protein matrix of a blood clot.

Muscle and Nerve Action. Calcium ions are required for muscle contraction and the release of neurotransmitters from neuron synapses.

Metabolic Reactions. Calcium is necessary for many general metabolic functions in the body. Such functions include the intestinal absorption of vitamin B_{12}, the activation of the fat-splitting enzyme pancreatic lipase, and the secretion of insulin by the β cells of the pancreas. Calcium also interacts with the cell membrane proteins that govern the cell membrane's permeability to nutrients.

Requirements

The Dietary Reference Intake (DRI) for calcium should provide sufficient calcium nourishment for the body while recognizing that a lower intake may be adequate for many individuals. For all infants who are up to 6 months old, the Adequate Intake (AI) level is 200 mg/day; for infants who are 7 to 12 months old, the AI is 260 mg/day. Calcium needs increase during the growth years of childhood and adolescence, during which the Recommended Dietary Allowances (RDAs) are as follows: 1 to 3 years, 700 mg/day; 4 to 8 years, 1000 mg/day; and 9 to 18 years, 1300 mg/day. For both men and women between the ages of 19 to 50 years, the RDA for desirable calcium retention is 1000 mg/day, with a rise to 1200 mg/day for women who are more than 50 years old. During pregnancy and lactation, the RDA is currently set as being equal to the level for the general age group, as follows: 1300 mg/day for up to the age of 18 years and 1000 mg/day for ages 19 years old and older.[1]

Deficiency States

Various bone deformities may occur if sufficient dietary calcium is unavailable during growth years. The deficiency disease rickets is related to an inadequate level of vitamin D to support the intestinal absorption of calcium. A decrease of blood calcium concentration (i.e., hypocalcemia) relative to blood phosphorus concentration results in tetany, which is a condition that is characterized by

---

thyroid-stimulating hormone (TSH) an anterior pituitary hormone that regulates the activity of the thyroid gland; also known as *thyrotropin*.

hypocalcemia a serum calcium level that is below normal.

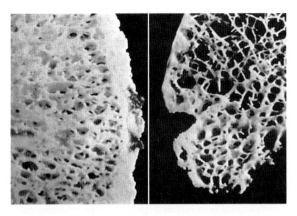

Figure 8-1 Osteoporosis. Normal bone *(left)* versus osteoporotic bone *(right)*. (Reprinted from Mahan LK, Escott-Stump S. *Krause's food & nutrition therapy.* 12th ed. Philadelphia: Saunders; 2008.)

muscle spasms. The most common calcium-related clinical issue today is osteoporosis. Osteoporosis is an abnormal decrease in bone density, especially in postmenopausal women, that is characterized by reduced bone mass, increased bone fragility, and a greater risk for the development of bone fractures (Figure 8-1). Such bone fractures are becoming more common among elderly men as well.[2] Each year in the United States, more than 1.5 million bone fractures and $17 to $20 billion in health care costs are linked to osteoporosis (see the Cultural Considerations box, "Bone Health in Gender and Ethnic Groups").[3]

Osteoporosis is not a primary calcium deficiency disease as such; rather, it results from a combination of factors that create chronic calcium deficiency. These factors include the following: (1) inadequate calcium intake; (2) poor intestinal calcium absorption related to deviations in the amounts of hormones that control calcium absorption and metabolism; and (3) a lack of physical activity, which stimulates muscle insertion into bones and significantly influences bone strength, shape, and mass. Insufficient physical activity contributes to the development of osteoporosis, and immobility after injury or disease can cause serious bone loss. Bone is a dynamic tissue, with both new bone formation and resorption occurring constantly. A portion of the skeleton is reabsorbed and replaced with new bone each year; this bone remodeling can affect up to 50% of total bone mass per year in young children and approximately 5% of bone mass in adults. Unfortunately, bone resorption often exceeds bone formation in postmenopausal women and in aging men. The interaction of factors in osteoporosis that result in bone calcium resorption outpacing bone calcium deposition are not fully understood. Increased calcium intake alone—be it via dietary calcium or

supplemental calcium—does not prevent osteoporosis in susceptible adults or successfully treat diagnosed cases of osteoporosis. Therapies that reduce bone loss in osteoporosis include combinations of the various factors that are involved in the building of bones: dietary calcium, the active hormonal form of vitamin D, estrogens, and weight-bearing physical activity.

Food intake studies report that the average calcium intakes of females from adolescence through adulthood are generally well below the DRI. The period of life during which bone density reaches its peak is also the period of life where teenage girls are likely to experience the largest dietary calcium deficit.[4] Teenage girls consume 878 mg/day of calcium on average, whereas the recommended RDA is 1300 mg/day. Deficiencies during this critical period of bone development may have long-term negative outcomes with regard to overall bone strength and risk for osteoporosis.[5]

Toxicity Symptoms

The toxicity of calcium from food sources is unlikely. However, a Tolerable Upper Intake Level (UL) for calcium has been set at 2000 to 3000 mg/day (depending on age) as a result of the negative effects of excessive calcium supplementation over time. Hypercalcemia is associated with the calcification of soft tissue and the decreased intestinal absorption of several other minerals. Calcium can interfere with the intestinal absorption of iron, magnesium, phosphorus and zinc, thereby reducing the bioavailability of these essential nutrients.

Food Sources

Milk and milk products are the most important sources of readily available calcium. Milk that is used in cooking (e.g., in soups, sauces, or puddings) or in milk products such as yogurt, cheese, and ice cream is an excellent source of dietary calcium (Figure 8-2). Calcium-fortified tofu, fruit juices, and other food products (e.g., cereals, cereal bars) are also high in bioavailable calcium. In

osteoporosis an abnormal thinning of the bone that produces a porous, fragile, lattice-like bone tissue of enlarged spaces that are prone to fracture or deformity.

resorption the destruction, loss, or dissolution of a tissue or a part of a tissue by biochemical activity (e.g., the loss of bone, the loss of tooth dentin).

hypercalcemia a serum calcium level that is above normal.

CULTURAL CONSIDERATIONS

BONE HEALTH IN GENDER AND ETHNIC GROUPS

The World Health Organization defines osteopenia as a bone mineral density (BMD) of between 1 and 2.5 standard deviations below the mean of a reference group. Osteoporosis involves a BMD of 2.5 standard deviations or more below the mean of the reference group.

Osteoporosis affects a significant number of older Americans. Currently, 2% of men (0.8 million) and 10% of women (4.5 million) who are 50 years old or older are living with osteoporosis.[1] An additional 34.5 million Americans have osteopenia, which is a significant risk factor for osteoporosis.

Osteoporosis often is thought of as a "white woman's disease." However, this debilitating bone disease is prevalent in men and other ethnic groups as well. It is well established that there is a disparity between genders. The National Institutes of Health estimates that one out of every two women (compared with one in four men) who are 50 years old or older will have bone fractures at some point during their lives as a result of osteoporosis.[2] With regard to differences among ethnic groups, a recent study found that non-Hispanic black men and women had the highest BMD and the lowest risk for osteoporosis throughout life compared with other ethnic groups. The same researchers found that non-Hispanic white men and women had significantly higher BMDs than Mexican Americans.[3] The reasons for these observed differences by race are unclear; however, ethnicity, gender, and age are all well accepted as important factors when calculating the risk for osteoporosis, which is the most common form of bone disease.

Many factors are involved in BMD and the relative risk for the development of fragile bones, including body weight, physical activity, hormonal influences, and dietary intakes of several vitamins and minerals (not just calcium). Nutrition affects bone health by providing the materials that are needed for tissue deposition, maintenance, and repair. Overall bone strength is determined by BMD and the collagen matrix formation. Collagen, which is a structural protein, accounts for more than 20% of the dry weight of total bone mass and 90% of the organic bone matrix. Collagen degradation is associated with osteoporosis. As such, the vitamins and minerals that are critical for a strong collagen and bone matrix also are integral to overall bone health. A delicate balance of several nutrients is important for healthy bone building, including protein; vitamins C, D, and K; calcium; phosphorus; copper; magnesium; manganese; potassium; and zinc.

Osteoporosis is currently costing Americans more than $17 billion annually in direct medical costs. Coupled with the general trends of an aging population, this bone disease is a serious national concern. Because BMD reaches a peak mass by the average age of 30 years, the years before this are vital for developing healthy bones and preventing the onset of osteoporosis. Establishing peak bone mass ensures a greater reserve of bone mineral and collagen so that, as age-associated degradation ensues, effects are essentially postponed or abated altogether. A healthy diet following the MyPlate guidelines should provide all of the essential nutrients, and it is imperative during the first three decades of life to establish healthy bones.

For more information about osteoporosis please see the Web site of the National Institutes of Health Osteoporosis and Related Bone Diseases National Resource Center at www.niams.nih.gov/health_info/bone/osteoporosis/.

1. Looker AC, Melton LJ 3rd, Harris TB, et al. Prevalence and trends in low femur bone density among older US adults: NHANES 2005-2006 compared with NHANES III. *J Bone Miner Res.* 2010; 25:64-71.
2. National Institutes of Health Osteoporosis and Related Bone Diseases National Resource Center. *Osteoporosis in men* (website): www. niams.nih.gov/Health_Info/Bone/Osteoporosis/men.asp. Accessed October 8, 2011.
3. Looker AC, Melton LJ 3rd, Harris T, et al. Age, gender, and race/ethnic differences in total body and subregional bone density. *Osteoporos Int.* 2009; 20:1141-1149.

addition, several plants provide a natural source of this important mineral. Calcium in low-oxalate greens such as bok choy, broccoli, collard greens, kale, and turnip greens is absorbed and can be an important source of calcium for vegetarians. Oxalic acid is a compound that is found in plants such as spinach, rhubarb, Swiss chard, beet greens, and certain other vegetables and nuts that forms an insoluble salt with calcium (calcium oxalate), thus interfering with the intestinal absorption of calcium. Phytate, which is another plant compound that is found in grains such as wheat, can bind with calcium and interfere with its intestinal absorption. Table 8-1 lists food sources of calcium.

In addition to food sources, calcium intake from supplements is widespread. Surveys show that almost 6% of women in the United States specifically take calcium supplements, whereas 22% of the total population takes a multivitamin and mineral supplement that contains some calcium.[6] The bioavailability of calcium from supplements depends on the dose and whether it is taken with a meal. Calcium is best absorbed in doses of 500 mg or less and when taken with food rather than on an empty stomach (see the For Further Focus box, "Calcium From Food or Supplements: Which Is Better?").

Phosphorus

Functions

The phosphorus atom in nature is most commonly found in combination with four oxygen atoms to form the

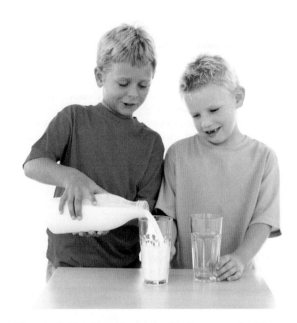

Figure 8-2 Milk is the major food source of calcium. (Copyright Photos.com.)

TABLE 8-1 **FOOD SOURCES OF CALCIUM**

Item	Quantity	Amount (mg)
Bread, Cereal, Rice, and Pasta		
Corn muffin, commercially prepared	1 medium (113 g)	84
Cream of Wheat cereal, cooked	¾ cup	86
English muffin, plain, enriched	1 muffin (57 g)	93
Oatmeal, instant, fortified, prepared with water	¾ cup	98
Whole-grain cereal, Total	¾ cup	1000
Vegetables		
Collard greens, boiled	¾ cup	140
Spinach, boiled*	¾ cup	122
Fruits		
Orange juice, fortified with calcium and vitamin D	8 fl oz	351
Meat, Poultry, Fish, Dry Beans, Eggs, and Nuts		
Salmon, pink, canned, drained solids with bone	3 oz	235
Sardines, canned in oil, solids with bone	3 oz	325
Soybeans, boiled	½ cup	88
Tofu, raw, firm, prepared with calcium sulfate	½ cup	861
Milk and Dairy Products or Their Substitutes		
Cheese, mozzarella, part skim milk	1 oz	222
Milk, skim	8 fl oz	301
Milk, whole	8 fl oz	276
Soy milk	8 fl oz	93
Soy milk, calcium fortified	8 fl oz	368
Tofu yogurt	8 fl oz	309
Yogurt, plain, low fat	8 fl oz	448

*Low bioavailability.
Data from the U.S. Department of Agriculture, Agricultural Research Service: Nutrient Data Laboratory. *USDA nutrient database for standard reference* (website): www.ars.usda.gov/ba/bhnrc/ndl. Accessed October 2010.

phosphate molecule. Phosphorus and calcium (in the form of hydroxyapatite) are critical to bone formation. In addition, phosphorus functions in the following metabolic processes.

Bone and Tooth Formation. The calcification of bones and teeth depends on the deposition of hydroxyapatite [$Ca_{10}(PO_4)_6(OH)_2$] by osteoblasts in bone's collagen matrix. The ratio of calcium to phosphorus in typical bone is approximately 1.5 : 1 by weight.

Energy Metabolism. Phosphorus in the form of phosphate (PO_4^{3-}) is necessary for the controlled oxidation of carbohydrate, fat, and protein to release the energy in their covalent bonds (as a component of thiamin pyrophosphate), and it captures energy for use in the body as a component of adenosine triphosphate. Phosphate is also involved in protein construction (as a component of RNA), cell function (as a component of cell enzymes activated by phosphorylation), and genetic inheritance (as a component of DNA).

Acid-Base Balance. Phosphate is an important chemical buffer that helps to maintain the pH homeostasis of body fluids.

Requirements

The typical American diet contains enough phosphorus to meet body needs. Surveys indicate that the mean daily phosphorus intake in the United States is approximately 1297 mg/day.[4] The AI level during the first 6 months of life is 100 mg/day, and, from the ages of 7 to 12 months, it is 275 mg/day. Healthy breast-fed infants receive adequate phosphorus. For children, the RDA varies with the stage of growth. Between the ages of 1 and 3 years, the RDA is 460 mg/day; between the ages of 4 and 8 years, it is 500 mg/day. From the ages of 9 to 18 years, which is a period of rapid bone growth, the RDA is 1250 mg/day. The established RDAs in the DRI guidelines for both men and women who are 19 years old and older is 700 mg/day, with no additional needs established for women who are pregnant or lactating.[7]

FOR FURTHER FOCUS

CALCIUM FROM FOOD OR SUPPLEMENTS: WHICH IS BETTER?

If only we could take a supplement to meet all of our nutrition needs, then we would not have to bother with eating healthy! Unfortunately, that is the type of thinking that fuels the continued search for the "magic pill." Good health is not a simple matter, and our bodies are no simple machines. They require lots of nutrients to function properly, and these must be provided by the diet. One of the major minerals that is needed by our body is calcium. According to the National Health and Nutrition Examination Study, relatively few women meet their Adequate Intakes for calcium through their diets. The graph below represents the average calcium intake for females by age group.

From the U.S. Department of Agriculture, Agricultural Research Service. *Nutrient intakes from food: mean amounts consumed per individual, by gender and age. What We Eat in America, NHANES 2007-2008* (website): www.ars.usda.gov/SP2UserFiles/Place/12355000/pdf/0708/Table_1_NIN_GEN_07.pdf. Accessed October 8, 2011; and Food and Nutrition Board, Institute of Medicine. *Dietary reference intakes for calcium, phosphorous, magnesium, vitamin D, and fluoride.* Washington, DC: National Academies Press; 1997.

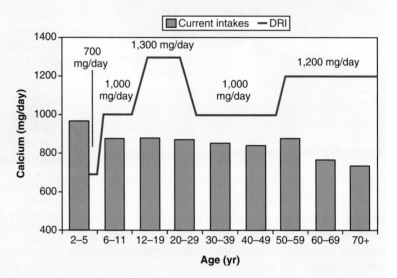

A variety of factors influence our dietary intake of calcium. Over the past decade, Americans' food choices have changed in ways that directly affect calcium-rich food consumption. For example, Americans are replacing milk with soft drinks; they are eating out more often at restaurants; they seem to be perpetually dieting (and dairy products are often one of the first foods to go); and they are largely unaware of the healthy link between calcium-rich foods and health.

Health organizations such as the National Institutes of Health, the Academy of Nutrition and Dietetics, the American Medical Association, and the National Academy of Sciences agree that the best source of calcium is dairy products. The primary reason for this is because, unlike calcium supplements, calcium-rich foods supply the body with other beneficial nutrients as well, including protein; vitamins A, B_{12}, and D (if fortified); magnesium; potassium; riboflavin; niacin; and phosphorus. Some nondairy foods naturally contain calcium, including salmon with bones, dried beans, turnip greens, mustard greens, kale, tofu, and broccoli. Most people find that meeting the Dietary Reference Intake for calcium exclusively from nondairy foods can be difficult, because the relative amount of calcium in these foods is significantly less than that found in dairy products. For example, half a cup of chopped kale has 47 mg of calcium, whereas 8 oz of skim milk contains 302 mg. In addition, many vegetables contain phytates and oxalates that form insoluble complexes with calcium and thus, decrease their bioavailability to the body.

Keller and colleagues analyzed the consumer cost and bioavailability of calcium from major sources. They found that Total cereal was the least expensive food source of calcium, with fluid milk and calcium-fortified orange juice being the next least expensive.[1] Calcium from supplements may be found in a variety of forms, including calcium carbonate, citrate, phosphate, lactate, and gluconate. The amount of calcium absorbed into the body from these sources varies considerably. Of the calcium supplements, calcium carbonate in a chewable form (e.g., Tums) or supplement provides the least expensive and most bioavailable source of calcium, with a 34% absorption fraction.[1]

The best way to improve one's overall diet is to consume a variety of foods that are high in calcium, preferably from dairy or fortified dairy substitute sources. However, calcium-fortified foods and supplements may be necessary for some people to meet their recommended intake of calcium. Calcium is best absorbed in doses of 500 mg or less at a time.

Regardless of where your calcium comes from, take a moment to consider the overall value of your diet, and assess whether improvements are warranted.

For more information about the fortification of calcium in the American food supply, please see Rafferty K, Walters G, Heaney RP. Calcium fortificants: overview and strategies for improving calcium nutriture of the U.S. population. *J Food Sci.* 2007; 72:R152-R158.

1. Keller JL, Lanou A, Barnard ND. The consumer cost of calcium from food and supplements. *J Am Diet Assoc.* 2002; 102(11): 1669-1671.

Deficiency States

Phosphate (the dietary form of phosphorus) is widely distributed in foods; thus, a deficiency is rare. A person must be completely deprived of food for an extended period to develop a dietary phosphorus deficiency. The only evidence of deficiency has been among people who consumed large amounts of antacids that contained aluminum hydroxide. The aluminum (Al^{3+}) binds with phosphate, thereby making the phosphate unavailable for intestinal absorption. Phosphorus deficiency (i.e., hypophosphatemia) results in bone loss; it is characterized by weakness, loss of appetite, fatigue, and pain.

Toxicity Symptoms

A toxicity of phosphorus (i.e., hyperphosphatemia) from food intake is equally rare. However, if phosphorus intake is significantly higher than calcium intake for a long period, bone resorption may occur. The DRI guidelines list the UL for phosphorus at 4 g/day for people between the ages of 9 and 70 years.[7]

Food Sources

Phosphorus is part of all living tissue, and it is found in all animal and plant cells; therefore, phosphorus is sufficient in the natural food supply of virtually all animals. High-protein foods are particularly rich in phosphorus, so milk and milk products, meat, fish, and eggs are the primary sources of phosphorus in the average diet. The bioavailability of phosphorus from plant seeds (e.g., cereal grains, beans, peas, other legumes, nuts) is much lower, because these foods contain phytic acid, which is a storage form of phosphorus in seeds that humans cannot directly digest. However, intestinal bacteria can make up to 50% of phosphorus from phytic acid available for intestinal absorption. Table 8-2 outlines some main food sources of phosphorus.

Sodium

Sodium is one of the most plentiful minerals in the body. Approximately 120 g (4.2 oz) is present in an adult body.

Functions

The main function of sodium is the maintenance of body water balance, which is discussed further in Chapter 9. Sodium also has important tasks in muscle action and nutrient absorption.

Water Balance. Ionized sodium concentration is the major influence on the volume of body water outside of the cells (i.e., extracellular) (Figure 8-3). Variations in sodium concentration largely control the movement of water across biologic membranes by osmosis. Sodium is

TABLE 8-2 FOOD SOURCES OF PHOSPHORUS

Item	Quantity	Amount (mg)
Vegetables		
Potato, baked, with skin	1 medium (173 g)	121
Meat, Poultry, Fish, Dry Beans, Eggs, and Nuts		
Almonds, roasted	1 oz (22 nuts)	139
Bacon, fried	3 medium slices	128
Beef, ground, 70% lean, pan browned	3 oz	172
Beef liver, pan fried	3 oz	412
Beef top round, lean, broiled	3 oz	173
Chicken, dark meat, roasted, without skin	3 oz	152
Chicken, white meat, roasted, without skin	3 oz	184
Chickpeas (garbanzo beans), boiled	½ cup	138
Clams, cooked, moist heat	3 oz	287
Cod, cooked, dry heat	3 oz	117
Crab, Alaskan king, cooked, moist heat	3 oz	238
Halibut, cooked, dry heat	3 oz	242
Ham, sliced, regular (11% fat)	3 oz	130
Lentils, boiled	½ cup	178
Lobster, cooked, moist heat	3 oz	157
Pinto beans, boiled	½ cup	126
Sirloin steak, lean, broiled	3 oz	184
Soybeans, boiled	½ cup	211
Tofu, raw, firm, prepared with calcium sulfate	½ cup	152
Trout, rainbow, cooked, dry heat	3 oz	226
Tuna, light, canned in water, drained solids	3 oz	139
Milk and Dairy Products		
Cheese, cheddar	1 oz	145
Cheese, mozzarella, part skim milk	1 oz	131
Cottage cheese, 1% milk fat	½ cup	151
Milk, 1% fat	8 fl oz	232
Yogurt, plain, low fat	8 fl oz	353

The food group that is composed of bread, cereal, rice, and pasta is not an important source of phosphorus. Whole-grain products are higher in phosphorus than are refined grain products, but the phosphorus, in the form of phytate, is not bioavailable to humans. Data from the U.S. Department of Agriculture, Agricultural Research Service: Nutrient Data Laboratory. *USDA nutrient database for standard reference* (website): www.ars.usda.gov/ba/bhnrc/ndl. Accessed October 2010.

hypophosphatemia a serum phosphorus level that is below normal.

hyperphosphatemia a serum phosphorus level that is above normal.

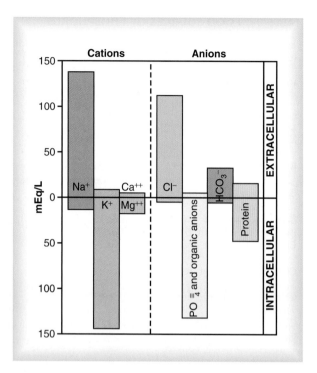

Figure 8-3 The ionic composition of the major body fluid compartments. (Reprinted from Guyton AC, Hall JE. *Textbook of medical physiology.* 12th ed. Philadelphia: Saunders; 2006.)

also an integral part of the digestive juices that are secreted into the gastrointestinal tract, most of which are reabsorbed by the intestinal cells.

Muscle Action. Sodium and potassium ions are necessary for the normal response of stimulated neurons, the transmission of nerve impulses to muscles, and the contraction of muscle fibers.

Nutrient Absorption. Sodium-dependent glucose transporters, which are a vital part of intestinal cells, allow for the passage of glucose and galactose from the intestinal lumen into the intestinal cells.

Requirements

The body is able to function on various amounts of dietary sodium through mechanisms that have been designed to conserve or excrete the mineral as needed. For that reason, no specific RDA for sodium exists. Individual sodium needs vary greatly depending on growth stage, sweat loss, and medical conditions (e.g., diarrhea, vomiting). The DRI standards include an AI for the three major electrolytes that are needed to maintain body fluid balance: sodium, chloride, and potassium. A sodium intake of 1.5 g/day should be adequate for healthy people who are not excessively losing sodium through extended

exercise and sweating. Adults between the ages of 50 and 70 years have a slightly reduced AI (1.3 g/day) that corresponds with decreased energy intake. The AI for individuals who are more than 71 years old is 1.2 g/day.[8]

Deficiency States

Sodium deficiencies are rare, because the body's need is low, and individual intake is typically high. An exception is during heavy sweating, such as by those who are engaged in heavy labor or strenuous physical exercise in a hot environment for an extended period of time (i.e., more than 2 hours). Commercial sports drinks, which replace sodium, glucose, and fluid, may be useful to restore losses. Although sweat is relatively low in sodium, drinking too much plain water during extended strenuous exercise can dilute blood sodium concentration and exacerbate sodium deficiency complications (see Chapter 16). Sodium deficiency (i.e., hyponatremia) can result in acid-base imbalances and muscle cramping.

Toxicity Symptoms

The sodium content of the average American diet, which contains a high amount of processed foods, usually far exceeds the recommended intake range. The National Health and Nutrition Examination Survey (NHANES) of 2007 to 2008 revealed that men consume an average of 4043 mg/day of sodium and that women have an average intake of 2884 mg/day.[4] Excessive sodium intake has been linked to hypertension in individuals who are salt sensitive (i.e., approximately 25% of hypertensive patients).[9] However, for most people with healthy kidneys and adequate water intake, the kidneys excrete excess sodium in the urine. The acute excessive intake of sodium chloride (i.e., table salt) causes the accumulation of sodium in the blood (i.e., hypernatremia) and extracellular spaces. This sodium can pull water out of cells into the extracellular space by osmosis, thereby causing edema. The current DRIs set the UL for sodium intake at 2.3 g/day but state that some individuals may have a much lower tolerance.[8]

Food Sources

Common table salt as used in cooking, seasoning, and processing foods is the main dietary source of sodium.

---

hyponatremia a serum sodium level that is below normal.

hypernatremia a serum sodium level that is above normal.

Sodium occurs naturally in foods, and it is generally most prevalent in foods of animal origin. Enough sodium is found in natural food sources to meet the body's needs. When food manufacturers add salt and other sodium compounds to processed foods as a preservative, sodium intake dramatically increases. For example, cured ham has approximately 20 times more sodium than raw pork. Natural unprocessed food sources of sodium include animal products such as milk, meat, and eggs and vegetables such as carrots, beets, leafy greens, and celery (see the Evolve site for the sodium and potassium content of foods and Appendix C for salt-free seasoning guides).

Potassium

The adult body contains approximately 270 g (9.5 oz) of potassium, which is nearly twice the amount of sodium.

Functions

Potassium is involved with sodium in the maintenance of the body water balance, and it also has many other metabolic functions.

Water Balance. Potassium is the major electrolyte inside cells (i.e., intracellular). Its osmotic effect holds water inside the cells and counterbalances the osmotic effect of sodium, which draws water out of the cells and into the extracellular fluid (see Figure 8-3).

Metabolic Reactions. Potassium plays a role in energy production, the conversion of blood glucose into stored glycogen, and the synthesis of muscle protein.

Muscle Action. Potassium ions also play a role in nerve impulse transmission to stimulate muscle action. Along with magnesium and sodium, potassium acts as a muscle relaxant that opposes the stimulating effect of calcium, which allows for muscle contraction. The heart muscle is sensitive to potassium levels; therefore, blood potassium concentration is regulated within narrow tolerances.

Insulin Release. Potassium is necessary for the release of insulin from pancreatic β cells in response to rising blood glucose concentrations.

Blood Pressure. Sodium is one of the main dietary factors that is associated with hypertension; however, hypertension may be more related to the sodium and potassium ratio (this is a molar ratio as opposed to a mass ratio) than to the amount of dietary sodium alone. A potassium intake that is equal to the sodium intake may help to prevent the development of hypertension; such is the basis for the Dietary Approaches to Stop Hypertension (DASH) diet (see www.nhlbi.nih.gov/hbp/prevent/h_eating/h_e_dash.htm for more information).

Requirements

As with sodium, the present DRI guidelines do not have an RDA for potassium, although potassium is essential in the diet. The AI of potassium is 4.7 g/day for all adults.[8] The National Research Council recommends an increase in potassium intake through the increased consumption of fruits and vegetables. The average American diet provides significantly less potassium than the established AI, with a median daily intake of 2 to 3 g/day.[4] The *Dietary Guidelines for Americans* committee identified potassium as a key nutrient that is lacking in the typical American diet, which led to the recommendation to increase the daily intake of fruits, vegetables, whole grains, and dairy products.[10]

Deficiency States

Symptoms of potassium deficiency are well defined but seldom related to inadequate dietary intake. Potassium deficiency (i.e., hypokalemia) is more likely to develop during clinical situations such as prolonged vomiting or diarrhea, the use of diuretics, severe malnutrition, or surgery. Hypokalemia also is a concern while a person is using antihypertensive medications, particularly diuretics that cause urinary potassium loss. Characteristic symptoms of potassium deficiency include heart muscle weakness with possible cardiac arrest, respiratory muscle weakness with breathing difficulties, poor intestinal muscle tone with resulting bloating, and overall muscle weakness.

Toxicity Symptoms

As with sodium, the kidneys normally excrete excess potassium so that toxicity does not occur. However, if oral potassium intake is excessive or if intravenous potassium is given that causes hyperkalemia, the heart muscle can weaken to the point at which it stops beating. A UL has not been established for potassium from food sources.

Food Sources

Potassium is an essential part of all living cells; thus, it is abundant in natural foods. The richest dietary sources of potassium are unprocessed foods: fruits such as oranges and bananas, vegetables such as broccoli and leafy green

---

hypokalemia a serum potassium level that is below normal.

hyperkalemia a serum potassium level that is above normal.

vegetables, fresh meats, whole grains, and milk products. Those who eat large amounts of fruits and vegetables have a high potassium intake. Plant sources of potassium are highly water soluble; therefore, much of the potassium is lost when fruits and vegetables are boiled or blanched (unless the water is retained). Table 8-3 lists food sources of potassium.

Chloride

Chloride is the chemical form of chlorine in the human body. Chloride accounts for approximately 3% of the body's total mineral content, and it is widely distributed throughout body tissues.

Functions

Chloride is predominantly found in the extracellular fluid compartments, where it helps to maintain the water and acid-base balances (see Figure 8-3). Its two significant functions involve digestion and respiration.

Digestion. Chloride (Cl^-) is one element of the hydrochloric acid (HCl) that is secreted in the gastric juices. The action of gastric enzymes requires that stomach fluids have a specific acid concentration (i.e., a pH of approximately 1.0).

Respiration. Carbon dioxide, which is a by-product of cellular metabolism, is transported by red blood cells (RBCs) to the lungs, where it is expelled during respiration. Within the RBCs, the enzyme carbonic anhydrase combines carbon dioxide (CO_2) with water (H_2O) to form carbonic acid (H_2CO_3). Carbonic acid then dissociates into a bicarbonate ion (HCO_3^-) and a proton (H^+). Bicarbonate ions move out of the RBCs and into the plasma, and chloride ions (Cl^-) move into the RBCs and out of the plasma, thereby maintaining the balance of negative charges on either side of the RBC membrane. The exchange of a bicarbonate ion with a chloride ion in the plasma is called the *chloride shift*.

Requirements

The AI for chloride for young adults is set at 2.3 g/day on the basis of a molecular equivalence to sodium.[8] Similar to sodium's AI, the need for chloride gradually declines after the age of 50 years.

Deficiency States

A dietary deficiency of chloride does not occur under normal circumstances. Because the normal intake and output of chloride from the body parallels that of sodium, conditions that lead to a sodium deficiency also can lead to a chloride deficiency. The primary reason for chloride deficiency is excessive loss through vomiting, which

TABLE 8-3 FOOD SOURCES OF POTASSIUM

Item	Quantity	Amount (mg)
Bread, Cereal, Rice, and Pasta		
Wheat germ, toasted cereal	¾ cup	803
Vegetables		
Avocado, raw	¼ medium	244
Brussels sprouts, boiled	½ cup	247
Potato, baked, with skin	1 medium (173 g)	926
Spinach, boiled	½ cup	419
Sweet potato, with skin, baked	1 medium (114 g)	542
Tomato, raw	1 medium	254
Fruits		
Banana	1 medium (118 g)	422
Dates, dried, pitted	¼ cup, chopped	292
Orange juice, fresh	8 fl oz	496
Orange, navel	1 medium (140 g)	232
Prunes, dried, pitted	½ cup (87 g)	637
Prune juice, canned	8 fl oz	707
Raisins, seedless	¼ cup	272
Meat, Poultry, Fish, Dry Beans, Eggs, and Nuts		
Beef liver, pan fried	3 oz	298
Beef top round, lean, broiled	3 oz	221
Chickpeas (garbanzo beans), boiled	½ cup	239
Clams, cooked, moist heat	3 oz	534
Crab, blue, cooked, moist heat	3 oz	275
Ground beef, 70% lean, pan browned	3 oz	279
Halibut, cooked, dry heat	3 oz	490
Ham, sliced, 11% fat	3 oz	244
Lentils, boiled	½ cup	365
Lima beans, boiled	½ cup	478
Pinto beans, boiled	½ cup	373
Salmon, cooked, dry heat	3 oz	352
Sirloin steak, lean, broiled	3 oz	348
Soybeans, boiled	½ cup	443
Milk and Dairy Products		
Milk, skim	8 fl oz	382
Milk, whole	8 fl oz	349
Yogurt, plain, low fat	8 fl oz	573
Sugar		
Molasses	1 Tbsp	293

Data from the U.S. Department of Agriculture, Agricultural Research Service: Nutrient Data Laboratory. *USDA nutrient database for standard reference* (website): www.ars.usda.gov/ba/bhnrc/ndl. Accessed October 2010.

results in metabolic alkalosis from disturbances in the acid-base balance (see Chapter 9).

Toxicity Symptoms

The only known dietary cause of chloride toxicity is as a result of severe dehydration, when the concentration of chloride is too great. No ULs are established for chloride.

Food Sources

Dietary chloride is almost entirely provided by sodium chloride, which is the chemical name of ordinary table salt. The kidneys efficiently reabsorb chloride when dietary intake is low.

Magnesium

An adult body contains 25 g (i.e., a little less than 1 oz) of magnesium on average. Sixty percent of this magnesium is present in the bones.

Functions

Magnesium has widespread metabolic functions, and it is found in all body cells. About 99% of body magnesium is intracellular, with the remaining 1% found in the extracellular space.

General Metabolism. Magnesium is a necessary cofactor for more than 300 enzymes that make use of nucleotide triphosphates (e.g., adenosine triphosphate) for activation or catalyzing reactions that produce energy, synthesize body compounds, or help to transport nutrients across cell membranes.

Protein Synthesis. Magnesium is a cofactor for enzymes that activate amino acids for protein synthesis and that synthesize and maintain DNA. When cells replicate, they must produce new proteins. The cell replication process requires magnesium to function correctly.

Muscle Action. Magnesium ions are involved in the conduction of nerve impulses that stimulate muscle contraction as part of magnesium adenosine triphosphate (MgATP). Calcium is pumped out of the myofibrillar spaces into the sarcoplasmic reticulum by pumps that require MgATP for energy.

Basal Metabolic Rate. MgATP is involved in the secretion of thyroxine, thus helping the body to maintain a normal metabolic rate and to adapt to cold temperatures.

Requirements

The DRI guidelines establish RDA amounts by age and gender. Requirements increase gradually with age. For those between the ages of 14 and 18 years, the RDA for magnesium is 410 mg/day for boys and 360 mg/day for girls. For those who are 19 to 30 years old, the RDA is 400 mg/day for men and 310 mg/day for women. For adults 31 years old and older, the RDA is 420 mg/day for men and 320 mg/day for women. The RDA is slightly higher during pregnancy.[7] The average American diet provides less magnesium than the established RDA, with a median daily intake of 334 mg/day for men and 258 mg/day for women.[4]

Deficiency States

A magnesium deficiency from a lack of dietary magnesium is quite rare among people who consume balanced diets. Symptoms of magnesium deficiency (i.e., hypomagnesemia) have been observed in clinical situations such as starvation, persistent vomiting or diarrhea with a loss of magnesium-rich gastrointestinal fluids, and most commonly as a result of renal disorders. Hypomagnesemia is also a symptom of various diseases that involve the cardiovascular and neuromuscular systems as well as in patients with diabetes mellitus, kidney disease, and alcoholism.[11] In severe cases, hypomagnesemia can be life threatening.[12] Deficiency symptoms include muscle weakness and cramps, hypertension, and blood vessel constriction in the heart and brain.

Toxicity Symptoms

Magnesium from food has not been observed to have adverse effects at high intake levels. Therefore, the DRI standards give a UL only for magnesium intake from supplements and pharmaceutical preparations. The UL from nonfood sources is 350 mg/day for people who are 9 years old and older; it is less for younger children.[7] Individuals who consume excessive amounts of magnesium from supplements or nonfood sources (e.g., medications) may experience nausea, vomiting, and diarrhea.

Food Sources

Although magnesium is relatively common in foods, the content is variable. Unprocessed foods have the highest concentrations of magnesium. Major food sources of magnesium include nuts, soybeans, cocoa, seafood, whole grains, dried beans and peas, and green vegetables. More than 80% of the magnesium in cereal grains is lost with the removal of the germ and outer layers. Significant

hypomagnesemia a serum magnesium level that is below normal.

amounts of magnesium may also be present in drinking water in regions that have hard water with a fairly high mineral content.

Sulfur

Functions

As part of the amino acids cysteine and methionine, sulfur is an essential part of protein structure, and it is present in all body cells. It participates in widespread metabolic and structural functions, and it is also a component of the vitamins thiamin and biotin.

Hair, Skin, and Nails. Disulfide bonds between cysteine residues in the protein keratin are essential to the structure of the hair, skin, and nails.

General Metabolic Functions. Sulfhydryl or thiol groups (i.e., sulfur that is covalently bonded to hydrogen) form high-energy bonds that make various metabolic reactions energetically favorable.

Vitamin Structure. Sulfur is a component of thiamin and biotin, which act as coenzymes in cell metabolism.

Collagen Structure. The disulfide bonding of cysteine residues is necessary for collagen superhelix formation, and it is therefore important in the building of connective tissue.

Requirements

Dietary requirements for sulfur are not stated as such, because sulfur is supplied by protein foods that contain the amino acids methionine and cysteine.

Deficiency States

Sulfur deficiency states have not been reported. Such conditions only relate to general protein malnutrition and the deficient intake of the sulfur-containing amino acids.

Toxicity Symptoms

Sulfur is unlikely to reach toxic concentrations in the body as a result of dietary intake; thus, no UL has been established.

Food Sources

A diet that contains adequate protein contains adequate sulfur. Sulfur is only available to the body as part of the amino acids methionine and cysteine and in the vitamins thiamin and biotin. Thus, animal protein foods are the main dietary sources of sulfur. Sulfur is widely available in meat, eggs, milk, cheese, legumes, and nuts.

Table 8-4 provides a summary of the major minerals.

TRACE MINERALS

Iron

Iron has the longest and best-described history of all of the micronutrients. The human body contains approximately 45 mg iron per kilogram of body weight. As with several other nutrients, iron is essential for life, but it can be toxic in excess. Thus, the body has developed exquisite systems for balancing iron intake and excretion and for efficiently transporting iron in and out of cells to maintain homeostasis. Iron is transported in the body bound to transferrin, and it is stored as ferritin in the liver, the spleen, and other tissues (Figure 8-4).

Functions

Iron serves as the functional part of hemoglobin, and it plays a role in the body's general metabolism.

Hemoglobin Synthesis. Approximately 70% of the body's iron is in hemoglobin within RBCs. Iron is a component of heme, which is the nonprotein part of hemoglobin. Hemoglobin carries oxygen to the cells, where it is used for oxidation and metabolism. Iron also is part of myoglobin, a protein that is found in muscle cells that is structurally and functionally analogous to hemoglobin in blood.

General Metabolism. Iron is necessary for glucose metabolism, antibody production, drug detoxification by the liver, collagen and purine synthesis, and the conversion of β-carotene to active vitamin A.

Requirements

Iron needs vary throughout life, depending on growth and development. The DRIs establish the recommended intakes of iron for children as follows: the AI for infants up to the age of 6 months is 0.27 mg/day; for the ages of 7 to 12 months, the RDA is 11 mg/day; for the ages of 1 to 3 years, the RDA is 7 mg/day; and for the ages of 4 to 8 years, the RDA is 10 mg/day. RDAs for iron for the age of 9 years old and older are between 8 and 11 mg/day for

transferrin a protein that binds and transports iron through the blood.

ferritin the storage form of iron.

TABLE 8-4 SUMMARY OF MAJOR MINERALS

Mineral	Functions	Recommended Intake (Adults)	Deficiency	Tolerable Upper Intake Level (UL) and Toxicity	Sources
Calcium (Ca)	Bone and teeth formation; blood clotting; muscle contraction and relaxation; nerve transmission	Between the ages of 19 and 50 years, 1000 mg; between the ages of 51 and 70 years, 1200 mg in women and 1000 mg in men; 70 years old or older, 1000 mg	Tetany, rickets, osteoporosis	UL: 2500 mg Increases the risk of kidney stones and constipation; interferes with the absorption of other nutrients	Dairy products, fish bones, fortified orange juice and cereals, legumes, green leafy vegetables
Phosphorus (P)	Bone and tooth formation; energy metabolism; DNA and RNA; acid-base balance	700 mg	Unlikely, but can cause bone loss, loss of appetite, and weakness	UL: 4g Bone resorption (loss of calcium)	High-protein foods (e.g., meat, dairy), soft drinks
Sodium (Na)	Major extracellular fluid control; water balance; acid-base balance; muscle action; transmission of nerve impulse and resulting contraction	Adequate intake: between the ages of 19 and 50 years, 1.5 g; between the ages of 51 and 70 years, 1.3 g; 71 years old or older, 1.2 g	Fluid shifts, acid-base imbalance, cramping	UL: 2.3 g Hypertension in salt-sensitive people; edema	Table salt, processed foods (e.g., luncheon meats, salty snacks)
Potassium (K)	Major intracellular fluid control; acid-base balance; regulation of nerve impulse and muscle contraction; blood pressure regulation	Adequate intake: 14 years old or older, 4.7 g	Irregular heartbeat, difficulty breathing, muscle weakness	UL not set Cardiac arrest	Fresh fruits and vegetables, meats, whole grains
Chloride (Cl)	Acid-base balance (chloride shift); hydrochloric acid (digestion)	Adequate intake: between the ages of 19 and 50 years, 2.3 g; between the ages of 51 and 70 years, 2.0 g; 71 years old or older, 1.8 g	Hypochloremic alkalosis with prolonged vomiting or diarrhea	UL not set Toxicity unlikely	Table salt, processed foods
Magnesium (Mg)	Coenzyme in metabolism, muscle and nerve action; helps with thyroid hormone secretion	Men, 400 to 420 mg; women, 310 to 320 mg	Tremor, spasm, low serum level after gastrointestinal losses or renal losses from alcoholism, convulsions	UL 350 mg (from supplements) Nausea; vomiting; diarrhea	Whole grains, nuts, legumes, green vegetables, seafood, cocoa
Sulfur (S)	Essential constituent of cell protein, hair, skin, nails, vitamin, and collagen structure; high-energy sulfur bonds in energy metabolism	Diets that are adequate in protein contain adequate sulfur	Unlikely	UL not set Toxicity unlikely	Meat, eggs, cheese, milk, nuts, legumes

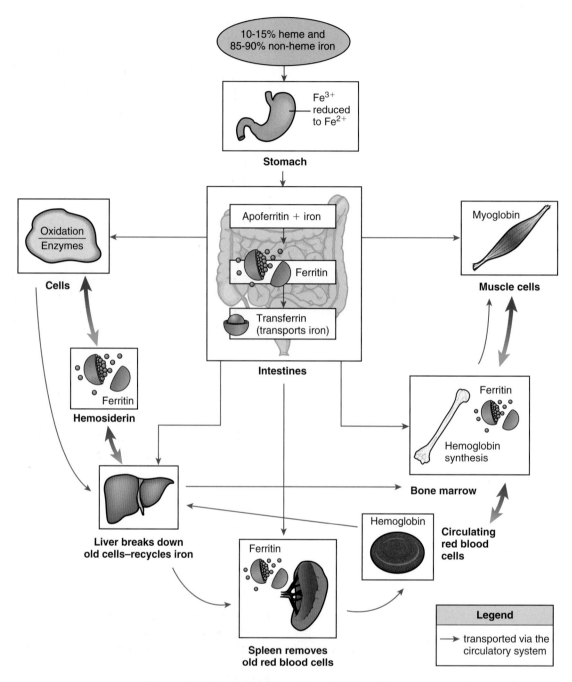

Figure 8-4 The absorption and metabolism of iron.

boys and between 8 and 18 mg/day for girls to accommodate growth spurts.[13] Women require more iron to cover the losses that occur during menstruation. Throughout pregnancy, a woman's RDA for iron increases to 27 mg/day. This increase usually requires an iron supplement, because neither the usual American diet nor the iron stores of many women can meet the increased iron demands of pregnancy. The average iron intake of women between the ages of 20 and 50 years is 13 mg/day, which is notably below the RDA.[4]

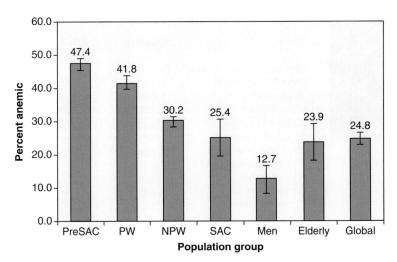

Figure 8-5 The global prevalence of anemia (%) and the number of individuals (in millions) affected in different population groups. *PreSAC,* Preschool-aged children (0 to 4.99 years old); *PW,* pregnant women; *NPW,* nonpregnant women (15 to 49.99 years old); *SAC,* school-aged children (5 to 14.99 years old); *Men* (15 to 59.99 years old); *Elderly* (includes men who are more than 60 years old and women who are more than 50 years old). (Reprinted from McLean E, Cogswell M, Egil I, et al. Worldwide prevalence of anaemia, WHO Vitamin and Mineral Nutrition Information System, 1993-2005. *Public Health Nutr.* 2009; 12(4):444-454.

Deficiency States

The major condition that indicates a deficiency of iron is anemia. Iron-deficiency anemia is usually evaluated biochemically by the percentage of packed RBCs (i.e., hematocrit), the RBC hemoglobin level, or the percentage of transferrin saturation. Iron-deficiency anemia is the most prevalent nutrition problem in the world today (Figure 8-5). The World Health Organization estimates that iron deficiency anemia affects 24.8% of the population worldwide, with a disproportionate prevalence seen among preschool-aged children and pregnant women.[14]

Iron-deficiency anemia may have several causes, including the following: (1) inadequate dietary iron intake; (2) excessive blood loss; (3) an inability to form hemoglobin as a result of a lack of factors such as vitamin B_{12} (i.e., pernicious anemia); (4) a lack of gastric hydrochloric acid, which liberates iron for intestinal absorption; (5) inhibitors of iron absorption (e.g., phytate, phosphate, tannin, oxalate); and (6) intestinal mucosal lesions that affect the absorptive surface area.

Toxicity Symptoms

Iron toxicity from a single large dose (20 to 60 mg per kilogram of body weight) can be fatal. The UL for iron is 45 g/day for adults.[13]

In the United States, iron overdose from supplements is one of the leading causes of poisoning among young children who are less than 6 years old. Symptoms include nausea, vomiting, and diarrhea. If these children are not immediately treated, several organ systems may be adversely affected, including the cardiovascular system, the central nervous system, the kidney, the liver, and the hematologic system.[15]

Chronic excessive iron intake through dietary supplements may impair the absorption of zinc, cause gastrointestinal upset, and increase the risk of the development of

heart disease and cancer. Hemochromatosis, an iron overload disease, may result from five types of genetic mutations, but it is most commonly the result of a mutation in the hemochromatosis (*HFE*) gene.[16] The congenital disease is an autosomal recessive disorder that results in iron overload even though iron intake is within the normal range. This disorder affects 1 in 200 to 1 in 300 individuals of northern European descent.[17] Afflicted individuals absorb excessive amounts of iron from food; over time (usually between the ages of 40 and 60 years), the iron accumulation causes widespread organ damage. Treatment involves frequent bloodletting (i.e., therapeutic phlebotomy) to reestablish normal serum iron levels. If treatment begins before widespread damage occurs, patients may have a normal life expectancy.

Food Sources

The typical Western diet provides an average of 6 mg of iron per 1000 kcal of energy intake. Iron is widely distributed in the U.S. food supply, primarily in meat, eggs, vegetables, and fortified cereals (Figure 8-6). Liver and fortified cereal products are especially good sources. The body absorbs iron more easily when it is taken along with vitamin C. Iron in food occurs in two forms: heme and nonheme. Heme iron is the most efficiently absorbed form of dietary iron, but it contributes the least to the total iron intake. Heme iron is found in only 40% of the animal food sources and in no plant foods (Table 8-5). Nonheme iron is less efficiently absorbed, because it is more tightly bound in foods, yet most of our food sources

---

anemia a blood condition that is characterized by a decreased number of circulating red blood cells, decreased hemoglobin, or both.

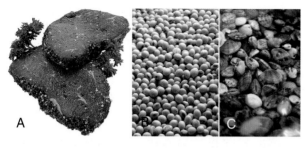

Figure 8-6 Food sources of dietary iron. **A,** Beef. **B,** Black-eyed peas. **C,** Oysters and clams. (Copyright JupiterImages Corporation.)

TABLE 8-5 **CHARACTERISTICS OF THE HEME AND NONHEME PORTIONS OF DIETARY IRON**

	Heme	Nonheme
Food sources	None in plant sources; 40% of iron in animal sources	All iron in plant sources; 60% of iron in animal sources
Absorption rate	Rapid; transported and absorbed intact	Slow; tightly bound in organic molecules

(i.e., 60% of the animal food sources and all the plant food sources) contain nonheme iron. To enhance the absorption of nonheme iron, food sources of vitamin C and moderate amounts of lean meats, fish, or poultry should be consumed in the same meal. Enriched and fortified cereal products are a good source of nonheme iron. Table 8-6 lists food sources of iron.

Iodine

The average adult body contains only 20 to 50 mg of iodine.

Functions

Iodine's basic function is as a component of thyroxine (T_4), a hormone that is synthesized by the thyroid gland and that helps to control the basal metabolic rate. T_4 synthesis is ultimately controlled by the hypothalamus and the pituitary gland. The hypothalamus excretes thyrotropin-releasing hormone (TRH). TRH, in turn, stimulates the release of TSH from the anterior pituitary gland. TSH controls the thyroid gland uptake of iodine from the bloodstream and the release of triiodothyronine (T_3) and T_4 into the circulation (Figure 8-7). Blood T_4 concentration determines how much TRH the hypothalamus releases and how much TSH the pituitary gland

TABLE 8-6 **FOOD SOURCES OF IRON**

Item	Quantity	Amount (mg)
Bread, Cereal, Rice, and Pasta		
Bran Flakes cereal	¾ cup	8.1
Bran muffin	1 medium (113 g)	4.75
Cream of Wheat, instant, cooked	¾ cup	8.98
Oatmeal, fortified, instant, prepared with water	¾ cup	7.26
Wheat Bran flakes cereal, Complete	¾ cup	17.98
Fruits and Vegetables		
Prune juice, canned	8 fl oz	3.02
Spinach, boiled, drained*	½ cup	3.21
Meat, Poultry, Fish, Dry Beans, Eggs, and Nuts		
Beef, ground, 70% lean, pan browned	3 oz	2.11
Beef liver, pan fried	3 oz	5.24
Beef top round, lean, broiled	3 oz	2.78
Chickpeas (garbanzo beans), boiled	½ cup	2.37
Clams, cooked, moist heat	3 oz	23.77
Lentils, boiled	½ cup	3.3
Lima beans, large, boiled	½ cup	6.74
Oysters, cooked, dry heat	3 oz	6.6
Shrimp, cooked, moist heat	3 oz	2.63
Soybeans, boiled	½ cup	4.42
Tofu, raw, firm, prepared with calcium sulfate	½ cup	2.03

*Low bioavailability
Data from the U.S. Department of Agriculture, Agricultural Research Service: Nutrient Data Laboratory. *USDA nutrient database for standard reference* (website): www.ars.usda.gov/ba/bhnrc/ndl. Accessed October 2010.

thyroxine (T_4) an iodine-dependent thyroid gland hormone that regulates the metabolic rate of the body.

thyrotropin-releasing hormone (TRH) a hormone that is secreted by the hypothalamus and that stimulates the release of thyroid-stimulating hormone by the pituitary.

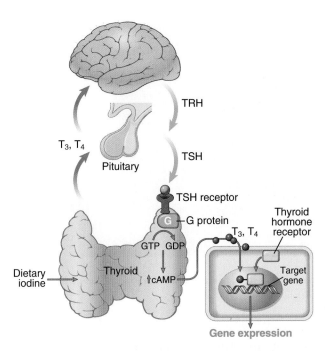

Figure 8-7 Uptake of iodine for triiodothyronine and thyroxine production. (Reprinted from Guyton AC, Hall JE. *Textbook of medical physiology.* 12th ed. Philadelphia: Saunders; 2006.)

releases. As blood T_4 concentration decreases, the hypothalamus and the pituitary gland are stimulated to release more TRH and TSH, respectively.

The transport form of iodine in the blood is called *serum protein-bound iodine.* T_3, T_4, and inorganic iodine are eventually disposed of by the liver in bile.

Requirements

The body's need for iodine has been extensively studied. To maintain desirable tissue levels of iodine, the adult body's minimal requirement is 50 to 75 mcg/day; therefore, to provide an extra margin of safety, the RDA is 150 mcg/day for all people who are 14 years of age and older; less is indicated for infants and children. During pregnancy, the need increases to 220 mcg/day; during lactation, it increases to 290 mcg/day.[13]

Deficiency States

The World Health Organization reports that iodine-deficiency disorders are the easiest and least expensive of all nutrient disorders to prevent; however, they remain the number one cause of preventable brain damage worldwide. Iodine-deficiency disorders are generally found in geographic locations with mountains or frequent flooding that result in poor soil iodine levels. Roughly 31% of the world's population has insufficient iodine intake; these

individuals are at high risk for the following deficiency diseases.[18]

Goiter. Goiter is characterized by an enlargement of the thyroid gland (Figure 8-8). When the thyroid gland is starved for iodine, it cannot produce a normal amount of T_4. Because of a low blood T_4 concentration, the pituitary gland continues to release more TSH. These large amounts of TSH overstimulate the nonproductive thyroid gland, thereby causing its size to increase greatly. An iodine-starved thyroid gland may weigh 0.45 to 0.67 kg (1 to 1.5 lb) or more. Although the thyroid is one of the larger endocrine glands, it normally only weighs 10 to 20 g in an adult.

Cretinism. Cretinism is characterized by physical deformity, dwarfism, and mental retardation. This serious condition occurs among children who are born to mothers who had limited iodine intake during adolescence and pregnancy. During pregnancy, the mother's need for iodine takes precedence over the iodine needs of the developing child. Thus, the fetus suffers from iodine deficiency and continues to do so after birth. The physical and mental development of these children is severely impeded and irreversible.[19]

Impaired Mental and Physical Development. Iodine deficiency at any stage in life may result in mental impairment. Studies indicate that there is a significant reduction in the intelligence quotient of people with chronic and severe iodine deficiency. Iodine deficiency during the adolescent and teen years delays growth as well as the onset of puberty.[19,20]

Hypothyroidism. An adult form of hypothyroidism called *myxedema* occurs when a poorly functioning thyroid gland does not make enough T_4, thereby greatly reducing the basal metabolic rate. The symptoms of this condition are thin, coarse hair; dry skin; poor cold tolerance; weight gain; and a low, husky voice.

Hyperthyroidism. Hyperthyroidism is a condition in adults in which the overstimulated thyroid gland releases excessive T_4, thereby greatly increasing the basal metabolic rate. Hyperthyroidism is known as *Graves' disease* or *exophthalmic goiter* because of its prominent symptom of protruding eyeballs. Other symptoms include weight loss, hand tremors, general nervousness, increased appetite, and an intolerance of heat.

goiter an enlarged thyroid gland that is caused by a lack of enough available iodine to produce the thyroid hormone thyroxine.

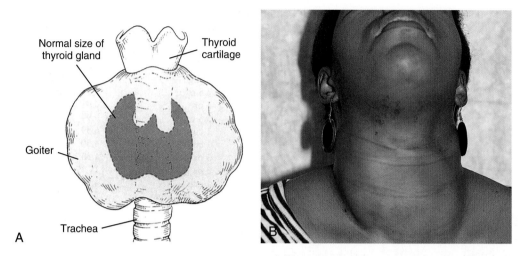

Figure 8-8 A, Illustration of a goiter. **B,** The extreme enlargement is a result of an extended duration of iodine deficiency. (**B,** Reprinted from Swartz MH. *Textbook of physical diagnosis.* 5th ed. Philadelphia: Saunders; 2006.)

Toxicity Symptoms

The incidental intake of iodine through supplementation or water contamination may result in toxicity. Excessive intake may cause iodine-excess goiter, autoimmune thyroiditis, hypothyroidism, elevated TSH, and ocular damage.[21]

Although the risk of iodine toxicity exists, the continued use of iodized salt is still widely practiced in several countries, including the United States. The risk for iodine deficiency far outweighs the small potential for iodine toxicity. The UL of iodine in healthy adults is 1100 mcg/day.[13]

Food Sources

The amount of iodine in natural food sources varies considerably depending on the iodine content of the soil in which the food was grown. Seafood consistently provides a good amount of iodine. However, the major reliable source of iodine in U.S. diets is iodized table salt, with each gram containing 76 mcg of iodine. Salt that is used in the preparation of processed food supplies iodine for those people who do not use table salt.

Zinc

Zinc is an essential trace mineral with wide clinical significance. The amount of zinc in the adult body is approximately 1.5 g (0.05 oz) in women and 2.5 g (0.09 oz) in men.

Functions

Zinc is especially important during growth periods such as pregnancy, lactation, infancy, childhood, and adolescence. Zinc is present in minute quantities in all body organs, tissues, fluids, and secretions. In these tissues, zinc participates in three different types of metabolic functions, as outlined in the following paragraphs.

Enzyme Constituent. Zinc's wide tissue distribution reflects its broad metabolic activity as an essential part of certain cell enzyme systems. More than 200 zinc-containing enzymes have been identified. Zinc's role in protein metabolism is associated with wound healing and healthy skin. Zinc greatly influences rapidly growing tissues, including those involved in fetal development during gestation.

Immune System. A considerable amount of protein-bound zinc is present in leukocytes (i.e., white blood cells). Zinc is integral in the health of the immune system as a result of its role in the synthesis of nucleic acids (DNA and RNA) and protein.[22] Zinc is also needed for lymphocyte transformation. Healthy lymphoid tissue, which gives rise to lymphocytes, is rich in zinc.

Other Functions. Zinc stabilizes the prohormone storage form of insulin in the pancreas. It is also involved in the protection of RBCs from oxidative damage and in taste and smell acuity.

Requirements

The DRIs establish an AI for infants of 2 to 3 mg/day during the first 3 years of life and of 5 mg/day for children between the ages of 4 and 8 years. The zinc requirement continues to rise until adulthood for both genders. Males who are 14 years old and older require 11 mg of zinc per day, whereas females need 8 mg/day, with the exception of 14- to 18-year-old girls, whose needs are slightly higher. Pregnant women require 11 mg/day to meet fetal growth needs and 12 mg/day for lactation. Pregnant or lactating girls who are younger than 18 years old require 2 mg/day more zinc than pregnant women older than 18 years old.[13] The average daily zinc intake for men and women in the United States is 14.4 mg and 9.9 mg, respectively.[4]

Deficiency States

Adequate zinc intake is imperative during periods of rapid tissue growth, such as childhood and adolescence. Stunted growth, especially in boys, has been observed in some populations in which dietary zinc intake is low.[23] Impaired taste and smell (i.e., hypogeusia and hyposmia, respectively) are improved with increased zinc intake if dietary zinc intake was previously inadequate. Zinc deficiency commonly causes poor wound healing, hair loss, diarrhea, skin irritation, and overall compromised immune function.[22] Patients with poor appetites, who subsist on marginal diets, or who have chronic wounds or illnesses with excessive tissue breakdown may be particularly vulnerable to developing zinc deficiency (see the For Further Focus box, "Zinc Barriers").

Acrodermatitis enteropathica (AE) is a rare autosomal recessive disorder that results in severe zinc deficiency and death if it is not treated. Patients with this condition are not able to absorb sufficient zinc from the gut. Classical symptoms of acrodermatitis enteropathica begin with skin lesions and progress to severely compromised immune function (Figure 8-9). This metabolic disorder is successfully treated with oral zinc supplements at high doses if it is diagnosed during infancy.

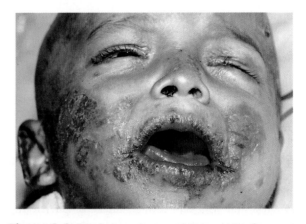

Figure 8-9 Skin lesions that are characteristic of severe zinc deficiency in a patient with acrodermatitis enteropathica. (Kumar V, Abbas AK, Fausto N. *Robbins and Cotran pathologic basis of disease.* 7th ed. Philadelphia: Saunders; 2005.)

FOR FURTHER FOCUS

ZINC BARRIERS

Are people eating more zinc but absorbing it less? Current trends toward a heart-healthy diet may be the reason why. Some Americans may be at risk for developing a zinc deficiency—not because they are avoiding zinc-rich foods but because they are choosing foods and supplements that reduce zinc's availability for absorption. Here are some examples:

- Animal foods, which are rich in readily available zinc, are consumed less by an increasingly cholesterol-conscious public.
- Dietary fiber may hinder absorption and create a negative zinc balance.
- Food processing may make zinc less available.
- Vitamin and mineral supplements may contain iron-to-zinc ratios of greater than 3 : 1 and thus, provide enough iron to inhibit zinc absorption.

Low levels of zinc can reduce the amount of protein that is available to carry iron and vitamin A to the target tissues. It can also reduce an individual's normal appetite and taste for certain foods.

The following suggestions may help to increase dietary zinc:

- Include some form of animal food (e.g., meat, milk, and eggs) or vegetarian-acceptable fortified food in the diet each day to ensure an adequate intake of zinc.
- Avoid the excessive use of alcohol.
- Avoid "crash" diets, which are typically low in micronutrients.

Signs of zinc deficiency are fairly rare in the United States, but they are becoming more apparent among at-risk people (e.g., older adults who are hospitalized with long-term chronic illnesses).[1] However, there is no need for the general public to take massive supplemental doses. These large doses may compete with other minerals (e.g., iron) and create other deficiency problems. Excess zinc can lead to nausea, abdominal pain, anemia, and immune system impairment. As with all other nutrients, too much of a good thing can sometimes be as bad as—or even worse than—too little.

1. Prasad AS. Impact of the discovery of human zinc deficiency on health. *J Am Coll Nutr.* 2009; 28(3):257-265.

Toxicity Symptoms

As with several other minerals, zinc toxicity from food sources alone is uncommon. However, prolonged supplementation that exceeds the recommended zinc intake can alter lymphocyte function and cause adverse symptoms such as nausea, vomiting, and epigastric pain.[24] The UL for zinc of 40 mg/day was established on the basis of the negative effects of excess zinc supplementation on copper metabolism.[13] Excessive zinc intake inhibits copper absorption, thereby resulting in a zinc-induced copper deficiency.

Food Sources

The greatest source of dietary zinc in the United States is meat, which supplies approximately 70% of the zinc that is consumed. Seafood (particularly oyster) is another excellent source of zinc. Legumes and whole grains are reasonable sources of zinc, but the zinc in these foods is less available for intestinal absorption as a result of phytate binding. A balanced diet usually meets adult needs for zinc. People who consume diets with little or no animal products and who have a high intake of phytate-rich unrefined grains may be at risk for developing marginal zinc deficiency.[25] Table 8-7 lists food sources of zinc.

Selenium

Functions

Selenium is present in all body tissues except adipose tissue. The highest concentrations of selenium are in the liver, kidneys, heart, and spleen. Selenium is an essential part of the antioxidant enzyme glutathione peroxidase, which protects the lipids in cell membranes from oxidative damage. An abundance of selenium may spare vitamin E to an extent, because both selenium and vitamin E protect against free radical damage. Selenium is also a component of many proteins in the body that are referred to as *selenoproteins.* One such selenoprotein is type 1 iodothyronine 5′ deiodinase, which is the enzyme that converts T_4 to T_3.

The DRI panel on antioxidants reviewed the current scientific research on selenium. The panel concluded that, although selenium intakes that are higher than the RDA may protect against cancer, further large-scale research is necessary to confirm such an effect.[26] However, several recent studies found no correlation between dietary selenium intake above recommended amounts and cancer prevention.[27,28]

Requirements

The recommendations for selenium intake are made by age group without specificity to gender. For both men and women who are 14 years old and older, the RDA is

TABLE 8-7 FOOD SOURCES OF ZINC

Item	Quantity	Amount (mg)
Bread, Cereal, Rice, and Pasta		
Bran Flakes cereal	¾ cup	1.5
Bran muffin	1 medium (113 g)	2.08
Wheat Bran flakes cereal, Complete	¾ cup	15.22
Meat, Poultry, Fish, Dry Beans, Eggs, and Nuts		
Almonds, roasted	1 oz	1
Beef, ground, 70% lean, pan browned	3 oz	5.06
Beef liver, pan fried	3 oz	4.45
Beef round top, lean, broiled	3 oz	3.83
Cashews, roasted	1 oz	1.59
Chicken, dark meat only, cooked, without skin	3 oz	1.81
Chickpeas (garbanzo beans), boiled	½ cup	1.25
Clams, cooked, moist heat	3 oz	2.32
Crab, Alaskan king, cooked, moist heat	3 oz	6.48
Ham, sliced, regular (11% fat)	3 oz	1.15
Lentils, boiled	½ cup	1.26
Lima beans, large, boiled	½ cup	2.68
Lobster, cooked, moist heat	3 oz	2.48
Oysters, cooked, dry heat	3 oz	38.4
Shrimp, cooked, moist heat	3 oz	1.33
Sirloin steak, lean, broiled	3 oz	4.84
Tofu, raw, firm, prepared with calcium sulfate	½ cup	1.05
Milk and Dairy Products		
Milk, skim	8 fl oz	1.03
Yogurt, plain, low fat	8 fl oz	2.18

Data from the U.S. Department of Agriculture, Agricultural Research Service: Nutrient Data Laboratory. *USDA nutrient database for standard reference* (website): www.ars.usda.gov/ba/bhnrc/ndl. Accessed October 2010.

55 mcg/day. The RDA decreases by age for children: it is 40 mcg/day for children who are 9 to 13 years old, 30 mcg/day for children who are 4 to 8 years old, and 20 mcg/day for children who are 1 to 3 years old. The DRI does not list an RDA for infants. On the basis of mean intakes of breast milk, an infant's observed AI level is 15 mcg/day for the first 6 months of life and 20 mcg/day from the ages of 7 to 12 months. The recommended selenium intake day during pregnancy is 60 mcg/day, and it is 70 mcg/day during lactation.[26]

Deficiency States

Inadequate selenium negatively alters immune function and increases the opportunity for oxidative stress, specifically within the thyroid gland. Selenium deficiency is generally only found in geographic areas with a poor soil content of selenium.[29] Research indicates that adequate selenium intake plays a role in preventing *Kashin-Bek disease* and *Keshan disease*. Kashin-Bek disease results in chronic arthritis and joint deformity. Keshan disease, which is named after the area in China where it was discovered, is a disease of the heart muscle that primarily affects young children and women of childbearing age and that can lead to heart failure as a result of cardiomyopathy (i.e., degeneration of the heart muscle).

Toxicity Symptoms

The most common symptom of selenium toxicity is hair loss, joint pain, nail discoloration and gastrointestinal upset (i.e., nausea, vomiting, and diarrhea). Most known cases of dietary selenium toxicity are in isolated regions of the world where the soil has extremely high levels of selenium. However, in 2008 a misformulated dietary supplement resulted in 201 cases of selenium poisoning in the United States, with symptoms that persisted for more than 3 months.[30] The UL for selenium is 400 mcg/day for people who are 14 years old and older.[26]

Food Sources

Most selenium in food is highly available for intestinal absorption. The amount of selenium in food depends on the quantity of selenium in the soil that is used to graze animals and grow plants. Seafood, kidney, and liver are consistently good sources of selenium. To a lesser extent, other meats also provide selenium. Grains and other seeds have variable selenium content, and fruits and vegetables generally contain little selenium. In the United States and Canada, the dietary intake of selenium can vary by the geographic region in which the fruits and vegetables are grown, but these local differences are mitigated by the national food distribution system. The average adult intake of selenium in the United States is 104.9 mcg/day.[4]

The following sections briefly review the remaining essential trace minerals.

Fluoride

Fluoride forms a strong bond with calcium; thus, it accumulates in calcified body tissues such as bones and teeth. Fluoride's main function in human nutrition is to prevent dental caries. Fluoride strengthens the ability of teeth to withstand the erosive effect of bacterial acids. To a great extent, the fluoridation of the public water supply (for which the optimal level is 1 ppm) is responsible for the remarkable decline in dental caries during recent decades. The use of fluoridated toothpaste (0.1% fluoride) and improved dental hygiene habits have also benefited dental health.

According to the DRI guidelines, research data are insufficient with regard to fluoride intake to support a specific RDA. Alternatively, the DRI lists observed AIs by age group. For adults who are 19 years old and older, the AI is 4 mg/day for men and 3 mg/day for women, with lower intakes for children. It is not recommended that fluoride intake increase during pregnancy and lactation. The DRI guidelines set the UL for fluoride at 10 mg/day for people who are 9 years old and older to avoid dental fluorosis (Figure 8-10).[7]

Fish, fish products, and tea contain the highest concentrations of fluoride. Cooking in fluoridated water raises the fluoride concentration in many foods. People who are using well water should periodically check the fluoride concentration of their water, because well water can contain excessively high natural sources of fluoride.

Copper

Copper has frequently been called the "iron twin," because both iron and copper are metabolized in much the same way, and both are components of cell enzymes. Both of these minerals are also involved in energy production and hemoglobin synthesis. Severe copper deficiency is rare, and it can be attributed to individual adaptation to somewhat lower intakes.

There are two severe inborn errors of metabolism that involve copper. The first is Menkes' disease, which is an X-linked genetic disease of copper metabolism that currently has no treatment or cure. Individuals who are affected with Menkes' disease progress through neurodegeneration and connective tissue deterioration, and they usually do not survive past childhood.[31] Wilson's disease is a rare autosomal recessive genetic disorder that causes an abnormally high storage of copper in the body. Without treatment, Wilson's disease can result in liver and nerve damage that leads to death. However, there are treatments for Wilson's disease that may stabilize or even reverse it.[32]

The adult RDA for dietary copper intake is 900 mcg/day. Pregnant and lactating women are recommended to increase their copper intake to 1 mg/day and 1.3 mg/day, respectively.[13] The average daily intake of dietary

---

fluorosis an excess intake of fluoride that causes the yellowing of teeth, white spots on the teeth, and the pitting or mottling of tooth enamel.

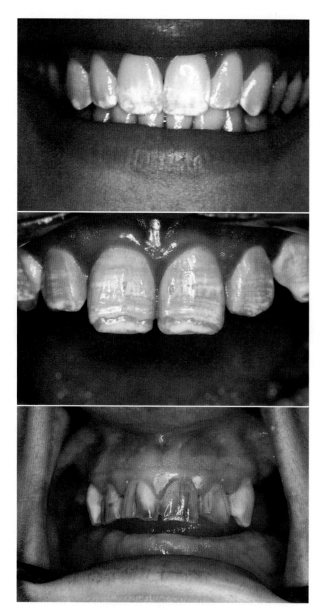

Figure 8-10 Fluorosis.

copper in the United States is 1.3 mg/day.[4] The UL for copper is 10 mg/day to avoid gastrointestinal upset and liver damage.[13] Copper is widely distributed in natural foods. Organ meats (especially liver), seafood, nuts, seeds, legumes, and grains are the richest food sources of copper.

Manganese

The adult body contains approximately 20 mg of manganese that is found primarily in the liver, pancreas, pituitary gland, and bones. Manganese functions like many other trace minerals: as a component of cell enzymes. Manganese-dependent enzymes catalyze many important metabolic reactions. In some magnesium-dependent enzymes, manganese may serve as a substitute for magnesium, depending on the availability of these two minerals. The intestinal absorption and bodily retention of manganese are associated with serum ferritin concentration.

Manganese deficiency has been documented in animal studies, but there are no known manganese deficiencies among humans who are consuming a free diet. Manganese toxicity occurs as an industrial occupation disease known as *inhalation toxicity* in miners and other workers who are exposed to manganese dust over long periods. The excess manganese accumulates in the liver and the central nervous system, thereby producing severe neuromuscular symptoms that are similar to those of Parkinson's disease. There is also a potential for manganese toxicity among patients who are receiving total parenteral nutrition, because the bioavailability is approximately 95% greater than if it is absorbed enterally. In addition, the normal elimination pathway is often impaired in these patients; thus, manganese accumulates in and damages the brain.[33] The UL from dietary sources is 11 mg/day for healthy adults.[13]

The DRIs estimate an AI of 2.3 mg/day for men and 1.8 mg/day for women who are older than 19 years of age. Needs gradually increase during and after childhood, and pregnant and lactating women need more manganese (2.0 mg/day and 2.6 mg/day, respectively).[13] The best food sources of manganese are of plant origin. Whole grains, cereal products, and teas are the richest food sources.

Chromium

The precise amount of chromium that is present in body tissues is uncertain, because analysis is difficult. Although large geographic variations occur, total body chromium is less than 6 mg. Chromium is an essential component of the organic complex glucose tolerance factor, which stimulates the action of insulin. Chromium supplements were previously thought to reduce insulin resistance (the cause of impaired glucose tolerance) and to improve lipid profiles for at-risk patients. However, a recent randomized double-blind study that examined the effects of chromium supplements in subjects with impaired glucose tolerance did not find significant improvements in glucose tolerance among those who took chromium compared with the control group.[34] For adults, the AI of chromium intake is 35 mcg/day for men and 25 mcg/day for women. Chromium needs gradually rise from infancy to adulthood and then decline after the age of 50 years. Pregnant and lactating women have an increased need of 30 mcg/day and 45 mcg/day, respectively. No UL has been established.[13] Brewer's yeast is a rich source of chromium, and most grains and cereal products contain significant amounts.

Molybdenum

Molybdenum is better absorbed than many minerals, and inadequate dietary intake is unlikely. The amount of molybdenum in the body is exceedingly small; it ranges from 0.1 to 1 mcg per gram of body tissue. Molybdenum is the functional catalytic component in several cell enzymes. For adults, the RDA of molybdenum is 45 mcg/day. Pregnant and lactating women need an additional 5 mcg/day. The National Academy of Sciences found it necessary to establish a UL of 2000 mcg/day for adults who are older than 19 years of age.[13] The amounts of molybdenum in foods vary considerably depending on the soil in which they are grown. Food sources include legumes, whole grains, milk, leafy vegetables, and organ meats.

Table 8-8 provides a summary of selected trace minerals.

Other Essential Trace Minerals

RDAs and AIs were not set for the remaining trace minerals: aluminum, arsenic, boron, nickel, silicon, tin, and vanadium. At the time of the 2002 DRIs, not enough data were available to establish such recommendations.[13] Most of these minerals are deemed essential to the nutrition of specific animals and probably are essential to human nutrition as well, although the complete process of their metabolism is not yet fully understood. Because these minerals occur in such small amounts, they are difficult to study, and dietary deficiency is highly unlikely.

The available research data regarding boron, nickel, and vanadium is sufficient to establish a tolerable UL level. The adult ULs for both boron and vanadium were set on the basis of data that were gathered from animal studies: for boron, the UL is 20 mg/day; for vanadium, it is 1.8 mg/day. The adult UL for arsenic was set at 1 mg/day.[13]

MINERAL SUPPLEMENTATION

The same principles that were discussed in Chapter 7 for vitamin supplementation apply to mineral supplementation as well. Special needs during growth periods and in clinical situations may require specific mineral supplements. Before taking supplements, potential nutrient-nutrient interactions and drug-nutrient interactions should be considered. Several situations can occur in which mineral bioavailability may be hindered (see the Drug-Nutrient Interaction box, "Mineral Depletion").

Life Cycle Needs

Mineral supplements may be needed during rapid growth periods throughout the life cycle.

DRUG-NUTRIENT INTERACTION

MINERAL DEPLETION

Medications interact with minerals through two major mechanisms: either by blocking absorption or by inducing renal excretion. The following are examples of common drug-nutrient interactions that specifically affect mineral status:

- *Diuretics:* People who require the long-term use of diuretic drugs for the treatment of hypertension may need to pay special attention to certain minerals that are also lost. The minerals that are usually excreted with excess water are sodium, potassium, magnesium, and zinc. The increased intake of foods that are high in these minerals is generally enough to regain homeostasis. Some diuretics (e.g., spironolactone) are potassium sparing and thus extra potassium should not need to be consumed.
- *Chelating agents:* Chelation therapy is used to remove excess metal ions from the body. Penicillamine is

used to treat Wilson's disease (i.e., the excess accumulation of copper in the body) and rheumatoid arthritis and to prevent kidney stones. It attaches to zinc and copper, thereby blocking absorption and leading to the excretion and possible depletion of these essential minerals.

- *Antacids:* The acidic environment of the stomach is required for the absorption of many drugs and nutrients, including minerals. When this environment is altered as a result of the chronic use of antacids, mineral deficiencies can occur. Phosphate deficiency is a concern for individuals who are chronically using over-the-counter antacids. In extreme cases, hypercalcemia may result, and damage to soft tissues can occur.

TABLE 8-8 SUMMARY OF SELECTED TRACE ELEMENTS

Mineral	Functions	Recommended Intake (Adults)	Deficiency	Tolerable Upper Intake Level (UL) and Toxicity	Sources
Iron (Fe)	Hemoglobin and myoglobin formation; cellular oxidation of glucose; antibody production	Men, 8 mg; women between the ages of 19 and 50 years, 18 mg; women who are 50 years old or older, 8 mg	Anemia, pale skin, impaired immune function	UL: 45 mg Nausea; vomiting; diarrhea; liver, kidney, heart, and central nervous system damage; hemochromatosis (iron overload disease)	Liver, meats, egg yolk, whole grains, enriched bread and cereal, dark green vegetables, legumes, nuts
Iodine (I)	Synthesis of thyroxine, which regulates cell oxidation and basal metabolic rate	150 mcg	Goiter, cretinism, hypothyroidism, hyperthyroidism	UL: 1100 mcg Goiter	Iodized salt, seafood
Zinc (Zn)	Essential enzyme constituent; protein metabolism; storage of insulin; immune system; sexual maturation	Men, 11 mg; women, 8 mg	Impaired wound healing and taste and smell acuity, retarded sexual and physical development	UL: 40 mg Nausea; vomiting; decreased immune function; impaired copper absorption	Meat, seafood (especially oysters), eggs, milk, whole grains, legumes
Selenium (Se)	Forms glutathione peroxidase; spares vitamin E as an antioxidant; protects lipids in cell membrane	55 mcg	Impaired immune function, Keshan disease, heart muscle failure	UL: 400 mcg Brittleness of hair and nails; gastrointestinal upset	Seafood, kidney, liver, meats, whole grains
Fluoride (Fl)	Constituent of bone and teeth; prevents dental caries	Adequate Intake: men, 4 mg; women, 3 mg	Increased dental caries	UL: 10 mg Dental fluorosis	Fluoridated water, toothpaste
Copper (Cu)	Associated with iron in energy production, hemoglobin synthesis, iron absorption and transport, and nerve and immune function	900 mcg	Anemia, bone abnormalities	UL: 10 mg Toxicity disease (Wilson's disease, which results in liver and nerve conduction damage)	Liver, seafood, whole grains, legumes, nuts
Manganese (Mn)	Activates reactions in urea synthesis, energy metabolism, lipoprotein clearance, and the synthesis of fatty acids	Adequate Intake: men, 2.3 mg; women, 1.8 mg	Clinical deficiency present only with protein-energy malnutrition	UL: 11 mg Inhalation toxicity in miners, which results in neuromuscular disturbances	Cereals, whole grains, soybeans, legumes, nuts, tea, vegetables, fruits
Chromium (Cr)	Associated with glucose metabolism	Adequate Intake: men, 35 mcg; women, 25 mcg	Impaired glucose metabolism	UL not set Toxicity unlikely	Whole grains, cereal products, brewer's yeast
Molybdenum (Mo)	Constituent of many enzymes	45 mcg	Unlikely	UL: 2 mg Toxicity unlikely	Organ meats, milk, whole grains, leafy vegetables, legumes

Pregnancy and Lactation

Women require additional chromium, copper, iodine, iron, magnesium, manganese, molybdenum, selenium, and zinc to meet the demands of rapid fetal growth during pregnancy. DRIs remain elevated for several minerals throughout lactation to meet both mother and infant needs. Not all women will require dietary supplements to meet these increased needs, because they will be met with a healthy, balanced diet. However, some nutrients (e.g., iron) are regularly supplemented, because it is sometimes challenging to meet the DRI recommendations through dietary intake alone during this time.

Adolescence

Rapid bone growth during adolescence requires increased calcium and phosphorus. If an adolescent's diet provides insufficient calcium, the risk for bone-density problems (e.g., osteoporosis) during the later adult years is increased. Too little dietary calcium may lead to the resorption of calcium from bone to maintain an appropriate blood calcium concentration. With the major increases in soft-drink consumption coupled with the decreased milk consumption per capita in the United States, concern has increased about poor bone growth during these critical years.

Supplements that combine iron with folate may be indicated for adolescent girls as they begin their menstrual cycles.

Adulthood

Healthy adults who consume well-balanced and varied diets do not require mineral supplements. A well-rounded and varied diet in combination with adequate physical activity and exercise maintains optimal bone health in most adults. Some studies do indicate that supplemental calcium and vitamin D may improve bone health and reduce the risk of fracture among postmenopausal women.[35] However, at any adult age, calcium supplementation alone neither prevents nor successfully treats osteoporosis, the cause of which is not clear and involves multiple factors. Calcium supplements may be used as part of a treatment program together with vitamin D, estrogen, and increased physical activity.

Clinical Needs

People with certain clinical problems or those who are at high risk for developing such problems may require mineral supplements.

Iron-Deficiency Anemia

One of the most prevalent health problems encountered in population surveys is iron-deficiency anemia. The need for increased iron intake has long been established for pregnant and breast-feeding women.[13] The following high-risk groups also may need to supplement their diets: adolescent girls and women who are in their child-bearing years who consume poor diets; people who are food insecure (i.e., those who are not able to secure enough food on a consistent basis); alcohol-dependent individuals; vegetarians; and elderly people who consume poor diets.

Zinc Deficiency

The increased popularity of vegetarian diets has amplified concern about possible zinc deficiency because of the low zinc content of plant foods. The position statement of the Academy of Nutrition and Dietetics and the Dietitians of Canada regarding vegetarian diets indicates that zinc requirements for individuals who consume high phytate diets may exceed the current DRIs.[25] Signs of zinc deficiency are slow growth, impaired taste and smell, poor wound healing, and skin irritation; however, 3 to 24 weeks may pass before symptoms appear. Others who are at risk for zinc deficiency include alcohol-dependent individuals; people on long-term, low-calorie diets; and elderly people in long-term institutional care.

SUMMARY

- Minerals are elements that are widely distributed in foods. They are absorbed by the intestines and used in building body tissue; activating, regulating, and controlling metabolic processes; and transmitting neurologic messages.
- Minerals are classified in accordance with their relative amounts in the body. Major minerals are necessary in larger quantities than trace minerals, and they make up 60% to 80% of all of the inorganic material in the body. Trace minerals, which are necessary in quantities as small as a microgram, make up less than 1% of the body's inorganic material.

- RDAs have not been set for all minerals because of a lack of scientific data. However, AIs or ULs have been set for almost all essential minerals without RDAs.
- Mineral supplementation—along with vitamin supplementation—continues to be a hot topic of research. There are periods that occur throughout the life cycle and specific disease states that may warrant supplementation. However, in most situations, a balanced diet provides an adequate supply of all of the essential nutrients.

CRITICAL THINKING QUESTIONS

1. List the seven major minerals. Describe their functions and the problems created by dietary deficiency or excess.
2. List the trace minerals that are essential to human nutrition. Which ones have established RDAs? Which ones have suggested AIs? Why is establishing an RDA for every mineral difficult?

3. Considering the normal dietary supply of minerals, would you recommend the taking of a multimineral dietary supplement? If so, to whom and for what reasons?

CHAPTER CHALLENGE QUESTIONS

True-False
Write the correct statement for each statement that is false.
1. *True or False:* Most of the phosphorus in the diet is absorbed and used by the body for bone formation.
2. *True or False:* The typical adult consumption of sodium is approximately 10 times the amount that the body actually requires for metabolic balance.
3. *True or False:* Potassium is the major electrolyte that controls the water outside of cells.

4. *True or False:* Chloride is a necessary component of stomach fluids.
5. *True or False:* Copper has many metabolic functions, the most important of which is its role in T_4 synthesis.
6. *True or False:* A high intake of selenium has been proved to prevent cancer in almost everyone.
7. *True or False:* Iodine is associated with iron functions in the body and is called the "iron twin."

Multiple Choice
1. Overall calcium balance is mostly maintained by which two balanced regulatory agents?
   a. Vitamin A and thyroid hormone
   b. Ascorbic acid and growth hormone
   c. Vitamin D and parathyroid hormone
   d. Phosphorus and TSH
2. Optimal levels of body iron are controlled at the point of absorption, which is interrelated with a system of transport and storage. Which of the following statements correctly describes this iron-regulating process?
   a. The iron form in food requires an acid medium to reduce it to the form that is necessary for absorption.
   b. 70% to 90% of the iron that is ingested in food is absorbed.

   c. Vitamin C acts as a binding and carrying agent to transport and store iron.
   d. When RBCs are destroyed, the iron that is used to make the hemoglobin is excreted.
3. A known function of fluoride in human nutrition is dental health. Which of the following statements correctly describes this relationship?
   a. Small amounts of fluoride produce mottled, discolored teeth.
   b. Fluoridation of the public water supply in very small amounts helps to prevent dental caries.
   c. The topical application of fluoride is not effective on young teeth.
   d. Fluoride works with vitamin A to build strong teeth.

4. Cretinism is a disorder in children who are born to mothers who had a deficiency of which mineral during adolescence and pregnancy?
   a. Calcium
   b. Phosphorus
   c. Iron
   d. Iodine

5. Which mineral has the following functions: blood clotting, muscle and nerve action, and bone and teeth formation?
   a. Calcium
   b. Phosphorus
   c. Magnesium
   d. Chloride

6. Which of the following minerals is a trace mineral?
   a. Potassium
   b. Iron
   c. Chloride
   d. Sulfur

⊖volve Please refer to the Students' Resource section of this text's Evolve Web site for additional study resources.

REFERENCES

1. Food and Nutrition Board, Institute of Health. *Dietary reference intakes for calcium and vitamin D.* Washington, DC: National Academy of Sciences; 2010.
2. Khosla S. Update in male osteoporosis. *J Clin Endocrinol Metab.* 2010;95(1):3-10.
3. Becker DJ, Kilgore ML, Morrisey MA. The societal burden of osteoporosis. *Curr Rheumatol Rep.* 2010;12(3):186-191.
4. U.S. Department of Agriculture, Agricultural Research Service. *Nutrient intakes from food: mean amounts consumed per individual, by gender and age, in the United States, 2007-2008. What we eat in America, NHANES 2007-2008* (website): www.ars.usda.gov/SP2UserFiles/Place/12355000/pdf/0708/Table_1_NIN_GEN_07.pdf. Accessed October 6, 2011.
5. Cooper C, Harvey N, Javaid K, et al. Growth and bone development. *Nestle Nutr Workshop Ser Pediatr Program.* 2008;61:53-68.
6. Ervin RB, Wright JD, Reed-Gillette D. Prevalence of leading types of dietary supplements used in the third national health and nutrition examination survey, 1988–94. *Adv Data.* 2004 Nov;9(349):1-7.
7. Food and Nutrition Board, Institute of Medicine. *Dietary reference intakes for calcium, phosphorous, magnesium, vitamin D, and fluoride.* Washington, DC: National Academies Press; 1997.
8. Food and Nutrition Board, Institute of Medicine. *Dietary reference intakes for water, potassium, sodium, chloride, and sulfate.* Washington, DC: National Academies Press; 2004.
9. Savica V, Bellinghieri G, Kopple JD. The effect of nutrition on blood pressure. *Annu Rev Nutr.* 2010;30:365-401.
10. U.S. Department of Agriculture, U.S. Department of Health and Human Services. *Dietary guidelines for Americans, 2010.* Washington, DC: U.S. Government Printing Office; 2010.
11. Musso CG. Magnesium metabolism in health and disease. *Int Urol Nephrol.* 2009;41(2):357-362.
12. Assadi F. Hypomagnesemia: an evidence-based approach to clinical cases. *Iran J Kidney Dis.* 2010;4(1):13-19.
13. Food and Nutrition Board, Institute of Medicine. *Dietary reference intakes for vitamin A, vitamin K, arsenic, boron, chromium, copper, iodine, iron, manganese, molybdenum, nickel, silicon, vanadium, and zinc.* Washington, DC: National Academies Press; 2001.
14. McLean E, Cogswell M, Egli I, et al. Worldwide prevalence of anaemia, WHO Vitamin and Mineral Nutrition Information System, 1993-2005. *Public Health Nutr.* 2009;12(4):444-454.
15. Anderson AC. Iron poisoning in children. *Curr Opin Pediatr.* 1994;6(3):289-294.
16. McLaren GD, Gordeuk VR. Hereditary hemochromatosis: insights from the Hemochromatosis and Iron Overload Screening (HEIRS) Study. *Hematology Am Soc Hematol Educ Program.* 2009;195-206.
17. Pietrangelo A. Hereditary hemochromatosis: pathogenesis, diagnosis, and treatment. *Gastroenterology.* 2010;139(2):393-408, 408.e1-408.e2.
18. World Health Organization. *Assessment of iodine deficiency disorders and monitoring their elimination.* Geneva: World Health Organization; 2007.
19. Zimmermann MB. Iodine deficiency. *Endocr Rev.* 2009;30(4):376-408.
20. Markou KB, Tsekouras A, Anastasiou E, et al. Treating iodine deficiency: long-term effects of iodine repletion on growth and pubertal development in school-age children. *Thyroid.* 2008;18(4):449-454.
21. Patrick L. Iodine: deficiency and therapeutic considerations. *Altern Med Rev.* 2008;13(2):116-127.
22. Prasad AS. Zinc in human health: effect of zinc on immune cells. *Mol Med.* 2008;14(5-6):353-357.
23. Gibson RS, Manger MS, Krittaphol W, et al. Does zinc deficiency play a role in stunting among primary school children in NE Thailand? *Br J Nutr.* 2007;97(1):167-175.
24. Plum LM, Rink L, Haase H. The essential toxin: impact of zinc on human health. *Int J Environ Res Public Health.* 2010;7(4):1342-1365.

25. Craig WJ, Mangels AR. Position of the academy of nutrition of dietetics: vegetarian diets. *J Am Diet Assoc.* 2009; 109(7):1266-1282.

26. Food and Nutrition Board, Institute of Medicine. *Dietary reference intakes for vitamin C, vitamin E, selenium, and carotenoids.* Washington, DC: National Academies Press; 2000.

27. Lippman SM, Klein EA, Goodman PJ, et al. Effect of selenium and vitamin E on risk of prostate cancer and other cancers: the Selenium and Vitamin E Cancer Prevention Trial (SELECT). *JAMA.* 2009;301(1):39-51.

28. Dunn BK, Richmond ES, Minasian LM, et al. A nutrient approach to prostate cancer prevention: The Selenium and Vitamin E Cancer Prevention Trial (SELECT). *Nutr Cancer.* 2010;62(7):896-918.

29. Steinnes E. Soils and geomedicine. *Environ Geochem Health.* 2009;31(5):523-535.

30. MacFarquhar JK, Broussard DL, Melstrom P, et al. Acute selenium toxicity associated with a dietary supplement. *Arch Intern Med.* 2010;170(3):256-261.

31. Tumer Z, Moller LB. Menkes disease. *Eur J Hum Genet.* 2010;18(5):511-518.

32. Gouider-Khouja N. Wilson's disease. *Parkinsonism Relat Disord.* 2009;15(Suppl 3):S126-S129.

33. Hardy G. Manganese in parenteral nutrition: who, when, and why should we supplement? *Gastroenterology.* 2009;137(5 Suppl):S29-S35.

34. Gunton JE, Cheung NW, Hitchman R, et al. Chromium supplementation does not improve glucose tolerance, insulin sensitivity, or lipid profile: a randomized, placebo-controlled, double-blind trial of supplementation in subjects with impaired glucose tolerance. *Diabetes Care.* 2005;28(3):712-713.

35. Bergman GJ, Fan T, McFetridge JT, Sen SS. Efficacy of vitamin D3 supplementation in preventing fractures in elderly women: a meta-analysis. *Curr Med Res Opin.* 2010;26(5):1193-1201.

FURTHER READING AND RESOURCES

World Health Organization. *Worldwide prevalence of anaemia 1993-2005, WHO Global Database on Anaemia* (website): www.who.int/nutrition/publications/micronutrients/anaemia_iron_deficiency/9789241596657/en/index.html.

The following Web sites are good sources for information about certain minerals in the diets and their role in general health. You can also go to the National Heart, Lung, and Blood Institute Web site to learn about the role of sodium and hypertension and to read more about how to follow a low-sodium diet. Examine the American Dental Association Oral Health Topics for more information about the protective role of fluoride in dental hygiene.

American Dental Association. www.ada.org/fluoride.aspx

National Digestive Diseases Information Clearinghouse, hemochromatosis. http://digestive.niddk.nih.gov/ddiseases/pubs/hemochromatosis/

National Heart, Lung, and Blood Institute. www.nhlbi.nih.gov/hbp/prevent/sodium/sodium.htm

National Osteoporosis Foundation. www.nof.org

CHAPTER 9

Water Balance

KEY CONCEPTS

- Water compartments inside and outside of the cells maintain a balanced distribution of total body water.
- The concentration of various solute particles in water determines the internal shifts and movement of water.

- A state of dynamic equilibrium among all parts of the body's water balance system sustains life.

Water is the most vital nutrient to human existence. Humans can survive far longer without food than without water. Only the continuous need for air is more demanding.

One of the most basic nutrition tasks is ensuring a balanced distribution of water to all body cells. Water is critical for the physiologic functions that are necessary to support life. This chapter briefly looks at the finely developed water balance system in the body, how this system works, and the various parts and processes that maintain it.

BODY WATER FUNCTIONS AND REQUIREMENTS

Water: The Fundamental Nutrient

Basic Principles

Three basic principles are essential to an understanding of the balance and uses of water in the human body.

A Unified Whole. The human body forms one continuous body of water that is contained by a protective envelope of skin. Water moves to all of the parts of the body, and it is controlled by solvents within the water and membranes that separate the compartments. Virtually every space inside and outside of the cells is filled with water-based body fluids. Within this environment, all processes that are necessary to life are sustained.

Body Water Compartments. The key word *compartment* is generally used in human physiology to refer to dynamic areas within the body. Body water can be discussed in terms of total body water as well as in separate individual locations throughout the body (i.e., intracellular or extracellular compartments). Membranes separate compartments of water. The body's dynamic mechanisms constantly shift water to places of greatest need and maintain equilibrium among all parts. Specific compartments are discussed later in this chapter.

Particles in the Water Solution. The concentration and distribution of particles in water (e.g., sodium, chloride, calcium, magnesium, phosphate, bicarbonate, protein) determine the internal shifts and balances among the compartments of body water.

Homeostasis

The body's state of dynamic balance is called homeostasis. W.B. Cannon, a physiologist, viewed these balance

---

homeostasis the state of relative dynamic equilibrium within the body's internal environment; a balance that is achieved through the operation of various interrelated physiologic mechanisms.

principles as "body wisdom."[1] Early in the twentieth century he applied the term *homeostasis* to the capacity that is built into the body to maintain its life systems, despite what enters the system from the outside. The body has a great capacity to use numerous finely balanced homeostatic mechanisms to protect its vital water supply.

Body Water Functions

The body water supply has the following characteristics: (1) it acts as a solvent; (2) it serves as a means of transport; (3) it regulates temperature control; and (4) it provides lubrication for the body.

Solvent. Water provides the basic liquid solvent for all chemical reactions within the body. The polarity of water effectively ionizes and dissolves many substances.

Transport. Water circulates throughout the body in the form of blood and various other secretions and tissue fluids. In this circulating fluid, the many nutrients, secretions, metabolites (i.e., products formed from metabolism), and other materials can be carried anywhere in the body to meet the needs of all body cells.

Thermoregulation. Water is necessary to help maintain a stable body temperature. As the body temperature rises, sweat is released and evaporates from the skin, thereby cooling the body.

Lubricant. Water also has a lubricating effect on moving parts of the body. For example, fluid within joints (i.e., synovial fluid) helps to provide smooth movement and prevents damage from friction.

Body Water Requirements

The Dietary Reference Intake for water, which was set for the first time by the National Academy of Sciences in 2004, is based on the median total water intake reported by participants in the Third National Health and Nutrition Examination Survey (NHANES), which took place from 1988 to 1994. The amount of total water includes water in both beverages and food. Set as Adequate Intakes, the Dietary Reference Intakes for water are the amounts that are required to meet the needs of healthy individuals who are relatively sedentary and living in temperate climates.[2] Recommendations are primarily established to prevent the harmful effects of dehydration, which include metabolic and functional abnormalities. To meet adult fluid needs and thus be hydrated, the average sedentary woman should consume 2.7 L (91 oz) of total water per day. Because approximately 19% of total water intake comes from food, a woman should aim for 74 fluid ounces (9 cups) of fluids in the form of beverages per day, with the rest being provided by food. A sedentary man should consume 3.7 L (125 oz) of total water per day.[2] Assuming that approximately 0.7 L of water is consumed within food, a man should aim for 101 fluid ounces (3 L) of fluid in the form of beverages per day. However, physical activity and alterations in climate require more fluid to offset losses. Table 9-1 lists the Adequate Intakes of fluid for all individuals.

The body's requirement for water varies in accordance with several factors: environment, activity level, functional losses, metabolic needs, age, and other dietary factors.

Surrounding Environment. As the temperature rises in the surrounding environment, body water is lost as sweat in an effort to maintain body temperature. Water intake must accommodate such losses in sweat. Increasing body temperatures may be caused by the natural climate or by the heat produced by physical work. On the opposite end of the spectrum, cold temperatures and altitude result in elevated respiratory water loss, hypoxia- or cold-induced diuresis, and increased energy expenditure, all of which increase water needs as well.[2]

Activity Level. Heavy work or extensive physical activity (e.g., participation in sports) increases the water requirement for two reasons: (1) more water is lost in sweat and respiration; and (2) more water is necessary for the increased metabolic demand that results from physical activity.

Athletes require a large increase in water intake, especially in hot weather. The American College of Sports Medicine, the Academy of Nutrition and Dietetics, and the Dietitians of Canada recommend drinking 5 to 7 mL per kilogram of body weight of water or sports drink at least 4 hours before exercise (see For Further Focus box entitled "Hydrating With Water or a Sports Drink" in Chapter 16 for more information about sports drinks). Fluid intake needs during activity will depend on body size, sweat rates, and type of activity. Athletes are encouraged to rehydrate by drinking at least 16 to 24 oz of fluid for every pound of body weight that is lost during exercise.[3]

Functional Losses. When any disease process interferes with the normal functioning of the body, water requirements are affected. For example, with gastrointestinal problems such as prolonged diarrhea, large amounts

---

polarity the interaction between the positively charged end of one molecule and the negative end of another (or the same) molecule.

TABLE 9-1 **ADEQUATE INTAKE OF WATER (LITERS PER DAY)**

Age	MALE			FEMALE		
	From Food	**From Beverages**	**Total Water**	**From Food**	**From Beverages**	**Total Water**
0 to 6 months	0.0	0.7	0.7	0.0	0.7	0.7
7 to 12 months	0.2	0.6	0.8	0.2	0.6	0.8
1 to 3 years	0.4	0.9	1.3	0.4	0.9	1.3
4 to 8 years	0.5	1.2	1.7	0.5	1.2	1.7
9 to 13 years	0.6	1.8	2.4	0.5	1.6	2.1
14 to 18 years	0.7	2.6	3.3	0.5	1.8	2.3
>19 years	0.7	3.0	3.7	0.5	2.2	2.7
Pregnancy, 14 to 50 years				0.7	2.3	3.0
Lactation, 14 to 50 years				0.7	3.1	3.8

1 L = 33.8 oz; 1 L = 1.06 qt; 1 cup = 8 oz.
Data from the Food and Nutrition Board, Institute of Medicine. *Dietary reference intakes for water, potassium, sodium, chloride, and sulfate.* Washington, DC: National Academies Press; 2004.

of water may be lost. Uncontrolled diabetes mellitus causes an excess loss of water through urine as a result of high blood glucose levels. In such cases, the replacement of lost water and electrolytes is vital to prevent dehydration.

Metabolic Needs. Body metabolism requires water. A general rule is that roughly 1000 mL of water is necessary for the metabolism of every 1000 kcal in the diet.

Age. Age plays an important role in determining water needs. High fluid intake (via breast milk or formula) is critical during infancy because an infant's body content of water is large (approximately 70% to 75% of the total body weight) and because a relatively large amount of this total body water is outside of the cells and thus is more easily lost.

Other Dietary Factors. Certain dietary additives and medications can affect water requirements because of their natural diuretic effects. Several medications contain diuretics specifically for the purpose of reducing overall body fluid, as in the case of antihypertensive medications (e.g., hydrochlorothiazide [Dyazide], furosemide [Lasix], bumetanide [Bumex], torsemide [Demadex]). Individuals who are taking medications that promote water loss should be monitored for dehydration and electrolyte imbalance. Other dietary factors that have long been viewed as diuretics are alcohol and caffeine. However, studies that have evaluated the hydration status of individuals consuming caffeinated and noncaffeinated beverages did not differ, which indicates that caffeine did not negatively affect the total water balance when it was consumed in moderation.[4] Although alcohol does acutely increase urine output after ingestion (i.e., within the first 3 hours), the long-term effect (i.e., up to 12 hours) is

antidiuretic. Thus, alcohol intake does not appear to cause total body fluid loss over a 24-hour period (see the Drug-Nutrient Interaction box, "Drug Effects on Water and Electrolyte Balance").

Dehydration

Dehydration is the excessive loss of total body water. Relative severity can be measured in terms of the percentage of total body weight loss, with symptoms apparent after 2% of normal weight is lost. Initial symptoms include thirst, headache, decreased urine output, dry mouth, and dizziness. As the condition worsens, symptoms can progress to visual impairment, hypotension, loss of appetite, muscle weakness, kidney failure, and seizures. Chronic or severe dehydration is known to increase the resting heart rate; to contribute to kidney infections, gallstones, and constipation; and to adversely influence cognitive function, exercise performance (particularly in untrained individuals), and the maintenance of body temperature (i.e., thermoregulation).[2,5-8] Without correction, dehydration can advance to coma and death (see the Clinical Applications box, "Adverse Effects of Progressive Dehydration"). Fluid losses of more than 10% of body weight usually require medical assistance for a complete recovery.

Dehydration presents special concerns among elderly adults. The hypothalamus is the regulatory center for thirst, hunger, body temperature, water balance, and

---

diuretic any substance that induces urination and subsequent fluid loss.

DRUG-NUTRIENT INTERACTION

DRUG EFFECTS ON WATER AND ELECTROLYTE BALANCE

Some medications can affect fluid and electrolyte balance. Anticholinergics such as amitriptyline (Elavil) and chlorpromazine (Thorazine) may result in a thickening of the saliva and dry mouth. Individuals who are using these medications should be advised to increase their fluid intake on a regular basis.

Antidepressants are divided into classes on the basis of their activity in the brain. Selective serotonin reuptake inhibitors (SSRIs such as Paxil, Zoloft, Prozac, Celexa), tricyclics, serotonin–norepinephrine reuptake inhibitors (SNRIs such as Effexor), and norepinephrine–dopamine reuptake inhibitors (NDRIs such as Wellbutrin) have oral and gastrointestinal side effects that include taste changes, nausea, vomiting, and dry mouth. Patients can avoid some of the negative side effects by drinking 2 to 3 L water per day and maintaining a consistent sodium intake.

Corticosteroids such as prednisone, methylprednisolone, and hydrocortisone increase the excretion of several nutrients, including potassium. Patients should be encouraged to increase their daily intake of fluids and of foods that are high in potassium to maintain an adequate body balance.

Loop diuretics (e.g., Lasix) and thiazide diuretics (e.g., hydrochlorothiazide) are both used to treat hypertension by increasing the urinary excretion of fluids. Minerals are lost in the urine along with fluid excretion. Patients who are taking these drugs should increase the amount of fresh fruits and vegetables in their diets and to eat other foods that are good sources of potassium. Although sodium and chloride also are lost in the urine, it is not necessary to increase the intake of these electrolytes, as long as the individual is consuming a normal varied diet.

Potassium-sparing diuretics (e.g., spironolactone) also work to rid the body of excess fluids, but they do so without wasting potassium in the urine. Therefore, patients should be careful to not use potassium-based salt substitutes so that they can avoid hyperkalemia (i.e., excessively high potassium levels in the blood).

Antipsychotics (e.g., phenothiazines, chlorpromazine) can cause a condition known as *psychogenic polydipsia*. Patients who are taking these drugs often experience dry mouth, and they will consume large amounts of water. If the patient's fluid consumption exceeds his or her capacity for excretion, this can result in hyponatremia and water intoxication. Symptoms of water intoxication include vomiting, ataxia, agitation, seizures, and coma.

CLINICAL APPLICATIONS

ADVERSE EFFECTS OF PROGRESSIVE DEHYDRATION

A loss of as little as 3% of total body weight from dehydration can result in impaired physical performance.[1] Physical performance is relative to the individual in question. A runner who is progressively losing body water in the form of sweat, without appropriate fluid replacements, will likely suffer from decreased speed or endurance. However, an elderly person who has also lost 3% of his or her body weight may suffer dramatically more complicated physical impairments (e.g., a fall that results in an injury).

Individuals with fever, diarrhea, and vomiting can lose body weight in the form of fluids quite rapidly. Likewise, the risk of dehydration increases in hot, humid environments and at altitudes of more than 8200 feet.[2] The figure shown in this box demonstrates the progressive complications that are associated with total body water loss. Note that the thirst response is not present until a loss of approximately 0.5% of the total body weight. This is why solely relying on thirst for an indication of fluid needs is not a sensitive indicator. By the time you are thirsty, you have already lost precious body water.

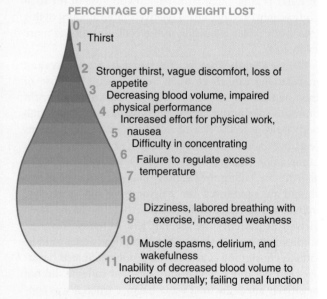

PERCENTAGE OF BODY WEIGHT LOST

0 — Thirst
1
2 — Stronger thirst, vague discomfort, loss of appetite
3 — Decreasing blood volume, impaired physical performance
4 — Increased effort for physical work, nausea
5 — Difficulty in concentrating
6 — Failure to regulate excess temperature
7
8 — Dizziness, labored breathing with exercise, increased weakness
9
10 — Muscle spasms, delirium, and wakefulness
11 — Inability of decreased blood volume to circulate normally; failing renal function

1. Kraft JA, Green JM, Bishop PA, et al. *Impact of dehydration on a full body resistance exercise protocol. Eur J Appl Physiol.* 2010;109(2): 259-267.
2. Rodriguez NR, DiMarco NM, Langley S. Position of the Academy of Nutrition and Dietetics, Dietitians of Canada, and the American College of Sports Medicine: Nutrition and athletic performance. *J Am Diet Assoc.* 2009;109(3):509-527.

blood pressure. However, physiologic changes in the hypothalamus naturally occur with age and, as a result, elderly individuals exhibit an overall decreased thirst sensation and reduced fluid intake when they are dehydrated compared with younger adults.[9,10] Other physiologic changes (e.g., diminishing kidney function) accompany the aging process and may exacerbate body fluid losses.

Water Intoxication

Although it is not nearly as common, water intoxication from overconsumption can occur. The excessive intake of plain water may result in the dangerous condition of hyponatremia (i.e., low serum sodium levels of less than 136 mEq/L). Under normal situations, excess water that is consumed is lost by increased urine output, and this is not likely to pose a problem for a normal healthy person who is eating an otherwise typical diet. However, individuals with renal insufficiency or neurologic disorders that affect the thirst mechanism and those who participate in heavy endurance exercise may not be able to dilute or excrete urine appropriately.

As blood volume is diluted with excess water, the water moves to the intracellular fluid (ICF) spaces to reestablish equilibrium with sodium concentrations there, thereby diluting ICF as well. This movement causes edema (Figure 9-1), lung congestion, and muscle weakness. Individuals who are at risk for hyponatremia from water intoxication are infants (if they are forced to drink by an adult), psychiatric patients with polydipsia, patients who are taking psychotropic drugs, and individuals who are participating

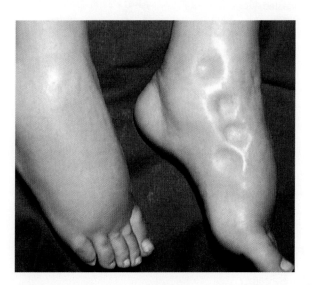

Figure 9-1 Edema. Note the finger-shaped depressions that do not rapidly refill after an examiner has exerted pressure. (From Thibodeau GA, Patton KT. *Anatomy & physiology.* 6th ed. St. Louis: Mosby; 2007.)

in prolonged endurance events without fluid and electrolyte replacement.[2]

WATER BALANCE

Body Water: The Solvent

Amount and Distribution

Normal body water content ranges from 45% to 75% of the total body weight in adults. Men usually have 10% more body water than women for an average of 60% and 50% of total body weight, respectively. Differences are generally attributable to a higher ratio of muscle to fat mass in males. Muscle contains significantly more water compared with adipose tissue.

Total body water is categorized into two major compartments (Figure 9-2).

Extracellular Fluid. The total body water outside of the cell is called the *extracellular fluid* (ECF). This water collectively makes up approximately 20% of the total body weight and 34% of the total body water. One fourth of the ECF (i.e., 4% to 5% of the total body weight) is contained in the blood plasma or the intravascular compartment. The remaining three fourths (i.e., 15% of the total body weight) is composed of the following: (1) water that surrounds the cells and bathes the tissues (i.e., interstitial fluid); (2) water within the lymphatic circulation; and (3) water that is moving through the body in various tissue secretions (i.e., transcellular fluid). Interstitial fluid circulation helps with the movement of materials in and out of body cells. Transcellular fluid is the smallest component of ECF (i.e., approximately 2.5% of total body water). Transcellular fluid consists of water within the gastrointestinal tract, cerebrospinal fluid, ocular and joint fluid, and urine within the bladder.

Intracellular Fluid. Total body water inside cells is called the *intracellular fluid*. This water collectively amounts to roughly twice the amount of water that is outside of the cells, thus making up approximately 40% to 45% of total body weight and 66% of total body water.

The relative amounts of water in the different body water compartments are compared in Table 9-2.

Overall Water Balance. Water enters and leaves the body by various routes that are controlled by basic mechanisms such as thirst and hormones. The average adult

polydipsia excessive thirst and drinking.

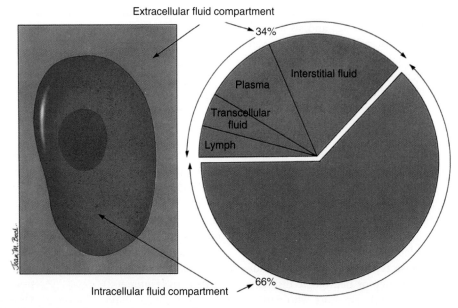

Figure 9-2 The distribution of total body water. (From Thibodeau GA, Patton KT. *Anatomy & physiology*. 6th ed. St. Louis: Mosby; 2007.)

TABLE 9-2 **VOLUMES OF BODY FLUID COMPARTMENTS AS A PERCENTAGE OF BODY WEIGHT**

Body Fluid	Infant	Adult Male	Adult Female
Extracellular Fluid			
Plasma	4	4	4
Interstitial fluid	26	16	11
Intracellular Fluid	45	40	35
Total	75	60	50

(Copyright JupiterImages Corp.)

Reprinted from Thibodeau GA, Patton KT. *Anatomy & physiology*. 6th ed. St. Louis: Mosby; 2007. Illustration copyright Rolin Graphics.

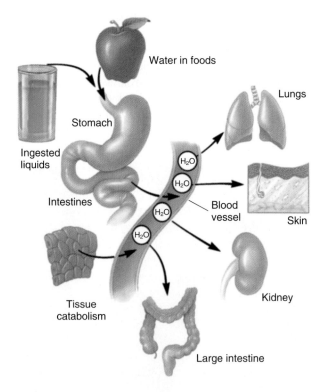

Figure 9-3 Sources of fluid intake and output. (From Thibodeau GA, Patton KT. *Anatomy & physiology*. 6th ed. St. Louis: Mosby; 2007.)

TABLE 9-3 **WATER CONTENT OF SELECTED FOOD**

Food	Water Content (%)
Apple, raw	86
Apricot, raw	86
Banana, raw	75
Bread, white	36
Bread, whole wheat	38
Broccoli, cooked	89
Cantaloupe, raw	90
Carrots, raw	88
Cheese, cheddar	37
Cheese, cottage	79
Chicken, roasted	64
Corn, cooked	70
Grapes, raw	81
Lettuce, iceberg	96
Macaroni/spaghetti, cooked	66
Mango, raw	82
Orange, raw	87
Peach, raw	89
Pear, raw	84
Pickle	92
Pineapple, raw	86
Potato, baked	75
Squash, cooked	94
Steak, tenderloin, cooked	50
Sweet potato, boiled	80
Turkey, roasted	62

Modified from the Food and Nutrition Board, Institute of Medicine. *Dietary reference intakes for water, potassium, sodium, chloride, and sulfate.* Washington, DC: National Academies Press; 2004.

metabolizes 2.5 to 3 L of water per day in a balance between intake and output.

Water Intake. Water enters the body in three main forms: (1) as preformed water in liquids that are consumed; (2) as preformed water in foods that are eaten; and (3) as a product of cell oxidation when nutrients are burned in the body for energy (i.e., metabolic water or "water of oxidation") (Figure 9-3). A variety of foods and their relative water content are listed in Table 9-3.

Older adults are at higher risk for dehydration as a result of inadequate intake and the physiologic changes that are associated with aging. Many older people suffer from xerostomia, which is caused by a severe reduction in the flow of saliva; this in turn negatively affects food intake. The condition may be associated with the use of certain medications, with certain diseases or conditions, or with radiation therapy of the head and neck. Conscious attention to adequate fluid intake (i.e., not less than the recommended minimum of 1500 to 2000 mL/day) is an important part of health maintenance and care in this population. Fluid intake should not depend on thirst, because the thirst sensation is an

TABLE 9-4 **AVERAGE DAILY ADULT INTAKE AND OUTPUT OF WATER**

Form of Water	Intake (mL/day)	Body Part	Output (mL/day)
Preformed		Lungs	350
In liquids	1500	Skin	
In foods	700	Diffusion	350
Metabolism (i.e.,	200	Sweat	100
the oxidation		Kidneys	1400
of food)		Anus	200
Total	2400	Total	2400

Modified from Thibodeau GA, Patton KT. *Anatomy & physiology.* 6th ed. St. Louis: Mosby; 2007.

indicator of present dehydration rather than an advance warning.

Water Output. Water leaves the body through the kidneys, skin, lungs, and feces (see Figure 9-3). Of these output routes, the largest amount of water exits through the kidneys. A certain amount of water must be excreted as urine to rid the body of metabolic waste. This is called *obligatory water loss,* because it is compulsory for survival. The kidneys may also put out an additional amount of water each day, depending on body activities, needs, and intake. This additional water loss varies in accordance with the climate, the physical activity level, and the individual's intake. On average, the daily water output from the body totals approximately 2400 mL, which balances the average intake of water.

Table 9-4 summarizes the comparative intake and output that affect body water balance.

Solute Particles in Solution

The solutes in body water are a variety of particles in varying concentrations. Two main types of particles control water balance in the body: electrolytes and plasma proteins.

Electrolytes

Electrolytes are small inorganic substances (i.e., either single-mineral elements or small compounds) that can dissociate or break apart in solution and that carry an

---

xerostomia the condition of dry mouth that results from a lack of saliva; saliva production can be hindered by certain diseases (e.g., diabetes, Parkinson's disease) and by some prescription and over-the-counter medications.

electrical charge. These charged particles are called *ions.* In any chemical solution, separate particles are constantly in balance between cations and anions to maintain electrical neutrality.

Cations. Cations are ions that carry a positive charge (e.g., sodium [Na^+], potassium [K^+], calcium [Ca^{2+}], magnesium [Mg^{2+}]).

Anions. Anions are ions that carry a negative charge (e.g., chloride [Cl^-], bicarbonate [HCO_3^-], phosphate [PO_4^{3-}], sulfate [SO_4^{2-}]).

The constant balance between electrolytes—specifically sodium and potassium—maintains the electrochemical and cell membrane potentials. Because of their small size, electrolytes can freely diffuse across most membranes of the body, thereby maintaining a constant balance between the intracellular and extracellular electrical charge. The fluid and electrolyte balances are intimately related, so an imbalance in one produces an imbalance in the other.

Electrolyte concentrations in body fluids are measured in terms of milliequivalents (mEq). Milliequivalents represent the number of ionic charges or electrovalent bonds in a solution. The number of milliequivalents of an ion in a liter of solution is expressed as mEq/L. Table 9-5 outlines the balance between cations and anions in the ICF and ECF compartments, which are exactly balanced.

Plasma Proteins

Plasma proteins—mainly in the form of albumin and globulin—are organic compounds of large molecular size.

They do not move as freely across membranes as electrolytes do, because the electrolytes are much smaller. Thus, plasma protein molecules are retained in the blood vessels, and they control water movement in the body and maintain blood volume by influencing the shift of water in and out of capillaries in balance with the surrounding water. In this function, plasma proteins are called *colloids,* which exert colloidal osmotic pressure (COP) to maintain the integrity of the blood volume. Cellular proteins help to guard cell water in a similar manner.

Small Organic Compounds

In addition to electrolytes and plasma protein, other small organic compounds are dissolved in body water. Their concentration is ordinarily too small to influence shifts of water; however, in some instances, they are found in abnormally large concentrations that do influence water movement. For example, glucose is a small particle that circulates in body fluids, but it can increase water loss from the body and result in a condition known as polyuria when it is in abnormally high concentrations (e.g., uncontrolled diabetes).

Separating Membranes

Two types of membranes separate and contain water throughout the body: capillary membranes and cell membranes.

Capillary Membranes

The walls of capillaries are thin and porous. Therefore, water molecules and small particles can move freely across them. Such small particles, having free passage across capillary walls, include electrolytes and various nutrient materials. However, larger particles such as plasma protein molecules cannot pass through the small pores of the capillary membrane. These larger molecules remain in the capillary vessel and exert COP to bring water and small molecules back into the capillary.

TABLE 9-5 BALANCE OF CATION AND ANION CONCENTRATIONS IN EXTRACELLULAR FLUID AND INTRACELLULAR FLUID*

Electrolyte	Extracellular Fluid (mEq/L)	Intracellular Fluid (mEq/L)
Cation		
Na^+	142	35
K^+	5	123
Ca^{2+}	5	15
Mg^{2+}	3	2
Total	155	175
Anion		
Cl^-	104	5
PO_4^{3-}	2	80
SO_4^{2-}	1	10
Protein	16	70
CO_3^{2-}	27	10
Organic acids	5	
Total	155	175

*This balance maintains electroneutrality within each compartment.

colloidal osmotic pressure (COP) the fluid pressure that is produced by protein molecules in the plasma and the cell; because proteins are large molecules, they do not pass through the separating membranes of the capillary walls; thus, they remain in their respective compartments and exert a constant osmotic pull that protects vital plasma and cell fluid volumes in these areas.

polyuria an excess water loss through urination.

Cell Membranes

Cell membranes are specially constructed to protect and nourish the cell's contents. Although water is freely permeable, other molecules or ions use channels within the phospholipid bilayer (see Figure 3-6) for passage across the membrane. The membrane channels are highly specific to the molecules that are allowed to pass. For example, sodium channels only allow sodium to pass, and chloride channels only allow chloride to pass.

Forces Moving Water and Solutes Across Membranes

A variety of forces are at work in the cell membrane to allow for the maintenance of dynamic equilibrium.

Osmosis

Osmosis is the movement of water molecules from an area with a low solute concentration to an area with a high solute concentration. When solutions of different concentrations exist on either side of selectively permeable membranes, the osmotic pressure moves water across the membrane to help equalize the solutions on both sides. Therefore, osmosis can be defined as the force that moves water molecules from an area of greater concentration of water molecules (i.e., with fewer particles in solution) to an area of lesser concentration of water molecules (i.e., with more particles in solution). Figure 9-4 illustrates how water will move from the 10% glucose solution across the semipermeable membrane to the 20% glucose solution to equalize

the solute concentrations. Because the membrane is permeable to glucose, the amount of glucose will also change on either side of the membrane to establish equilibrium.

Diffusion

As osmosis applies to water molecules, diffusion applies to the particles in solution. Simple diffusion is the force by which these particles move outward in all directions from an area of greater concentration of particles to an area of lesser concentration of particles (see Chapter 5). The relative movement of water molecules and solute particles by osmosis and diffusion effectively balances solution concentrations—and hence pressures—on both sides of the membrane. Again, refer to Figure 9-4, in which the two balancing forces of osmosis and diffusion are shown.

Facilitated Diffusion

Facilitated diffusion follows the same principles of simple diffusion in that particles passively move down a concentration gradient. The only difference is that, with facilitated diffusion, membrane transporters assist particles

---

osmosis the passage of a solvent (e.g., water) through a membrane that separates solutions of different concentrations and that tends to equalize the concentration pressures of the solutions on either side of the membrane.

osmotic pressure the pressure that is produced as a result of osmosis across a semipermeable membrane.

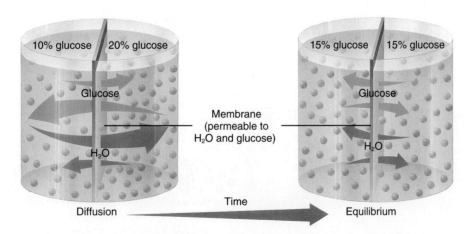

Figure 9-4 Osmosis and diffusion through a membrane. Note that the membrane that separates a 10% glucose solution from a 20% glucose solution allows both glucose and water to pass. The container on the left shows the two solutions separated by the membrane at the start of osmosis and diffusion. The container on the right shows the results of osmosis and diffusion after some time. (From Thibodeau GA, Patton KT. *Anatomy & physiology*. 6th ed. St. Louis: Mosby; 2007.)

with the crossing of the membrane. Some molecules (e.g., glucose) can diffuse across the cell membrane by either simple diffusion or facilitated diffusion, but they move much faster with the help of a transporter.

Filtration

Water is forced or filtered through the pores of membranes when the pressure outside of the membrane is different. This difference in pressure results from the differences in the particle concentrations of the two solutions, which cause water and small particles to move back and forth between capillaries and cells according to shifting pressures to establish homeostasis.

Active Transport

Particles in solution that are vital to body processes must move across membranes throughout the body at all times, even when the pressures are against their flow. Thus, energy-driven active transport is necessary to carry these particles "upstream" across separating membranes. Such active transport mechanisms usually require a carrier to help ferry the particles across the membrane (see Chapter 5).

Pinocytosis

Sometimes larger particles (e.g., proteins, fats) enter absorbing cells by the process of pinocytosis (Figure 9-5). In this process, larger molecules attach themselves to the thicker cell membrane, and they are then engulfed by the cell. In this way, they are encased in a vacuole, which is a small space or cavity that is formed in the protoplasm of the cell. In this small cavity, nutrient particles are carried across the cell membrane and into the cell. Once inside the cell, the vacuole opens, and cell enzymes metabolize the particles. Pinocytosis is one of the basic mechanisms by which fat is absorbed from the small intestine.

Tissue Water Circulation: The Capillary Fluid Shift Mechanism

One of the body's most important controls in maintaining overall water balance is the capillary fluid shift mechanism. This mechanism performs a balancing act between opposing fluid pressures to nourish the life of the cell.

Purpose

Water and other nutrients constantly circulate through the body tissues by way of blood vessels. However, to nourish cells, the water and nutrients must get out of the blood vessels (i.e., the capillaries) and into the cells. Water and cell metabolites, which are the products of metabolism that are leaving the cell, must then get back into the capillaries to circulate throughout the body. In other words, essential water, nutrients, and oxygen must be pushed out of the blood circulation and into the tissue circulation to distribute their goods throughout the body; at this point, water, cell metabolites, and carbon dioxide must be pulled back into the blood circulation to dispose of metabolic wastes through the kidneys or the lungs. The body maintains this constant flow of water through the tissues and carries materials to and from the cells by means of opposing fluid pressures: (1) hydrostatic pressure, which is an intracapillary blood pressure from the contracting heart muscle pushing blood into circulation; and (2) COP, which is pressure from the plasma proteins drawing tissue fluids back into the ongoing circulation. A filtration process operates according to the differences in osmotic pressure on either side of the capillary membrane.

Process

When blood first enters the capillary system from the larger vessels that come from the heart (i.e., the

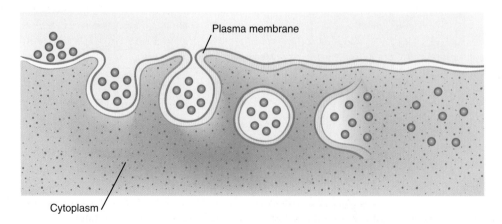

Plasma membrane

Cytoplasm

Figure 9-5 Pinocytosis; the engulfing of a large molecule by the cell.

arterioles), the greater blood pressure from the heart forces water and small particles (e.g., glucose) into the tissues to bathe and nourish the cells. This force of blood pressure is an example of hydrostatic pressure. However, plasma protein particles are too large to go through the pores of capillary membranes. When the circulating tissue fluids are ready to reenter the blood capillaries, the initial blood pressure has diminished. The COP of the concentrated protein particles that remain in the capillary vessel is now the greater influence. COP draws water and its metabolites back into the capillary circulation after having served the cells and carries them to larger vessels for blood circulation back to the heart. A small amount of normal turgor pressure from the resisting tissue of the capillary membrane remains the same and operates throughout the system. This fundamental fluid shift mechanism constantly controls water balance through its capillary and tissue circulation to nourish cells all over the body. This vital fluid flow through tissue is maintained by the balance between the blood pressure and the osmotic pressure of the plasma protein particles.

Organ Systems Involved

In addition to blood circulation, two other major organ systems help to protect the homeostasis of the body water: gastrointestinal circulation and renal circulation.

Gastrointestinal Circulation

Secretions that help with the process of digestion and absorption include saliva, gastric juice, bile, pancreatic juice, and intestinal juice. Of these secretions, all but bile are predominantly water. In the latter portion of the intestine, most of the water and electrolytes are then reabsorbed into the blood to circulate over and over again. This constant movement of a large volume of water and its electrolytes among the blood, the cells, and the gastrointestinal tract is called the *gastrointestinal circulation*. The sheer magnitude of this vital gastrointestinal circulation, as shown in Table 9-6, indicates the seriousness of fluid loss from the upper or lower portion of the gastrointestinal tract. This circulation is maintained in isotonicity with the surrounding extracellular water, and it carries a risk for clinical imbalances.

Law of Isotonicity. The gastrointestinal fluids are part of the ECF compartments, which also includes the blood. These fluids are isotonic, which means that they are in a state of equal osmotic pressure that results from equal concentrations of electrolytes and other solute particles. For example, when a person drinks plain water without any solutes or accompanying food, electrolytes and salts enter the intestine from the surrounding blood

TABLE 9-6 APPROXIMATE TOTAL VOLUME OF DIGESTIVE SECRETIONS*

Secretion	Volume (mL)
Saliva	1500
Gastric secretions	2500
Bile	500
Pancreatic secretions	700
Intestinal secretions	3000
Total	8200

*As produced over the course of 24 hours by an adult of average size.

TABLE 9-7 APPROXIMATE CONCENTRATION OF CERTAIN ELECTROLYTES IN DIGESTIVE FLUIDS (MEQ/L)

Secretion	Na^+	K^+	Cl^-	HCO_3^-
Saliva	10	25	10	15
Gastric secretions	40	10	145	0
Pancreatic secretions	140	5	40	110
Jejunal secretions	135	5	110	30
Bile	140	10	110	40

supply to equalize pressures. If a concentrated solution of food is ingested, additional water is then drawn into the intestine from the surrounding blood to dilute the intestinal contents. In each instance, water and electrolytes move among the parts of the ECF compartment to maintain solutions that are isotonic in the gastrointestinal tract with the surrounding fluid (see the Clinical Applications box, "Principles of Oral Rehydration Therapy").

Clinical Applications. Because of the large amounts of water and electrolytes involved, upper and lower gastrointestinal losses are the most common cause of clinical fluid and electrolyte problems. Such problems exist, for example, in cases of persistent vomiting or prolonged diarrhea, in which large amounts of water and electrolytes are lost. The large concentration of electrolytes involved in the gastrointestinal circulation is shown in Table 9-7.

Renal Circulation

The kidneys maintain appropriate levels of all constituents of the blood by filtering the blood and then selectively reabsorbing water and needed materials to be carried throughout the body. Through this continual "laundering" of the blood by the millions of nephrons in the kidneys, water balance and the proper solution of blood are maintained. When disease occurs in the kidneys and this filtration process does not operate normally, water imbalances occur (see Chapter 21).

CLINICAL APPLICATIONS

PRINCIPLES OF ORAL REHYDRATION THERAPY

Diarrhea is usually considered a trivial problem in developed countries, however; it is the second leading cause of death among children who are younger than 5 years old worldwide (pneumonia is the leading cause).[1] Although 90% of the deaths from diarrhea are associated with fluid loss, the mere provision of water alone can be dangerous. The principles of electrolyte absorption dictate appropriate rehydration methods for children with diarrhea.

Intravenous therapy, which was developed by Darrow in the 1940s, provided sodium chloride (a base) and potassium in water and proved to be very successful. Unfortunately, intravenous therapy is not readily available to those who need it most. A large number of isolated, poor, rural families in both developed and developing countries do not have access to health care facilities. Fortunately, the World Health Organization has developed a means of oral rehydration therapy that is much less expensive and that is being used in the United States as well as in developing countries. If safe drinking water is available, the oral rehydration salt solution packet can be mixed at home and administered by a care provider. The ingredients of the oral rehydration salt packets are 2.6 g of sodium chloride (table salt), 2.9 g of trisodium citrate dihydrate, 1.5 g of potassium chloride (or a salt substitute such as Diamond Crystal or Morton Salt Substitute), and 13.5 g of glucose.[2] These salts are mixed with 1 L of safe water. (A premade formula such as Pedialyte [Abbott Laboratories, Abbott Park, Ill] is also appropriate.)

This combination is based on the principles of sodium absorption that have been observed in the small intestine.

Transport of Metabolic Compounds
A number of metabolic compounds—principally glucose but also certain amino acids, dipeptides, and disaccharides—depend on sodium to allow them to cross the intestinal wall.

Additive Effects
The rate at which sodium is absorbed depends on the presence of substances such as glucose or other protein metabolic products. The more substances that are present, the better the absorption of sodium will be.

Water Absorption
The rate of water absorption is enhanced as sodium absorption improves. Thus, a solution of sodium and potassium salts plus glucose can be given orally.

In addition to oral rehydration therapy, infants and older children with acute diarrhea should continue to eat well-tolerated foods. Fasting practices were based on the former belief that recovery is more effective if the bowel is allowed to rest and heal. To the contrary, children should be fed their regular age-appropriate diets (i.e., breast milk, formula, or solid foods), allowed to determine the amount of food that they need, and given extra food as the diarrhea subsides to recover nutritional deficits. Food choices should be guided by individual tolerances. The use of the BRAT diet (**b**ananas, **r**ice, **a**pplesauce, and **t**ea or **t**oast) is not recommended, because it does not include typical foods that are consumed by infants and small children and only worsens the energy and nutrient decline.

1. World Health Organization. *Diarrhoea: why children are still dying and what can be done.* World Health Organization: Geneva; 2009.
2. World Health Organization. *Oral Rehydration Salts: Production of the new ORS.* World Health Organization: Geneva; 2006.

Hormonal Controls

Two hormonal systems help to maintain constant body water balance.

Antidiuretic Hormone Mechanism. Antidiuretic hormone, which is also called *vasopressin,* is synthesized by the hypothalamus and stored in the pituitary gland for release. Antidiuretic hormone conserves water, and it works on the kidneys' nephrons to induce the reabsorption of water. In any stressful situation with a threatened or real loss of body water, this hormone is released to conserve body water and to reestablish the normal blood volume and osmotic pressure (Figure 9-6).

Renin-Angiotensin-Aldosterone System. As blood flow through the kidneys drops below normal, the enzyme renin is released into the blood. Renin acts to convert angiotensinogen, which is produced by the liver and circulates within the blood, to angiotensin I. Angiotensin I travels to the lungs, where angiotensin-converting enzyme (ACE) converts it into angiotensin II. Angiotensin II results in vasoconstriction and triggers the release of aldosterone from the adrenal glands, which are located on top of each kidney. Aldosterone stimulates the kidneys' nephrons to reabsorb sodium (Figure 9-7). Therefore, the renin-angiotensin-aldosterone system is primarily a sodium-conserving mechanism, but it also exerts a secondary control over water reabsorption, because water follows sodium. Both antidiuretic hormone and aldosterone may be activated by stressful situations (e.g., body injury, surgery).

ACID-BASE BALANCE

The optimal degree of acidity or alkalinity must be maintained in body fluids to support human life. This vital balance is achieved with the use of chemical and physiologic buffer systems.

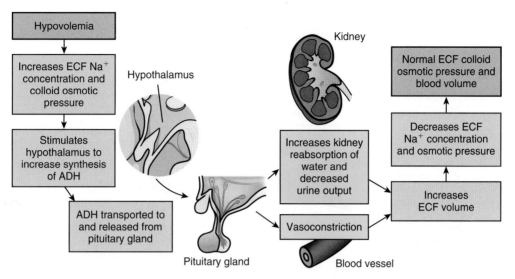

Figure 9-6 The antidiuretic hormone (ADH) mechanism. The ADH mechanism helps to maintain the homeostasis of extracellular fluid (ECF) colloid osmotic pressure by regulating its volume and electrolyte concentration.

Acids and Bases

The concept of acids and bases relates to hydrogen ion concentration. Acidity is expressed in terms of pH. The abbreviation *pH* is derived from a mathematical term that refers to the power of the hydrogen ion concentration. A pH of 7 is the neutral point between an acid and a base. Because pH is a negative mathematic factor, the higher the hydrogen ion concentration (i.e., the more acid), the lower the pH number. Conversely, the lower the hydrogen ion concentration (i.e., the less acid), the higher the pH number. Substances with a pH of less than 7 are acidic, and substances with a pH of more than 7 are alkaline.

Acids

An acid is a compound that has more hydrogen ions and that also has enough to release extra hydrogen ions when it is in solution.

Bases

A base is a compound that has fewer hydrogen ions. Thus, in solution, it accepts hydrogen ions, thereby effectively reducing the solution's acidity.

Acids and bases are the normal by-products of nutrient absorption and metabolism. As such, mechanisms to reestablish equilibrium within the body are constantly at work. Box 9-1 lists various sources of acids and bases.

Buffer Systems

The body deals with degrees of acidity by maintaining buffer systems to handle an excess of either acid or base.

BOX 9-1   SOURCES OF ACIDS AND BASES

Acids
Carbonic acid and lactic acid: the aerobic and anaerobic metabolism of glucose
Sulfuric acid: the oxidation of sulfur-containing amino acids
Phosphoric acid: the oxidation of phosphoproteins for energy
Ketone bodies: the incomplete oxidation of fat for energy
Minerals: chlorine, sulfur, and phosphorus

Bases
Minerals: potassium, calcium, sodium, and magnesium
Sodium bicarbonate
Calcium carbonate

The human body contains many buffer systems, because only a relatively narrow range of pH (i.e., 7.35 to 7.45) is compatible with life.

Chemical Buffer System

A chemical buffer system is a mixture of acidic and alkaline components. It involves an acid and a base partner that together protect a solution from wide variations in its pH, even when strong bases or acids are added to it. For example, if a strong acid is added to a buffered solution, the base partner reacts with the acid to form a weaker acid. If a strong base is added to the solution, the acid partner combines with it to form a weaker base. The carbonic acid (H_2CO_3)/bicarbonate ($NaHCO_3$) buffer system is the body's main buffer system for the following reasons.

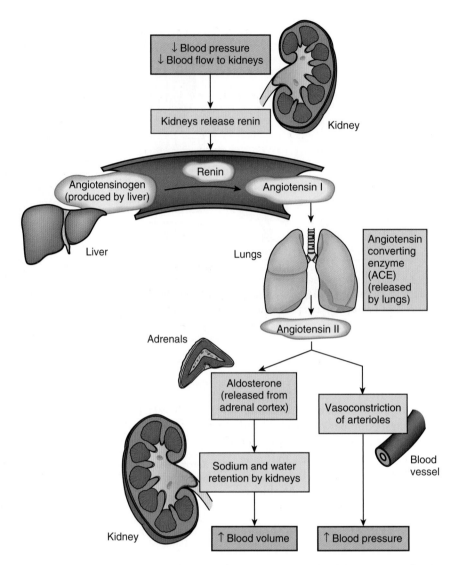

Figure 9-7 The renin-angiotensin-aldosterone mechanism. The renin-angiotensin-aldosterone mechanism restores normal extracellular fluid (ECF) volume when that volume decreases to less than normal by retaining sodium and water in the kidneys and vasoconstriction.

Available Materials. The raw materials for producing carbonic acid (H_2CO_3) are readily available: these are water (H_2O) and carbon dioxide (CO_2).

Base-to-Acid Ratio. The bicarbonate buffer system is able to maintain this essential degree of acidity in the body fluids because the bicarbonate (base) is approximately 20 times more abundant than the carbonic acid. This 20:1 ratio is maintained even though the absolute amounts of the two partners may fluctuate during adjustment periods. Whether or not additional base or acid enters the system, as long as the 20:1 ratio is maintained, over time, the ECF pH is held constant.

Physiologic Buffer Systems

When chemical buffers cannot reestablish equilibrium, the respiratory and renal systems will respond.

Respiratory Control of pH. With every breath, CO_2 (an acid) leaves the body. Therefore, changes in respiration rates can either increase or decrease the loss of acids. Hyperventilation (i.e., increasing the depth and rate of breathing) increases the release of CO_2, thereby combating acidosis. Conversely, hypoventilation (i.e., slowing down the depth and pace of breathing) retains CO_2, which ultimately increases the acidity of blood to alleviate alkalosis.

Urinary Control of pH. In the event that chemical buffer systems and the respiratory buffer system do not reestablish blood pH, the kidneys can adapt by excreting more or less hydrogen ions. If blood pH is too acidic, the kidneys will accept more hydrogen ions from the blood in exchange for a sodium ion. Because sodium ions are basic, blood is losing an acid (i.e., H^+) while gaining a base, thereby increasing blood pH back to normal.

Chemical and physiologic buffer systems are critical for maintaining the blood pH within an acceptable range for life.

acidosis a blood pH of less than 7.35; respiratory acidosis is caused by an accumulation of carbon dioxide (an acid); metabolic acidosis may be caused by a variety of conditions that result in the excess accumulation of acids in the body or by a significant loss of bicarbonate (a base).

alkalosis a blood pH of more than 7.45; respiratory alkalosis is caused by hyperventilation and an excess loss of carbon dioxide; metabolic alkalosis is seen with extensive vomiting in which a significant amount of hydrochloric acid is lost and bicarbonate (a base) is secreted.

SUMMARY

- The human body is approximately 45% to 75% water. The primary functions of body water are to provide the water environment that is necessary for cell work, to act as a transporter, to control body temperature, and to lubricate moving parts.
- Body water is distributed in two collective body water compartments: ICF and ECF. The water inside of the cells is the larger portion, which accounts for approximately 40% to 45% of the total body weight. The water outside of the cells consists of the fluid that is in spaces between cells (e.g., interstitial and lymph fluid), blood plasma, secretions in transit (e.g., the gastrointestinal circulation), and a smaller amount of fluid in cartilage and bone.

- The overall water balance of the body is maintained by fluid intake and output.
- Two types of solute particles control the distribution of body water: (1) electrolytes, which are mainly charged mineral elements; and (2) plasma proteins, which are chiefly albumin. These solute particles influence the movement of water across cell or capillary membranes, thereby allowing for the tissue circulation that is necessary to nourish cells.
- The acid-base buffer system, which is mainly controlled by the lungs and kidneys, makes use of electrolytes and hydrogen ions to maintain a normal ECF pH of approximately 7.4. This pH level is necessary to sustain life.

CRITICAL THINKING QUESTIONS

1. If a large amount of dietary sodium were consumed in one day, what effect would that likely have on the total body water level, and which compartment would be the most affected?
2. Define the term *homeostasis*. Give examples of how this state is maintained in the body.

3. Describe five factors that influence water requirements. List and describe four functions of body water.
4. Apply your knowledge of the capillary fluid shift mechanism to account for the gross body edema that is seen in malnourished individuals.

CHAPTER CHALLENGE QUESTIONS

Matching
Match the terms provided with the corresponding items listed below.

DEFINITIONS
1. The chief electrolyte that guards the water outside of cells
2. An ion that carries a negative electrical charge
3. A sodium-conserving mechanism or control agent

4. The simple passage of water molecules through a membrane that separates solutions of different concentrations from the side of a lower concentration of solute particles to the side of a higher concentration of particles, thereby tending to equalize the solutions
5. A substance (i.e., an element or compound) that, in solution, conducts an electrical current and that is dissociated into cations and anions

CHAPTER CHALLENGE QUESTIONS—cont'd

6. Particles in solution (e.g., electrolytes, protein)
7. The state of dynamic equilibrium that is maintained by an organism among all of its parts and that is controlled by many finely balanced mechanisms
8. The chief electrolyte that guards the water inside of cells
9. The major plasma protein that guards and maintains blood volume
10. The fluid that is located inside the cell wall
11. An ion that carries a positive electrical charge
12. The body's method of maintaining tissue water circulation by opposing fluid pressures
13. The force that is exerted by a contained fluid (e.g., blood pressure)
14. The movement of particles throughout a solution and across membranes outward from an area of a denser concentration of particles to all surrounding spaces
15. A type of fluid that exists outside of cells
16. The movement of particles in solution across cell membranes and against normal osmotic pressures that involves both a carrier and energy for the work

TERMS

a. Osmosis
b. Solutes
c. Diffusion
d. Cation
e. Interstitial fluid
f. Homeostasis
g. Anion
h. Potassium
i. Albumin
j. Hydrostatic pressure
k. Sodium
l. Electrolyte
m. Active transport
n. Aldosterone
o. Capillary fluid shift mechanism
p. Intracellular fluid

⊖volve Please refer to the Students' Resource section of this text's Evolve Web site for additional study resources.

REFERENCES

1. Cannon WB. *The wisdom of the body*. New York: WW Norton; 1932.
2. Food and Nutrition Board, Institute of Medicine. *Dietary reference intakes for water, potassium, sodium, chloride, and sulfate*. Washington, DC: National Academies Press; 2004.
3. Rodriguez NR, DiMarco NM, Langley S. Position of the academy of nutrition and dietetics, dietitians of canada, and the American college of sports medicine: nutrition and athletic performance. *J Am Diet Assoc*. 2009;109(3):509-527.
4. Maughan RJ, Griffin J. Caffeine ingestion and fluid balance: a review. *J Hum Nutr Diet*. 2003;16(6):411-420.
5. Manz F, Wentz A. The importance of good hydration for the prevention of chronic diseases. *Nutr Rev*. 2005;63(6 Pt 2):S2-S5.
6. Manz F. Hydration and disease. *J Am Coll Nutr*. 2007;26(5 Suppl):535S-541S.
7. Kraft JA, Green JM, Bishop PA, et al. Impact of dehydration on a full body resistance exercise protocol. *Eur J Appl Physiol*. 2010;109(2):259-267.
8. Merry TL, Ainslie PN, Cotter JD. Effects of aerobic fitness on hypohydration-induced physiological strain and exercise impairment. *Acta Physiol (Oxf)*. 2010;198(2):179-190.
9. Kenney WL, Chiu P. Influence of age on thirst and fluid intake. *Med Sci Sports Exerc*. 2001;33(9):1524-1532.
10. Farrell MJ, Zamarripa F, Shade R, et al. Effect of aging on regional cerebral blood flow responses associated with osmotic thirst and its satiation by water drinking: a PET study. *Proc Natl Acad Sci U S A*. 2008;105(1):382-387.

FURTHER READING AND RESOURCES

The following organizations provide up-to-date recommendations regarding water and electrolyte balance in addition to a plethora of other health information.

American College of Sports Medicine. www.acsm.org (search for fluid requirements)

Mayo Clinic, Food and Nutrition. www.mayoclinic.com/health/water/NU00283

Jequier E, Constant F. Water as an essential nutrient: the physiological basis of hydration. *Eur J Clin Nutr*. 2010;64(2):115-123.
Popkin BM, D'Anci KE, Rosenberg IH. Water, hydration, and health. *Nutr Rev*. 2010;68(8):439-458.
These two recent reviews address the importance of maintaining adequate hydration.

Robinson JR. Water, the indispensable nutrient. *Nutr Today*. 1970;5(1):16-23, 28-29.
This classic article by a New Zealand physician who is a world authority in this field clearly describes the processes that are involved in body water balance. This article is filled with excellent charts and diagrams to illustrate key principles.

CHAPTER **10**

Nutrition during Pregnancy and Lactation

KEY CONCEPTS

- The mother's food habits and nutritional status before conception—as well as during pregnancy—influence the outcome of her pregnancy.
- Pregnancy is a prime example of physiologic synergism in which the mother, the fetus, and the placenta collaborate to sustain and nurture new life.

- Through the food that a pregnant woman eats, she gives her unborn child the nourishment that is required to begin and support fetal growth and development.
- Through her diet, a breast-feeding mother continues to provide all of her nursing baby's nutrition needs.

Healthy body tissues depend directly on the essential nutrients in food. This is especially true during pregnancy, because a whole new body is being formed. The tremendous growth of a baby from the moment of conception to the time of birth depends entirely on nourishment from the mother. The complex process of rapid human growth and lactation demands a significant increase in nutrients from the mother's diet.

This chapter explores the nutrition needs of pregnancy and the lactation period that follows and recognizes the vital role that each plays to produce a healthy infant.

NUTRITIONAL DEMANDS OF PREGNANCY

Years ago, traditional practices and diet during pregnancy were highly restrictive in nature. They were built on assumptions and folklore of the past, and they had little or no basis in scientific fact. Early obstetricians even supported the notion that semistarvation of the mother during pregnancy was a blessing in disguise, because it produced a small, lightweight baby who was easy to deliver. To this end, physicians recommended a diet that was restricted in kilocalories, protein, water, and salt for pregnant women.

Developments in both nutrition and medical science have refuted these ideas and laid a sound base for positive nutrition in current maternal care. It is now known that the mother's and child's health depend on the pregnant woman eating a well-balanced diet with

 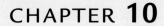

increased amounts of essential nutrients. In fact, women who have always eaten a well-balanced diet are in a good state of nutrition at conception, even before they know that they are pregnant. Such women have a better chance of having a healthy baby and remaining in good health compared with women who have been undernourished.

The nine months between conception and the birth of a fully formed baby is a spectacular period of rapid growth and intricate functional development. Such activities require increased energy and nutrient support to produce a positive, healthy outcome. General guidelines for these increases are provided in the comprehensive Dietary Reference Intakes (DRIs) issued by the National Academy of Sciences.[1-6]

The DRIs are based on the general needs of healthy populations. Some women (e.g., those who are poorly nourished when becoming pregnant or those with additional risks) require more nutrition support. The *Dietary Guidelines for Americans* also outline specific recommendations for pregnant and lactating women (Box 10-1).[7] This chapter reviews the basic nutrition needs for the

---

BOX 10-1 **DIETARY GUIDELINES FOR AMERICANS, 2010, FOR SPECIFIC POPULATIONS REGARDING PREGNANCY AND LACTATION**

General Recommendations
- Maintain an appropriate calorie balance during each stage of life, including childhood, adolescence, adulthood, pregnancy and breast-feeding, and older age.

For Women Who Are Capable of Becoming Pregnant
- Choose foods that supply heme iron, which is more readily absorbed by the body; additional iron sources; and enhancers of iron absorption, such as vitamin C-rich foods.
- Consume 400 micrograms per day of synthetic folic acid from fortified foods or supplements in addition to food forms of folate from a varied diet.

For Women Who Are Pregnant or Breast-Feeding
- Consume 8 to 12 ounces of seafood per week from a variety of seafood types.
- Because of their high methyl mercury content, limit white (albacore) tuna to 6 ounces per week and do not eat the following four types of fish: tilefish, shark, swordfish, and king mackerel.
- If pregnant, take an iron supplement as recommended by an obstetrician or another health care provider.

From the U.S. Department of Agriculture, U.S. Department of Health and Human Services. *Dietary guidelines for Americans, 2010.* Washington, DC: U.S. Government Printing Office; 2009.

---

positive support of a normal pregnancy, with emphasis placed on critical energy and protein requirements as well as on key vitamin and mineral needs.

Energy Needs

Reasons for Increased Need

During pregnancy, the mother needs more energy in the form of kilocalories for two important reasons: (1) to supply the increased fuel demanded by the metabolic workload for both the mother and the fetus; and (2) to spare protein for the added tissue-building requirements. For these reasons, the mother must include more nutrient-dense food in her diet.

Amount of Energy Increase

The national standard recommends an increase of 340 kcal/day during the second trimester of pregnancy and of approximately 450 kcal/day during the third trimester.[5] This brings the total kilocalorie recommendation to about 2200 to 2800 kcal/day for most women starting with the second trimester of pregnancy, which is an increase of about 15% to 20% over the energy needs of nonpregnant women. Active, large, or nutritionally deficient women may require even more energy. The emphasis always should be on adequate kilocalories to secure the nutrient and energy needs of a rapidly growing fetus. Sufficient weight gain is vital to a successful pregnancy; however, excess weight gain can pose risks and should be avoided. Increased complex carbohydrates, monounsaturated, and polyunsaturated fats, and protein in the diet are the preferred sources of energy, especially during late pregnancy and lactation.

Protein Needs

Reasons for Increased Need

Protein serves as the building blocks for the tremendous growth of body tissues during pregnancy, as follows:

- *Development of the placenta.* The placenta is the fetus's lifeline to the mother. The mature placenta requires sufficient protein for its complete development as a vital and unique organ to sustain, support, and nourish the fetus during growth.
- *Rapid growth of the fetus.* The mere increase in size of the fetus from one cell to millions of cells in a 3.2-kg (7-lb) infant in only 9 months indicates the relatively large amount of protein that is required for such rapid growth.
- *Growth of maternal tissues.* To support pregnancy and lactation, the increased development of uterine and breast tissue is required.

- *Increased maternal blood volume.* The mother's plasma volume increases by 40% to 50% during pregnancy. More circulating blood is necessary to nourish the fetus and to support the increased metabolic workload. However, with extra blood volume comes a need for the increased synthesis of blood components, especially hemoglobin and plasma protein, which are proteins that are vital to pregnancy. An increase in hemoglobin helps to supply oxygen to the growing number of cells. Meanwhile, plasma protein (albumin) production increases to regulate blood volume through osmotic pressure. Adequate albumin prevents an abnormal accumulation of water in tissues beyond the normal edema of pregnancy.
- *Amniotic fluid.* Amniotic fluid, which contains various proteins, surrounds the fetus during growth and guards it against shock or injury.
- *Storage reserves.* Increased storage reserves of tissue are needed in the mother's body to prepare for the large amount of energy that is required during labor, delivery, the immediate postpartum period, and lactation.

Amount of Protein Increase

Protein intake during pregnancy should increase by 25 g/day above nonpregnancy needs.[5] This increase is approximately 50% more than the average woman's protein requirement. However, high-risk or active pregnant women may require even more protein.

Food Sources

The only complete protein foods of high biologic value are eggs, milk, cheese, soy products, and meat (e.g., beef, poultry, fish, pork). Certain other incomplete proteins from plant sources such as legumes and grains contribute additional secondary amounts. Protein-rich foods also contribute other nutrients, such as calcium, iron, and B-complex vitamins. The amount of food from each food group that supplies the needed nutrients is indicated in the sample food plan given in Table 10-1 (see Chapter 4 for a discussion of dietary sources of protein and protein quality).

Key Mineral and Vitamin Needs

Increases in several minerals and vitamins are needed during pregnancy to meet the greater structural and metabolic requirements. These increases are indicated in the DRI tables that are inside this text's front cover. Because a growing fetus cannot be protected from the poor diet of the mother, special attention to the nutrients that pose a specific risk for deficiency is warranted.

Minerals

Calcium. A good supply of calcium—along with phosphorus, magnesium, and vitamin D—is essential for the fetal development of bones and teeth as well as for the mother's own body needs. Calcium is also necessary for blood clotting. A diet that includes at least 3 cups of milk or milk substitute daily plus dairy or dairy substitute products (e.g., calcium-fortified soy products) and generous amounts of green vegetables and enriched or whole grains usually supplies enough calcium. During pregnancy, physiologic changes occur in the mother's absorption capacity to help meet the needs of some nutrients; for example, calcium and zinc are both more bioavailable during pregnancy. The body's enhanced capability to absorb and retain these nutrients from the diet during pregnancy helps the mother to meet her nutrient needs as well as those of the growing fetus. Calcium supplements may be indicated for cases of poor maternal intake or pregnancies that involve more than one fetus. Because food sources of the two major minerals (i.e., calcium and phosphorus) are almost the same, a diet that is sufficient in calcium also provides enough phosphorus.

Iron. Particular attention is given to iron intake during pregnancy. Iron is essential for the increased hemoglobin synthesis that is required for the greater maternal blood volume as well as for the baby's necessary prenatal storage of iron. Iron deficiency anemia affects about 30% of low-income pregnant women and increases the risk of preterm delivery and low birth weight infants.[8] Because iron occurs in small amounts in food sources and because much of this intake is not in a readily absorbable form, the maternal diet alone rarely meets requirements, despite increased absorptive capacity during pregnancy. The current standards recommend a daily iron intake of 27 mg/day, which is significantly more than a woman's nonpregnant need of 18 mg/day.[4] Consuming foods that

---

hemoglobin a conjugated protein in red blood cells that is composed of a compact, rounded mass of polypeptide chains that forms globin (the protein portion) and that is attached to an iron-containing red pigment called *heme;* hemoglobin carries oxygen in the blood to cells.

plasma protein any of a number of protein substances that are carried in the circulating blood; a major one is *albumin,* which maintains the fluid volume of the blood through colloidal osmotic pressure.

TABLE 10-1 **DAILY FOOD PLAN FOR PREGNANT WOMEN**

This particular food plan is based on the average needs of a pregnant woman who is 30 years old, who is 5 feet and 5 inches tall, who weighs 125 pounds before pregnancy, and who is physically active between 30 and 60 minutes each day. Plans provided by the MyPlate.gov site are specific to each individual woman; however, this is an example for a woman of the described stature and activity level.

	First Trimester	Second Trimester	Third Trimester
	2200 kcal	2400 kcal	2600 kcal
▶Grains[1]	7 ounces	8 ounces	9 ounces
▶Vegetables[2]	3 cups	3 cups	3½ cups
Fruits	2 cups	2 cups	2 cups
▶Milk	3 cups	3 cups	3 cups
▶Meat & Beans	6 ounces	6½ ounces	6½ ounces
Make half of your grains whole.			
Aim for at least this amount of whole grains per day.	3½ ounces	4 ounces	4½ ounces
[2] **Vary your veggies.**			
		Aim for this much weekly	
Dark green vegetables	3 cups	3 cups	3 cups
Orange vegetables	2 cups	2 cups	2½ cups
Dry beans and peas	3 cups	3 cups	3½ cups
Starchy vegetables	6 cups	6 cups	7 cups
Other vegetables	7 cups	7 cups	8½ cups
Oils and Discretionary Calories			
Aim for this amount of oils per day.	6 teaspoons	7 teaspoons	8 teaspoons
Limit extras (extra fats and sugars) to this amount per day.	290 calories	360 calories	410 calories

These plans are based on 2200-, 2400-, and 2600-calorie food-intake patterns. The recommended nutrient intake increases throughout the pregnancy to meet changing nutritional needs.
From the U.S. Department of Agriculture, Center for Nutrition Policy and Promotion. *USDA's MyPlate home page* (website): www.choosemyplate.gov. Accessed August 23, 2011.

are high in vitamin C along with dietary sources of iron enhances the body's ability to absorb and use iron with a low bioavailability. In addition, avoiding foods that inhibit iron absorption (e.g., whole-grain cereals, unleavened whole-grain breads, legumes, tea, coffee) within meals that provide significant iron is recommended.

Because the increased pregnancy requirement is difficult to meet with the iron content of a typical American diet, daily iron supplements are often recommended. As with most supplemental forms of nutrients, bioavailability is suboptimal compared with food sources; thus, the encouragement of a balanced diet with ample iron is preferable (see Table 8-6 for a list of foods that are high in iron). Although there is limited research available regarding dietary supplement use in pregnant women, one report noted that adherence to iron supplementation is correlated with ethnicity and socioeconomic status.[9] Thus, additional encouragement and education for African-American, Mexican-American, and low-income women to continue taking appropriate iron supplements

during pregnancy may benefit both the mother and the fetus.

Many women believe that iron supplements will result in unpleasant gastrointestinal side effects. Historically, iron supplements given to pregnant women were in excessively high doses (e.g., 100 to 200 mg/day), in which cases some negative side effects were experienced. However, studies show that iron supplements that are taken between meals or at bedtime in doses of 20 to 80 mg/day are adequate to prevent iron-deficiency anemia with no clinical gastrointestinal side effects.[10]

Vitamins

Increased attention to most all vitamins is needed to support a healthy pregnancy. Vitamins A and C are needed in higher amounts during pregnancy, because they are both important elements in tissue growth. The need for B vitamins is increased because of the vital role of these vitamins as coenzyme factors for energy production and protein metabolism.

Folate. Folate builds mature red blood cells throughout pregnancy, and it is also particularly needed during the early periconceptional period (i.e., from approximately 2 months before conception to week 6 of gestation) to ensure healthy embryonic tissue development and to prevent the malformation of the neural tube. The neural tube forms during the critical period from 17 to 30 days' gestation, and it grows into the mature infant's spinal column and its network of nerves. Although the exact mechanism by which folate helps thwart neural tube defects (NTDs) is unknown, it is estimated that 46% to 70% of NTD cases could be prevented with adequate folate supplementation during and immediately before pregnancy.[11,12] Spina bifida and anencephaly are the two most common forms of NTDs, which are defined as any malformation of the embryonic brain or spinal cord. The Centers for Disease Control and Prevention estimates that, before the national fortification of grains with folic acid, there was an annual average of 4130 NTD-affected pregnancies in the United States. Following the 1998 federally mandated food fortification, the national average of NTD-affected pregnancies has declined by 27%.[13]

Spina bifida occurs when the lower end of the neural tube fails to close (see Figure 7-6). As a result, the spinal cord and backbone do not develop properly. The severity of spina bifida varies in accordance with the size and location of the opening in the spine. Disability ranges from mild to severe, with limited movement and function. Anencephaly occurs when the upper end of the neural tube fails to close. In this case, the brain fails to develop or is entirely absent. Pregnancies that are affected by anencephaly end in miscarriages or death soon after delivery.

The current DRIs recommend a daily folate intake of 600 mcg/day during pregnancy and of 400 mcg/day for nonpregnant women during their childbearing years.[2] Women who are unable to achieve such dietary recommendations by eating foods that are fortified with folate may do so with a dietary supplement. All enriched flour and grain products as well as fortified cereals contain a well-absorbed form of dietary folic acid. Other natural sources of folate include liver; dark green leafy vegetables; legumes (e.g., pinto beans, black beans, kidney beans); soybeans; wheat germ; orange juice; asparagus; and broccoli.

Vitamin D. As was mentioned in Chapter 7, vitamin D deficiency is a common worldwide problem, including among pregnant women. Vitamin D deficiency during pregnancy is linked with many adverse outcomes for both the mother and the fetus, including preeclampsia, gestational diabetes, and impaired growth of the fetus.[14-16]

Increased vitamin D needs to ensure the absorption and use of calcium and phosphorus for fetal bone growth can be met by the mother's intake of at least 3 cups of fortified milk (or milk substitute) in her daily food plan. Fortified milk contains 10 mcg (400 IU) of cholecalciferol (i.e., vitamin D) per quart, which is twice the Adequate Intake amount. The mother's exposure to sunlight increases her endogenous synthesis of vitamin D as well. Lactose-intolerant women or vegetarians can obtain adequate vitamin D from fortified soymilk or rice milk products.

Registered dietitians are an excellent resource for pregnant women who need help planning a well-accepted balanced diet. DRI tables that are inside this text's front cover list all nutrient recommendations for pregnant and lactating women. Many important nutrients are needed in higher quantities during pregnancy; only the ones that pose a significant risk for deficiency have been discussed here.

Weight Gain during Pregnancy

Amount and Quality

The mother's optimal weight gain during pregnancy, which should be sufficient to support and nurture both herself and her fetus, is essential. Appropriate weight gain is a positive reflection of good nutritional status, and it contributes to a successful course and outcome of pregnancy. The average weight gained is approximately 29 lb (Table 10-2). The Institute of Medicine recommends setting weight gain goals together with the pregnant woman in accordance with her prepregnancy nutritional status and her body mass index (BMI), as follows[17]:

- Underweight women (BMI of ≤ 18.5 kg/m^2): 28 to 40 lb
- Normal-weight women (BMI of 18.5 to 24.9 kg/m^2): 25 to 35 lb
- Overweight women (BMI of 25 to 29.9 kg/m^2): 15 to 25 lb

---

spina bifida a congenital defect in the embryonic fetal closing of the neural tube to form a portion of the lower spine, which leaves the spine unclosed and the spinal cord open to various degrees of exposure and damage.

anencephaly the congenital absence of the brain that results from the incomplete closure of the upper end of the neural tube.

TABLE 10-2 APPROXIMATE WEIGHT GAIN DURING A NORMAL PREGNANCY

Product	Weight (lb)
Fetus	7.5
Placenta	1.5
Amniotic fluid	2
Uterus (weight increase)	2
Breast tissue (weight increase)	2
Blood volume (weight increase)	3
Maternal stores: fat, protein, water, and other nutrients	11
Total	29

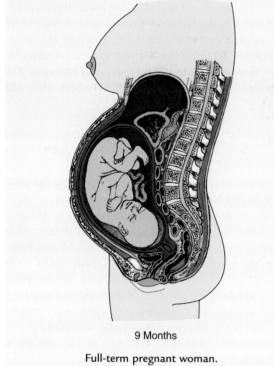

9 Months

Full-term pregnant woman.

(Reprinted from Lowdermilk DL, Perry SE. *Maternity & women's health care.* 9th ed. St. Louis: Mosby; 2007.)

- Obese women (BMI of ≥ 30 kg/m²): 11 to 20 lb
- Teenage girls: 35 to 40 lb (this is the upper end of the recommended range)
- Women who are carrying twins or triplets: 25 to 54 lb

Important considerations in each case are the quantity and quality of weight gain as well as the foods consumed to bring it about, which should involve a nourishing, well-balanced diet. Inappropriate weight gain (i.e., too much or too little) on the basis of the prepregnancy BMI is strongly associated with adverse pregnancy outcomes for both the mother and the infant (e.g., gestational hypertension; delivery complications, low or high birth weight).[18]

Severe caloric restriction during pregnancy is potentially harmful to the developing fetus and the mother. Such a restricted diet cannot supply all of the energy and nutrients that are essential to the growth process. Thus, weight reduction never should be undertaken during pregnancy. Special care for pregnant women who are suffering from eating disorders (e.g., anorexia nervosa, bulimia nervosa) is essential for the health of both the mother and the fetus.

Rate of Weight Gain

Approximately 1 to 2 kg (2 to 4 lb) is the average amount of weight gain that occurs during the first trimester (i.e., the first 3 months) of pregnancy. Thereafter, approximately 0.5 kg (1 lb) per week during the remainder of the pregnancy is typical, although there are exceptions. Only unusual patterns of gain (e.g., a sudden sharp increase in weight after the twentieth week of pregnancy, which may indicate abnormal water retention) must be watched. Alternatively, an insufficient or low maternal weight gain during the second or third trimester increases the risk for intrauterine growth restriction (IUGR). One study found that maternal weight changes from the first to second trimester were strongly associated with fetal femur and tibia lengths and infant length at birth, thus indicating a sensitive period during gestation for linear growth.[19] Increased energy demand is normal during late pregnancy and helps to prepare for full infant growth needs and the mother's approaching delivery and lactation. As always, carbohydrates selected from enriched or whole-grain breads and cereals, fruits, vegetables, and legumes are the preferred energy sources.

Daily Food Plan

General Plan

Ideally, some form of a food plan will be established for the pregnant woman on an individual basis to meet her increased nutrition needs. Such a core plan (see Table 10-1) can serve as a guideline, with additional amounts of foods used as needed to meet her caloric needs. This core food plan is built on basic foods that are available in American markets and designed to supply necessary nutrient increases. Energy needs increase as the pregnancy progresses, and the recommended addition of 340 to 450 kcal/day applies to the second and third trimesters.[5] However, adolescent, underweight, or

---

intrauterine growth restriction (IUGR) a condition that occurs when a newborn baby weighs less than 10% of predicted fetal weight for gestational age.

malnourished women require special attention to be paid to increased energy needs from the onset of the pregnancy.

Alternative Food Patterns

The core food plan provided here may be only a starting point for women with alternate food patterns. Such food patterns may occur among women with different ethnic backgrounds, belief systems, and lifestyles, thereby making individual diet counseling important. Specific nutrients (not specific foods) are required for successful pregnancies, and these may be found in a variety of foods. Wise health care providers encourage pregnant women to use foods that serve both their personal and nutrition needs. Many resources have been developed to serve as guides for a variety of alternative food patterns (e.g., ethnic, vegetarian). If the mother's vegetarian pattern includes dairy products and eggs (i.e., if she is a lacto-ovo vegetarian), achieving a sound diet to meet pregnancy needs is not a problem. Strict vegans can meet their dietary protein needs through the use of soy foods (e.g., tofu, soy milk, soy yogurt, soybeans) and complementary proteins (see Chapter 4 for additional information and resources that address planning a vegetarian diet).

Specific counseling about avoiding alcohol, caffeine, tobacco, and recreational drug use during pregnancy is also important. Information about the direct effects of poor nutrition on the fetus—especially related to brain development and developmental delays—helps to motivate many pregnant women to choose a well-selected diet of optimal nutritional value.

Basic Principles

Whatever the food pattern, two important principles govern the prenatal diet: (1) pregnant women should eat a sufficient quantity of high-quality food; and (2) pregnant women should eat regular meals and snacks and avoid fasting and skipping meals, especially breakfast.

GENERAL CONCERNS

Functional Gastrointestinal Problems

Nausea and Vomiting

"Morning sickness" (which actually has nothing to with the morning and can happen at any time throughout the day) affects about 75% of women during early pregnancy; it can be distressing and disruptive. It is most likely caused by hormonal adaptations to human chorionic gonadotropin during the first trimester, and it generally peaks at about 9 weeks' gestation.[20] Although pregnant women often resort to alternative treatments (e.g., acupuncture) for the relief of symptoms, to date these methods do not appear to be effective for treating nausea and vomiting in this population.[21] Some studies show improvements in symptoms with the dietary supplementation of vitamin B_6 and ginger, although findings are not consistent.[21-23] The following actions may help with the relief of symptoms: (1) eating small frequent meals and snacks that are fairly dry and bland and that consist of high-protein foods; (2) consuming liquids between (rather than with) meals; and (3) avoiding odors, foods, or supplements that trigger nausea.[20]

If nausea and vomiting persist past the first trimester and become severe and prolonged, then the woman may have a condition called hyperemesis gravidarum, and medical treatment is required. Approximately 1% of pregnant women develop hyperemesis gravidarum, and women who have experienced this condition with their first pregnancy are at a much greater risk for recurrence during any additional pregnancies (15.2%).[24] Patients with hyperemesis gravidarum should be closely followed for hydration, electrolyte balance, and appropriate weight gain. Prescription antiemetic medication may benefit some women in this situation (see the Drug-Nutrient Interaction box, "Antiemetic Medications").

Constipation

Although it is usually a minor complaint, constipation may occur during the latter part of pregnancy as a result of the increasing pressure of the enlarging uterus and the muscle-relaxing effect of progesterone on the gastrointestinal tract, thereby reducing normal peristalsis. Helpful remedies include adequate exercise, increased fluid intake, and high-fiber foods such as whole grains, vegetables, dried fruits (especially prunes and figs), and other fruits and juices. Pregnant women should avoid artificial and herbal laxatives.

Hemorrhoids

Hemorrhoids are enlarged veins in the anus that often protrude through the anal sphincter, and they are not uncommon during the latter part of pregnancy. This vein enlargement is usually caused by the increased weight of the baby and the downward pressure that this weight produces. Hemorrhoids may cause considerable

---

hyperemesis gravidarum a condition that involves prolonged and severe vomiting in pregnant women, with a loss of more than 5% of body weight and the presence of ketonuria, electrolyte disturbances, and dehydration.

discomfort, burning, and itching; they may even rupture and bleed under the pressure of a bowel movement, thereby causing the mother more anxiety. Hemorrhoids are usually controlled by the dietary suggestions given for constipation. Sufficient rest during the latter part of the day may also help to relieve some of the downward pressure of the uterus on the lower intestine. Hemorrhoids resolve spontaneously after delivery in many women, in which case long-term treatment is not necessary.

Heartburn

Pregnant women sometimes have heartburn or a "full" feeling. These discomforts occur especially after meals, and they are caused by the pressure of the enlarging uterus crowding the stomach. The gastric reflux of food may occur in the lower esophagus, thereby causing irritation and a burning sensation. This common symptom has nothing to do with the heart, but it is called "heartburn" because of the close proximity of the lower esophagus to the heart. The full feeling comes from general gastric pressure, the lack of normal space in the area, a large meal, or the formation of gas. Dividing the day's food intake into a series of small meals and avoiding large meals at any time usually help to relieve these issues. Comfort is sometimes improved by the wearing of loose-fitting clothing.

High-Risk Mothers and Infants

Identifying Risk Factors

Pregnancy-related deaths claim the lives of 500 to 600 women in the United States annually.[25] Identifying risk factors and addressing them early are critical to the promotion of a healthy pregnancy. Nutrition-related risk

---

DRUG-NUTRIENT INTERACTION

ANTIEMETIC MEDICATIONS

Antiemetics are prescribed to control nausea in a number of situations, including migraine headaches, chemotherapy, and postoperative nausea. Occasionally excessive nausea and vomiting during early pregnancy (i.e., hyperemesis gravidarum) can compromise the nutritional status of both the mother and the fetus as a result of food aversions or inadequate nutrient intake. In severe cases, a physician may opt to prescribe an antiemetic medication.[1]

One of these medications, Reglan (metoclopramide), may also be prescribed during lactation to stimulate the secretion of prolactin and thus increase the milk supply. Some nutritional implications of taking antiemetics include dry mouth, diarrhea, abdominal pain, and constipation. Phenergan (promethazine), which is another antiemetic option, may increase the patient's need for riboflavin.[2]

Kelli Boi

1. Flake ZA, Scalley RD, Bailey AG. Practical selection of antiemetics. *Am Fam Physician.* 2004;69(5):1169-1174.
2. Pronsky Z. *Food-medication interactions.* 15th ed. Birchrunville, Penn: Food-Medication Interactions; 2008.

CLINICAL APPLICATIONS

NUTRITIONAL RISK FACTORS DURING PREGNANCY

Risk Factors at the Onset of Pregnancy
- Age: 18 years old or younger or 35 years old or older
- Frequent pregnancies: three or more during a 2-year period
- Poor obstetric history or poor fetal performance
- Poverty, food insecurity, or both
- Bizarre or trendy food habits or eating disorder
- Abuse of tobacco, alcohol, or drugs
- Therapeutic diet that is required for a chronic disorder
- Poorly controlled preexisting condition (e.g., diabetes, hypertension)
- Weight: either less than 85% or more than 120% of ideal weight

Risk Factors during Pregnancy
- Anemia: low hemoglobin level (i.e., less than 12 g) or hematocrit level (i.e., less than 34%)
- Inadequate weight gain: any weight loss or weight gain of less than 1 kg (2 lb) per month after the first trimester
- Excessive weight gain: more than 1 kg (2 lb) per week after the first trimester
- Substance abuse (i.e., alcohol, tobacco, drugs)
- Gestational diabetes, pregnancy-induced hypertension, hyperemesis gravidarum, pica, or another pregnancy-related condition
- Poor nutritional status, especially involving folic acid, iron, or calcium
- Multifetal gestation

factors are listed in the Clinical Applications box, "Nutritional Risk Factors During Pregnancy."

To avoid the compounding results of poor nutrition during pregnancy, mothers who are at risk for complications should be identified as soon as possible. These nutrition-related factors are based on clinical evidence of inadequate nutrition. Do not wait for clinical symptoms of poor nutrition to appear. The best approach is to identify poor food patterns and to prevent nutrition problems from developing. Three types of dietary patterns that do not support optimal maternal and fetal nutrition are as follows: (1) insufficient food intake; (2) poor food selection; and (3) poor food distribution throughout the day.

Teenage Pregnancy

The United States has one of the highest teenage pregnancy rates seen among industrialized nations. The Centers for Disease Control and Prevention reports an annual rate of 70.6 pregnancies for every 1000 girls between the ages of 15 and 19 years.[26] Pregnancy at this early age is physically and emotionally difficult. From a nutrition standpoint, special care must be given to support the adequate growth of both the mother and the fetus. The current DRIs distinguish specific vitamin and mineral needs for pregnant females who are younger than 18 years old. See the For Further Focus box, "Pregnant Teenagers," for more information about health and nutrition for adolescent mothers.

FOR FURTHER FOCUS

PREGNANT TEENAGERS

Few situations are as life-changing for a single teenage girl and her family as an unintended pregnancy. Depending on how she and her family—as well as her partner—deal with the situation, lifelong consequences may occur for them as well as for the broader community. Adolescent pregnancy rates have historically been higher among African-American and Hispanic teens than among Caucasians in the United States, but rates are gradually declining in all ethnic groups[1] (see Figure).

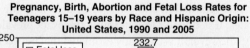

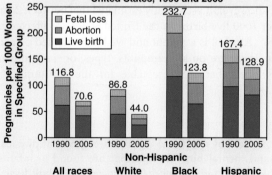

Pregnancy, Birth, Abortion and Fetal Loss Rates for Teenagers 15–19 years by Race and Hispanic Origin: United States, 1990 and 2005

From Ventura SJ, Abma JC, Mosher WD, Henshaw SK. *Estimated pregnancy rates for the United States, 1990-2005: an update* (website): www.cdc.gov/nchs/data/nvsr/nvsr58/nvsr58_04.pdf. Accessed October 9, 2011.

Pregnant teenagers are at high risk for pregnancy complications and poor outcomes, with increased rates of low birth weight and infant mortality. The following problems contribute to these complications: the physiologic demands of the pregnancy, which compromise the teenager's needs for her own unfinished growth and development; the psychosocial influences of a low income; inadequate diet; and experimentation with alcohol, smoking, and other drugs. Little or no access to appropriate prenatal care may also significantly contribute to a lack of nutrition support for the pregnancy. Early nutrition intervention is essential, and it can change the course of events and the pregnancy outcome. Changes from the inconsistent and often poor food pattern of teenagers may be difficult to achieve, and the care of these individuals is challenging. Experienced and sensitive health care workers in teen clinics emphasize the need for supportive individual and group nutrition counseling. The following suggestions may help to secure a positive and healthy environment for the teen.

Know Each Client Personally
All nutrition services must be tailored to the unique needs and characteristics of each pregnant teenager. Many of these girls have lower educational levels and even limited reading skills to which educational material must be adapted. Low-income teens lack the financial resources to maintain an adequate diet, and those who are living at home may have little control over the food that is available to them. Personal stress regarding the pregnancy is paramount, and nutrition concerns are often not a priority. Skipping meals and snacking instead is common, and even dieting is frequent.

Seek Ways to Motivate Clients
Schedule appointments on days that clients are coming in to pick up their food packages from the Women, Infant, and Children (WIC) Food and Nutrition Services program. Invite the teen's mother and her friends to accompany her to group counseling sessions so that they can support the recommendations that are made. Make each recommendation concrete and reasonable. Avoid scare tactics.

FOR FURTHER FOCUS—cont'd

PREGNANT TEENAGERS

Make Appropriate Assessments

Use simple and concrete forms to evaluate dietary intake (e.g., the basic food groups of the MyPlate.gov guidelines). A traditional model can be used, with increased amounts indicated for pregnancy, as both an educational and assessment tool.

Make Practical Interventions

Plan short, enjoyable, and active learning sessions. Use positive reinforcement liberally. Provide specific suggestions for carrying out changes at home. Review progress during follow-up sessions, and always maintain a positive and supportive atmosphere.

Support the Teenager's Responsibility

Help the teenager learn to be responsible. Pregnant teenagers must take on responsibility, often for the first time, for their own nourishment and the nourishment of others. Helping them in a supportive manner to understand and carry out this responsibility—which ultimately only they can do—is a primary objective of nutrition counseling. Nutrition consultants must be skillful so that they can establish the kind of rapport and relationship in which these responsibilities can develop and grow.

1. National Center for Health Statistics. *NCHS data on teen pregnancy.* Atlanta: Centers for Disease Control and Prevention; 2009.

Recognizing Special Counseling Needs

Every pregnant woman needs personalized care and support during pregnancy. However, women with risk factors such as those listed here have special counseling needs. In each case, the clinician must work with the mother in a sensitive and supportive manner to help her to develop a healthy food plan that is both practical and nourishing. Dangerous practices (e.g., fad dieting, extreme macrobiotic diets, attempted weight loss) should be identified early and corrected. In addition to avoiding dangerous practices, several special needs require sensitive counseling, including those related to age and parity, detrimental lifestyle habits, and socioeconomic problems.

Age and Parity. Pregnancies at either age extreme of the reproductive cycle carry special risks. Adolescent pregnancy adds many social and nutritional risks as its social upheaval and physical demands are imposed on an immature teenage girl. Sensitive counseling must involve both information and emotional support with good prenatal care throughout. Alternatively, pregnant women who are older than 35 years old and having their first child also require special attention. Pregnancy rates among women who are more than 35 years old continue to rise in the United States.[26] These women may be more at risk for high blood pressure and gestational diabetes, and they need guidance about the appropriate rate of weight gain and an effective dietary plan. In addition, women with a high parity rate (i.e., those who have had several pregnancies within a limited number of years) may be at increased risk for poor pregnancy outcomes,

because they enter each successive pregnancy drained of nutrition resources and usually facing the increasing physical and economic pressures of child care.

Alcohol. Alcohol use during pregnancy can lead to the well-documented fetal alcohol spectrum disorders (FASD), of which fetal alcohol syndrome (FAS) is the most severe form (Figure 10-1). Fetal alcohol spectrum disorders comprise the leading causes of preventable mental retardation and other birth defects in the United States. It is difficult to determine the exact prevalence of FAS; however, it is currently estimated that between 2 and 7 per 1000 live births in the United States are affected by FAS.[27] Alcohol is a potent and well-documented teratogen. There are no safe amounts, types, or times during pregnancy that are acceptable for the consuming of

---

fetal alcohol spectrum disorders a group of physical and mental birth defects that are found in infants who are born to mothers who used alcohol during pregnancy; the physical and mental disabilities vary in severity, and there is no cure.

fetal alcohol syndrome (FAS) a combination of physical and mental birth defects that are found in infants who are born to mothers who used alcohol during pregnancy; this is the most severe of the fetal alcohol spectrum disorders, and there is no cure.

teratogen a drug or substance that causes a birth defect.

CLINICAL APPLICATIONS

WHO WILL HAVE A LOW BIRTH WEIGHT BABY?

Infants who weigh less than 2500 g (5 lb 8 oz) at birth often present with medical complications and require special care in the newborn intensive care unit. Poor weight gain during pregnancy is a significant contributor to this problem.

Factors That Influence the Trend Toward More Low Birth Weight Babies
- Premature delivery
- Intrauterine growth restriction
- Health complications of the mother, including disease or infection
- Material use of cigarettes, alcohol, and drugs
- Inadequate maternal weight gain
- Poor socioeconomic factors

Reducing the Risk of Low Birth Weight Infants
- Maintain regular eating patterns throughout pregnancy, and be sure to consume an adequate amount of energy and nutrients.
- Take a multivitamin that contains 400 mcg of folic acid before becoming pregnant and one that contains 600 mcg while pregnant.
- Stop using cigarettes, alcohol, and drugs.
- Get early and regular prenatal care.
- Carefully control any preexisting conditions (e.g., diabetes, hypertension).
- Contact your health care providers immediately if preterm labor is suspected.[1]

March of Dimes, *Low Birthweight*. 2008, Access November 2010; Available from: http://www.marchofdimes.com/professionals/medicalresources_lowbirthweight.html.

alcohol. FAS is 100% preventable by abstaining from alcohol during gestation.[28] A study that compared the risk of FAS among different ethnic and socioeconomic groups of women found that the relative risk for FAS varies among populations and that it is influenced by environmental and behavioral conditions in addition to prepregnancy BMI and nutrition status; however, no ethnic or socioeconomic group is without incidence.[29]

Nicotine. Cigarette smoking or exposure to environmental tobacco smoke during pregnancy is associated with placental abnormalities and fetal damage, including

prematurity and low birth weight (see the Clinical Applications box, "Who Will Have a Low Birth Weight Baby?").[30-32] An estimated 18% of pregnant women continue to smoke cigarettes during pregnancy, which contributes to complications and poor fetal outcome.[33]

Drugs. Drug use, whether medicinal or recreational, poses many problems for both the mother and the fetus, especially when it involves the use of illegal drugs. Self-medication with over-the-counter drugs also may present adverse effects. Drugs cross the placenta and enter the fetal circulation, thereby creating a potential addiction in the unborn child. Dangers come from the drugs themselves, the use of contaminated needles, and the impurities that are contained in street drugs.

Vitamin abuse from megadosing with basic nutrients such as vitamin A during pregnancy also may cause fetal damage. Drugs made from vitamin A compounds (e.g., retinoids such as tretinoin [Accutane], which are prescribed for severe acne) have caused the spontaneous abortion of malformed fetuses by women who conceived during acne treatment. Thus, the use of these drugs without contraception is contraindicated.

Caffeine. Caffeine use is common during pregnancy. However, caffeine can cross the placenta and enter the fetal circulation. One cup of coffee contains approximately 100 mg of caffeine, and caffeinated soft drinks range between 10 and 50 mg of caffeine per 12-oz serving. Caffeine stays in the bloodstream longer in pregnant women than other adults.[34] Studies have found conflicting results regarding the effects of caffeine on pregnancy

Microcephaly

Epicanthal folds

Small palpebral fissure

Retrognathia

Figure 10-1 Fetal alcohol syndrome. (Reprinted from Thibodeau GA, Patton KG. *Anatomy & physiology*. 6th ed. St.: Mosby; 2007.)

outcome. A recent study of 2643 pregnant women in the United Kingdom found an increase in the prevalence of miscarriage and stillbirth among women who consumed more than 100 mg caffeine per day.[35] However, another large-scale meta-analysis concluded that moderate amounts of caffeine throughout the day do not have negative effects on reproduction or fetal health.[36]

Pica. Pica is the craving for and the purposeful consumption of nonfood items (e.g., chalk, laundry starch, clay). It is a practice that is sometimes seen in pregnant or malnourished individuals. Although the mechanism is not known, pica is significantly associated with iron-deficiency anemia as well as other contributing factors.[37] Although pica may occur in any population group, worldwide it is most common among pregnant women. The practice of eating nonfood substances can introduce pathogens (e.g., bacteria, worms) and inhibit micronutrient absorption, thereby resulting in various deficiencies. Most patients do not readily report the practice of pica; therefore, practitioners should always ask patients directly about their consumption of any nonfood substances.

Socioeconomic Problems. Special counseling is often needed for women and young girls who live in low-income situations. Poverty especially puts pregnant women in grave danger, because they need resources for financial assistance and food supplements. Dietitians and social workers on the health care team can provide special counseling and referrals. Community resources include programs such as the Special Supplemental Nutrition Program for Women, Infants and Children, known as *WIC,* which has helped to improve the health and well-being of many children in the United States (Figure 10-2). WIC also provides nutrition education counseling regarding the nutrition needs of both the mothers and their babies.

Complications of Pregnancy

Anemia

Iron-deficiency anemia is the most common nutritional deficiency worldwide. Although a disproportionate amount of these cases occur in underdeveloped countries, approximately 42% of pregnant women worldwide experience iron-deficiency anemia. The prevalence ranges greatly, from 6.1% in North America to 55.8% in Africa.[38] Anemia is more prevalent among poor women, many of whom live on marginal diets that lack iron-rich foods, but it is by no means restricted to lower socioeconomic groups. Dietary intake must be improved and supplements used as necessary to avoid the long-term detrimental effects on the fetus of nutritional deficiencies during

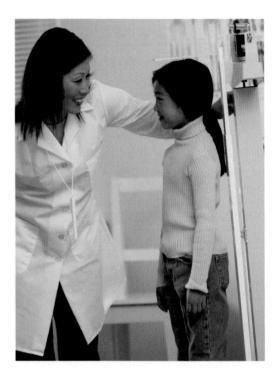

Figure 10-2 Measuring a child's growth at a Women, Infant, and Children Food and Nutrition Services appointment. (Copyright Photos.com.)

gestation. As a result of the severe complications of both iron- and folate-deficiency anemia, the World Health Organization currently recommends a weekly iron and folic acid dietary supplement as a safe, effective, and inexpensive way to prevent nutritional deficiencies during pregnancy.[39]

Neural Tube Defects

As previously discussed, the DRIs of 400 mcg/day of folate for women who are capable of becoming pregnant is increased to 600 mcg/day during pregnancy.[2] This is especially important when individual dietary adequacy is doubtful or if there is a genetic risk for NTDs in the family. Women who do not take folate supplements or who do not frequently consume fruit, juices, whole-grain or fortified cereals, or green leafy vegetables are more likely to have less-than-optimal folate intake.

Intrauterine Growth Restriction

IUGR occurs when an infant weighs less than the 10th percentile of the predicted fetal weight for gestational age. Women with high-risk pregnancies have an elevated risk of IUGR. A fetus with IUGR is at risk for preterm birth, being small for gestational age, and having a low birth weight.[40] Many factors may contribute to IUGR, but low prepregnancy weight, inadequate weight gain during pregnancy, and the use of cigarettes, alcohol, and other drugs are strong factors. Furthermore, infants who suffer from IUGR are at higher risk for the development of several chronic diseases as adults, including cardiovascular disease, type 2 diabetes, and obesity.

Hypertensive Disorders of Pregnancy

The etiology of pregnancy-induced hypertension is unknown, but it is a leading cause of pregnancy-related death. Pregnancy-induced hypertension includes several classifications:

- *Gestational hypertension:* blood pressure of more than 140/90 mmHg
- *Preeclampsia:* gestational hypertension plus proteinuria
- *Eclampsia:* preeclampsia plus seizures
- *HELLP syndrome:* **h**emolysis, **e**levated **l**iver enzymes, and **l**ow **p**latelets

Complications of pregnancy-induced hypertension often require hospitalization and induced labor. Studies have shown that calcium supplementation reduced the risk for hypertension in women who were pregnant for the first time and especially in those with low calcium intake to begin with, although the disorder is not thought to be exclusively associated with diet.[41] Specific treatment varies according to individual symptoms and needs; however, in any case, optimal nutrition is important, and prompt medical attention is required. Early and consistent prenatal care is imperative to identify risks early during the pregnancy. The only cure for severe cases is termination or the delivery of the infant.

Gestational Diabetes

Gestational diabetes is defined as any degree of glucose intolerance with onset during pregnancy, and the definition applies regardless of whether insulin or only diet modification is used for treatment. The prevalence of gestational diabetes in the United States is approximately 7% of all pregnancies (roughly 200,000) annually.[42] Prenatal clinics routinely screen pregnant women between 24 and 28 weeks' gestation with a 50-g oral glucose challenge. Careful follow-up is provided for those who show glucosuria or who meet the following diagnostic criteria: they have a random blood glucose level of more than 200 mg/dL (11.1 mmol/L) or a fasting blood glucose level of more than 126 mg/dL (7.0 mmol/L), or they fail to clear glucose from the bloodstream within the specified time after an oral glucose tolerance test. Particular attention is given to women who are at higher risk for the development of gestational diabetes, including those who are 30 years old and older who are overweight (i.e., those with a

BMI of ≥ 26 kg/m^2) and who have a history of any of the following predisposing factors:

- Previous history of gestational diabetes
- Family history of diabetes or ethnicity associated with a high incidence of diabetes
- Glucosuria
- Obesity
- Previous delivery of a large baby weighing 4.5 kg (10 lb) or more

Gestational diabetes occurs more frequently among African Americans, Hispanic and Latino Americans, Asian Americans, Pacific Islanders, and Native Americans. From 20% to 50% of women with gestational diabetes subsequently develop type 2 diabetes later in life, and they are more likely to develop cardiovascular disease and metabolic syndrome at an early age, especially those who also have a family history of type 2 diabetes.[43,44] Therefore, identifying and providing close follow-up testing and treatment with a well-balanced diet, exercise, and insulin (as needed) are important interventions. These women are at higher risk for fetal damage (i.e., birth defects or stillbirth), prematurity, macrosomia, and neonatal hypoglycemia. Children who are born to women with gestational diabetes are at greater risk for having impaired glucose tolerance, being overweight, and developing metabolic syndrome during adolescence.[45]

Preexisting Disease

Preexisting diseases (e.g., cardiovascular diseases, hypertension, type 1 or 2 diabetes) can cause complications during pregnancy. Inborn errors of metabolism (e.g., phenylketonuria) and food allergies or intolerances (e.g., celiac disease, lactose intolerance) must also be taken into consideration and maintained under good control to mitigate any flare-ups or compromised nutrient intake. All potential preexisting diseases will not be discussed here, because pregnant women may have any combination of preexisting conditions.

In each case, a woman's pregnancy is managed—usually by a team of specialists—in accordance to the principles of care related to pregnancy and the particular disease involved. See Chapters 18 through 23 for major

---

pregnancy-induced hypertension the development of hypertension during pregnancy after the twentieth week of gestation.

stillbirth the death of a fetus after the twentieth week of pregnancy.

macrosomia an abnormally large baby.

nutrition-related diseases that require medical nutrition therapy.

LACTATION

The World Health Organization states that breast-feeding is "an unequalled way of providing ideal food for the healthy growth and development of infants."[46] Breast-feeding is recommended as the exclusive source of nutrition for infants who are up to 6 months old. After 6 months, iron-fortified complementary foods should be added to the basic diet of breast milk. The *Healthy People 2020* goals for breast-feeding are as follows[47]:

- 82% or more of mothers initiate breast-feeding during the early postpartum period
- 44.3% or more of mothers exclusively breast-feed through the first 3 months
- 60.5% or more of mothers continue to breast-feed through the first 6 months, and 23.7% or more exclusively breast-feed for the first 6 months
- 34% or more of mothers continue to breast-feed at 1 year

Trends

Approximately 79% of infants worldwide are breast-fed for the first year compared with 21.4% in the United States. Although the rates are still very low in the United States compared with other countries, breast-feeding here has been on the rise since the 1970s[48] (Figure 10-3). Breast-feeding initiation and continuation are higher among well-educated, older, married women of a higher socioeconomic status (see the Cultural Considerations box, "Breast-Feeding Trends in the United States").[49] The American Academy of Pediatrics recommends breast-feeding for at least the first 12 months postpartum.[50] However, only 43% of American mothers continue any form of breast-feeding past 6 months postpartum.[49] Most women report discontinuing breast-feeding because of difficulties such as sore nipples, the infant spitting up, and engorged breasts. With proper instruction and a caring environment, most of these difficulties can be overcome.

The Baby-Friendly Hospital Initiative

The Baby-Friendly Hospital Initiative, which was launched by the World Health Organization and the United Nations Children's Fund, has increased breast-feeding rates worldwide.[51] Box 10-2 outlines the 10 steps for successful breast-feeding that are recommended by the Baby-Friendly Hospital Initiative. Almost all women who choose to breast-feed their infants can do so. Well-nourished mothers who breast-feed exclusively provide adequate nutrition, with solid foods usually added to the baby's diet when the baby is approximately 6 months old.

Physiologic Process of Lactation

Mammary Glands and Hormones

The female breasts are highly specialized secretory organs (Figure 10-4). Throughout pregnancy, the mammary glands are preparing for lactation. The mammary glands are capable of extracting certain nutrients from the maternal blood in addition to synthesizing other compounds.

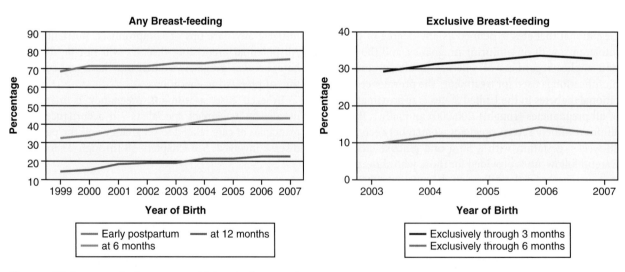

Figure 10-3 Breast-feeding among children in the United States. (Adapted from the Centers for Disease Control and Prevention. *Percent of U.S. children who were breastfed, by birth year, National Immunization Survey, United States, 2010* (website): www.cdc.gov/breastfeeding/ data/NIS_data/. Accessed October 9, 2011.)

CULTURAL CONSIDERATIONS

BREAST-FEEDING TRENDS IN THE UNITED STATES

Increasing the prevalence of breast-feeding continues to be a health goal both nationally and internationally, as is seen in the objectives of *Healthy People 2020* and the goals of the World Health Organization. The most recent report from the National Center for Health Statistics shows that the percentage of mothers who initiate breast-feeding has increased from 54.1% in 1986 to 75% in 2007.[1,2] The current national estimates for the percentage of U.S. children who were breast-fed at 6 months is 43%, and it is 22.4% at 12 months; this is just short of the current national goals.[2]

In the United States, breast-feeding is most common among women who are older than 30 years old; are Asian, Hispanic, and Latino; and have higher educations. A higher prevalence of breast-feeding is also noted among married women, and it is more common in the Western states (see map).[2]

PREVALENCE OF BREAST-FEEDING IN THE UNITED STATES

Selected Characteristics of Mother	Percentage Breast-Feeding at 6 Months
Total	43.0
Mother's Age at Baby's Birth	
≤ 20 years	22.2
20 to 29 years	33.4
≥ 30 years	50.5

Selected Characteristics of Mother	Percentage Breast-Feeding at 6 Months
Race or Ethnicity	
American Indian or Alaska Native	42.4
Asian	58.6
Black or African American	27.9
Hispanic or Latino	46.0
Native Hawaiian or Pacific Islander	45.3
White	45.1
Education	
Not a high school graduate	37.0
High school graduate	31.4
Some college	41.0
Collage graduate	59.9
Poverty Income Ratio*	
< 100%	34.7
100% to 184%	36.9
185% to 349%	45.0
≥ 350%	54.0

As a health care provider, be sure to note the perceived obstacles to the initiation and continuation of breast-feeding so that education and alternatives may be presented at the appropriate time (i.e., before delivery). The American

Percent of Children Exclusively Breast-fed Through 6 Months of Age among Children Born in 2007 (provisional)

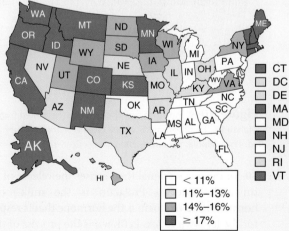

From the Centers for Disease Control and Prevention. *Percent of U.S. children who were breastfed, by birth year, National Immunization Survey, United States 2010,* Atlanta: Centers for Disease Control and Prevention; 2010.

CULTURAL CONSIDERATIONS—cont'd

BREAST-FEEDING TRENDS IN THE UNITED STATES

Academy of Pediatrics notes the following potential obstacles[3]:

- Insufficient prenatal education about breast-feeding
- Disruptive hospital policies and practices
- Inappropriate interruption of breast-feeding
- Early hospital discharge in some populations
- Lack of timely routine follow-up care and postpartum home health visits
- Maternal employment (especially in the absence of workplace facilities that support breast-feeding)

- Lack of family and broad societal support
- Media portrayal of bottle-feeding as normative
- Commercial promotion of infant formula through the distribution of hospital discharge packs
- Coupons for free or discounted formula
- Misinformation about what medical conditions may be contraindications for breast-feeding
- Lack of guidance and encouragement from health care professionals

*The poverty income ratio is the self-reported family income compared with the federal poverty threshold value. It depends on the number of people in the household.

References
1. National Center for Health Statistics. *Health, United States, with chartbooks on trends in the health of Americans*. National Center for Health Statistics: Hyattsville, Md; *2005*.
2. Centers for Disease Control and Prevention. *Percent of U.S. children who were breastfed, by birth year, National Immunization Survey, United States*. Centers for Disease Control and Prevention: Atlanta; 2010.
3. Gartner, LM, et al. *Breastfeeding and the use of human milk*. Pediatrics. 2005;115(2):496-506.

BOX 10-2   TEN STEPS TO SUCCESSFUL BREAST-FEEDING

1. Have a written breast-feeding policy that is routinely communicated to all health care staff.
2. Train all health care staff in the skills that are necessary to implement this policy.
3. Inform all pregnant women about the benefits and management of breast-feeding.
4. Help mothers to initiate breast-feeding within 30 minutes after birth.
5. Show mothers how to breast-feed and maintain lactation, even if they may be separated from their infants.
6. Give newborn infants no food or drink other than breast milk unless it is medically indicated to do so.
7. Practice rooming in: allow mothers and infants to remain together 24 hours a day.
8. Encourage breast-feeding on demand.
9. Give no artificial teats or pacifiers to breast-feeding infants.
10. Foster the establishment of breast-feeding support groups, and refer mothers to these groups when they are discharged from the hospital or clinic.

From the World Health Organization; United Nations Children's Fund. *The Baby-Friendly Hospital Initiative* (website): www.unicef.org/programme/breastfeeding/baby.htm. Accessed June 2011.

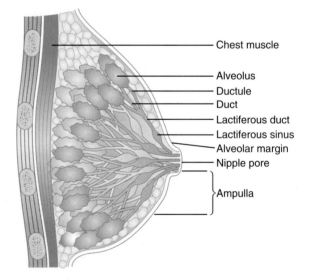

Figure 10-4 **Anatomy of the breast.** (Reprinted from Mahan LK, Escott-Stump S. *Krause's food & nutrition therapy*. 12th ed. Philadelphia: Saunders; 2008.)

The combined effort results in the nutrient-complete breast milk. After the delivery of the baby, milk production and secretion are stimulated by the two hormones prolactin and oxytocin.

The stimulation of the nipple from infant suckling sends nerve signals to the brain of the mother (Figure 10-5); this nerve signal then causes the release of prolactin and oxytocin. Prolactin is the milk-producing hormone, and oxytocin is the hormone that is responsible for the letdown reflex. Letdown is the process of the milk moving from the upper milk-producing cells down to the nipple for infant suckling.

Supply and Demand

Milk production is a supply-and-demand procedure. The mammary glands are stimulated to produce milk each

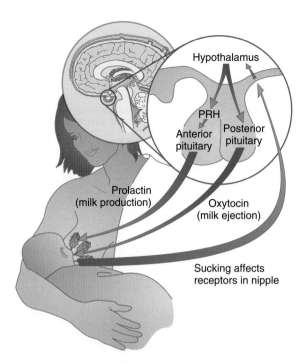

Figure 10-5 Physiology of milk production and the letdown reflex. *PRH,* Prolactin-releasing hormone. (Reprinted from Mahan LK, Escott-Stump S. *Krause's food & nutrition therapy.* 12th ed. Philadelphia: Saunders; 2008.)

time that the infant feeds. Therefore, the more milk that is taken from the breast (i.e., during breast-feeding or pumping), the more milk the mother produces, thereby always meeting the infant's needs. As a result of this supply-and-demand production, mothers of multiple infants (e.g., twins, triplets) are able to produce more milk with the additional stimulation. Some mothers of multiples find it easier to pump and then bottle-feed the infants the breast milk so that other members of the family can help with feedings.

Composition

Breast milk changes in composition to meet the specific needs of infants as they grow. Colostrum is the first milk that is produced after birth. It is a yellowish fluid that is rich in antibodies, and it gives the infant his or her first immune boost. Mature breast milk comes in within a few days after delivery, and the composition changes throughout each feeding as a result of the combination of fore, mid, and hind milk (hind milk is the highest in essential fatty acids). As you can see from Table 10-3, the composition of mature human milk is quite different from that of cow's milk. Cow's milk is an inappropriate food source for infants younger than 1 year old because of its high protein and electrolyte levels.

Nutrition Needs

The basic diet followed during pregnancy as well as the prenatal nutrient supplements used should be continued through the lactation period. The MyPlate food guide system provides specific nutrient information for pregnant and lactating moms at www.choosemyplate.gov/mypyramidmoms/index.html. The Daily Food Plan for Moms takes into account the mother's age, height, weight, and physical activity level; the infant's age; and how much breast milk the mom is producing to offer individualized recommendations. The Web site also provides help with menu planning for mothers with an easy-to-use interactive site.

Diet

Energy and Nutrients. Lactation requires energy for both the process and the product. Some of this energy may be met by the extra fat that is stored during pregnancy. The increased calorie recommendations are 330 kcal/day (plus 170 kcal/day from maternal stores) during the first 6 months of lactation and 400 kcal/day during the second 6 months of lactation compared with the woman's nonpregnant, nonlactating energy requirements. The requirement for protein during lactation is 25 g/day more than a woman's average need of 46 g/day (i.e., 0.8 g per kilogram of body weight body weight per day) for a total of 71 g/day (i.e., 1.1 g/kg body weight per day).[5] An example of a core food plan for meeting the nutrient needs of pregnant and lactating women is presented in Table 10-1.

Fluids. Because milk is a fluid, breast-feeding mothers need ample fluids for adequate milk production; their fluid intake should be approximately 3 L/day. Water and other sources of fluid such as juices, milk, and soup contribute to the fluid that is necessary to produce milk. Beverages that contain alcohol and caffeine should be avoided, because these substances pass into the breast milk.

Rest and Relaxation

In addition to the increase in diet and the adequate fluid intake, breast-feeding mothers require rest, moderate exercise, and relaxation. Because the production and letdown reflexes of lactation are hormonally controlled, negative environmental and psychologic factors contribute to the early cessation of breast-feeding.[52,53] Such factors are called *prolactin inhibitors,* and they include stress, fatigue, medical complications, lack of support, poor self-efficacy, and irregular breast-feeding. A lactation specialist can help by counseling mothers about their new family situations and by helping them to develop a plan to meet their personal needs.

TABLE 10-3 **NUTRITION COMPOSITION OF HUMAN MILK VERSUS COW'S MILK***

| Nutrient | HUMAN MILK | | | Cow's Milk |
	Colostrum	Transitional	Mature	
Kilocalories	67	72	74	70
Protein (g)	2.7	1.6	0.9	3.3
Carbohydrate (g)†	5.3	6.6	7.2	4.8
Fat (g)	2.9	3.6	4.5	3.7
Lactalbumin (g)		0.8	0.3	0.4
Fat-Soluble Vitamins				
A (IU)	296	283	240	303
D (IU)	—	—	5	4
E (mg)	0.8	1.32	0.2	0.06
K (mcg)	—	—	2.3	—
Water-Soluble Vitamins				
Thiamin (mg)	0.015	0.006	0.014	0.042
Riboflavin (mg)	0.029	0.033	0.035	0.16
Niacin (mg)	0.075	0.15	0.2	0.085
Pantothenic acid (mg)	0.183	0.288	0.18	0.3
Vitamin C (mg)	4.4	5.4	4.3	0.9
Folate (mcg)	0.05	0.02	0.52	0.23
Minerals				
Calcium (mg)	31	34	30	125
Phosphorus (mg)	14	17	15	96
Iron (mg)	0.09	0.04	0.03	0.04
Zinc (mg)	0.5	0.4	0.16	0.37
Magnesium (mg)	4.2	3.5	4	13
Iodine (mcg)	6	—	6	11
Electrolytes				
Sodium (mg)	5	19	17	76
Potassium (mg)	74	63	53	152
Chloride (mg)	58	30	37	108

Modified from Mitchell MK. *Nutrition across the life span.* 2nd ed. Philadelphia: Saunders; 2003.
*Per 100 mL.
†Lactose.

Long-Term Results of Feeding Methods

Risks of Formula Feeding

Medical professionals agree that breast-feeding is the normal means by which an infant should be fed and that other feeding methods carry risks for the infant. For decades, the literature has presented many benefits of breast-feeding. However, many researchers believe that it is more useful to present the risks of formula feeding as opposed to the benefits of feeding in a normal manner.[54] Another way to look at it is to assume that the many benefits of breast-feeding are only the normal expectations of infant feeding; therefore, infants who are receiving other forms of feeding would suffer the losses of such normal advantages. Because most research to date has focused on the benefits of breast-feeding instead of the

risks of formula feeding, it is only appropriate to present the scientific findings in the manner in which they were studied.

Advantages of Breast-Feeding

Many physiologic and practical advantages of breast-feeding are gained by both the mother and the infant; these are listed in Box 10-3. In a policy statement from the American Academy of Pediatrics, the authors cited the health benefits of breast-feeding for the infant, which include decreasing the incidence or severity of infectious diseases; increasing cognitive performance; and decreasing rates of sudden infant death syndrome, type 1 and 2 diabetes, lymphoma, leukemia, Hodgkin's disease, obesity, hypercholesterolemia, and asthma.[50] In addition, the mother receives many health benefits as well. Some noted

---

BOX 10-3   BENEFITS OF BREAST-FEEDING COMPARED WITH FORMULA FEEDING

BENEFITS FOR INFANTS

- Optimal nutrition for infant
- Strong bonding with mother
- Safe, fresh milk
- Enhanced immune system
- Reduced risk for acute otitis media, nonspecific gastro-enteritis, severe lower respiratory tract infections, and asthma
- Protection against allergies and intolerances
- Promotion of the correct development of the jaw and teeth
- Association with higher intelligence quotient and school performance through adolescence
- Reduced risk for chronic diseases such as obesity, type 1 and 2 diabetes, heart disease, hypertension, hypercholesterolemia, and childhood leukemia
- Reduced risk for sudden infant death syndrome
- Reduced risk for infant morbidity and mortality

BENEFITS FOR MOTHERS

- Strong bonding with infant
- Increased energy expenditure, which may lead to faster return to prepregnancy weight
- Faster shrinking of the uterus
- Reduced postpartum bleeding
- Delayed return of the menstrual cycle
- Decreased risk for chronic diseases such as type 2 diabetes and breast and ovarian cancer
- Improved bone density and decreased risk for hip fracture
- Decreased risk for postpartum depression; enhances self-esteem in the maternal role
- Time saved by not having to prepare and mix formula
- Money saved by not buying formula and from not having to pay the increased medical expenses associated with formula feeding

From James DC, Lessen R. Position of the Academy of Nutrition and Dietetics: promoting and supporting breastfeeding. *J Am Diet Assoc.* 2009; 109(11):1926-1942.

---

advantages of breast-feeding for the mother are decreased bleeding; an earlier return to prepregnancy weight; and decreased risks of breast cancer, ovarian cancer, and osteoporosis.[50]

The antibodies in human milk that are passed to the nursing infant make a significant contribution to the infant's immune system. In addition, a large-scale meta-analysis that was published by the World Health Organization concluded that breast-feeding is "associated with increased cognitive development in childhood, in studies that controlled for confounding by socioeconomic status and stimulation at home."[55] This means that breast-fed infants are cognitively advanced compared with formula-fed infants, despite differences in environmental influences, with a positive relationship seen between the duration of breast-feeding and the intelligence quotient of the child.[56]

Additional Resources

The Academy of Nutrition and Dietetics and the American Academy of Pediatrics encourage and strongly support breast-feeding for all able mothers for the first 12 months of life and continued thereafter for as long as mutually desired.[48,50] The American Academy of Pediatrics keeps updated breast-feeding information available for the public at www.aap.org/healthtopics/breastfeeding.cfm.

The World Health Organization has written and posted an entire chapter entitled "Infant and Young Child Feeding" for medical students and allied health professionals that is freely available online at whqlibdoc.who.int/publications/2009/9789241597494_eng.pdf. A multitude of additional resources about this topic are available from the World Health Organization at www.who.int/topics/breastfeeding/en/index.html.

SUMMARY

- Pregnancy involves the fundamental interaction of the following three distinct yet unified biologic entities: the placenta, the fetus, and the mother. Maternal needs also reflect the increasing nutrition needs of the fetus and the placenta.
- Optimal weight gain during pregnancy varies with the normal nutritional status and weight of the woman, with a goal of 25 to 35 lb for a woman of average weight. Sufficient weight gain is important during pregnancy to support the rapid growth that

is taking place. However, the nutritional quality of the diet is as significant as the actual amount of weight gain.

- Common problems during pregnancy include first-trimester nausea and vomiting associated with hormonal adaptations and, later, constipation, hemorrhoids, or heartburn that result from the pressure of the enlarging uterus. These problems are usually relieved without medication by simple and often temporary changes in the diet.

Continued

SUMMARY—cont'd

- Unusual or irregular eating habits, age, parity, pre-pregnancy weight status, and low income are among the many related conditions that put pregnant women at risk for complications.

- The ultimate goal of prenatal care is a healthy infant and a healthy mother who can breast-feed her child if she chooses to do so. Breast milk provides essential nutrients in quantities that are uniquely suited for optimal infant growth and development.

CRITICAL THINKING QUESTIONS

1. Which nutrients are required in larger amounts during pregnancy? Plan a 1-day diet that would meet the nutrient needs of a pregnant women during her third trimester.
2. Identify two common gastrointestinal problems that are associated with pregnancy, and describe the diet management of each.

3. Discuss the major nutritional factors that are needed to support lactation. What additional nonnutrition needs does the breast-feeding mother have, and what suggestions can you give to help her meet them?
4. Why is additional fluid needed for lactation?

CHAPTER CHALLENGE QUESTIONS

True-False
1. *True or False:* The development of the fetus is directly related to the diet of the mother.
2. *True or False:* Strict weight control during pregnancy is necessary to avoid complications.
3. *True or False:* Fat should be removed from the pregnant woman's diet to prevent edema.
4. *True or False:* A higher risk for pregnancy complications occurs among teenagers and older women.
5. *True or False:* A woman's diet before pregnancy has little effect on the outcome of her pregnancy.

6. *True or False:* No woman should ever gain more than 15 to 20 lb during pregnancy.
7. *True or False:* The rapid growth of the fetal skeleton requires increased calcium in the mother's diet.
8. *True or False:* Inadequate vitamin D intake during pregnancy contributes to skeletal development issues in the fetus.
9. *True or False:* Anemia is common during pregnancy.
10. *True or False:* Additional kilocalories and fluids are needed during lactation.

Multiple Choice
1. Maternal blood volume during pregnancy
   a. increases.
   b. decreases.
   c. remains unchanged.
   d. fluctuates widely.
2. Pregnant mothers are often prescribed supplemental iron. Studies show that iron supplements are effective for the prevention of
   a. edema.
   b. gestational diabetes.
   c. anemia.
   d. nausea and vomiting.
3. Women with gestational diabetes have an increased risk of developing what condition later in life?
   a. Osteoporosis
   b. Type 1 diabetes
   c. Type 2 diabetes
   d. Pregnancy-induced hypertension

4. Breast-feeding is the normal method of feeding an infant. Research shows that the benefits that breast-fed infants enjoy over their formula-fed counterparts include
   a. a decreased risk of obesity.
   b. a decreased risk of type 1 and 2 diabetes.
   c. a decreased risk of infectious disease.
   d. All of the above
5. Which of the following hormones is responsible for milk letdown during lactation?
   a. Prolactin
   b. Estrogen
   c. Oxytocin
   d. Human growth hormone
6. The World Health Organization and the American Academy of Pediatrics recommend breast-feeding for at least
   a. 3 months.
   b. 8 months.
   c. 12 months.
   d. 3 years.

⊜volve Please refer to the Students' Resource section of this text's Evolve Web site for additional study resources.

REFERENCES

1. Food and Nutrition Board, Institute of Medicine. *Dietary reference intakes for calcium, phosphorous, magnesium, vitamin D, and fluoride.* Washington, DC: National Academies Press; 1997.
2. Food and Nutrition Board, Institute of Medicine. *Dietary reference intakes for thiamin, riboflavin, niacin, vitamin B6, folate, vitamin B12, pantothenic acid, biotin, and choline.* Washington, DC: National Academies Press; 2000.
3. Food and Nutrition Board, Institute of Medicine. *Dietary reference intakes for vitamin C, vitamin E, selenium, and carotenoids.* Washington, DC: National Academies Press; 2000.
4. Food and Nutrition Board, Institute of Medicine. *Dietary reference intakes for vitamin A, vitamin K, arsenic, boron, chromium, copper, iodine, iron, manganese, molybdenum, nickel, silicon, vanadium, and zinc.* Washington, DC: National Academies Press; 2001.
5. Food and Nutrition Board, Institute of Medicine. *Dietary reference intakes for energy, carbohydrate, fiber, fat, fatty acids, cholesterol, protein, and amino acids.* Washington, DC: National Academies Press; 2002.
6. Food and Nutrition Board, Institute of Medicine. *Dietary reference intakes for water, potassium, sodium, chloride, and sulfate.* Washington, DC: National Academies Press; 2004.
7. U.S. Department of Agriculture, U.S. Department of Health and Human Services. *Dietary guidelines for Americans, 2010,* Washington, DC: U.S. Government Printing Office; 2010.
8. Kaiser L, Allen LH. Position of the academy of nutrition and dietetics: nutrition and lifestyle for a healthy pregnancy outcome. *J Am Diet Assoc.* 2008;108(3):553-561.
9. Picciano MF, McGuire MK. Use of dietary supplements by pregnant and lactating women in north America. *Am J Clin Nutr.* 2009;89(2):663S-667S.
10. Milman N, Bergholt T, Eriksen L, et al. Iron prophylaxis during pregnancy – how much iron is needed? A randomized dose-response study of 20-80 mg ferrous iron daily in pregnant women. *Acta Obstet Gynecol Scand.* 2005;84(3):238-247.
11. Beaudin AE, Stover PJ. Insights into metabolic mechanisms underlying folate-responsive neural tube defects: a minireview. *Birth Defects Res A Clin Mol Teratol.* 2009;85(4):274-284.
12. Blencowe H, Cousens S, Modell B, Lawn J. Folic acid to reduce neonatal mortality from neural tube disorders. *Int J Epidemiol.* 2010;39(Suppl 1):i110-i121.
13. Centers for Disease Control and Prevention. Spina bifida and anencephaly before and after folic acid mandate–United States, 1995-1996 and 1999-2000. *MMWR Morb Mortal Wkly Rep.* 2004;53(17)362-365.
14. Lewis S, Lucas RM, Halliday J, Ponsonby AL. Vitamin D deficiency and pregnancy: from preconception to birth. *Mol Nutr Food Res.* 2010;54(8):1092-1102.
15. Barrett H, McElduff A. Vitamin D and pregnancy: an old problem revisited. *Best Pract Res Clin Endocrinol Metab.* 2010;24(4):527-539.
16. Dror DK, Allen LH. Vitamin D inadequacy in pregnancy: biology, outcomes, and interventions. *Nutr Rev.* 2010;68(8):465-477.
17. National Academy of Sciences, Committee on Nutritional Status During Pregnancy and Lactation, Food and Nutrition Board. *Nutrition during pregnancy.* Washington, DC: National Academies Press; 1990.
18. Crane JM, White J, Murphy P, et al. The effect of gestational weight gain by body mass index on maternal and neonatal outcomes. *J Obstet Gynaecol Can.* 2009;31(1):28-35.
19. Neufeld LM, Haas JD, Grajéda R, Martorell R. Changes in maternal weight from the first to second trimester of pregnancy are associated with fetal growth and infant length at birth. *Am J Clin Nutr.* 2004;79(4):646-652.
20. Niebyl JR. Clinical practice. Nausea and vomiting in pregnancy. *N Engl J Med.* 2010;363(16):1544-1550.
21. Matthews A, Dowswell T, Haas DM, et al. Interventions for nausea and vomiting in early pregnancy. *Cochrane Database Syst Rev.* 2010;(9):CD007575.
22. Ensiyeh J, Sakineh MA. Comparing ginger and vitamin B6 for the treatment of nausea and vomiting in pregnancy: a randomised controlled trial. *Midwifery.* 2009;25(6):649-653.
23. Chittumma P, Kaewkiattikun K, Wiriyasiriwach B. Comparison of the effectiveness of ginger and vitamin B6 for treatment of nausea and vomiting in early pregnancy: a randomized double-blind controlled trial. *J Med Assoc Thai.* 2007;90(1):15-20.
24. Trogstad LI, Stoltenberg C, Magnus P, et al. Recurrence risk in hyperemesis gravidarum. *BJOG.* 2005;112(12):1641-1645.
25. National Center for Health Statistics. *Health, United States, 2010: with special feature on death and dying.* Hyattsville, Md: U.S. Government Printing Office; 2011.
26. Ventura SJ, Abma JC, Mosher WD, Henshaw SK. Estimated pregnancy rates for the United States, 1990-2005: an update. *Natl Vital Stat Rep.* 2009;58(4):1-14.
27. May PA, Gossage JP, Kalberg WO, et al. Prevalence and epidemiologic characteristics of FASD from various research methods with an emphasis on recent in-school studies. *Dev Disabil Res Rev.* 2009;15(3):176-192.
28. Centers for Disease Control and Prevention. *Fetal alcohol spectrum disorders (FASDs)* (website): www.cdc.gov/ncbddd/fasd/facts.html. Accessed November 2010.
29. May PA, Gossage JP, White-Country M, et al. Alcohol consumption and other maternal risk factors for fetal alcohol syndrome among three distinct samples of women before, during, and after pregnancy: the risk is relative. *Am J Med Genet C Semin Med Genet.* 2004;127C(1):10-20.
30. Leonardi-Bee J, Smyth A, Britton J, Coleman T. Environmental tobacco smoke and fetal health: systematic review and meta-analysis. *Arch Dis Child Fetal Neonatal Ed.* 2008;93(5):F351-F361.
31. Ward C, Lewis S, Coleman T. Prevalence of maternal smoking and environmental tobacco smoke exposure during pregnancy and impact on birth weight: retrospective study using Millennium Cohort. *BMC Public Health.* 2007;7:81.

32. Einarson A, Riordan S. Smoking in pregnancy and lactation: a review of risks and cessation strategies. *Eur J Clin Pharmacol*. 2009;65(4):325-330.

33. Substance Abuse and Mental Health Services Administration. *Results from the 2004 National survey on drug use and health: national findings, tobacco use*. Rockville, Md: Substance Abuse and Mental Health Services Administration, Office of Applied Studies; 2005.

34. Christian MS, Brent RL. Teratogen update: evaluation of the reproductive and developmental risks of caffeine. *Teratology*. 2001;64(1):51-78.

35. Greenwood DC, Alwan N, Boylan S, et al. Caffeine intake during pregnancy, late miscarriage and stillbirth. *Eur J Epidemiol*. 2010;25(4):275-280.

36. Maslova E, Bhattacharya S, Lin SW, Michels KB. Caffeine consumption during pregnancy and risk of preterm birth: a meta-analysis. *Am J Clin Nutr*. 2010;92(5):1120-1132.

37. Young SL. Pica in pregnancy: new ideas about an old condition. *Annu Rev Nutr*. 2010;30:403-422.

38. McLean E, Cogswell M, Egli I, et al. Worldwide prevalence of anaemia, WHO Vitamin and Mineral Nutrition Information System, 1993-2005. *Public Health Nutr*. 2009;12(4):444-454.

39. World Health Organization. *Weekly iron–folic acid supplementation (WIFS) in women of reproductive age: its role in promoting optimal maternal and child health. Position statement*. Geneva: World Health Organization; 2009.

40. Mook-Kanamori DO, Steegers EA, Eilers PH, et al. Risk factors and outcomes associated with first-trimester fetal growth restriction. *JAMA*. 2010;303(6):527-534.

41. Hofmeyr GJ, Lawrie TA, Atallah AN, Duley L. Calcium supplementation during pregnancy for preventing hypertensive disorders and related problems. *Cochrane Database Syst Rev*. 2010;(8):CD001059.

42. American Diabetes Association. Diagnosis and classification of diabetes mellitus. *Diabetes Care*. 2011;34(Suppl 1):S62-S69.

43. Carr DB, Utzschneider KM, Hull RL, et al. Gestational diabetes mellitus increases the risk of cardiovascular disease in women with a family history of type 2 diabetes. *Diabetes Care*. 2006;29(9):2078-2083.

44. Retnakaran R. Glucose tolerance status in pregnancy: a window to the future risk of diabetes and cardiovascular disease in young women. *Curr Diabetes Rev*. 2009;5(4):239-244.

45. Tam WH, Ma RC, Yang X, et al. Glucose intolerance and cardiometabolic risk in adolescents exposed to maternal gestational diabetes: a 15-year follow-up study. *Diabetes Care*. 2010;33(6):1382-1384.

46. World Health Organization. *Global strategy for infant and young child feeding*. Geneva: World Health Organization; 2003.

47. U.S. Department of Health and Human Services. *Healthy People 2020*. Washington, DC: U.S. Government Printing Office; 2010.

48. James DC, Lessen R. Position of the academy of nutrition and dietetics: promoting and supporting breastfeeding. *J Am Diet Assoc*. 2009;109(11):1926-1942.

49. Centers for Disease Control and Prevention. *Percent of U.S. children who were breastfed, by birth year, National Immunization Survey, United States 2010*. Atlanta: Centers for Disease Control and Prevention; 2010.

50. Gartner LM, Morton J, Lawrence RA, et al. Breastfeeding and the use of human milk. *Pediatrics*. 2005;115(2):496-506.

51. Perez-Escamilla R. Evidence based breast-feeding promotion: the Baby-Friendly Hospital Initiative. *J Nutr*. 2007;137(2):484-487.

52. Li J, Kendall GE, Henderson S, et al. Maternal psychosocial well-being in pregnancy and breastfeeding duration. *Acta Paediatr*. 2008;97(2):221-225.

53. O'Brien M, Buikstra E, Fallon T, Hegney D. Exploring the influence of psychological factors on breastfeeding duration, phase 1: perceptions of mothers and clinicians. *J Hum Lact*. 2009;25(1):55-63.

54. McNiel ME, Labbok MH, Abrahams SW. What are the risks associated with formula feeding? A re-analysis and review. *Birth*. 2010;37(1):50-58.

55. Horta BL, Bahl R, Martines JC, Victora CG. *Evidence on the long-term effects of breastfeeding: systematic reviews and meta-analyses*. Geneva: World Health Organization; 2007.

56. Kramer MS, Aboud F, Mironova E, et al; Promotion of Breastfeeding Intervention Trial (PROBIT) Study Group. Breastfeeding and child cognitive development: new evidence from a large randomized trial. *Arch Gen Psychiatry*. 2008;65(5):578-584.

FURTHER READING AND RESOURCES

Each of the following organizations has an earnest interest in the health care of pregnant women and their children. For information about a variety of topics involving pregnancy and lactation, explore their Web sites.

American Academy of Pediatrics. www.aap.org

Birth Defect Research for Children, Inc.. www.birthdefects.org

Canadian Paediatric Society. www.cps.ca

La Leche League International, Inc.. www.llli.org

March of Dimes Birth Defects Foundation. www.modimes.org

U.S. Department of Agriculture WIC Program. www.fns.usda.gov/wic

World Health Organization, Breastfeeding. www.who.int/topics/breastfeeding/en

Kramer MS, Aboud F, Mironova E, et al; Promotion of Breastfeeding Intervention Trial (PROBIT) Study Group. Breastfeeding and child cognitive development: new evidence from a large randomized trial. *Arch Gen Psychiatry*. 2008;65(5):578-584.

Researchers outline and discuss one of the largest randomized trials addressing the benefits of breast-feeding for child cognitive development.

Ornoy A, Ergaz Z. Alcohol abuse in pregnant women: effects on the fetus and newborn, mode of action and maternal treatment. *Int J Environ Res Public Health*. 2010;7(2):364-379.

CHAPTER 11

Nutrition during Infancy, Childhood, and Adolescence

KEY CONCEPTS

- The normal growth of individual children varies within a relatively wide range of measures.
- Human growth and development require both nutritional and psychosocial support.

- A variety of food patterns and habits supply the energy and nutrient requirements of normal growth and development, although basic nutritional needs change with each growth period.

n any culture, food nurtures both the physical and emotional process of "growing up" for each infant, child, and adolescent. Food and eating during these significant years of childhood do not exist apart from the broader overall process of growth and development. The entire process ultimately has a hand in creating and shaping the whole person.

This chapter considers food and feeding to be a basic part of an individual's growing up. It then relates the various age groups' nutritional needs and food patterns to individual psychosocial development and physical growth.

NUTRITION FOR GROWTH AND DEVELOPMENT

Life Cycle Growth Pattern

The normal human life cycle follows four general stages of overall growth, with individual variation along the way.

Infancy

Growth is rapid during the first year of life, with the rate tapering off somewhat during the latter half of the year. Most infants double their birth weight by the time that they are 6 months old, and they triple it between 12 and 15 months of age. Growth in length is not quite as rapid, but infants generally increase their birth length by 50% during the first year and double it by 4 years of age.

Childhood

Between infancy and adolescence, the childhood growth rate slows and becomes irregular. Growth occurs in small spurts during which children have increased appetites and eat accordingly. Appetites usually taper off during periodic plateaus. Parents who recognize the ebb and flow of normal growth patterns during the latent period of childhood can relax and enjoy this time. Alternatively, unawareness of or inexperience with this normal flux in growth and appetite can result in stress and battles over food between parents and children.

Adolescence

The onset of puberty begins the second stage of rapid growth, which continues until adult maturity. Growth hormone and sex hormones rise, which brings multiple and often bewildering body changes to young adolescents. During this period, long bones grow quickly, sex characteristics develop, and fat and muscle mass increase.

Adulthood

With physical maturity comes the final phase of a normal life cycle. Physical growth levels off during adulthood and then gradually declines during old age. However, mental and psychosocial development lasts a lifetime.

Measuring Childhood Growth

Individual Growth Rates

Children grow at widely varying rates. Therefore, the best counsel for parents is that children are individuals. A child's growth is not inadequate because the rate does not equal that of another child. General measures of growth in children relate to physical development as well as mental, emotional, social, and cultural growth.

Physical Growth

Growth charts, such as those developed by the World Health Organization (WHO) and the Centers for Disease Control and Prevention (CDC), provide an assessment tool for measuring growth patterns in infants, children, and adolescents. These charts are based on large numbers of well-nourished children who represent the national population. They are used as guides to follow an individual child's pattern of physical growth in relation to the general percentile growth curves of the population. The current recommendation is for clinicians to use the WHO growth charts for infants who are up to 2 years old and the CDC growth charts for children who are older than 2 years old.[1] The combined use of the WHO and CDC growth charts allows practitioners to plot the growth patterns for height (or length), weight, and head circumference from birth to the age of 20 years. The body mass index (BMI)-for-age charts for children can be used continuously from 2 years of age into adulthood. Because the BMI during childhood is an indicator of the adult BMI, the risk of obesity can be identified and addressed early.

There are specific growth charts for boys and girls and for infants from birth to the age of 24 months; a separate set of growth charts has been created for children and adolescents between the ages of 2 and 20 years. Figure 11-1 demonstrates two examples of the growth charts. See the Evolve site for this book for the full set of the WHO and CDC growth charts. An accurate reading depends on using the appropriate growth chart. Special growth charts are available for several diseases or conditions that affect childhood growth; these are more appropriate to use for affected children than the standard WHO or CDC charts. Some examples of conditions for which specialty growth charts are available include low or very low birth weight infants, achondroplasia, Down syndrome, fragile X syndrome, Prader-Willi syndrome, sickle cell disease, and spastic quadriplegia. See the Clinical Applications box, "Use and Interpretation of the Centers for Disease Control

and Prevention Growth Charts" for a step-by-step demonstration of how to accurately use the standard charts.

Individual measures of physical growth for children include weight and height, head circumference, general signs of health, and laboratory tests. Accurate measurements are critical to the assessment process. Small errors in measurement can easily lead to a false alarm regarding a child's growth pattern.

Psychosocial Development

Various assessments can be used to measure mental, emotional, social, and cultural growth and development. Food is intimately related to these aspects of psychosocial development as well as to physical growth. The growing child does not learn food attitudes and habits in a vacuum but rather as a part of close personal and social relationships.

NUTRITIONAL REQUIREMENTS FOR GROWTH

Energy Needs

Kilocalories

The demand for energy as measured in kilocalories per kilogram (kg) of body weight is relatively large during childhood. During the first 3 years of life, children need somewhere between 80 and 120 kcal/kg body weight per day to support rapid growth.[2] This is significantly higher than adult needs of 30 to 40 kcal/kg per day. Although the exact energy needs of premature infants are highly variable and not well defined, they are thought to range from 110 to 130 kcal/kg per day.[3,4] The Dietary Reference Intake values in Table 11-1 present general recommendations for energy and protein needs at different ages. However, specific individual needs vary with age and condition. For example, the total daily caloric intake of an average 5-year-old child is spent in the following way:

- Basal metabolism: 50%
- Physical activity: 25%
- Tissue growth: 12%
- Fecal loss: 8%
- Metabolic effect of food: 5%

However, some children are more physically active than others and have a higher kcal/kg per day

---

body mass index the body weight in kilograms divided by the square of the height in meters (kg/m^2); this measurement correlates with body fatness and the health risks associated with obesity.

USE AND INTERPRETATION OF THE CENTERS FOR DISEASE CONTROL AND PREVENTION GROWTH CHARTS

Purpose

This guide instructs health care providers regarding how to use and interpret the Centers for Disease Control and Prevention and World Health Organization growth charts. With the use of these charts, health care providers can assess growth in infants, children, and adolescents and compare it with a nationally representative reference that is based on children of all ages and ethnic groups.

During a routine screening, health care providers assess physical growth by using the child's weight, stature, length, and head circumference. When plotted correctly, a series of measurements offers important information about a child's growth pattern and possible nutrition risks. Contributing factors such as parental stature and the presence of acute or chronic illness should also be considered when making health and nutrition assessments.

Step 1: Obtain Accurate Weights and Measures

When weighing and measuring children, follow procedures that yield accurate measurements, and use equipment that is well maintained.

Step 2: Select the Appropriate Growth Chart

Select the growth chart to use on the basis of the age and gender of the child:

- Use the World Health Organization growth standards to monitor growth for infants and children who are between the ages of 0 and 2 years.
- Use the Centers for Disease Control and Prevention growth charts for children who are 2 years old and older.

Step 3: Record Data

First, record information about factors obtained at the initial visit that influence growth.

- Enter the child's name and the record number, if appropriate.
- Enter the mother's and father's statures, as reported.
- Enter the child's gestational age in weeks.
- Enter the date of birth (omit this step when using growth charts for children who are between the ages of 2 and 20 years).
- Enter the child's birth weight, length, and head circumference.
- Add any notable comments (e.g., breast-feeding).

Record information obtained during the current visit.

- Enter today's date.
- Enter the child's age.
- Enter the child's weight, stature, and head circumference (if appropriate) immediately after taking the measurement.
- Add any notable comments (e.g., was not cooperative).

Step 4: Calculate the Body Mass Index

The body mass index (BMI) is calculated by using weight and stature measurements; it compares a child's weight relative to stature with that of other children of the same age and gender.

- Determine the BMI with the following calculation:

$$BMI = Weight\ (kg)/Stature\ (m)^2$$

or

$$BMI = (Weight\ [lb] \times 703)/Stature\ (in)^2$$

Weight and stature measurements must be converted to the appropriate decimal value.

Example: 37 lb 4 oz = 37.25 lb; $41\frac{1}{2}$ in = 41.5 in

Enter the BMI to one place after the decimal point (e.g., 15.204 = 15.2).

Step 5: Plot the Measurements

On the appropriate growth chart, plot the measurements recorded in the data entry table for the current visit.

- Find the child's age on the horizontal axis. When plotting weight for length, find the length on the horizontal axis. Use a straight edge or a right-angle ruler to draw a vertical line up from that point.
- Find the appropriate measurement (i.e., weight, length, stature, head circumference, or BMI) on the vertical axis. Use a straight edge or a right-angle ruler to draw a horizontal line across from that point until it intersects the vertical line.
- Make a small dot where the two lines intersect.

Step 6: Interpret the Plotted Measurements

The curved lines on the growth chart show selected percentiles that indicate the rank of the child's measurement. For example, when the dot is plotted on the 95th percentile line for BMI for age, it means that 5% children of the same age and gender in the reference population have a higher BMI for age.

1. Determine the percentile rank.
2. Determine if the percentile rank suggests that the anthropometric index is indicative of nutritional risk on the basis of the percentile cutoff value.
3. Compare today's percentile rank with the rank from previous visits to identify any major shifts in the child's growth pattern and the need for further assessment.

Anthropometric Index	Nutritional Percentile Cutoff Value	Status Indicator
BMI for age	≥95th	Overweight
Weight for length	≥95th	Overweight
BMI for age	≥85th and ≤95th	At risk of overweight
Weight for length	≤5th	Underweight
Stature/length for age	≤5th	Short stature
Head circumference for age	≤5th or ≥95th	Developmental problems

TABLE 11-1 **DIETARY REFERENCE INTAKES OF ENERGY AND PROTEIN FROM BIRTH TO 18 YEARS OF AGE**

	Age	Estimated Energy Requirement	Protein (g)
Infants	0 to 3 months	(89 × Weight [kg] − 100) + 175 kcal	9.1
	4 to 6 months	(89 × Weight [kg] − 100) + 56 kcal	9.1
	7 to 12 months	(89 × Weight [kg] − 100) + 22 kcal	11
	13 to 36 months	(89 × Weight [kg] − 100) + 20 kcal	13
Boys	3 to 8 years	88.5 − (61.9 × Age [y]) + PA × (26.7 × Weight [kg] + 903 × Height [m]) + 20 kcal	19
	9 to 18 years	88.5 − (61.9 × Age [y]) + PA × (26.7 × Weight [kg] + 903 × Height [m]) + 25 kcal	34 to 52
Girls	3 to 8 years	135.3 − (30.8 × Age [y]) + PA × (10.0 × Weight [kg] + 934 × Height [m]) + 20 kcal	19
	9 to 18 years	135.3 − (30.8 × Age [y]) + PA × (10.0 × Weight [kg] + 934 × Height [m]) + 25 kcal	34 to 46

PA, Physical activity level. Data from the Food and Nutrition Board, Institute of Medicine. *Dietary reference intakes for energy, carbohydrate, fiber, fat, fatty acids, cholesterol, protein, and amino acids (macronutrients)*. Washington, DC: National Academies Press; 2002.

expenditure. Likewise, a child who is growing rapidly has higher tissue growth needs and a higher basal metabolism compared with a similar child who is not going through a growth spurt.

Macronutrients

Carbohydrates are the main energy source of total kilocalories. Carbohydrates also spare protein so that the protein that is vital for building tissue during childhood growth is not diverted for energy needs. Fat is a backup energy source, and it supplies the essential fatty acids that are necessary for growth.

Protein Needs

Protein is the fundamental tissue-building substance of the body. It supplies the essential amino acids for tissue growth and maintenance. As a child grows, the protein requirements per kg of body weight gradually decline. For example, for the first 6 months of life, the protein requirements of an infant are 1.52 g/kg of body weight; however, the protein needs of a fully grown adult are only 0.8 g/kg.[2] A healthy, active, growing child usually eats enough of a variety of foods to supply the necessary protein and kilocalories for overall growth.

Water Requirements

Water is an essential nutrient that is second only to oxygen for life. Metabolic needs, especially during periods of rapid growth, demand adequate fluid intake. For example, compare infant and adult water needs. Infants require more water per unit of body weight than adults for three important reasons: (1) a greater percentage of the infant's total body weight is composed of water; (2)

TABLE 11-2 **APPROXIMATE DAILY FLUID NEEDS DURING GROWTH YEARS**

Age	Males and Females (L/day)	Age	Males (L/day)	Females (L/day)
0 to 6 months	0.7	9 to 13 years	2.4	2.1
7 to 12 months	0.8	14 to 18 years	3.3	2.3
1 to 3 years	1.3	> 19 years	3.7	2.7
4 to 8 years	1.7			

Data from the Food and Nutrition Board, Institute of Medicine. *Dietary reference intakes for water, potassium, sodium, chloride, and sulfate*, Washington, DC: National Academies Press; 2004.

a larger proportion of the infant's total body water is in the extracellular spaces; and (3) infants have a larger proportional body surface area and metabolic rate compared with adults. In one day, an infant generally consumes an amount of water that is equivalent to 10% to 15% of his or her body weight, whereas an adult consumes a daily amount that is equivalent to 2% to 4% of his or her body weight. Table 11-2 provides a summary of the estimated daily fluid needs during the years of growth.

Mineral and Vitamin Needs

Although they yield no energy themselves, minerals and vitamins have important roles in tissue growth and maintenance as well as in overall energy metabolism. Positive childhood growth depends on adequate amounts of all essential substances. Some nutrients of special interest are discussed in the following sections.

Birth to 24 months: Girls
Head circumference-for-age
and Weight-for-length percentiles

NAME _____

RECORD # _____

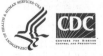

AGE (MONTHS)

HEAD CIRCUMFERENCE

WEIGHT

LENGTH

Date	Age	Weight	Length	Head Circ.	Comment

Published by the Centers for Disease Control and Prevention, November 1, 2009
SOURCE: WHO Child Growth Standards (http://www.who.int/childgrowth/en)

A

Figure 11-1 Example of a Centers for Disease Control and Prevention and World Health Organization growth chart.
(Courtesy National Center for Health Statistics, National Center for Chronic Disease Prevention and Health Promotion, Hyattsville, Md.)
Continued

2 to 20 years: Boys
Body mass index-for-age percentiles

Date	Age	Weight	Stature	BMI*	Comments

*To Calculate BMI: Weight (kg) ÷ Stature (cm) ÷ Stature (cm) × 10,000
or Weight (lb) ÷ Stature (in) ÷ Stature (in) × 703

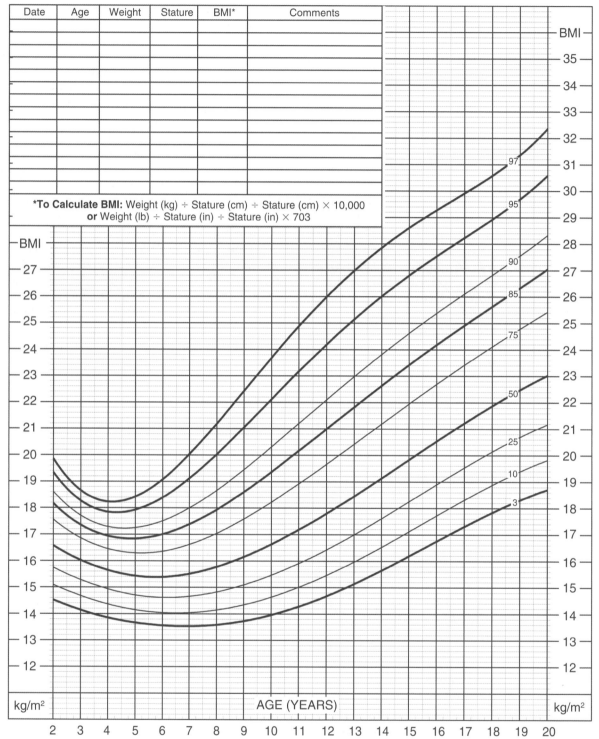

AGE (YEARS)

kg/m²

Published May 30, 2000 (modified10/16/00).
SOURCE: Developed by the National Center for Health Statistics in collaboration with
the National Center for Chronic Disease Prevention and Health Promotion (2000).
http://www.cdc.gov/growthcharts

B

SAFER · HEALTHIER · PEOPLE™

Figure 11-1, cont'd

Calcium

Calcium needs are critical during the most rapid growth periods of infancy through adolescence. During infancy, the mineralization of the skeleton is taking place while the bones are growing larger and the teeth are forming. Many factors influence bone development in infants and toddlers, including the maternal nutritional status during pregnancy, the type of infant feeding, the calcium and phosphorus content of breast milk or of a breast milk alternative formula, the introduction of solid foods, and the diet during the toddler and preschool years.[5]

Approximately 40% of adult peak bone mineral density is deposited during the short period of adolescence. Bone density—particularly in the long bones and the vertebrae—demands adequate calcium, phosphorus, vitamin D, protein, and several other nutrients. In fact, both research and clinical experience indicate that as a preventive measure to reduce the risk for fractures and osteoporosis, weight-bearing activity and appropriate calcium must be emphasized during adolescence more so than at any other time throughout the life span.[6,7]

Calcium absorption, calcium deposition in bone, and calcium retention in adolescent girls peaks just before menarche. In addition, calcium retention declines as sexual maturity progresses, and researchers have found significant differences in calcium retention among ethnic groups.[8] The Cultural Considerations box entitled "Racial Differences in Calcium Retention and Peak Bone Mass" discusses this issue further.

Iron

Iron is essential for hemoglobin formation and cognitive development during the early years of life. Infants of mothers with diabetes or preeclampsia, growth-restricted newborns, and preterm infants are at a greater risk for iron-deficiency anemia.[9] The presence of iron deficiency during this critical time is negatively associated with cognitive and behavioral performance in children.[10] The iron content of breast milk is highly absorbable and fully meets the needs of an infant for the first 6 months of life.[11] At that point, the infant's nutrition needs for iron typically exceed that provided exclusively by breast milk, and the addition of solid foods (e.g., enriched cereal, egg yolk, meat) at approximately 6 months of age helps to supply additional iron. Infants who are not breast-fed need iron-fortified infant formula. Cow's milk, which is very low in iron, should be entirely avoided for the first year of life.

VITAMIN SUPPLEMENTS

Much debate has occurred over the years about dietary supplementation of vitamins and minerals for infants.

The American Academy of Pediatrics recognizes only two vitamins that are potentially needed in supplemental form: vitamins K and D.[12] Nearly all infants who are born in the United States and Canada receive a prophylactic shot of 1 mg of vitamin K, and no further supplementation is recommended for breast- or formula-fed infants. Vitamin K is critical for blood clotting. A major contributor to the daily supply of vitamin K is provided by bacterial production in the gut. Because infants are born without bacterial flora, their vitamin K synthesis and stores are minimal. Oral vitamin D drops (200 IU) are recommended for breast-fed infants beginning during the first 2 months of life and continuing until the infant is drinking 500 mL (16 oz) of vitamin-D–fortified milk, or dairy alternative, daily.[12] Formula-fed infants receive supplemental vitamin D in the formula.

Excessive supplementation in infants and children is not unheard of, and, as with adults, toxicity is a danger. Excess amounts of vitamins A and D (hypervitaminosis) are of special concern in children (see Chapter 7). Excess intake may occur over prolonged periods as a result of ignorance, carelessness, or misunderstanding. Parents should provide only the amount that they are directed to give and no more.

AGE-GROUP NEEDS

Infancy

Food is intimately related to each stage of development, because physical growth and personal psychosocial development go hand in hand.

Immature Infants

Special care is crucial for tiny immature babies, who are categorized into two primary groups that are defined by weight or gestational age.

Weight. As defined by birth weight, low birth weight infants weigh less than 2500 g (5 lb 8 oz); very low birth weight infants weigh less than 1500 g (3 lb 5 oz); extremely low birth weight babies weigh less than 990 g (2 lb 3 oz).

Gestational Age. As defined by gestational age, premature infants are born preterm at less than 270 days' gestation and weigh less than 2500 g (5 lb 8 oz). Infants that are small for gestational age (SGA) are born at full term, but they have had some degree of intrauterine growth restriction before birth, and they have general growth limitations and low weight.

Immature infants are subject to problems with growth and nutrition. Because their bodies are not fully formed, they differ from term infants of normal weight in the following ways: (1) they have more body water, less protein,

CULTURAL CONSIDERATIONS

RACIAL DIFFERENCES IN CALCIUM RETENTION AND PEAK BONE MASS

As discussed in the Cultural Considerations box in Chapter 8, "Bone Health in Gender and Ethnic Groups," noted disparities exist among the genders and ethnic groups regarding bone density. African Americans have significantly higher bone mineral density than their Caucasian counterparts throughout life. Two studies that involved adolescent girls provided insight into the mechanism responsible for racial differences in peak bone mass. Bryant and colleagues found that, during the period of peak calcium retention and development of bone mass, African-American girls were able to retain 57% more dietary calcium than Caucasian girls (see figure), and they had a higher rate of bone formation.[1]

The authors concluded from this finding that adult differences in bone mass originate during adolescence, thereby making the dietary intake of calcium-rich foods throughout the teen years a critical component of lifelong bone health. A follow-up study that compared calcium retention with a range of calcium intake in a similar cohort of subjects obtained similar results: African-American girls retain more calcium at all intake levels than do their Caucasian counterparts, and retention peaks for both ethnic groups just before the onset of puberty.[2] This difference in calcium retention is apparent despite the lower vitamin D status found among African-American girls, which was historically thought to influence calcium absorption efficiency.[3]

Because adolescence is such a pivotal point for bone health through calcium retention, factors that affect the body's ability to maintain dietary calcium are equally as important. Dietary sodium promotes the loss of calcium through urinary excretion. Wigertz and colleagues were interested in comparing the differences in this effect between adolescent African-American and Caucasian girls.[4] Those authors found that urinary calcium excretion increased along with increased sodium intake among Caucasian girls

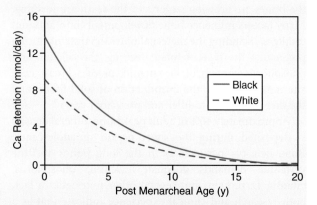

Model for calcium retention as a function of postmenarchal age in African-American and Caucasian girls. *Solid line,* African-American girls; *dashed line,* Caucasian girls. The cumulative racial difference in bone mass on the basis of calcium accretion from the onset of menarche to 20 years after menarche is predicted to be 12%. (Reprinted from Bryant RJ, Wastney ME, Martin BR, et al. Racial differences in bone turnover and calcium metabolism in adolescent females. *J Clin Endocrinol Metab.* 2003;88:1043-1047.)

much more so than among African-American girls. This indicates that high intakes of sodium in Caucasian girls will intensify the loss of calcium and further weaken potential bone mass.

Health care providers should impress upon adolescent girls—especially Caucasian girls—that high calcium intake with limited sodium consumption will have long-lasting benefits for their bone health.

1. Bryant RJ, Wastney ME, Martin BR, et al. Racial differences in bone turnover and calcium metabolism in adolescent females. *J Clin Endocrinol Metab.* 2003;88(3):1043-1047.
2. Bruan M, Palacios C, Wigertz K, et al. Racial differences in skeletal calcium retention in adolescent girls with varied controlled calcium intakes. *Am J Clin Nutr.* 2007;85(6):1657-1663.
3. Weaver CM, McCabe LD, McCabe GP, et al. Vitamin D status and calcium metabolism in adolescent black and white girls on a range of controlled calcium intakes. *J Clin Endocrinol Metab.* 2008;93(10):3907-3914.
4. Wigertz K, Palacios C, Jackman LA, et al. Racial differences in calcium retention in response to dietary salt in adolescent girls. *Am J Clin Nutr.* 2005;81(4):845-850.

and fewer minerals; (2) there is little subcutaneous fat to maintain body temperature; (3) they have poorly calcified bones; (4) their nerve and muscle development are incomplete, thus making their sucking reflexes weak or absent; (5) they have a limited ability for digestion, absorption, and renal function; and (6) they have immature livers that lack developed metabolic enzyme systems or adequate iron stores. To survive, these tiny babies require special feeding.

Type of Milk. The American Academy of Pediatrics recommends the normal feeding of breast milk to

premature and other high-risk infants. Very low birth weight infants may benefit from human milk fortifier in addition to breast milk. Infants of mothers who are not able to breast-feed are encouraged to consider using human milk from milk banks.[12] Mothers of preterm infants produce milk that is significantly higher in energy, carbohydrates, protein, and fat to meet the elevated needs of preterm infants.[13]

Methods of Feeding. Tube feeding and peripheral vein feeding are used in special cases, but both carry hazards and are to be avoided if possible. For most immature infants, bottle feeding or nursing can be successful with care and support. Infants who have not yet developed the sucking reflex, which is acquired at approximately 32 weeks' gestation, can still benefit from breast milk, provided that the mother is willing and able to pump her breast milk for delivery to the baby by tube or cup feeding.

Term Infants

Mature newborns have more finely developed body systems and grow rapidly; they gain approximately 168 g (6 oz) per week during the first 6 months. The feeding process is an important component of the bonding relationship between the parent and the child. Iron-fortified solid foods should be added to the infant's basic diet of breast milk (or formula) at approximately 6 months of age.

Breast-Feeding

Human milk is the ideal first food for infants, and it is the primary recommendation of pediatricians and dietitians.[12,14] During pregnancy, the breasts prepare for lactation; toward term, they produce colostrum. Mature breast milk comes in 3 to 5 days after delivery. As the infant grows, breast milk adapts in composition to match the needs of the developing child, and the fat content of breast milk changes from the beginning to the end of a single feeding. Foremilk, which is the first mature milk to let down, is the lowest in fat content; midmilk has progressively more fat content; and hindmilk, which is the milk that comes at the end of the feeding, has the highest fat content. Thus, fully emptying at least one breast at every feeding is important to provide the infant with the energy-dense hindmilk.

The newborn's rooting reflex, his or her oral needs for sucking, and basic hunger help to facilitate breast-feeding for healthy, relaxed mothers (Figure 11-2). Working mothers who want to breast-feed their babies can do so by using manual expression or a breast pump while at work as well as freezing and storing milk in sealed plastic baby bottle liners for later use. Child-care facilities provided in some business and industry settings support breast-feeding by employed mothers. Breast-feeding mothers can find support and guidance through local groups of the national La Leche League or professional certified lactation counselors. For additional information about breast-feeding, see Chapter 10.

Bottle-Feeding

If a mother chooses not to breast-feed or if some condition in either the mother or the baby prevents it, bottle-feeding of an appropriate formula is an acceptable alternative. Research shows that many mothers do not

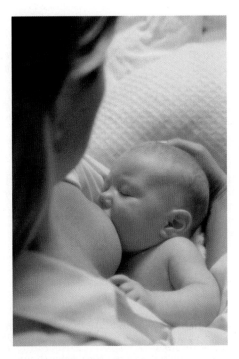

Figure 11-2 Breast-feeding the newborn infant. Note that the mother avoids touching the infant's outer cheek so as not to counteract the infant's natural rooting reflex at the touch of the breast. (Copyright JupiterImages Corp.)

adhere to recommended safety precautions when preparing infant formula, which can increase the risk for infant food-borne illness and scalding.[15] Sterile procedures in formula preparation, the amount of formula consumed, and weaning from the bottle are some aspects that must be addressed to ensure the health of the child.

Choosing a Formula. Most mothers who bottle-feed their infants use a standard commercial formula. In some cases of milk allergy or intolerance, a soy-based formula (not soy milk) is used. For infants who are allergic to cow's milk and soy-based formulas, amino-acid–based formulas may be medically advised. Examples include Nutramigen (Mead Johnson Nutrition, Evansville, Ind), EleCare (Abbott Nutrition, Columbus, Ohio), and Neocate (Nutricia North America, Gaithersburg, Md). Table 11-3 compares the nutrient composition of breast milk with that of standard and specialty formulas.

colostrum a thin yellow fluid that is first secreted by the mammary glands a few days after childbirth, preceding the mature breast milk; it contains up to 20% protein, including a large amount of lactalbumin, more minerals, and less lactose and fat than mature milk as well as immunoglobulins that represent the antibodies that are found in maternal blood.

TABLE 11-3 **NUTRITIONAL VALUE OF HUMAN MILK AND FORMULA**

NUTRITIONAL COMPONENT PER LITER	HUMAN MILK	STANDARD FORMULAS*	SPECIAL FORMULAS FOR INFANTS THAT ARE NOT BREAST-FED OR THAT CANNOT TOLERATE STANDARD FORMULAS	
	Mature	Enfamil, Similac, and Good Start	Nutramigen (casein hydrolysate and free amino acids)	EleCare (free amino acids)
Kilocalories	700	672	670	676
Protein (g)	10.3	14.2	18.6	20.4
Fat (g)	44	35.3	35.3	32.2
Carbohydrate (g)	69	73.5	69	72.4
Calcium (mg)	320	492.3	627	730
Phosphorus (mg)	140	270.6	420	548
Sodium (mg)	7.4	7.6	13.5	13.2
Potassium (mg)	13	18.3	18.6	25.9
Iron (mg)	0.3	11.5[†]	12	12

*Most standard formulas are very similar. This represents an average of Enfamil (Mead Johnson Nutrition, Evansville, Ind); Similac (Abbott Nutrition, Columbus, Ohio); and Good Start (Nestle Infant Nutrition, Fremont, Mich).
[†]With added iron.

Preparing the Formula. With any commercial formula, the manufacturer's instructions for mixing concentrated or powdered formula with water should be precisely and consistently followed, and the formula should be refrigerated until use. Throughout the process, scrupulous cleanliness and accurate dilution are essential to prevent infection and illness. A ready-to-feed formula only requires a sterile nipple and bypasses many problems, but it is substantially more expensive. Bottles should be heated in a bowl of warm water (not in a microwave) to prevent the burning of the infant's mouth.

Feeding the Formula. Babies usually drink formula either cold or warm; they simply want it to be consistent. Tilting the bottle to keep the nipple full of milk can prevent air swallowing, and the baby's head should be slightly elevated during feeding to facilitate the passage of milk into the stomach. Caregivers should be encouraged to never prop the bottle or leave the baby alone to feed, especially as a pacifier at sleep time. This practice deprives the infant of the cuddling that is a vital part of nurturing, and it also allows milk to pool in the mouth, which can cause choking, earache, or baby bottle tooth decay. Children should never be put to sleep with a bottle of milk or fruit juice or any other caloric liquid that is capable of pooling in the mouth. Natural bacteria found in the mouth feeds on carbohydrates, thereby producing enamel-damaging acid. Baby bottle tooth decay (Figure 11-3) is a serious and completely avoidable problem that results from this practice.

Cleaning Bottles and Nipples. Whether preparing a single bottle for each feeding or an entire day's batch, scrub, rinse, and sterilize all equipment with the use of the terminal sterilization method. Rinse bottles and

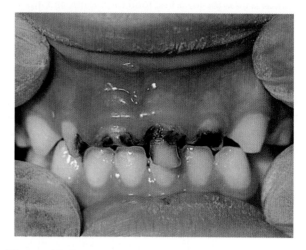

Figure 11-3 Baby bottle tooth decay. (From Swartz MH. *Textbook of physical diagnosis, history, and examination.* 5th ed. Philadelphia: Saunders; 2006.)

nipples after each feeding with special bottle and nipple brushes that force water through nipple holes to prevent milk from crusting in them.

Weaning

Throughout the feeding process, observant parents quickly learn to recognize their baby's signs of hunger and satiety and to follow the baby's lead. Babies are individuals

baby bottle tooth decay the decay of the baby teeth as a result of inappropriate feeding practices such as putting an infant to bed with a bottle; also called *nursing bottle caries, bottle mouth,* and *bottle caries.*

who set their own particular needs according to age, activity level, growth rate, and metabolic efficiency. A newborn has a very small stomach that holds only 1 to 2 fl oz, but he or she will gradually take in more as his or her stomach capacity enlarges relative to overall body growth. The amounts of increased intake during the first 6 months vary and reflect growth patterns. By 6 to 9 months of age, as increasing amounts of other foods are introduced, weaning from bottle-feeding takes place. For some children, growing physical capacities and the desire for independence lead to self-weaning, but many children need a little added encouragement from their parents.

Cow's Milk

An infant should never be fed cow's milk during the first year of life. Unmodified cow's milk is not suitable for infants; its concentration may cause gastrointestinal bleeding, and it provides too heavy a load of solutes for the infant's renal system. Infants and toddlers who are younger than 2 years old should also not be fed reduced-fat cow's milk (e.g., skim or low-fat milk), because insufficient energy is provided and because linoleic acid, which is the essential fatty acid for growth that is found in the fat portion of the milk, is lacking. To meet infant needs during the first year of life, the American Academy of Pediatrics recommends breast milk supplemented by vitamin D (if the mother is deficient and if the child has inadequate exposure to sunlight), with the gradual addition of iron-fortified foods beginning at approximately 6 months of age.[12] Infant formula is appropriate in place of breast milk if the mother so chooses.

Solid Food Additions

When to Introduce. Age is one of the basic indicators of readiness for solid foods. Solid foods are not recommended before 6 months of age, because the infant's immature gastrointestinal system cannot use them well before then. An expert group on pediatrics concluded that the most effective prevention regimen against allergic disease is to provide breast milk and to avoid solid foods and cow's milk for at least 4 to 6 months after birth.[16]

Another indicator of readiness for solid foods is the development of certain motor skills, such as keeping the head upright when unsupported and controlled movement of the tongue. It is equally important that parents and other caregivers are able to understand feeding cues from the infant (e.g., hunger, satiety) for a mutually pleasant experience.

What to Introduce. When solid foods are started, no specific sequence of food additions must be followed. However, some organizations promote the introduction of vegetables or even meat before fruits or grains. The root

TABLE 11-4 GUIDELINE FOR ADDING SOLID FOODS TO AN INFANT'S DIET DURING THE FIRST YEAR

When to Add	Foods Added*
6 months	Iron-fortified infant cereal made from rice, barley, or oats (these are offered one at a time) Pureed baby food (vegetables or strained fruit)
8 months	Whole-milk yogurt Pureed baby food (meats)
8 to 10 months	Introduce more grain products one at a time, including wheat, various crackers and breads, pasta, and cereal Add more vegetables and fruits in various textures (e.g., chopped, mashed, cooked, raw) Egg yolk, beans, and additional types of pureed meats Cottage cheese and hard cheeses (e.g., cheddar, Colby Jack)
10 to 12 months	Infants should be able to tolerate a large variety of grain products and textures Chopped fruits and vegetables Finger foods
12 months	Whole eggs Whole milk

*Semisolid foods should be given immediately before milk feeding. First, 1 or 2 tsp should be given. If the food is accepted and tolerated well, then the amount should be increased 1 to 2 Tbsp per feeding.

of this recommendation lies in two theories: (1) fruits are much sweeter than vegetables, and infants may develop a preference for a sweet taste first and then not take kindly to the more bitter taste of vegetables (although this theory lacks strong support); and (2) infants who were given meat before cereal had better zinc intake.

Table 11-4 provides a general schedule for the introduction of solid foods, but individual needs and responses vary, and the suggestions of individual practitioners should be the guide for a specific child. Introduce foods one at a time (starting with iron-fortified cereal) and in small amounts so that, if an adverse reaction occurs, the offending food can be easily identified. Over time, the child is introduced to a variety of foods and comes to enjoy many of them. Children's eating behaviors are complex and continue to change with age.

weaning the process of gradually acclimating a young child to food other than the mother's milk or a bottle-fed substitute formula as the child's natural need to suckle wanes.

Commercial or Homemade. Some mothers prefer to prepare their own baby food. Baby food can be prepared at home by cooking and straining vegetables and fruits, freezing a batch at a time in ice cube trays, and then storing the cubes in plastic bags in the freezer. A single cube can later be reheated for feeding. A variety of commercial baby foods are also available and are now prepared without added sugar, salt, or monosodium glutamate. Throughout the early feeding period, whatever plan is followed, there are a few basic principles that should guide the feeding process: (1) necessary nutrients —not any specific food or sequence—are needed; (2) food is a basis for learning; and (3) normal physical development guides an infant's feeding behavior (see the For Further Focus box, "How Infants Learn to Eat"). Good food habits begin early during life and continue as the child grows. By 8 or 9 months of age, infants should be able to eat table foods (i.e., cooked, chopped, and simply seasoned foods) without requiring special infant foods.

Summary Guidelines

The Nutrition Committee of the American Academy of Pediatrics has provided the following recommendations to guide infant feeding:

- *Breast-feeding* provides the ideal first food for the infant. It should be continued for at least the first full year of life, and it should be supplemented with a vitamin K shot at birth and daily vitamin D drops (if lifestyle factors indicate a need).
- *Iron-fortified formula* should be used for any infant who is not breast-feeding or for an infant who is older than 6 months old who does not consume a significant portion of his or her kilocalories from added solid foods. Fluoride supplements may be mixed in after 6 months of age only if the local water supply is not fluoridated.
- *Water and juice* are unnecessary for breast-fed infants during the first 6 months of life.
- *Solid foods* may be introduced at approximately 6 months of age, after the extrusion reflex of early infancy disappears and the ability to swallow solid food is established.
- *Whole cow's milk* , or milk substitute, may be introduced at the end of the first year (if the infant is consuming one third of his or her kilocalories as a balanced mixture of solid foods, including cereals, vegetables, fruits, and other foods) to supply adequate sources of vitamin C and iron. Reduced-fat or fat-free cow's milk is not recommended until after the age of 2 years.
- *Allergens* such as wheat, egg white, citrus juice, nuts, and chocolate should not be given as early

solid foods but rather added later, after tolerance has been established through their gradual introduction. (See Chapter 18 for more information about food allergies and intolerances).

- *Honey* should not be given to an infant who is younger than 1 year old, because botulism spores have been reported in honey, and the immune system capacity of the young infant cannot resist this infection.
- *Foods with a high risk for choking and aspiration* such as hot dogs, nuts, grapes, carrots, popcorn, cherries, peanut butter, and round candy are best delayed for careful use only with the older child and not given to an infant.

Throughout the first year of life, the requirements for physical growth and psychosocial development are met by human milk or formula, a variety of solid food additions, and a loving and trusting relationship between the parents and the child.

Childhood

Toddlers (1 to 3 Years Old)

When children learn to walk at approximately 1 year of age, these toddlers are off and running, exploring everything and learning new skills. This dawning sense of self, which is a fundamental foundation for ultimate maturity, carries over into many areas, including that of food. After parents become accustomed to the rapid growth and resulting appetite of the first year of life, they may be concerned when they see their toddler eating less food and at times having little appetite while being easily distracted from food to another activity (see the Clinical Applications box, "Feeding Made Simple"). Increasing the variety of foods available helps children to develop good food habits. The food preferences of young children grow directly from the frequency of a food's use in pleasant surroundings and the increased opportunity to become familiar with a number of foods. Sweets should be reserved for special occasions and not used habitually or as bribes.

Energy and protein needs are still high per each kilogram of body weight compared with adult needs (see

---

extrusion reflex the normal infant reflex to protrude the tongue outward when it is touched.

allergens food proteins that elicit an immune system response or an allergic reaction; symptoms may include itching, swelling, hives, diarrhea, and difficulty breathing as well as anaphylaxis in the worst cases.

FOR FURTHER FOCUS

HOW INFANTS LEARN TO EAT

Guided by reflexes and the gradual development of muscle control during their first year of life, infants learn many things about living in their particular environments. A basic need is food, which infants obtain through a normal developmental sequence of feeding behaviors during the process of learning to eat.

1 to 3 Months
Rooting, sucking, and swallowing reflexes are present at birth in term infants, along with the tonic neck reflex. Infants secure their first food, milk, with a suckling pattern in which the tongue is projected during a swallow. In the beginning, head control is poor, but it develops by the third month of life.

4 to 6 Months
The early rooting and biting reflex fades, and the tonic neck reflex has faded by 16 weeks. Infants now change from a suckling pattern with a protruded tongue to a mature and stronger suck with liquids, and a munching pattern begins. Infants are now able to grasp objects with a palmar grip, bring them to the mouth, and bite them.

7 to 9 Months
The gag reflex weakens as infants begin chewing solid foods. They develop a normal controlled gag along with control of the choking reflex. A mature munching increases their intake of solid foods while chewing with a rotary motion. These infants can sit alone, secure items, release and resecure them, and hold a bottle alone. They begin to develop a pincer grasp to pick up small items between the thumb and forefinger and put the items into the mouth.

10 to 12 Months
Older infants can now reach for a spoon. They bite nipples, spoons, and crunchy foods; they can grasp a bottle or food and bring it to the mouth; and, with assistance, they can drink from a cup. These infants have tongue control to lick food morsels off of the lower lip, and they can finger-feed themselves with a refined pincer grasp. These normal developmental behaviors are the basis for the progressive pattern of introducing semisolid and table foods to older infants.

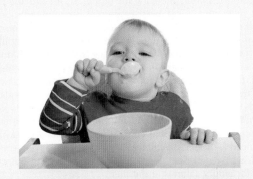

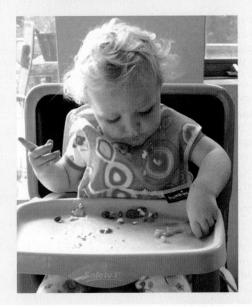

Table 11-1). Toddlers have a wide range of energy needs during this time, and these are directly related to their level of physical activity. Muscle mass, bone structure, and other body tissues continue to grow rapidly and require an adequate dietary supply of protein, minerals, and vitamins. The Food and Nutrition Board recommends a daily intake of 19 g of fiber to prevent constipation and to promote a healthy gastrointestinal tract.[2]

Preschool-Aged Children (3 to 5 Years Old)

Physical growth and appetite continue in spurts during this period. Mental capacities develop, and the expanding environment is gradually explored. Children continue to form patterns, attitudes, and basic eating habits as a result of social and emotional experiences. These varying experiences frequently lead to food jags (i.e., brief sprees or binges of eating one particular food) that last a few days

CLINICAL APPLICATIONS

FEEDING MADE SIMPLE

Birth to 2 Years Old

A study of parental adherence to infant and toddler feeding recommendations—the Feeding Infant and Toddlers Study (FITS)—found that, in a random national sample of more than 3000 children, the early introduction of solid foods, cow's milk, and juices persists despite recommendations from the American Academy of Pediatrics to delay the introduction of such foods until infants are developmentally ready (approximately 6 months of age for solid foods and juices and 1 year of age for cow's milk). The FITS study also found that high-calorie foods with low nutrient densities (e.g., french fries, soda) were consumed on any given day by 10% of children younger than 1 year old.[1] Parents should be reminded that both healthy and unhealthy eating habits develop early and that children's eating behaviors are heavily influenced by the food choices and eating habits of their caregivers. The nutrient needs of children this young do not allow for empty calories in the diet.

Toddlers 2 to 5 Years Old

Some parents waste a lot of time coaxing, arguing, begging, and even threatening their 2- to 5-year-old children to eat more than two peas at dinnertime. You can help save parents' time, tears, and energy by helping them to develop child-feeding strategies that are based on the normal developmental needs of their children. Parents should be reminded of the following:

- Children are not growing as fast as they did during the first year of life. Consequently, they need less food.
- Children's energy needs are irregular. Note their activity level, and provide food as needed to help their bodies keep up with the many activities planned for each day.

The following suggestions may make feeding children easier:

- *Offer a variety of foods.* After a taste, put a new food aside if it is not taken, and then try it again later to help the child develop broad tastes.
- *Serve small portions.* Let children ask for seconds if they are still hungry.
- *Guide children to serve themselves small portions.* Like adults, children's eyes tend to be bigger than their stomachs. Constant gentle reminders help them learn when to stop.
- *Avoid overseasoning.* Let a child's tastes develop gradually. If a food is too spicy, no amount of cajoling will make him or her eat it.
- *Do not force foods that the child dislikes.* Individual food dislikes usually do not last long. If the child shuns

one food, offer a similar one if it is available at that meal (e.g., offer a fruit if the child rejects a vegetable) so that little chance of nutrient deficiency occurs.

- *Do not put away the main meal before serving dessert.* If children are still hungry, some will ask for more food from the main meal after finishing dessert.
- *Keep quick-fix nutritious foods around for off-hour meals.* To keep parents from turning into permanent short-order cooks, keep foods such as fresh and dried fruit, 100% fruit or vegetable juice, cheese, peanut butter, whole-grain bread, and crackers available to serve between meals to provide essential nutrients.
- *Respect eating schedules in a nursery school or preschool program.* Because food is not always available in the classroom, young students learn to eat at regular times. They also tend to try foods that they rejected at home, probably because of peer pressure or a desire to impress a new authority figure such as a teacher.
- *Be patient.* Remember that, although adults may discuss world events over broccoli, toddlers are just now learning how to pick up food with a fork.

Toddlers may take longer to eat, or they may not even eat at all. Nevertheless, with flexibility, time, patience, and a sense of humor, most parents find that they can get enough nutrients into their children to keep them healthy and happy throughout the preschool years. When presented with nutritious food choices, preschoolers tend to self-regulate their intake to meet energy needs without adult intervention. Children's food preferences are strongly influenced by familial and environmental factors, which can create either a healthy or an unhealthy eating dynamic.[2]

For more information about typical feeding patterns for children, see the following resources:

- Satter E. *How to get your kid to eat . . . but not too much.* Boulder, Colo: Bull Publishing; 1997.
- Satter E. *Child of mine: feeding with love and good sense.* 3rd ed. Boulder, Colo: Bull Publishing; 2000.
- Satter E. *Your child's weight: helping without harming.* Madison, Wisc: Kelcy Press; 2005.
- American Academy of Pediatrics. *Pediatric Nutrition Handbook.* 6th ed. Elk Grove Village, Ill: American Academy of Pediatrics; 2009.
- Shield J, Mullen M. *The American Dietetic Association guide to healthy eating for kids: how your children can eat smart from five to twelve.* Indianapolis, Ind: Wiley Publishing; 2002.

1. Briefel, R.R., et al. Feeding infants and toddlers study: Improvements needed in meeting infant feeding recommendations. *J Am Diet Assoc.* 2004;104(1 Suppl 1):S31-S37.

2. Scaglioni, S., M. Salvioni, and C. Galimberti. Influence of parental attitudes in the development of children eating behaviour. *Br J Nutr.* 2008;99 (Suppl 1):S22-S25.

or weeks but that are usually short lived and of no major concern. Again, the key to happy and healthy eating is food variety and appropriately sized portions.

Group eating becomes a significant means of socialization. For example, during preschool, food preferences grow according to what the group is eating. In such situations, a child learns a variety of different food habits and forms new social relationships. The U.S. Department of Agriculture developed a child-friendly version of MyPlate, with dietary and physical activity recommendations and messages designed to appeal to young children (Figure 11-4). The U.S. Department of Agriculture's Food and Nutrition Information Center's "Lifecycle Nutrition" page has resources that are specifically for child nutrition and health (fnic.nal.usda.gov and click on "Lifecycle Nutrition"). This site has information for educators, families, parents, and kids as well as much more information about improving the overall nutritional health of children.

School-Aged Children (5 to 12 Years Old)

The generally slow and irregular growth rate continues during the early school years, and it is accompanied by overall body changes. During the year or two before adolescence in particular, reserves are being laid for the rapid growth period ahead. This is the last lull before the storm. By this time, body types are established, and growth rates vary widely. Girls' development usually bypasses that of boys during the latter part of this period. With the stimulus of school and a variety of learning activities, children experience increasing mental and social maturity, they develop the ability to work out problems, and they participate in competitive activities. They begin moving from dependence on parental patterns to the standards of peers in preparation for coming independence.

Food preferences are the product of earlier years, but school-aged children are increasingly exposed to new stimuli, including television, which is correlated to long-term negative influences on food habits.[17] The relationship between sound nutrition and intellectual learning has long been recognized, and it has established breakfast as a particularly important meal for school-aged children. The school breakfast and lunch programs provide nourishing meals that meet the Dietary Guidelines recommendations for many children who otherwise would lack balanced meals. The Academy of Nutrition and Dietetics has voiced concerns about the lack of such standards with a la carte and competitive foods currently offered at many schools.[18] Competitive foods contribute to the overconsumption of calories, they increase the plate waste of nutritionally balanced school lunches, and they decrease the intake of nutrients by students.[19] Although such programs (e.g., vending machines, fast-food services) can be quite lucrative for schools, the nutrition integrity and sacrifice of health must be considered.[20]

The classroom also provides positive learning opportunities, particularly when parents provide support at home. An interested and motivated teacher can integrate nutrition into many other learning activities. Community nutrition programs such as school breakfast and lunch programs, which have a large effect on a child's health, are discussed further in Chapter 13.

Common Nutrition Problems During Childhood

Failure to Thrive. The term *failure to thrive* has been used in pediatrics to describe infants, children, or adolescents who do not grow and develop normally. Failure to thrive most commonly affects young children between the ages of 1 and 5 years of both sexes. Sometimes pediatricians use a brief hospital stay to identify the cause. Careful nutrition assessment is essential for identifying underlying feeding problems. The following factors may be involved:

- *Clinical disease:* central nervous system disorders, endocrine disease, congenital defects, or partial intestinal obstruction (see the Drug-Nutrient Interaction box, "Anticonvulsants and Increased Nutrient Metabolism").
- *Neuromotor problems:* poor sucking or abnormal muscle tone from the retention of primitive reflexes that should have already faded; eating, chewing, and swallowing problems.

---

school breakfast and lunch programs federally assisted meal programs that operate in public and nonprofit private schools and residential child-care institutions; these programs provide nutritionally balanced, low-cost, or free meals to children each school day.

competitive foods any food or beverage that is served outside of a federal meal program in a food-program setting, regardless of nutritional value.

nutrition integrity as defined by the School Nutrition Association, "a level of performance that assures all foods and beverages available in schools are consistent with the Dietary Guidelines for Americans, and, when combined with nutrition education, physical activity, and a healthful school environment, contributes to enhanced learning and development of lifelong, healthful eating habits."

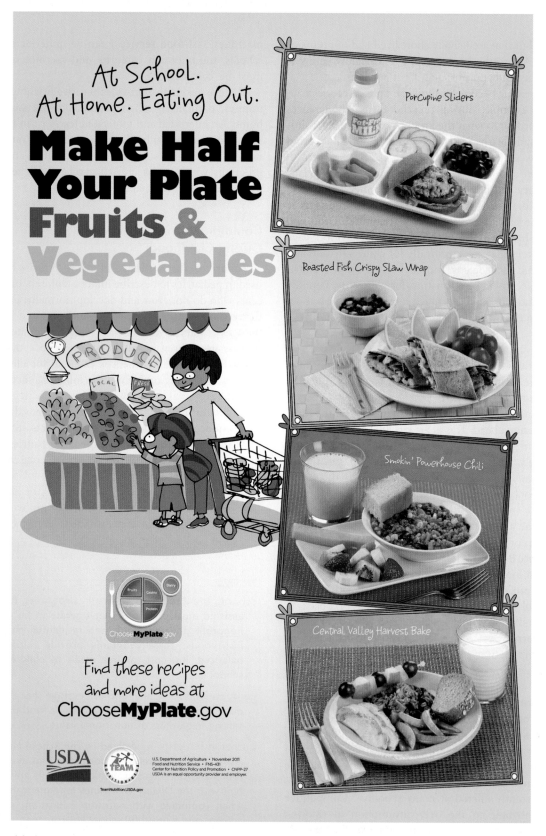

Figure 11-4 ChooseMyPlate for Kids. (Reprinted from the U.S. Department of Agriculture, Food and Nutrition Service, Center for Nutrition Policy and Promotion, Washington, DC: U.S. Government Printing Office; 2011. www.choosemyplate.gov.)

DRUG-NUTRIENT INTERACTION

ANTICONVULSANTS AND INCREASED NUTRIENT METABOLISM

Epilepsy is a chronic neurologic condition that affects 2.5 million people in the United States, with about 200,000 new cases diagnosed each year. Children who are younger than 2 years old and adults older than the age of 65 years are most likely to be affected by epilepsy.[1] Carbamazepine (Tegretol) is a first-line medication that is used for the treatment of generalized tonic-clonic and focal seizures.

Carbamazepine increases the metabolism of vitamin D, calcium, folate, and biotin, which means that the nutrients are used more quickly than normal. Patients who are receiving this drug should make adjustments to their diets to ensure adequate nutrition. This can be accomplished by eating more foods that are rich in these nutrients, including fortified dairy products, or dairy substitutes, for calcium and vitamin D and green leafy vegetables for folate and biotin. For those who require the long-term use of carbamazepine, dietary supplements—especially of calcium and vitamin D—may be necessary.[2]

Kelli Boi

1. Centers for Disease Control and Prevention. *Targeting epilepsy: improving the lives of people with one of the nation's most common neurological conditions: at a glance 2010* (website): www.cdc.gov/chronicdisease/resources/publications/AAG/epilepsy.htm. Accessed November 2010.
2. Pronsky Z. *Food-medication interaction.* 15th ed. Birchrunville, Penn: Food-Medication Interactions; 2008.

- *Dietary practices:* parental misconceptions or inexperience regarding what constitutes a normal diet for infants; inappropriate formula feeding or improper dilutions when mixing formula.
- *Unusual nutrient needs or losses:* adequate diet for growth but inadequate nutrient absorption and thus excessive fecal loss; hypermetabolic state that requires increased dietary intake.
- *Psychosocial problems:* family environment and relationships that result in emotional deprivation of the child that requires medical and nutritional intervention. (Similar problems also may occur later [e.g., between 2 and 4 years of age] when parents and children have conflicts about normal changes caused by slowed childhood growth and energy needs that result in changing food patterns, food jags, erratic appetites, reduced milk intake, and disinterest in eating.)

Failure to thrive is often caused by the complex interaction of factors, and no easy solutions exist. Vigilant history taking, supportive nutritional guidance, and warm personal care are necessary to influence growth patterns in these infants. The careful and sensitive correction of the social and environmental issues that surround the problem is crucial.

Anemia. Although the fortification of cereals and breads with iron has drastically reduced the number of cases of iron-deficiency anemia in the United States, it is still a common problem among children who follow certain eating trends. Children who are most often deficient in overall iron stores are formula-fed infants who are not receiving iron-fortified formula and older infants (i.e., those who are 6 months old and older) who are not consuming iron-fortified cereals and foods. *Milk anemia* is a term that is sometimes used for toddlers (i.e., children who are older than 1 year old) who excessively consume cow's milk. Milk is a poor source of iron, and it displaces other iron-rich foods. These toddlers and their parents are relying on cow's milk for the majority of nutrient intake. Although these children may eat iron-fortified foods, their high calcium intake can inhibit the absorption of iron. Iron-deficiency anemia has been linked to delayed cognitive development in children, and it can have irreversible long-term effects.[10]

Obesity. Childhood and adolescent obesity has been on the rise since the 1970s, and it continues to climb. High blood pressure, metabolic syndrome, and type 2 diabetes are health concerns that have historically been associated with older, overweight adults; however, they are increasingly becoming a problem among school-aged children.[21] Although there are many issues involved, some factors during gestation and early infancy that significantly increase the risk for childhood obesity include maternal overnourishment or undernourishment, gestational diabetes, maternal smoking, and formula feeding.[22,23]

Both genetics and environment play major roles in the risk for obesity and are likely covariables. Although overweight parents are more likely to have overweight kids, these families are also self-selecting environments that promote the development of obesity.[24] Such environmental factors include high-fat food selection or a restrictive feeding practice that ultimately leads to overeating and binging coupled with low physical activity. Infants and children are quite capable of recognizing satiety and self-regulating energy needs. However, this innate awareness seems to decline between the ages of 3 and 5 years, when "super-sized" meal servings start to influence the amount of food eaten, despite satiety. It is well accepted that the attitudes and behaviors of parental figures are key determinants of the development of childhood eating habits. In addition to the guidelines for feeding children given earlier in the Clinical Applications box entitled "Feeding Made Simple," the following recommendations are helpful for guiding parents toward appropriate eating environments and for helping them to lower the risk of obesity in their children[25]:

- Choose specific meal times.
- Provide a wide variety of nutrient-dense foods (e.g., fruits, vegetables) rather than "junk" foods with high energy density and poor nutrient content.
- Offer an age-appropriate portion size.
- Limit non-nutritive snacking and the use of juice or sweetened beverages.
- Permit children with normal body mass indices to self-regulate their total caloric intake.
- Have regular family meals to promote social interaction and to role model food-related behavior.
- Limit non-nutritive video and television watching to less than 2 hours daily.

Physical activity is an important part of a healthy lifestyle from birth to death. By developing an appreciation for and an enjoyment of regular physical activity during childhood, the risk for obesity may be reduced along with the health problems associated with it (Box 11-1). Alternatively, long hours in front of a television, unnecessary snacking, and no involvement in physical activity are habits that start young, die hard, and set the stage for an overweight or obese childhood.

Lead Poisoning. Lead poisoning in children can be extremely damaging to the central nervous system, and it can negatively alter both cognitive and motor skills. The CDC estimates that more than 250,000 American children between the ages of 1 and 5 years have health problems associated with lead poisoning each year.[26] Approximately 70% of lead exposure among children is the result of lead-based paint. Lead-containing paint chips from deteriorating buildings or renovations result in high levels of lead-contaminated dust. Children explore with their hands and mouths at this age, thereby making the oral intake and inhalation of lead highly likely. Lead-based paint was banned in the United States in 1978; however, many millions of homes still contain

---

BOX 11-1   CHILDHOOD OVERWEIGHT AND OBESITY FACTS

Prevalence of Obesity

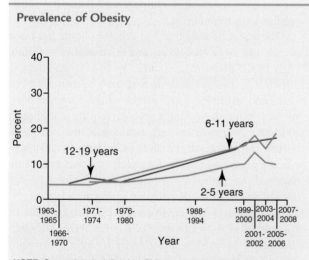

NOTE: Overweight is defined as BMI greater than or equal to sex- and age-specific 95th percentile from the 2000 CDC Growth Charts.
SOURCES: CDC/NCHS, National Health Examination Surveys II (ages 6-11), III (ages 12-17), and National Health and Nutrition Examination Surveys (NHANES) I-III, and NHANES 1999-2000, 2001-2002, 2003-2004, 2005-2006, and 2007-2008.

Ogden C, Carroll M. *Prevalence of obesity among children and adolescents: United States, Trends 1963-1965 through 2007-2008* (website): www.cdc.gov/nchs/data/hestat/obesity_child_07_08/obesity_child_07_08.htm. Accessed June 2011.

Contributing Factors
- Genetics
- Behavioral factors
  - Energy intake
  - Physical activity
  - Sedentary behaviors
- Environmental factors
  - Parental role models
  - Positive or negative child-care atmosphere
  - Exposure to health, wellness, and nutrition in school

Consequences
- Health risks
  - Asthma
  - Cardiovascular disease
  - Hepatic steatosis
  - Sleep apnea
  - Type 2 diabetes
- Psychosocial risks
  - Low self-esteem
  - Social discrimination

The Centers for Disease Control and Prevention's Web site about childhood obesity (www.cdc.gov/obesity/childhood/index.html) has up-to-date information regarding the condition's prevalence, current treatment recommendations, and information about state-based programs to help alleviate the health burden of childhood overweight and obesity.

Data from the Centers for Disease Control and Prevention. *Childhood overweight and obesity* (website): www.cdc.gov/nccdphp/dnpa/obesity/childhood/index.htm. Accessed June 2011.

lead paint. Children who live below the poverty line and in homes built before 1950 are at the greatest risk.[27] One of the *Healthy People 2020* targets is the complete elimination of lead exposure in children.[28]

Adolescence (12 to 18 Years Old)

Physical Growth

The final growth spurt of childhood occurs with the onset of puberty. This rapid growth is evident in increasing body size and the development of sex characteristics in response to hormonal influences. The rate of change varies widely among individual boys and girls, but particularly distinct growth patterns do emerge. Girls store more subcutaneous fat in the abdominal area. The pelvis widens in preparation for future childbearing, and the size of the hips also increase, which causes much anxiety for many figure-conscious young girls. In boys, physical growth is seen more in increased muscle mass and long-bone growth. At first a boy's growth spurt is slower than that of a girl, but he soon surpasses her in both weight and height.

There is an association with the timing of sexual maturation and the risk of adult onset chronic disease (e.g., cancer, metabolic syndrome).[29] Girls who reach sexual maturation early are more likely to become overweight or

---

CULTURAL CONSIDERATIONS

GROWTH CHARTS: CAN YOU USE THEM FOR ALL CHILDREN?

To assess a child's growth accurately, three things are essential: (1) an appropriate growth reference; (2) an accurate measurement; and (3) an accurate calculation of the child's age. Growth charts are not used to identify "short" or "tall" children. They are used as a means for the continuous assessment of a child's growth rate. Children are identified with a percentile of the population in terms of a specific anthropometric measurement. For example, if a child has a height for age at the 70th percentile, then 29% of the children of the same age and gender are taller, and 69% are shorter. With adequate nutrition and in the absence of disease, this child should continue to grow on the 70th percentile curve.

Health professionals use the 5th and 95th percentiles as cutoff points at which children who fall outside of this range are screened for potential health- or nutrition-related problems. Children and adolescents with a body mass index (BMI) for age above the 85th percentile are at risk for being overweight as adults. The cutoff point of the 95th percentile on the BMI-for-age charts correlates with a BMI of 30 in adults, which is considered obese. Because the BMI-for-age charts correlate with the adult BMI index, they can be used from childhood into adulthood, thereby providing a lifelong assessment tool that indicates risk factors for chronic disease associated with obesity.

Human Milk or Alternative Feeding Formula
Breast-fed infants have a slightly different growth curve from formula-fed infants. Breast-fed infants grow slightly more rapidly than formula-fed infants during the first 2 months of life, and then the rate of growth declines to a rate that is slower than that of formula-fed infants. The previous growth charts were predominantly based on formula-fed infants. The updated World Health Organization charts used infants

that were exclusively breast-fed in accordance with feeding recommendations (i.e., breast-feed for at least 12 months, with solid foods introduced between 4 and 6 months) to obtain the standards.

Growth Charts in Relation to Variations in Sexual Maturation
With regard to charting the growth patterns of an adolescent, practitioners should be aware of the racial differences in the timing of sexual maturation and how that relates to overall weight and body fat. A study that analyzed sexual maturation rates found that non-Hispanic African-American girls and boys begin the process of sexual maturity before Mexican-American or non-Hispanic Caucasian children do.[1] The median age at menarche was 12.06 years for the non-Hispanic African-American girls, 12.25 years for the Mexican-American girls, and 12.55 years for the non-Hispanic Caucasian girls. The timing of menarche in girls also was assessed in 1973; when compared with that data, the average onset of menarche does not appear to have changed over the past 30 years.[2] Such differences between racial groups are potentially important when assessing growth on a growth chart, because more mature children are likely to be taller and heavier than their less mature peers.

Using Growth Charts for Various Ethnic Groups
Not enough individuals participated in the data collection to create charts that were specific to racial or ethnic groups. Therefore, the Centers for Disease Control and Prevention and the World Health Organization promote the use of the standard growth charts for all racial and ethnic groups. Future studies will determine if significant differences exist and warrant the development of charts that are specific to different cultural backgrounds.

1. Sun SS, Schubert CM, Chumlea WC, et al. National estimates of the timing of sexual maturation and racial differences among US children. *Pediatrics.* 2002;110(5):911-919.
2. Sun SS, Schubert CM, Liang R, et al. Is sexual maturity occurring earlier among U.S. children? *J Adolesc Health.* 2005;37(5):345-355.

obese than girls who do not mature until later.[30] However, this association is the opposite for boys; boys who mature earlier are more likely to be thinner than their counterparts.[31] Racial differences also exist: non-Hispanic African-American girls and boys begin the process of sexual maturation before Mexican-American or non-Hispanic Caucasian children.[32] Such differences are specifically important when assessing growth on a growth chart. The age and stage of sexual maturation are associated with body fat and overall weight (see the Cultural Considerations box, "Growth Charts: Can You Use Them for All Children?").

Eating Patterns

Teenagers' eating habits are greatly influenced by their rapid growth as well as by self-consciousness and peer pressure. Teenagers tend to skip lunch more often than breakfast, to derive a great deal of their energy from snacks, to eat at fast-food restaurants, and to eat any kind of food at any time of day. Unfortunately, some teenagers begin to experiment with alcohol. Even a mild form of alcohol abuse in combination with the elevated nutrition demands of adolescence can easily affect a teen's nutritional status. In general overall nutrition, boys usually fare better than girls. Their larger appetite and the sheer volume of food consumed usually ensure an adequate intake of nutrients. Alternatively, because they are under a greater social pressure for thinness, girls may tend to restrict their food and have an inadequate nutrient intake.

Eating Disorders

Social, family, and personal pressures concerning figure control strongly influence many young girls and an increasing number of young boys. As a result, they sometimes follow unwise self-imposed crash diets for weight loss. In some cases, self-starvation occurs, and complex eating disorders such as anorexia nervosa and bulimia nervosa may develop. Psychologists have traditionally identified mothers as the main source of family pressure to remain thin. However, fathers may also contribute to the problem if they are emotionally distant and do not provide important feedback to build self-worth and self-esteem in their young children. Parents must help their children to see themselves as loved no matter what they weigh so that these children are not as vulnerable to social influences that equate extreme thinness with beauty.

Eating disorders involve a distorted body image and a morbid and irrational pursuit of thinness. Such disordered eating often begins during the early adolescent years, when many girls see themselves as fat even though their average weight is often below the normal weight for their height. The longer the duration of the illness, the less likely it is that a full recovery will be achieved. Thus, early detection and intervention are critical for restoration of overall health. Warning signs, treatment options, and diagnostic criteria are discussed further in Chapter 15.

SUMMARY

- The growth and development of healthy children depend on optimal nutrition support. In turn, good nutrition depends on many social, psychologic, cultural, and environmental influences that affect individual growth potential throughout the life cycle.
- From birth, the nutrition needs of children change with each unique growth period.
- *Infants* experience rapid growth. Human milk is the natural first food, with solid foods being delayed until approximately 6 months of age, when digestive and physiologic processes have matured.
- *Toddlers, preschoolers, and school-aged children* experience slowed and irregular growth. During this period, their energy demands are less per kilogram of body weight, but they require a well-balanced diet for continued growth and health.
- *Adolescents* undergo a large growth spurt before adulthood. This rapid growth involves both physical and sexual maturation.
- Social and cultural factors influence the developing food habits of all children.
- Boys usually obtain their increased caloric and nutrient demands because they eat larger amounts of food.
- Girls (and some boys) often feel social and peer pressure to restrict their food to control their weight, thereby causing some to develop severe eating disorders.

CRITICAL THINKING QUESTIONS

1. Preterm and term infants have different nutrition needs. Explain why immature infants have special dietary needs.
2. Why is breast-feeding the preferred method of feeding infants? Compare breast-feeding with the alternative commercial formulas that are available for bottle-fed babies.
3. Outline an appropriate schedule for new parents to use as a guide for adding solid foods to their baby's diet during the first year of life. What foods are not appropriate at this age and why?
4. Compare the changes in the growth and development of toddlers, preschoolers, and school-aged children. What factors influence their nutrition needs and eating habits?
5. Consider the factors that influence the changing nutrition needs and eating habits of adolescents. Who is usually at greater nutritional risk during this period, boys or girls? Why? What suggestions do you have for reducing the nutritional risk at this vulnerable age?

CHAPTER CHALLENGE QUESTIONS

True-False

Write the correct statement for each statement that is false.

1. *True or False:* A good way to keep infants and toddlers (i.e., from birth to the age of 2 years) from being overweight is to use nonfat milk in their diets.
2. *True or False:* A variety of protein foods in a child's diet helps to provide all of the essential amino acids for growth.
3. *True or False:* Failure to thrive is a condition in some infants and children who do not grow and develop normally; it is often associated with parental inexperience.
4. *True or False:* The rooting and sucking reflexes must be learned before a newborn infant can obtain breast milk.
5. *True or False:* A toddler needs the same food variety as an adult, according to the MyPlate guidelines, but with larger serving sizes.

Multiple Choice

1. Fat is needed in the child's diet to supply
   a. minerals.
   b. water-soluble vitamins.
   c. essential amino acids.
   d. essential fatty acids.
2. Iron deficiency in childhood is associated with which of the following diseases?
   a. Scurvy
   b. Rickets
   c. Anemia
   d. Pellagra
3. The growth and development of a school-aged child (i.e., 5 to 12 years old) are characterized by
   a. a rapid increase in physical growth with increased food requirements.
   b. the more rapid growth of girls during the latter part of the period.
   c. food jags and a refusal to eat.
   d. increased dependence on parental standards or habits.

⊖volve Please refer to the Students' Resource section of this text's Evolve Web site for additional study resources.

REFERENCES

1. Grummer-Strawn LM, Reinold C, Krebs NF; Centers for Disease Control and Prevention. Use of World Health Organization and CDC growth charts for children aged 0-59 months in the United States. *MMWR Recomm Rep.* 2010;59(RR-9):1-15.
2. Food and Nutrition Board, Institute of Medicine. *Dietary reference intakes for energy, carbohydrate, fiber, fat, fatty acids, cholesterol, protein, and amino acids.* Washington, DC: National Academies Press; 2002.
3. Herrmann KR. Early parenteral nutrition and successful postnatal growth of premature infants. *Nutr Clin Pract.* 2010;25(1):69-75.
4. Fusch C, Bauer K, Böhles HJ, et al; Working group for developing the guidelines for parenteral nutrition of The German Society for Nutritional Medicine. Neonatology/ paediatrics—guidelines on parenteral nutrition, Chapter 13. *Ger Med Sci.* 2009;7:Doc15.
5. Specker B. Nutrition influences bone development from infancy through toddler years. *J Nutr.* 2004;134(3): 691S-695S.
6. Rizzoli R, Bianchi ML, Garabédian M, et al. Maximizing bone mineral mass gain during growth for the prevention of fractures in the adolescents and the elderly. *Bone.* 2010;46(2):294-305.
7. Pitukcheewanont P, Punyasavatsut N, Feuille M. Physical activity and bone health in children and adolescents. *Pediatr Endocrinol Rev.* 2010;7(3):275-282.

8. Braun M, Palacios C, Wigertz K, et al. Racial differences in skeletal calcium retention in adolescent girls with varied controlled calcium intakes. *Am J Clin Nutr.* 2007;85(6): 1657-1663.

9. Riggins T, Miller NC, Bauer PJ, et al. Consequences of low neonatal iron status due to maternal diabetes mellitus on explicit memory performance in childhood. *Dev Neuropsychol.* 2009;34(6):762-779.

10. McCann JC, Ames BN. An overview of evidence for a causal relation between iron deficiency during development and deficits in cognitive or behavioral function. *Am J Clin Nutr.* 2007;85(4):931-945.

11. Food and Nutrition Board, Institute of Medicine. *Dietary reference intakes for vitamin A, vitamin K, arsenic, boron, chromium, copper, iodine, iron, manganese, molybdenum, nickel, silicon, vanadium, and zinc.* Washington, DC: National Academies Press; 2001.

12. Gartner LM, Morton J, Lawrence RA, et al; American Academy of Pediatrics Section on Breastfeeding. Breastfeeding and the use of human milk. *Pediatrics.* 2005;115(2): 496-506.

13. Bauer J, Gerss J. Longitudinal analysis of macronutrients and minerals in human milk produced by mothers of preterm infants. *Clin Nutr.* 2010;30(2):215-220.

14. James DC, Lessen R. Position of the American Dietetic Association: promoting and supporting breastfeeding. *J Am Diet Assoc.* 2009;109(11):1926-1942.

15. Labiner-Wolfe J, Fein SB, Shealy KR. Infant formula-handling education and safety. *Pediatrics.* 2008;122(Suppl 2):S85-S90.

16. Høst A, Halken S, Muraro A, et al. Dietary prevention of allergic diseases in infants and small children. *Pediatr Allergy Immunol.* 2008;19(1):1-4.

17. Harris JL, Bargh JA. Television viewing and unhealthy diet: implications for children and media interventions. *Health Commun.* 2009;24(7):660-673.

18. Bergman EA, Gordon RW. Position of the American Dietetic Association: local support for nutrition integrity in schools. *J Am Diet Assoc.* 2010;110(8):1244-1254.

19. Ralston K, Newman C, Clauson A, et al. *The national school lunch program: background, trends, and issues* (website): www.ers.usda.gov/publications/err61/err61.pdf. Accessed October 13, 2011.

20. Briggs M, Mueller CG, Fleischhacker S. Position of the American Dietetic Association, School Nutrition Association, and Society for Nutrition Education: comprehensive school nutrition services. *J Am Diet Assoc.* 2010;110(11): 1738-1749.

21. Spiotta RT, Luma GB. Evaluating obesity and cardiovascular risk factors in children and adolescents. *Am Fam Physician.* 2008;78(9):1052-1058.

22. Olstad DL, McCargar L. Prevention of overweight and obesity in children under the age of 6 years. *Appl Physiol Nutr Metab.* 2009;34(4):551-570.

23. Koletzko B, von Kries R, Closa R, et al. Can infant feeding choices modulate later obesity risk? *Am J Clin Nutr.* 2009; 89(5):1502S-1508S.

24. Dehghan M, Akhtar-Danesh N, Merchant AT. Childhood obesity, prevalence and prevention. *Nutr J.* 2005;4:24.

25. Scaglioni S, Salvioni M, Galimberti C. Influence of parental attitudes in the development of children eating behaviour. *Br J Nutr.* 2008;99(Suppl 1):S22-S25.

26. Centers for Disease Control and Prevention: *Lead* (website): www.cdc.gov/nceh/lead/. Accessed October 13, 2011.

27. Vivier PM, Hauptman M, Weitzen SH, et al. The important health impact of where a child lives: neighborhood characteristics and the burden of lead poisoning. *Matern Child Health J.* 2011;15(8):1195-1202.

28. U.S. Department of Health and Human Services. *Healthy People 2020.* Washington, DC: U.S. Government Printing Office; 2010.

29. Golub MS, Collman GW, Foster PM, et al. Public health implications of altered puberty timing. *Pediatrics.* 2008;121 (Suppl 3):S218-S230.

30. Himes JH, Obarzanek E, Baranowski T, et al. Early sexual maturation, body composition, and obesity in African-American girls. *Obes Res.* 2004;12(Suppl):64S-72S.

31. Wang Y. Is obesity associated with early sexual maturation? A comparison of the association in American boys versus girls. *Pediatrics.* 2002;110(5):903-910.

32. Sun SS, Schubert CM, Chumlea WC, et al. National estimates of the timing of sexual maturation and racial differences among US children. *Pediatrics.* 2002;110(5):911-919.

FURTHER READING AND RESOURCES

Food and Nutrition Service. School Meals: www.fns.usda.gov/cnd

Kidnetic. www.kidnetic.com

KidsHealth. www.kidshealth.org

MyPlate tools for kids (6 to 11 years old). http://www.choosemyplate.gov/children-over-five.html

MyPlate tools for preschoolers. http://www.choosemyplate.gov/preschoolers.html

National Center for Education in Maternal and Child Health. www.ncemch.org

World Health Organization child growth standards. www.who.int/childgrowth/en/

These Web sites are excellent resources for childhood nutrition information. One of the most important parts of working with parents and children on feeding and health issues is to have access to up-to-date information and ideas. Explore these sites to discover current topics that address the health and nutrition issues that face youth today.

Ogden CL, Carroll MD, Curtin LR, et al. Prevalence of high body mass index in US children and adolescents, 2007-2008. *JAMA.* 2010;303(3):242-249.

This article explores the prevalence and contributing factors of childhood obesity and prevention practices that may help to alleviate this growing health risk.

CHAPTER 12

Nutrition for Adults: The Early, Middle, and Later Years

KEY CONCEPTS

- Gradual aging throughout the adult years is a unique process that is based on an individual's genetic heritage and life experience.

- Aging is a total life process that involves biologic, nutritional, social, economic, psychologic, and spiritual aspects.

The rapid growth and development of adolescence leads to physical maturity as adults. Physical growth in size levels off, but the constant cell growth and reproduction that are necessary to maintain a healthy body continue. Other aspects of growth and development—mental, social, psychologic, and spiritual—continue for a lifetime.

Food and nutrition continue to provide essential support during the adult aging process. Life expectancy is increasing; thus, health promotion and disease prevention are even more important to ensure quality of life throughout these extended years.

This chapter explores the ways in which positive nutrition can help adults to lead healthier and happier lives.

ADULTHOOD: CONTINUING HUMAN GROWTH AND DEVELOPMENT

Coming of Age in America

Americans are experiencing tremendous change with regard to the composition of the population. The report from the U.S. Department of Health and Human Services entitled *Healthy People 2020* presents national goals for helping all people to make informed decisions about their health. One of the primary goals set for 2020 is to attain high-quality, longer lives that are free of preventable disease, disability, injury, and premature death.[1]

Population and Age Distribution

By the year 2050, according to the U.S. Census Bureau, the total U.S. population will grow to 439 million people, which is up 41.5% from 2010.[2] Older segments of the population will grow significantly during this period; the number of people who are older than 65 years old will more than double, with 21.5% of that age group being older than 85 years old[3] (Table 12-1). The median age will increase from 36.9 years to 39 years for the total population by 2050. Figure 12-1 shows population growth and projections from 1900 to 2050 for older adults. Growth rates for various ethnic subgroups continue to rise as well (see the Cultural Considerations box, "Racial and Ethnic Composition of the U.S. Population"). A changing age

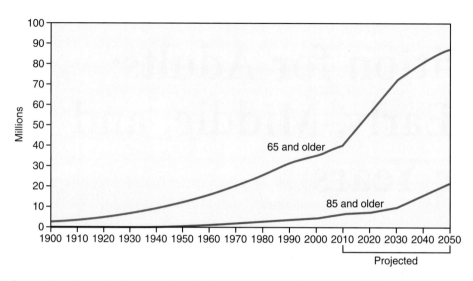

Figure 12-1 The number of people 65 years old and older by age group for the years 1900 to 2000 and projected to 2010 to 2050. Reference population data refer to the resident population. (Reprinted from the Federal Interagency Forum on Aging-Related Statistics. *Older Americans update 2006: key indicators of well being.* Washington, DC: U.S. Government Printing Office; 2006.)

TABLE 12-1 **POPULATION PROJECTIONS FOR ADULTS FROM 2010 TO 2050 BY AGE GROUP**

Male and Female Age (Years)	2010	Projection for 2050	Percent Increase
20 to 24	21,779,000	28,171,000	29.3
25 to 29	21,418,000	28,039,000	30.9
30 to 34	20,400,000	28,126,000	37.9
35 to 39	20,267,000	27,799,000	37.2
40 to 44	21,010,000	26,897,000	28.0
45 to 49	22,596,000	25,933,000	14.8
50 to 54	22,109,000	24,445,000	10.6
55 to 59	19,517,000	24,621,000	26.2
60 to 64	16,758,000	23,490,000	40.2
65 to 69	12,261,000	21,543,000	75.7
70 to 74	9,202,000	18,570,000	101.8
75 to 79	7,282,000	15,964,000	119.2
80 to 84	5,733,000	13,429,000	134.2
≥85	5,751,000	19,042,000	231.1

Data from the U.S. Census Bureau, Population Division. *Projections of the population by age and sex for the United States: 2010 to 2050.* Washington, DC: U.S. Government Printing Office; 2008.

distribution in the population results in changes in the health care system as well as job demands in geriatric health care.

Life Expectancy and Quality of Life

Life expectancy has dramatically increased during the past century, from only 47 years in 1900 to a projected average of 79.5 years in 2020 (77.1 years for men and 81.9 for women).[4] However, there are notable differences in life expectancy among various population groups and among those with different household incomes. Americans consistently value health-related quality of life, which is one's personal sense of physical and mental health and ability to act within the environment. Quality of life is a major focus of the *Healthy People 2020* initiative.[1]

Impact on Health Care

Career opportunities in the fields of disease prevention and health promotion are at an all-time high. Community and private classes about healthy lifestyles and nutrition target the prime concerns for a growing adult population. Weight management and diabetes management are two of the most popular topics. Dietitians, nurses, life coaches, personal trainers, psychologists, and other members of the health care team may be involved at various levels of such programs. A dire need exists for the health care system in America to prevent disease development in the adult population rather than relying on treatment.

Shaping Influences on Adult Growth and Development

The overall process of human aging has the unique potential for growth and fulfillment at every stage. The periods of adulthood (i.e., the young, middle, and older years) are

life expectancy the number of years that a person of a given age may expect to live; this is affected by environment, lifestyle, gender, and race.

Shifting racial and ethnic patterns continue to reshape the American population as a whole (see figure). The non-Hispanic population of the United States that is 65 years old or older is expected to almost double by 2050. Meanwhile, the Hispanic population that is 65 years old or older in the United States is expected to increase by a factor of six, from 2.9 million to 17.5 million.[1]

The estimated life expectancy varies among ethnic groups as well. For example, Caucasians have a life expectancy of 78.9 years, whereas African Americans have a life expectancy of 73.8 years.[2] Living arrangements, household income, educational attainment, type of medical insurance, and many other variables fluctuate among ethnic groups.

Health care providers should understand and address the cultural and ethnic needs of an elderly individual when providing nutrition education. All areas of social, socioeconomic, and available health care play significant factors when designing the best care plan. Cookie-cutter meal plans for one ethnic group are not particularly useful for another culturally diverse population. Given the rapidly changing ethnic diversity of the elderly population in the United States, it will be increasingly important to understand and practice cultural sensitivity.

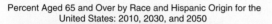

Percent Aged 65 and Over by Race and Hispanic Origin for the United States: 2010, 2030, and 2050

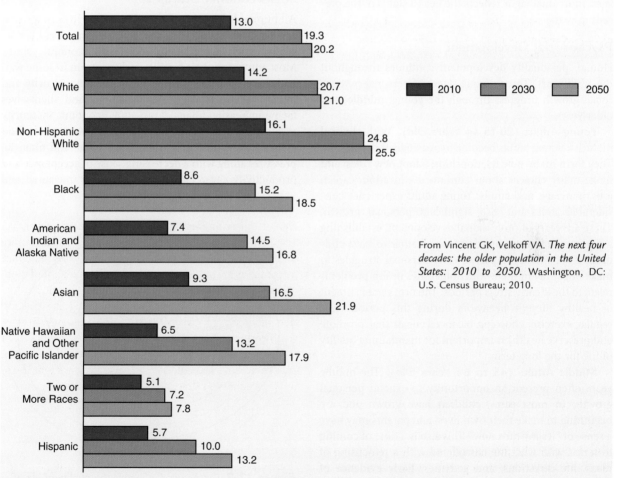

From Vincent GK, Velkoff VA. *The next four decades: the older population in the United States: 2010 to 2050.* Washington, DC: U.S. Census Bureau; 2010.

Note: Unless otherwise specified, data refer to the population who reported a race alone.
Populations for each race group include both Hispanics and non-Hispanics, unless otherwise specified. Hispanics may be of any race.

1. Vincent GK, Velkoff VA. *The next four decades: the older population in the United States: 2010 to 2050.* Washington, DC: U.S. Census Bureau; 2010.
2. Heron MP, Hoyert DL, Murphy SL, et al. Deaths: final data for 2006. National vital statistics reports; vol 57 no 14. Hyattsville, Md: National Center for Health Statistics; 2009.

no exception. Many individual and group events mark the course; however, at each stage, the four basic areas of adult life—physical, psychosocial, socioeconomic, and nutritional—shape general growth and development.

Physical Growth

The overall physical growth and maturity of the human body, which are governed by the genetic potential, level off during the early adult years. Physical growth is no longer a process of increasing numbers of cells and body size; rather, it involves the vital growth of new cells to replace old ones. After physical maturity is established, energy requirements decrease. Adjustment to a gradually declining metabolic rate and thus the need for fewer kilocalories is important for weight management. At older ages, individual vigor reflects the health status of the preceding years.

Psychosocial Development

Human personality development continues throughout the adult years. Three unique stages of personal psychosocial growth progress through the young, middle, and older years.

Young Adults (20 to 44 Years Old). With physical maturity, young adults become increasingly independent. They form many new relationships; adopt new roles; and make many choices about continued education, career, jobs, marriage, and family. Young adults experience considerable stress but also significant personal growth. These are years of professional development, establishing a home community, and deciding whether to have children, all of which are part of early personal struggles to make one's way in the world. Sometimes health problems relate to these early stress periods. The firm establishment of healthy lifestyle behaviors during this period (e.g., regular exercise, choosing balanced meals that promote and preserve health) is important for maintaining quality of life for the long term.

Middle Adults (45 to 64 Years Old). The middle years often present an opportunity to expand personal growth. In most cases, children have grown and are beginning to make their own lives, and parents may have a sense of "it's my turn now." This also is a time of coming to terms with what life has offered with a refocusing of ideas, life directions, and activities. Early evidence of chronic disease appears in some middle-aged adults. Wellness, health promotion, and the reduction of disease risks continue to be major focuses of health care.

Older Adults (65 Years Old and Older). Adults vary widely with regard to their personal and physical resources for dealing with older age. They may have a sense of wholeness and completeness, or they may increasingly withdraw from life. If the outcome of their life experiences is positive, they arrive at an older age rich in the wisdom of their years; they enjoy life and health, and they enrich the lives of those around them. However, some elderly people arrive at these years poorly equipped to deal with the adjustments associated with aging and the health problems that may arise. As this population continues to grow, the subdivision of young-old (65 to 74 years old), elderly (75 to 84 years old), and old-old (85 years old and older) has become a popular way to characterize individuals as general health and quality of life continue to improve. Many factors that influence perceived and actual quality of life are integrally associated with nutritional status (Figure 12-2).

Socioeconomic Status

All human beings grow up and live their lives in a social and cultural context. The rapidly changing world is currently experiencing major social and economic shifts. Most adults and their families feel the strain in some way, and these pressures directly influence food security and health. As people age, many seniors find themselves facing increasing financial pressure. Economic insecurity creates added stress and often leads to the need for food assistance (Figure 12-3). Sometimes social and financial pressures along with a decreasing sense of acceptance and productivity cause elderly people to feel unwanted and

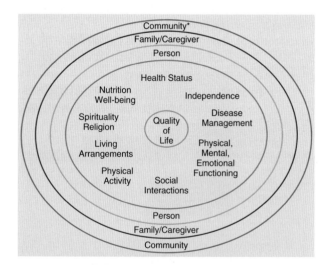

Figure 12-2 Factors that influence the quality of life of adults who are 60 years old and older. *The term *community* includes health and supportive services at local, state, and federal levels as well as health professionals and researchers. (Reprinted from Kuczmarski MF, Weddle DO; American Dietetic Association. Position paper of the American Dietetic Association: nutrition across the spectrum of aging, *J Am Diet Assoc.* 2005;105:616-630.)

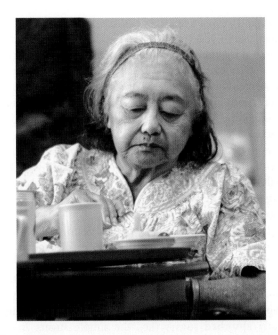

Figure 12-3 Elderly woman assisted by the Supplemental Nutrition Assistance Program (SNAP) to obtain needed food. (Copyright JupiterImages Corp.)

unworthy. Depression is a clinical syndrome that is not part of normal aging, and it is closely related to poor overall health, increased cost of health care, poor financial resources, and loneliness.[5,6] Elderly patients with declining health are particularly susceptible to depression, which is the most common psychiatric condition seen in the elderly population and a leading cause of unintended weight loss. Failure to thrive in the geriatric population, which is generally multifactorial in etiology and caused by a combination of chronic diseases, is associated with impaired physical function, malnutrition, depression, and cognitive impairment.[7] All people need a sense of belonging, achievement, and self-esteem. Unfortunately, many elderly people suffer from loneliness, uncertainty, and depression, all of which increase mortality.

Some basic needs that are common to all people are economic security, adequate nutrition, personal effectiveness, suitable housing, constructive and enjoyable activities, satisfying social relationships, and spiritual freedom. An increasing number of healthy, motivated, young-old adults are contributing to the productive workforce; they are redefining what it means to be a senior citizen.

Nutrition Needs

The energy and nutrient needs of individual adults in each age group vary in accordance with living and working situations. The Dietary Reference Intake (DRI) recommendations for healthy adults meet most needs, but the aging process influences individual nutritional requirements. Only in the most recent DRIs have scientists distinguished the nutrient needs of the 50- to 70-year-old adults from those who are 71 years old and older. One reason for this is that previously not a large enough population of healthy elderly adults was available to study their nutrient requirements and thus determine if needs continue to change throughout the life span.

THE AGING PROCESS AND NUTRITION NEEDS

General Physiologic Changes

Biologic Changes

Throughout life, every experience makes an imprint on one's individual heritage. Everyone ages in different ways, depending on his or her personal makeup and available resources.

Metabolism. Beginning at about the age of 30 years, a gradual loss of functioning cells occurs, which results in reduced cell metabolism. This change in metabolic rate reflects both lean muscle mass loss as well as a loss of high metabolically active organ tissues such as the brain, liver, heart, and kidneys.[8] The rate of this decline accelerates during later life. Not all skeletal muscle mass loss is mandatory, however. A major contributing factor to this loss is a lack of physical activity. Approximately 25% of Americans do not participate in any leisure-time physical activity.[9] The Institute of Medicine recommends 60 minutes of moderate exercise every day to maintain a healthy weight.[10] In addition, the *2008 Physical Activity Guidelines for Americans* recommend 150 minutes of moderate-intensity physical activity (or 75 minutes of vigorous-intensity physical activity) per week to reduce the risk of chronic disease (see Chapter 16). For more extensive health benefits, adults should participate in twice as much activity per week (i.e., 300 minutes of moderate-intensity activity or 150 minutes of vigorous-intensity activity).[11]

Hormones. Hormonal changes during the aging process have many repercussions in general health. The common decline in insulin production or insulin sensitivity often results in elevated blood glucose levels and diabetes. Decreases in melatonin, which is the hormone that is responsible for regulating body rhythms, may interfere with normal sleep cycles. Part of the normal changes in body composition is attributed to decreases in growth hormone and the sex hormones estrogen and testosterone. Menopause, which marks the end of a woman's childbearing years, involves the cessation of estrogen and progesterone production by the ovaries. This dramatic change in a woman's life, which usually occurs between the ages of 45 and 55 years, represents the most significant hormonal change associated with age. Menopause is accompanied by an increase in body fat, a decrease in lean tissue, and an increase in the risk of chronic disease (specifically heart disease and osteoporosis). Despite these changes, women today are better equipped than ever before with both social and medical support to embrace this period of life and to maintain health for many decades to come.

Effect on Food Patterns

Some of the physical changes of aging affect food patterns. For example, the secretion of digestive juices and the motility of gastrointestinal muscles gradually diminish, which causes decreased absorption and use of nutrients. Decreased taste, smell, thirst, and vision also affect appetite and reduce food and fluid intake. Several other conditions that commonly afflict elderly adults are not so obviously related to food intake but should be considered. For example, decreased hand function, which is especially common in the elderly, can reduce hand–eye coordination and the ability to cook and prepare food. Older people often have increased concern about body functions, more social stress, personal losses, and fewer social opportunities to maintain self-esteem; all of these concerns can affect food intake. A lack of sufficient nourishment is the primary nutrition problem of older adults.

Individuality of the Aging Process

Although the biologic changes of senescence are generally similar, each person is unique, and people show a wide variety of individual responses. Individuals age at different rates and in different ways, depending on their genetic heritage and the health and nutrition resources of their prior years. For example, some individuals are in the best shape of their lives after retirement. Thus, specific needs vary with functional ability.

Nutrition Needs

Macronutrients and Fluids

The basal metabolic rate declines an average of 1% to 2% per decade, with a more rapid decline occurring at approximately age 40 years of age for men and 50 years of age for women.[10] This correlates with a gradual loss of functioning body cells and reduced physical activity. The current national standard is based on estimates of 5% decreased metabolic activity during the middle and older years. The mean energy expenditure for women with a body mass index of 18.5 to 25 who are between the ages

of 51 and 70 years is 2066 kcal/day; for women who are older than 71 years old, it is 1564 kcal/day. For men of the same age and body mass index, energy expenditure averages 2469 kcal/day and 2238 kcal/day, respectively.[10] These recommendations are based on the averages of the population, and they may vary greatly among individuals. Physical and health statuses as well as living situations influence overall energy and nutrient requirements. Obesity during the adult years has a significant association with an increased prevalence of disability.[12] Thus, health promotion that includes weight control and disease prevention are important aspects of healthy living throughout the entire life span.

The basic fuels that are necessary to supply these energy needs are the same as they are for all stages of life: primarily carbohydrate, along with moderate fat.

Carbohydrate. Approximately 45% to 65% of total kilocalories should come from carbohydrate, with an emphasis on complex carbohydrates (e.g., whole grains). Easily absorbed sugars (i.e., the simple sugars in soft drinks, candy, and sweets) may also be used for energy, but they should be used in limited amounts and make up no more than 10% of total kilocalorie intake. The National Academy of Sciences has determined that an absolute minimum of 130 g of carbohydrates per day is necessary to maintain normal brain function in both children and adults.[10]

Fat. Fats usually contribute approximately 30% of total kilocalories and provide a backup energy source, important fat-soluble vitamins, and essential fatty acids. A reasonable goal is to avoid large quantities of fat and to emphasize the quality of the fat used. Fat digestion and absorption may be delayed in elderly people, but these functions are not greatly disturbed. Sufficient fat for helping food taste better aids appetite and in some cases provides needed kilocalories to prevent excessive weight loss.

Protein. The current national standard recommends an adult protein intake of 0.8 g per kilogram of body weight for a total protein intake of 56 g/day for an average-weight man (154 lb) and of 46 g/day for an average-weight woman (127 lb). Protein should provide approximately 10% to 35% of the total kilocalories (see Chapter 4).[10] The requirement for protein may increase during illness or convalescence or in the presence of a

---

menopause the end of a woman's menstrual activity and capacity to bear children.

senescence the process or condition of growing old.

wasting disease. In any case, protein needs are related to two basic factors: (1) the protein quality (i.e., the quantity and ratio of its amino acids); and (2) an adequate number of total kilocalories in the diet. Healthy adults who consume a balanced diet do not need supplemental amino acid preparations, which are an expensive and inefficient source of available nitrogen.

Fluid. Physiologic changes in the hypothalamus naturally occur with age, and, as a result, elderly individuals exhibit an overall decreased thirst sensation and reduced fluid intake compared with younger adults.[13,14] In addition, other physiologic changes associated with aging (e.g., diminishing kidney function) may exacerbate losses of body fluid and increase fluid intake requirements. See Table 9-1 for fluid intake recommendations for adults.

Micronutrients and Health Concerns

A diet that includes a variety of foods should supply adequate amounts of most vitamins and minerals for healthy adults. However, some essential nutrients may require special attention because of their relationship with possible health problems in the aging adult and morbidity or medication interactions.

Vitamin D and calcium are essential nutrients for growth and for the maintenance of healthy bone tissue. Osteoporosis (porous bone) is a disorder in which bone mineral density is low and bones become brittle, with a high risk of breaking (Figure 12-4). Approximately 10 million Americans currently have osteoporosis, and an additional 34 million have osteopenia. The prevalence of low bone density and osteoporosis, along with resultant disability, increases significantly with age (Figure 12-5). Race and sex are also influential factors in overall bone health. The risk for fracture is highest among Caucasian women, with African Americans and Hispanics having lower incidence rates.[15,16] Contributing factors for all populations include the following: (1) inadequate calcium and vitamin D intake; (2) physical inactivity; (3) smoking and alcohol use; (4) decreased estrogen after menopause in women; (5) thin build; and (6) certain medical conditions and the use of certain medications. Although the exact mechanism is not well understood, researchers also propose major depressive disorder as a risk factor for osteoporosis.[17]

The DRI standards state the Recommended Dietary Allowance level for vitamin D is 600 IU for both men and women between the ages of 51 and 70 years and 800 IU for individuals who are older than 70 years old.[18] To meet the dietary recommendation for vitamin D, elderly individuals should consume foods that are fortified with vitamin D or take a dietary supplement to overcome the

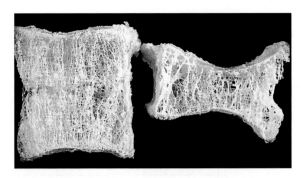

Figure 12-4 Osteoporotic vertebral body *(right)* shortened by compression fractures compared with a normal vertebral body. Note that the osteoporotic vertebra has a characteristic loss of horizontal trabeculae and a thickened vertical trabeculae. (Reprinted from Kumar V, Abbas AK, Fausto N, Mitchell R. *Robbins basic pathology.* 8th ed. Philadelphia: Saunders; 2007.)

reduced ability to endogenously synthesize vitamin D. Chapters 7 and 8 present good food sources of calcium and vitamin D.

Nutrient Supplementation

The use of dietary supplements by elderly adults—usually on a self-prescribed basis—is common. Although such routine use may not be necessary, supplements are often recommended for people in debilitated states or who have malabsorption conditions. In addition, the DRIs specify that individuals who are older than 50 years old should consume vitamin B_{12} in supplemental form or through fortified foods because of the high risk of deficiency that results from decreased gastric acid.[19] Hydrochloric acid is secreted from the gastric mucosal cells, and it is necessary for vitamin B_{12} digestion, along with intrinsic factor. However, as people age, the production and secretion of hydrochloric acid often decreases and may result in inadequate vitamin B_{12} absorption. In this case, subcutaneous vitamin B_{12} injections are necessary.

Many researchers worldwide believe that about half of the elderly population is deficient in vitamin D and warrants supplementation.[20] However, expert committees from the United States and Canada reported in the

osteoporosis a disease of the skeletal system that is characterized by a bone mineral density value that is more than 2.5 standard deviations below a 20-year-old sex-matched healthy person's average.

osteopenia a condition that involves a low bone mass and an increased risk for fracture.

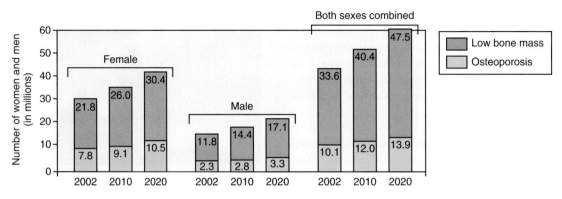

Figure 12-5 Projected prevalence of osteoporosis and low bone mass of the hip among women, men, and both sexes who are 50 years old or older. Note that the National Health and Nutrition Examination Survey is conducted by the National Center for Health Statistics, which is a part of the Centers for Disease Control and Prevention. This survey is conducted on a nationally representative sample of Americans. As a part of the study, bone mineral density of the hip was measured in 14,646 men and women who were 20 years old or older throughout the United States from 1988 until 1994. These values were compared with the World Health Organization definitions to derive the percentage of individuals who were older than 50 years old who have osteoporosis and low bone mass. These percentages were then applied to the total population of men and women who were older than 50 years old to estimate the absolute number of men and women in the United States with osteoporosis and low bone mass. Projections for 2010 and 2020 are based on population forecasts for these years; they are significantly higher than current figures because of the expected growth in the overall population and the expected aging of the population. (Reprinted from the U.S. Department of Health and Human Services. *Bone health and osteoporosis: a report of the surgeon general.* Rockville, Md: U.S. Department of Health and Human Services; 2004.)

updated DRIs for vitamin D and calcium that the majority of Americans receive adequate intake of these nutrients and that there is a risk of toxicity from excessive supplementation.[18] Individuals who live in nursing homes or other situations with little to no sunlight exposure or who avoid dairy products (which are good sources of vitamin D) may benefit from vitamin D evaluation to determine the need for supplementation.

CLINICAL NEEDS
Health Promotion and Disease Prevention
Reducing Risk for Chronic Disease

The emphasis of adult health care is on reducing individual risks for chronic disease as people grow older. This approach has always been used for development of the *Dietary Guidelines for Americans* and the national health objectives. These guidelines outline lifestyle changes that people can make to live healthier lives (see Figure 1-4, *Dietary Guidelines for Americans, 2010*). The guidelines emphasize individual needs and good eating habits that are based on moderation and variety. Health care providers are encouraged to promote healthy lifestyles among all patients and to relay the importance of disease prevention rather than treatment.

Nutritional Status

Many of the health problems of older adults result from general aging and states of malnutrition. Approximately 23% of older adults suffer from malnutrition,[21] which may develop for the following reasons:
- Poor food habits
  - Lack of appetite or loneliness and not wanting to eat alone
  - Lack of food availability as a result of economic or social issues
- Poor oral health (e.g., missing teeth, poorly fitting dentures)
- General gastrointestinal problems
  - Declining salivary secretions and dry mouth, with diminished thirst and taste sensations
  - Inadequate hydrochloric acid secretion in the stomach
  - Decreased enzyme and mucus secretion in the intestines
  - General decline in gastrointestinal motility

Individual medical symptoms range from vague indigestion or irritable colon to specific diseases such as peptic ulcer or diverticulitis (see Chapter 18). The Mini Nutritional Assessment (Figure 12-6) is one of the standard assessment tools that is routinely used to evaluate nutritional risk in elderly individuals.[22,23] The Mini Nutritional Assessment is a reliable tool that is highly sensitive

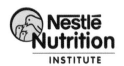

Mini Nutritional Assessment
MNA®

Last name:	First name:	Sex:	Date:

Age:	Weight, kg:	Height, cm:	I.D. Number:

Complete the screen by filling in the boxes with the appropriate numbers.
Add the numbers for the screen. If score is 11 or less, continue with the assessment to gain a Malnutrition Indicator Score.

Screening

A Has food intake declined over the past 3 months
due to loss of appetite, digestive problems,
chewing or swallowing difficulties?
0 = severe loss of appetite
1 = moderate loss of appetite
2 = no loss of appetite ☐

B Weight loss during last months
0 = weight loss greater than 3 kg (6.6 lbs)
1 = does not know
2 = weight loss between 1 and 3 kg (2.2 and 6.6 lbs)
3 = no weight loss ☐

C Mobility
0 = bed or chair bound
1 = able to get out of bed/chair but does not go out
2 = goes out ☐

D Has suffered psychological stress or acute
disease in the past 3 months
0 = yes   2 = no ☐

E Neuropsychological problems
0 = severe dementia or depression
1 = mild dementia
2 = no psychological problems ☐

F Body Mass Index (BMI) (weight in kg) / (height in m)²
0 = BMI less than 19
1 = BMI 19 to less than 21
2 = BMI 21 to less than 23
3 = BMI 23 or greater ☐

Screening score (subtotal max. 14 points) ☐ ☐

12 points or greater   Normal – not at risk –
no need to complete assessment

11 points or below   Possible malnutrition – continue assessment

Assessment

G Lives independently (not in a nursing home or hospital)
0 = no   1 = yes ☐

H Takes more than 3 prescription drugs per day
0 = yes   1 = no ☐

I Pressure sores or skin ulcers
0 = yes   1 = no ☐

J How many full meals does the patient eat daily?
0 = 1 meal
1 = 2 meals
2 = 3 meals ☐

K Selected consumption markers for protein intake
• At least one serving of dairy products
(milk, cheese, yogurt) per day?   yes ☐   no ☐
• Two or more servings of legumes
or eggs per week?   yes ☐   no ☐
• Meat, fish or poultry every day   yes ☐   no ☐
0.0 = if 0 or 1 yes
0.5 = if 2 yes
1.0 = if 3 yes ☐ ☐

L Consumes two or more servings
of fruits or vegetables per day?
0 = no   1 = yes ☐

M How much fluid (water, juice, coffee, tea, milk…)
is consumed per day?
0.0 = less than 3 cups
0.5 = 3 to 5 cups
1.0 = more than 5 cups ☐ ☐

N Mode of feeding
0 = unable to eat without assistance
1 = self-fed with some difficulty
2 = self-fed without any problem ☐

O Self view of nutritional status
0 = view self as being malnourished
1 = is uncertain of nutritional state
2 = views self as having no nutritional problem ☐

P In comparison with other people of the same age,
how do they consider their health status?
0.0 = not as good
0.5 = does not know
1.0 = as good
2.0 = better ☐.☐

Q Mid-arm circumference (MAC) in cm
0.0 = MAC less than 21
0.5 = MAC 21 to 22
1.0 = MAC 22 or greater ☐.☐

R Calf circumference (CC) in cm
0 = CC less than 31   1 = CC 31 or greater ☐

Assessment (max. 16 points) ☐ ☐.☐

Screening score ☐ ☐

Total Assessment (max. 30 points) ☐ ☐.☐

Ref.:   Vellas B, Villars H, Abellan G, et al. Overview of the MNA® - Its History and Challenges. J Nut
Health Aging 2006;10:456-465.
Rubenstein LZ, Harker JO, Salva A, Guigoz Y, Vellas B. Screening for Undernutrition in Geriatric
Practice: Developing the Short-Form Mini Nutritional Assessment (MNA-SF). J. Geront 2001;56A:
M366-377.
Guigoz Y. The Mini-Nutritional Assessment (MNA®) Review of the Literature - What does it tell us?
J Nutr Health Aging 2006; 10:466-487.

® Société des Produits Nestlé S.A., Vevey, Switzerland, Trademark Owners.

Malnutrition Indicator Score

17 to 23.5 points   at risk of malnutrition ☐

Less than 17 points   malnourished ☐

08.98 USA

Figure 12-6 Mini Nutritional Assessment. (Copyright Nestle USA, Inc., Glendale, Calif, 2009.)

and can detect the risk of malnutrition early. Other assessment tools that are appropriate for use in the geriatric population include the DETERMINE Nutrition Checklist (which was developed by the American Academy of Family Physicians, the Academy of Nutrition and Dietetics, and National Council on the Aging, Inc.) and the Nutrition Risk Assessment (which was developed by the Academy of Nutrition and Dietetics).[24]

Dental status should be a consideration when evaluating an individual's nutritional condition and as a possible cause of malnutrition. Oral health (i.e., the number of healthy teeth, the ability to chew, the perception of oral health) of older adults is significantly associated with nutritional status and Mini Nutritional Assessment scores.[25,26] Elderly individuals who are institutionalized and have no remaining teeth (i.e., edentulous) have a specific need for individualized nutrition care (see the Clinical Applications box, "Feeding Older Adults With Sensitivity").

Dehydration, which can be a problem in any age group, is common in the elderly population. Reduced thirst sensation coupled with the declining function of the kidneys can lead to an overall decline in body water status. Individuals who need assistance with getting water or getting to the bathroom may choose to not drink as much to avoid getting up as often. Water needs (relative to total energy needs) do not decline with age.

Weight Management

Both excessive weight loss and excessive weight gain can be signs of malnutrition. Many of the same depressed living situations and emotional factors that result in unhealthy weight loss also may lead to excessive weight gain. Overeating or undereating may be a coping mechanism for the stressful conditions that are encountered by some individuals. Obesity among adults has been on the rise in all subgroups of the adult population[27] (Figure 12-7).

As stated, physical activity is generally lacking in the American adult population. Physical activity is a major factor in weight management, and it can help prevent many of the debilitating conditions of old age. The American Cancer Society, the American Heart Association, the Academy of Nutrition and Dietetics, and the U.S. Department of Health and Human Services all recommend regular physical activity as a means of disease prevention that should be continued throughout life. The *Physical Activity Guidelines and Dietary Guidelines for Americans* specifically note the long-term benefits of regular cardiovascular and strength-training exercises in adults.[11,28] As the population continues to age, health care facilities are adapting to the increased need for aerobic and stretching classes that are aimed specifically at older adults who enjoy and benefit from daily exercise (Figure 12-8). Box 12-1 discusses the benefits of physical activity as indicated by the Centers for Disease Control and Prevention.

The prevalence of diabetes and impaired fasting glucose tolerance increases with aging.[29] Decreased glucose tolerance is the prediabetes syndrome in which the insulin response to glucose in the bloodstream is inadequate to maintain blood glucose levels within a

---

CLINICAL APPLICATIONS

FEEDING OLDER ADULTS WITH SENSITIVITY

Many older adults have eating problems that lead to malnutrition. Each person is a unique individual with particular needs, and he or she requires sensitive support to meet his or her nutritional and personal requirements.

Basic Guidelines
- *Analyze food habits carefully.* Learn about the attitudes, situations, and desires of the older person. Nutrition needs can be met with a variety of foods, so make suggestions in a practical, realistic, and supportive manner.
- *Never moralize.* Never say, "Eat this because it is good for you." This approach has little value for anyone, especially for those who are struggling to maintain their personal integrity and self-esteem in a youth-oriented, age-fearing culture.
- *Encourage food variety.* Mix new foods with familiar comfort foods. New tastes and seasonings often

encourage appetite and increase interest in eating. Many people think that a bland diet is best for all elderly persons, but this is not necessarily true. The decreased taste sensitivity of aging necessitates added attention to variety and seasoning. Smaller amounts of food and more frequent meals may also encourage better nutrition.

Assisted Feeding Suggestions
- Make no negative remarks about the food that is served.
- Identify the food that is being served.
- Allow the person to have at least three bites of the same food before going on to another food to allow time for the taste buds to become accustomed to the food.
- Give sufficient time for the person to chew and swallow.
- Give liquids throughout the meal and not just at the beginning and end.

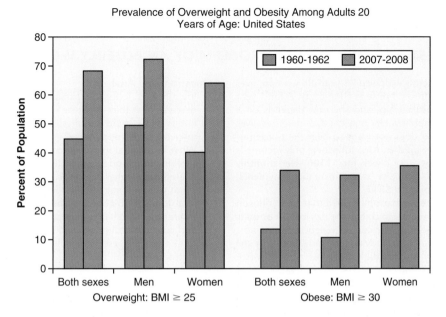

Prevalence of Overweight and Obesity Among Adults 20 Years of Age: United States

Overweight: BMI ≥ 25

Obese: BMI ≥ 30

Figure 12-7 Prevalence of overweight and obesity among adults between the ages of 20 and 74 years in the United States. (Data from the National Center for Health Statistics. *Health, United States, 2010: with special feature on death and dying.* Hyattsville, Md: U.S. Government Printing Office 2011.)

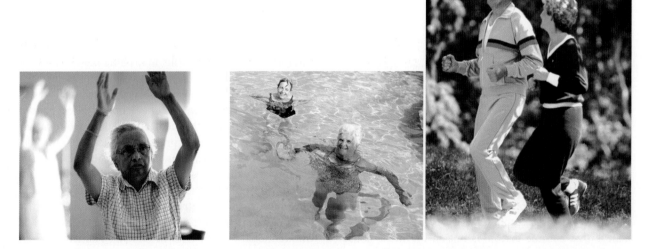

Figure 12-8 Healthy older adults enjoying a variety of physical activities. (Copyright JupiterImages Corp.)

normal range but not high enough for a diagnosis of diabetes. Weight management through regular physical activity along with balanced meals and snacks that include carbohydrate, fat, and protein can help individuals to avoid excessively high blood glucose concentrations and potentially delay or avoid the onset of diabetes.

Individual Approach

Individual and realistic planning is essential. All personalities and problems are unique, and individual needs vary widely. A malnourished older person needs much personal and sensitive support to build improved eating habits (see the Clinical Applications box, "Case Study: Situational Problem of an Elderly Woman").

CLINICAL APPLICATIONS

CASE STUDY: SITUATIONAL PROBLEM OF AN ELDERLY WOMAN

Mrs. Johnson, a recently widowed 78-year-old woman, lives alone in a three-bedroom house in a large city. A fall 1 year ago resulted in a broken hip, and she now depends on a walker for limited mobility. Her only child, a daughter, lives in a distant city and does not want to bear the burden of responsibility for her mother. Mrs. Johnson's only income is a monthly Social Security check for $1106. Her monthly mortgage payment, property taxes, insurance payments, and utility bills amount to $817.

A recent medical examination revealed that Mrs. Johnson has iron-deficiency anemia and that she has lost 12 pounds during the past 3 months. Her current weight is 80 pounds, and she is 5 feet, 2 inches tall. Mrs. Johnson states that she has not been hungry, and her daily diet is repetitious: broth, a little cottage cheese and canned fruit, saltine crackers, and hot tea. She lacks energy, she rarely leaves the house, and she appears to be emaciated and generally distraught.

Questions for Analysis

1. Identify Mrs. Johnson's personal problems, and describe how they might be influencing her eating habits. How could her physical problems have influenced her food intake?
2. What nutritional improvements could she make in her diet (include food suggestions), and how are these related to her physical needs at this stage of her life?
3. What practical suggestions do you have for helping Mrs. Johnson to cope with her physical and social environment? What resources, income sources, food, and companionship can you suggest? How do you think these suggestions would benefit her nutritional status and overall health?

BOX 12-1 BENEFITS OF PHYSICAL ACTIVITY

Physical activity has the following health benefits:
- Achieving weight control
- Reducing risk of cardiovascular disease
- Strengthening bones and muscles
- Improving mental health and mood
- Improving one's ability to perform daily activities and preventing falls, especially among older adults
- Increasing the chance of living longer

From the Centers for Disease Control and Prevention. *Benefits of physical activity* (website): www.cdc.gov/physicalactivity/everyone/health/index.html. Accessed June 2011.

Chronic Diseases of Aging

Chronic diseases of aging (e.g., hypertension, heart disease, stroke, emphysema, diabetes, cancer, arthritis, asthma) occur more frequently with advancing age, but they may present at a younger age with a strong family history. About 70% of deaths in the United States result from chronic disease annually. However, health experts believe that chronic disease is not an inevitable consequence of aging and estimate that the 80% of all cases of heart disease, stroke, and type 2 diabetes and 40% of cancer cases could have been prevented by lifestyle modifications.[30,31] The Centers for Disease Control and Prevention recommends the following lifestyle changes to promote health and prevent chronic disease in adulthood: (1) get regular physical activity; (2) maintain a healthy weight by choosing a balanced diet rich in fruits and vegetables; (3) stop smoking; and (4) limit alcohol intake.

Diet Modifications

In the presence of chronic disease, diet modifications and nutrition support are an important part of therapy. Details of these modified diets per disease are given in Chapters 17 through 23. In any situation, individual needs and food plans are essential for successful therapy.

Medications

Because people are living longer (many with one or more chronic disease), older adults may be taking several prescription drugs in addition to over-the-counter medications. Polypharmacy can affect overall nutritional status, because many drug-nutrient interactions can occur (see Chapter 17). Many of the medications that are often used by the elderly (e.g., blood pressure medication, antacids, anticoagulation medications, laxatives, diuretics, decongestants) can directly affect fluid balance, appetite, and the absorption and use of nutrients, thereby possibly contributing to malnutrition or dehydration (see the Drug-Nutrient Interaction box, "Medications Related to Unintentional Weight Loss in Nursing Homes"). When questioning patients about medication use, health care providers should specifically ask about the use of dietary supplements and herbs. Toxicities from supplements can be dangerous, even though many of these products are

---

polypharmacy the use of multiple medications by the same patient.

DRUG-NUTRIENT INTERACTION

MEDICATIONS RELATED TO UNINTENTIONAL WEIGHT LOSS IN NURSING HOMES

Physiologic, social, and environmental factors all play a role in increasing nutritional risk in the elderly population. Polypharmacy is very common among seniors: because the risk for several illnesses increases with age, older adults are often taking multiple medications for chronic conditions. Studies show that more than 50% of adults who are 65 years old and older take more than five medications per day.[1] Many medications have side effects that can affect appetite, weight, or the ability to absorb nutrients from food. Residents in skilled nursing facilities are at higher risk for polypharmacy and nutrition-related effects. Weight changes are closely monitored in nursing homes, so early nutritional interventions may be put in place to prevent malnutrition. It is crucial for the multidisciplinary team to communicate openly about changes in the patient's appetite, eating habits, and medication regimen so that potential risks can be identified.

The following medications are commonly prescribed among residents of skilled nursing facilities and should be appropriately monitored[2]:

- *Antidepressants:* Sertraline (Zoloft), which is a select serotonin reuptake inhibitor, can directly reduce appetite. Common side effects are anorexia, nausea, dry mouth, dyspepsia, and diarrhea. Tricyclic antidepressants such as amitriptyline (Elavil) can cause dry mouth and a sour or metallic taste.

Another antidepressant medication, mirtazapine (Remeron), is often used at a low dose as an appetite stimulant, although side effects like dry mouth and nausea may still occur.

- *Narcotic pain medications:* Narcotics tend to slow peristalsis and lead to chronic constipation with long-term use. Nausea and vomiting may also be present. Eating foods that are high in fiber and drinking plenty of fluids helps to alleviate these symptoms.
- *Thiazide diuretics:* These can cause nausea, vomiting, dry mouth, and gastrointestinal irritation. Weight loss related to fluid losses is often seen among patients who are taking diuretics. Nutrient intake should be monitored to ensure that weight loss is not related to a reduced appetite.
- *Nonsteroidal anti-inflammatory drugs:* These drugs often irritate the stomach mucosa and cause gastrointestinal distress, nausea, vomiting, bleeding, and ulcers. The overuse of these medications can lead to sudden and severe gastric bleeding. In serious cases of gastric bleeding, bowel rest may be indicated and parenteral nutrition required to maintain an individual's nutritional status.

Kelli Boi

1. Hajjar ER, Cafiero AC, Hanlon JT. Polypharmacy in elderly patients. *Am J Geriatr Pharmacther.* 2007;5(4):345-351.
2. Pronsky Z. *Food-medication interactions..* 15th ed. Birchrunville, Penn: Food-Medication Interactions; 2008.

considered to be "natural." Each person requires the careful evaluation of all of his or her drug use and instructions about how to take his or her medications in relation to meals (see the Drug-Nutrient Interaction box, "Medication Use in the Adult").

COMMUNITY RESOURCES

Government Programs for Older Americans

Poverty has a direct association with the prevalence of chronic disease. According to the National Center for Health Statistics, adults who are living below the national poverty level had a higher incidence of multiple chronic diseases than any other socioeconomic group for most age groups[32] (Figure 12-9). Health care providers must be aware of community resources and refer patients when appropriate. Many older adults who are at risk for malnutrition and who are eligible for nutrition assistance programs are not participating in them.

Older Americans Act

The Administration on Aging of the U.S. Department of Health and Human Services (www.aoa.gov) administers programs for older adults. Nutrition Services Incentive Programs provide cash and/or commodities to supplement meals. These services include both congregate and home-delivered meals, with related nutrition education and food service components.

Congregate Nutrition Services. This program provides adults who are older than 60 years of age and their spouses (particularly those with low incomes) with nutritionally sound meals in senior centers and other public or private community facilities. In these settings, older adults can gather for a hot noon meal and have access to both good food and social support. In addition to meals, other services include nutrition screening, education, assessment, and counseling, as needed.

Home-Delivered Meals. For those older adults who are ill or disabled and who cannot travel to the community centers, meals are delivered by couriers to their homes (i.e., Meals on Wheels). This service meets

DRUG-NUTRIENT INTERACTION

MEDICATION USE IN THE ADULT

Polypharmacy is common in the United States. As the table indicates, a significant proportion of the population takes at least one prescription medication, and a large percentage of people who are 45 years old and older are taking three or more prescription drugs at one time. During the last decade, the use of statin drugs, which are used to treat high cholesterol, has increased almost 10-fold among those 45 to 64 years old and 65 years old and older. In addition, antidiabetes drug use has increased by 50% in the same time frame.[1] This is indicative of the importance of diet to prevent chronic conditions in adults.

PERCENTAGE OF POPULATION TAKING PRESCRIPTION MEDICATIONS[2]

Age Group	Percentage of Population Taking At Least One Prescription Drug in the Past Month	Percentage of Population Taking Three or More Prescription Drugs in the Past Month
18 to 44 years old	38%	11%
45 to 64 years old	65%	35%
≥ 65 years old	89%	63%

In addition to prescription drugs, nonprescription (i.e., over-the-counter) medications, dietary supplements (i.e., vitamins and minerals), and herbal supplements are also commonly used by these individuals. Several potential drug-nutrient interactions may occur with the most commonly used medications (i.e., antidepressants, antihyperlipidemics, hypertensive medications, nonsteroidal anti-inflammatory drugs, and antihistamines). Because such a high percentage of patients are taking at least one medication, diet interactions with common medications must be considered. Foods and nutrients that should be avoided when taking these medications are listed below.

Drug Class	Food/Nutrient Interaction	How to Avoid an Adverse Reaction
Certain antidepressants (i.e., monoamine oxidase inhibitors)	Alcohol and foods that contain tyramine	Avoid beer, red wine, and tyramine-containing foods such as cheese, yogurt, sour cream, liver, cured meats, caviar, dried fish, avocados, bananas, raisins, soy sauce, miso soup, ginseng, and caffeine-containing products
	Fluids	Drink 2 to 3 L of water per day and take the drugs with food; keep sodium intake consistent
Antihyperlipidemics	Food and alcohol	Take with the evening meal, and avoid more than one alcoholic drink per day
	Fat-soluble vitamins, folate, B_{12}, and iron	Include rich sources of these vitamins and minerals in the diet
	Grapefruit juice	Avoid grapefruit juice
Antihypertensives	Licorice and tyramine-rich foods	Avoid licorice and tyramine-containing foods
	Grapefruit juice	Avoid taking with grapefruit juice
Nonsteroidal anti-inflammatory drugs	Alcohol	Limit alcohol intake
	Vitamin C, folate, and vitamin K	Increase intake of foods that are high in these vitamins and minerals
	Fluid balance	Take with water
Antihistamines	Alcohol	Avoid alcohol
	Grapefruit juice	Avoid taking with grapefruit juice

1. National Center for Health Statistics, *Health, United States, 2009: With Special Feature on Medical Technology.* 2010, U.S. Government Printing Office: Hyattsville, MD.
2. National Center for Health Statistics, *NCHS Data on Prescription Drugs Factsheet.* 2009, National Center for Health Statistics: Hyattsville, MD.

nutrition needs and provides human contact and support. The couriers are usually volunteers who are concerned about other people and their needs. A courier is often the only person a homebound individual may interact with during the day.

United States Department of Agriculture

The U.S. Department of Agriculture provides both research and services for older adults.

Research Centers. Research centers for studies on aging have been established in various areas of the United

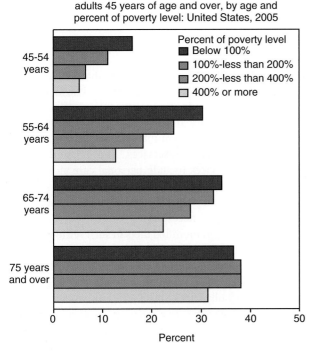

Figure 12-9 Three or more chronic conditions among adults 45 years old and older by age and percentage of poverty level. Note that this is a population of adults who have been told by a physician that they had three or more of the following conditions: hypertension, heart disease, stroke, emphysema, diabetes, cancer, arthritis and related diseases, or current asthma. The percentage of the poverty level is based on family income, family size, and family composition with the use of U.S. Census Bureau poverty thresholds. (Reprinted from the National Center for Health Statistics. *Health, United States, 2007: with chartbook on trends in the health of Americans.* Hyattsville, Md: U.S. Government Printing Office; 2007.)

States and are supported by the U.S. Department of Agriculture. For example, a Human Nutrition Research Center on Aging was built at Tufts University in Boston; this is the largest research facility in the world to be dedicated to the study of nutrition in aging. Studies there involve research on topics such as nutrition and its interactions with bone metabolism, cardiovascular health, cancer, sarcopenia, neurocognition, and vision. Much more knowledge about the nutritional requirements of older adults is needed to provide better care.

Extension Services. The U.S. Department of Agriculture operates agricultural extension services in state land grant universities, including food and nutrition education services. County home advisers help communities with practical materials and counseling for elderly people and community workers.

Supplemental Nutrition Assistance Program (SNAP). SNAP, which was formerly known as the Food Stamp Program, issues electronic benefits transfer cards to the primary care provider in households with a monthly income at or below 130% of the federal poverty line, regardless of age. The cards are similar to debit cards, and they can be used at authorized food retail outlets to purchase eligible food items. As of 2010, about 40 million low-income people benefit from SNAP every month, and 8% of participants are older than 60 years old.[33,34] SNAP promotes the consumption of fruits, vegetables, whole grains, fat-free or low-fat milk products, lean meats, poultry, and fish.

Commodity Supplemental Food Program. Individuals who are older than 60 years of age with a household income at or below 130% of the federal poverty line are eligible for assistance in the form of food packages. These food packages are not intended to provide a complete diet but rather to supplement the diet with foods that are high in the nutrients that are typically lacking in the diet of an elderly person. This program also serves other eligible groups, such as pregnant and breast-feeding women and children who meet the financial need qualifications.

Senior Farmers' Market Nutrition Program. This is a grant-based program that provides low-income older adults (i.e., individuals who are older than 60 years of age with an income that is not more than 185% of the federal poverty income guidelines) with coupons that they can exchange for fresh fruits, vegetables, and herbs obtained from farmers' markets, community-supported agriculture programs, and roadside stands. This program has increased the average servings of fruits and vegetables among participants, and it helps with the development of local farmers' markets.

Public Health Departments

Public Health Departments throughout the United States are an outreach division of the U.S. Department of Health and Human Services. Skilled health professionals work in the community through local and state public health departments. Public health nutritionists are important members of this health care team; they provide nutrition counseling and education, and they help with various food assistance programs.

state land grant universities an institution of higher education that has been designated by the state to receive unique federal support as a result of the Morrill Acts of 1862 and 1890.

Professional Organizations and Resources

National Groups

The American Geriatric Society and the Gerontological Society of America are national professional organizations of physicians, nurses, dietitians, and other interested health care workers. These societies publish journals and promote community and government efforts to meet the needs of aging individuals.

Community Groups

Local medical societies, nursing organizations, and dietetic associations sponsor various programs to help meet the needs of elderly people. An increasing number of qualified registered dietitians also are in private practice in most communities, and they can supply a variety of individual and group services. Senior centers in local communities are valuable resources for both well and disabled adults.

Volunteer Organizations

Many volunteer activities of health organizations (e.g., the American Heart Association, the American Diabetes Association) relate to the needs of older people and may serve as both rewarding opportunities for young-old adults and important sources of health-sustaining activities and information for old-old adults.

Chapter 13 discusses additional resources for nutritional assistance.

ALTERNATIVE LIVING ARRANGEMENTS

A multitude of alternative living arrangements exist for seniors. For example, independent living facilities are for independently functioning individuals who do not need medical attention and who enjoy recreational and social events with other seniors. Other housing options provide more services, may be staffed with health care workers, and provide different levels of care in accordance with needs. Examples include congregate care, continuing care retirement communities, and assisted living facilities. Nursing homes are fully staffed with medical professionals and are able to provide for most medical needs in the absence of an acute episode that requires hospitalization. The next sections of this chapter discuss only the types of alternative living arrangements that provide food and health care (i.e., not independent living facilities). Several organizations that provide helpful information about alternative living arrangements for seniors are listed under the Further Reading and Resources section of this chapter.

Congregate Care Arrangements

Congregate care arrangements are focused on keeping the elderly living in their own homes for as long as possible with outside assistance for specific needs. Some congregate care arrangements were discussed previously: congregate community meals, nutrition education through extension services, and home-delivered meals. Other services include personal care aides, adult day services, transportation, respite care, and more. Personal care aides may shop for groceries, cook, and even help with feeding, if necessary.

The emphasis on modified diets in such settings varies. Congregate meals and home-delivered meals are not likely to be specific to diets for individuals with highly particular needs. For example, individuals with diabetes who count carbohydrates, those with food intolerances or allergies, or those who have difficulty swallowing certain food consistencies (e.g., dysphagia) may require additional assistance. Most congregate care programs are regulated at the state level. Public programs (e.g., congregate meals and home-delivered meals) are required to offer meals that meet the *Dietary Guidelines for Americans, 2010,* and each meal should provide one third of the DRIs for select nutrients.

Continuing Care Retirement Communities

Continuing care retirement communities provide a continuum of residential long-term care, from independent living with community-organized events to nursing care facilities. Dietary assistance varies by the needs of the resident. Seniors can move into the community as independent living residences and participate in community activities and meals as they so choose. When their functional statuses indicate, seniors receive more care. Continuing care retirement communities usually have assisted living facilities and nursing homes in a campus-style setting. Nutritional involvement within these facilities is discussed in the next sections of this chapter, and it applies within this continuum-of-care approach as well.

Assisted Living Facilities

Assisted living facilities can go by several names, including *board and care, domiciliary care, sheltered housing, residential care,* and *personal care.* Assisted living arrangements may also exist within continuing care communities. Individual state governments regulate licensure for assisted living facilities. Most assisted living facilities provide all meals and snacks; housekeeping; laundry; and help with dressing, bathing, and personal hygiene. Some facilities provide social activities, limited transportation, and basic medication administration, but they may not provide medical or nursing care. Living areas vary from full apartments with kitchens to studio-type apartments with small kitchenettes to rooms with baths. The functional status of the individual helps to determine the most appropriate setting.

Meals are generally served in a cafeteria or restaurant setting. Some facilities provide menus with several options at each meal, and others serve a set menu for all residents, with attention given to special needs. Most assisted care facilities cater to basic dietary requests and the therapeutic diet needs of their residents. States vary widely with regard to regulations and standards for nutrition policies and services. Some states require that a registered dietitian review meal plans.

Nursing Homes

Nursing homes or long-term care facilities provide the most medical, nursing, and nutrition support of the alternative living arrangements. Approximately 13 million people who are 65 years old or older reside in nursing homes in the United States.[32] Many nursing homes also provide a residential rehabilitation site outside of the hospital for patients to recover from injuries, acute illnesses, and operations. Most patients in nursing homes need help with activities of daily living (e.g., bathing, toileting, transferring), and half of all residents need assistance with eating. Approximately half of the residents are older than 85 years old.

Nursing homes have dietitians on staff and are able to meet specific dietary requirements. However, much less emphasis on therapeutic diets is given for this population, because a least-restrictive diet model is likely to be more beneficial at this life stage.[35] Recent studies have found that family-style eating arrangements (e.g., a cafeteria with a server) benefit individuals who are at high risk for malnutrition, especially those with cognitive impairment and below-optimal body mass indices.[36] Researchers believe that the social interaction and feel of autonomy of family-style eating (compared with plated tray delivery) contribute to the significant increase in energy and nutrient intake. Many of these factors are depicted in Figure 12-2, which demonstrates how such issues relate to overall quality of life.

SUMMARY

- Meeting the nutrition needs of adults—especially older adults—is a challenge for several reasons. Current and past social, economic, and psychologic factors influence needs, and the biologic process of aging differs widely among individuals.
- As the average life expectancy continues to increase, research and recommendations regarding the needs of an aging population are updated.
- Many illnesses in older adults are the result of malnutrition rather than the effects of aging. Health promotion and disease prevention during early adulthood are key elements to sustain functionality throughout the later years.
- When working with older people, health care professionals must analyze food habits carefully and approach clients with encouragement for positive changes to be made. Individual supportive guidance and patience are necessary when using all appropriate nutrition resources.
- A variety of assisted living arrangements and nutrition services are available for seniors of all functional levels.

CRITICAL THINKING QUESTIONS

1. Mr. Jones is a healthy and active 82-year-old man. He exercises regularly, and he enjoys a variety of foods. Recently, he has started gaining weight. He says he eats exactly the same amount of food that he ate when he was 30 years younger. How would you explain this weight gain to Mr. Jones, and what suggestions would you make to him to prevent any additional unwanted weight gain?

2. Identify and describe three major factors that contribute to malnutrition in older adults. How do these factors influence the nutrition counseling process?

3. Your client is on a limited budget and has poor vision and shaky hands. Knowing that fresh fruit and vegetables are often expensive and require washing and cutting, what suggestions would you make for your client to meet the suggested servings of five fruits and vegetables per day?

CHAPTER CHALLENGE QUESTIONS

True-False

Write the correct statement for each statement that is false.

1. *True or False:* Total energy needs slowly decline with age, but water needs decline rapidly.
2. *True or False:* Beginning at approximately 30 years of age, a gradual decrease occurs in the performance capacity of most organ systems that lasts throughout adulthood.
3. *True or False:* An extensive research base of knowledge currently exists about the nutrition needs of elderly people, and it provides information about specific energy and nutrient requirements.
4. *True or False:* The simplest basis for judging the adequacy of kilocalorie intake is the maintenance of a normal weight.
5. *True or False:* Fat requirements increase with age.
6. *True or False:* Exercise is not recommended for elderly individuals.

Multiple Choice

1. The basic biologic changes of old age include
   a. an increase in the number of cells.
   b. a decreasing need for water.
   c. an increased basal metabolic rate.
   d. a gradual loss of functioning cells and reduced cell metabolism.

2. The Mini Nutrition Assessment is designed to identify signs of
   a. physical fitness.
   b. emotional stability.
   c. malnutrition.
   d. specific vitamin deficiencies.

3. Which of the following is an example of a physiologic change associated with aging? *(Circle all that apply.)*

   a. Increased cell metabolism to meet increased aging needs
   b. Decreased gastrointestinal motility
   c. A gradual increase in the body's muscle mass
   d. Decreased digestive secretions

4. Which of the following actions would help elderly persons find solutions to their health problems? *(Circle all that apply.)*

   a. Carefully analyzing individual living situations and food habits
   b. Reinforcing good habits, leaving harmless ones alone, and suggesting needed changes that are practical within the individual's living situation
   c. Encouraging variety in foods and seasonings
   d. Exploring and using available community resources for assistance

---

⊖volve Please refer to the Students' Resource section of this text's Evolve Web site for additional study resources.

REFERENCES

1. U.S. Department of Health and Human Service. *Healthy people 2020.* Washington, DC: U.S. Government Printing Office; 2010.
2. U.S. Census Bureau, Population Division. *Projections of the population and components of change for the United States: 2010 to 2050.* Washington, DC: U.S. Government Printing Office; 2009.
3. U.S. Census Bureau, Population Division. *Projections of the population by selected age groups and sex for the United States: 2010 to 2050.* Washington, DC: U.S. Government Printing Office; 2008.
4. Heron MP, Hoyert DL, Murphy SL, et al. *Deaths: final data for 2006.* National vital statistics reports; Vol 57 No 14. Hyattsville, MD: National Center For Health Statistics; 2009.
5. Borg C, Hallberg IR, Blomqvist K. Life satisfaction among older people (65+) with reduced self-care capacity: the relationship to social, health and financial aspects. *J Clin Nurs.* 2006;15(5):607-618.
6. Pitkala KH, Routasalo P, Kautiainen H, Tilvis RS. Effects of psychosocial group rehabilitation on health, use of health care services, and mortality of older persons suffering from loneliness: a randomized, controlled trial. *J Gerontol A Biol Sci Med Sci.* 2009;64(7):792-800.
7. Robertson RG, Montagnini M. Geriatric failure to thrive. *Am Fam Physician.* 2004;70(2):343-350.
8. St-Onge MP, Gallagher D. Body composition changes with aging: the cause or the result of alterations in metabolic rate and macronutrient oxidation? *Nutrition.* 2010;26(2):152-155.
9. Centers For Disease Control and Prevention. *1988-2008 no leisure-time physical activity trend chart* (Website): www.cdc.gov/nccdphp/dnpa/physical/stats/leisure_time.htm. Accessed October 16, 2011.
10. Food and Nutrition Board, Institute of Medicine. *Dietary reference intakes for energy, carbohydrate, fiber, fat, fatty acids, cholesterol, protein, and amino acids.* Washington, DC: National Academies Press; 2002.
11. U.S. Department of Health and Human Services. *2008 physical activity guidelines for Americans.* Washington, DC: U.S. Department of Health and Human Services; 2008.
12. Walter S, Kunst A, Mackenbach J, et al. Mortality and disability: the effect of overweight and obesity. *Int J Obes (Lond).* 2009;33(12):1410-1418.
13. Kenney WL, Chiu P. Influence of age on thirst and fluid intake. *Med Sci Sports Exerc.* 2001;33(9):1524-1532.

14. Farrell MJ, Zamarripa F, Shade R, et al. Effect of aging on regional cerebral blood flow responses associated with osmotic thirst and its satiation by water drinking: a pet study. *Proc Natl Acad Sci U S A.* 2008;105(1):382-387.

15. Burge R, Dawson-Hughes B, Solomon DH, et al. Incidence and economic burden of osteoporosis-related fractures in the United States, 2005-2025. *J Bone Miner Res.* 2007;22(3): 465-475.

16. U.S. Department of Health and Human Services. *Bone health and osteoporosis: a report of the surgeon general.* Rockville, Md: U.S. Department of Health and Human Services; 2004.

17. Cizza G, Primma S, Csako G. Depression as a risk factor for osteoporosis. *Trends Endocrinol Metab.* 2009;20(8): 367-373.

18. Food and Nutrition Board, Institute of Medicine. *Dietary reference intakes for calcium and vitamin D.* Washington, DC: National Academy of Sciences; 2010.

19. Food and Nutrition Board, Institute of Medicine. *Dietary reference intakes for thiamin, riboflavin, niacin, vitamin B6, folate, vitamin B12, pantothenic acid, biotin, and choline.* Washington, DC: National Academies Press; 2000.

20. Norman AW, Bouillon R. Vitamin D nutritional policy needs a vision for the future. *Exp Biol Med (Maywood).* 2010;235(9):1034-1045.

21. Kaiser MJ, Bauer JM, Rämsch C, et al. Mini nutritional assessment international group: frequency of malnutrition in older adults: a multinational perspective using the mini nutritional assessment. *J Am Geriatr Soc.* 2010;58(9): 1734-1738.

22. DiMaria-Ghalili RA, Guenter PA. The mini nutritional assessment. *Am J Nurs.* 2008;108(2):50-59; Quiz 60.

23. Agency for healthcare research and quality: nutrition. In: *Evidence-based geriatric nursing protocols for best practice.* Rockville, Md: U.S. Department of Health and Human Services; 2008.

24. American Dietetic Association. *ADA nutrition care manual.* Chicago, Ill: American Dietetic Association; 2010.

25. Okada K, Enoki H, Izawa S, et al. Association between masticatory performance and anthropometric measurements and nutritional status in the elderly. *Geriatr Gerontol Int.* 2010;10(1):56-63.

26. Gil-Montoya JA, Subirá C, Ramón JM, González-Moles MA. Oral health-related quality of life and nutritional status. *J Public Health Dent.* 2008;68(2):88-93.

27. Flegal KM, Caroll MD, Ogden CL, Curtin LR. Prevalence and trends in obesity among us adults, 1999-2008. *JAMA.* 2010;303(3):235-241.

28. U.S. Department of Agriculture, U.S. Department of Health and Human Services. *Dietary guidelines for Americans, 2010.* Washington, DC: U.S. Government Printing Office; 2010.

29. Karve A, Hayward RA. Prevalence, diagnosis, and treatment of impaired fasting glucose and impaired glucose tolerance in nondiabetic U.S. adults. *Diabetes Care.* 2010; 33(11):2355-2359.

30. Centers For Disease Control and Prevention. *The power of prevention: chronic disease. ... the public health challenge of the 21st century.* Atlanta: Centers for Disease Control and Prevention, National Center for Chronic Disease Prevention and Health Promotion; 2009.

31. World Health Organization. *Preventing chronic diseases: a vital investment.* Geneva: World Health Organization; 2005.

32. National Center For Health Statistics. *Health, United States, 2007: with chartbook on trends in the health of Americans.* Hyattsville, Md: U.S. Government Printing Office; 2007.

33. Leftin J, Gothro A, Eslami E. *Characteristics of supplemental nutrition assistance program households: fiscal year 2009.* Alexandria, Va: U.S. Department of Agriculture, Food and Nutrition Service, Office of Research and Analysis; 2010.

34. U.S. Department of Agriculture and Food and Nutrition Services. *Program data: supplemental nutrition assistance program* (Website): www.fns.usda.gov/pd/snapmain.htm. Accessed December 2010.

35. Dorner B, Friedrich EK, Posthauer ME. Position of the american dietetic association: individualized nutrition approaches for older adults in health care communities. *J Am Diet Assoc.* 2010;110(10):1549-1553.

36. Desai J, Winter A, Young KW, Greenwood CE. Changes in type of foodservice and dining room environment preferentially benefit institutionalized seniors with low body mass indexes. *J Am Diet Assoc.* 2007;107(5):808-814.

FURTHER READING AND RESOURCES

Administration on Aging. www.aoa.gov

American Society on Aging. www.asaging.org

Assisted Living Federation of America: www.alfa.org

Centers for Medicare & Medicaid Services. www.cms.hhs.gov

The Gerontological Society of America. www.geron.org

LeadingAge. www.leadingage.org/

National Council on Aging. www.ncoa.org

National Institute on Aging. www.nia.nih.gov

National Osteoporosis Foundation. www.nof.org

Nutrition Screening Initiative and the DETERMINE Checklist. www.gndpg.org/index_392.cfm

U.S. Department of Agriculture, Food and Nutrition Service, Commodity Supplemental Food Program. www.fns.usda.gov/fdd/programs/csfp/about-csfp.htm

These organizations are excellent sources of information about nutrition, health, and community services for the elderly.

Centers for Disease Control and Prevention. *The power of prevention: chronic disease....the public health challenge of the 21st century* (website): www.cdc.gov/chronicdisease/pdf/2009-Power-of-Prevention.pdf. Accessed October 16, 2011.

Dorner B, Friedrich EK, Posthauer ME. Position of the American Dietetic Association: individualized nutrition approaches for older adults in health care communities. *J Am Diet Assoc.* 2010;110(10):1549-1553.

Hoffmann AT. Quality of life, food choice and meal patterns—field report of a practitioner. *Ann Nutr Metab.* 2008; 52(Suppl 1):20-24.

CHAPTER 13

Community Food Supply and Health

KEY CONCEPTS

- Modern food production, processing, and marketing have both positive and negative influences on food safety.
- Many organisms in contaminated food transmit disease.
- Poverty often prevents individuals and families from having adequate access to their community food supply.

The health of a community largely depends on the safety of its available food and water supply. The American system of government control agencies and regulations, along with local and state public health officials, works diligently to maintain a safe food supply. The food supply in the United States has undergone dramatic changes during the past few decades.

This chapter explores the factors that influence the safety of food. Potential health problems related to the food supply can arise from several sources, such as lack of sanitation, food-borne disease, and poverty.

FOOD SAFETY AND HEALTH PROMOTION

Government Control Agencies

The food supply in the United States has exploded in recent years, and keeping the food supply safe is no small task. Several federal agencies help to control food safety and quality. The U.S. Food and Drug Administration (FDA) is the primary governing body of the American food supply, with the exception of meat and poultry. The Food Safety and Inspection Service of the U.S. Department of Agriculture (USDA) is responsible for the food safety of both domestic and imported meat

and poultry (Figure 13-1), and the National Marine Fisheries Service governs the safety of seafood and fisheries. The Environmental Protection Agency regulates the use of pesticides and other chemicals and ensures the safety of public drinking water. The regulation of advertising and of the truthful marketing of food products is a large job that is the duty of the Federal Trade Commission. The Centers for Disease Control and Prevention monitors and investigates cases of food-borne illness, and it is proactive with regard to education and prevention. Multiple other federal, state, and local agencies participate in education and research to promote the safety of the food supply.

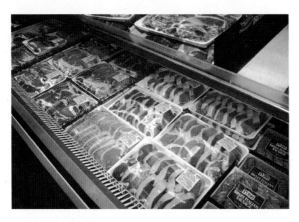

Figure 13-1 The safety of pork and other meat products is the responsibility of the U.S. Department of Agriculture and the Food Safety and Inspection Service. (Courtesy Ken Hammond, Agricultural Research Service, U.S. Department of Agriculture, Washington, DC.)

The U.S. Food and Drug Administration

Although several agencies are involved in the overall food safety of products sold in the United States, only the diverse roles of the FDA are discussed here.

Enforcement of Federal Food Safety Regulations. The FDA is a law-enforcement agency that has been charged by the U.S. Congress with ensuring that America's food supply is safe, pure, and wholesome. The agency enforces federal food safety regulations through various activities, including the following: (1) enforcing food sanitation and quality control; (2) controlling food additives; (3) regulating the movement of foods across state lines; (4) maintaining the nutrition labeling of foods; (5) ensuring the safety of public food service; and (6) ensuring the safety of most food products. The agency's methods of enforcement are recall, seizure, injunction, and prosecution. The use of recall is the most common method, and this is followed by seizures of contaminated food. Injunction involves a court order to stop the sale and production of a food item. This procedure is not common, and it generally occurs in response to a claim that a food item is potentially harmful or that it has not undergone appropriate testing or acquired adequate approval for sale.

Consumer Education. The FDA's division of consumer education conducts an active program of protection through consumer education and general public information. Special attention is given to nutrition misinformation. Pamphlets, books, posters, and other materials are prepared and distributed to individuals, students, and community groups. Consumer specialists work in all FDA district offices. The Web site www.foodsafety.gov is an organization that serves as the liaison between the public and all government agencies that are involved in food safety.

Research. Along with the USDA's Agricultural Research Service, FDA scientists continually evaluate foods and food components through their own research. For a more health-conscious public and a changing marketplace, the FDA is developing nutrition guidelines for a variety of food products, including main dishes, meat substitutes, fruit juices and fruit drinks, and snack foods. The FDA has a long history of food-safety activities, research, programs, and initiatives.

Development of Food Labels

Early Development of Label Regulations

During the mid-1960s, the FDA established "truth in packaging" regulations that dealt mainly with food standards. As food processing developed and the number of items grew, the labels included more nutrition information. Both types of label information—standards and nutrition facts—are important to consumers.

Food Standards. The basic standard of identity requires that labels on foods that do not have an established reference standard must list all of the ingredients in order of relative amount found in the product. Other food standard information on labels relates to food quality, fill of container, and enrichment.

Nutrition Information. Under regulations that were adopted in 1973, the FDA began developing a labeling system that describes a food's nutritional value. Some producers began to add limited information on their own to meet this increasing market demand. Many people became concerned that nutrition labeling was inadequate, but the real problem was what and how much was being labeled and in what format. Information about nutrients and food constituents that consumer groups believed should be listed on labels included the amount of macronutrients (i.e., carbohydrate, protein, and fat) and their total energy value (i.e., calories), key micronutrients (e.g., calcium, iron, vitamin A), sodium, cholesterol, trans fat, and saturated fat. Concerned public and professional groups also want nutrients to be identified in terms of percentages of the current Dietary Reference Intake standards per defined portion. Surveys indicate that 60% to 80% of shoppers consult the food label before purchasing a new product and that 30% to 40% of those individuals make their decision to buy on the basis of the information provided.[1]

Background of Present U.S. Food and Drug Administration Label Regulations

Over the past 20 years, two factors have fueled rapid progress toward better food labels: (1) an increase in the variety of food products entering the U.S. marketplace; and (2) changing patterns of American eating habits. Both factors led many health-conscious consumers and professionals alike to rely increasingly on nutrition labeling to help with the meeting of health goals. A number of labeling problems persisted, including a lack of uniformity, misleading health claims, and imprecise terms such as "natural" and "light."

These problems indicated a need to reorganize and coordinate the entire food-labeling system. This need had been reinforced by three previous landmark reports that related nutrition and diet to national health goals: *The Surgeon General's Report on Nutrition and Health,* the National Research Council's *Diet and Health Report,* and the Public Health Service's national health goals and objectives, *Healthy People 2000.* On the basis of these reports, the Institute of Medicine of the National Academy of Sciences established a Committee on the Nutrition Components of Food Labeling to study and report on the scientific issues and practical needs involved in food-labeling

reform. The committee's report provided basic guidelines for the rule-making process conducted by the FDA, the USDA, and the U.S. Department of Health and Human Services for submission to Congress to achieve the needed reforms (see the For Further Focus box, "Nutrition Labeling: Recommendations for a New Century"). Three areas of concern formed the basis of the recommendations from the Institute of Medicine: (1) foods for mandatory regulations; (2) the format of label information; and (3) the education of consumers. This report became the basic guideline for the final law and regulations that were enacted by the U.S. Congress in 1994.

Current Food Label Format

Nutrition Facts Label. The food label format that is so familiar now is quite different from the one used during the 1970s and 1980s. The title "Nutrition Facts" is printed in bold, eye-catching letters (Figure 13-2). Manufacturers may choose to include additional information, such as calories from saturated fat, polyunsaturated fat, monounsaturated fat, potassium, soluble and insoluble fiber, sugar alcohol (e.g., sorbitol), other carbohydrates, or other vitamins and minerals.

Another key term is *percent daily value* (%DV). The FDA set 2000 calories as the reference amount for

---

FOR FURTHER FOCUS

NUTRITION LABELING: RECOMMENDATIONS FOR A NEW CENTURY

The U.S. government is committed by law to the food-labeling reform mandated by a health-conscious public. A proliferation of new health-related food products and concerned health professionals have created a demand for accurate information on the foods that are sold in the United States. Nutrition is a strong selling point in today's consumer market.

The initial report and recommendations of the Institute of Medicine's Committee on the Nutrition Components of Food Labeling formed the foundation for the final implementation of the Nutrition Labeling and Education Act. This baseline focus resulted from a 1-year study requested by the U.S. Department of Health and Human Services and the U.S. Department of Agriculture. The committee made several recommendations that are embodied in the Nutrition Labeling and Education Act law.

Foods Covered by Nutrition Labeling
- Nutrition labeling should be mandatory on most packaged foods.
- Nutrition labeling should be provided at the point of purchase for produce, seafood, meats, and poultry.
- Restaurants should make the nutrient content of menu items available to customers on request.

Label Presentation
- The U.S. Food and Drug Administration and the U.S. Department of Agriculture set the standardized serving sizes.
- More complete ingredient listings should be provided on all foods.
- A modified regulatory scheme should be established for the development and approval of lower-fat alternative foods that currently have standards of identity.

Educating Consumers
- A well-designed nutrition labeling program should be fashioned as one part of a comprehensive education program, concurrent with the adoption of regulations for the labeling of nutrition content and its format, to help consumers make wise dietary choices.

From the beginning of the process, Congress wanted to develop legislative proposals to clarify the legal basis for these reforms. The food industry, health professionals, and consumer groups wanted to promote changes in nutrition labeling that reflect the current Dietary Reference Intakes and related product development. The recommendations of the committee have provided a helpful foundation for all concerned.

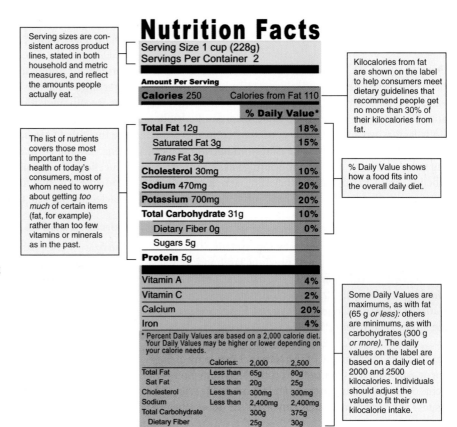

Figure 13-2 An example of a food product label showing the Nutrition Facts box that details nutrition information and that is mandated by the U.S. Food and Drug Administration under the Nutrition Labeling and Education Act. (Courtesy the U.S. Food and Drug Administration, Washington, DC.)

calculating the %DV, although individuals may vary greatly with regard to their specific needs. As a reference tool, the %DVs can be used to determine the overall value of a specific nutrient in the food (see the For Further Focus box, "Glossary of Terms for Current Labels"). For example, if the %DV for fiber in one serving of whole grain bread is 10%, a person who is eating the bread acquires one tenth of the recommended total fiber intake for his or her day.

In addition, the serving size (i.e., the amount of the food that is customarily consumed at one time) must be given and expressed in household measures; this is followed by the metric weight in parentheses and the total number of servings per container.[2]

Health Claims. Health claims that link nutrients or food groups with a risk for disease are strictly regulated. To make an association between a food product and a specific disease, the FDA must approve the claim, the food must meet the criteria set forth for that specific claim, and the wording used on the package must be approved. A list of nutrients that are currently approved for use in the United States and the specific diseases that they are associated with is given in the For Further Focus box entitled "Glossary of Terms for Current Labels." An

example of such a health claim would be the link between a diet that is low in saturated fat and cholesterol and a reduced risk of coronary heart disease. For a food to carry this label, it must be low in saturated fat, low in cholesterol, and low in total fat. If the food is fish or game meat, it must be deemed "extra lean." The specific wording of this example claim must include the following: *saturated fat and cholesterol, coronary heart disease,* or *heart disease;* there must also be a physician's statement about the claim that defines high or normal total cholesterol. The FDA also provides model claim statements from which food producers may choose. For this specific claim, the model statement is as follows: "Although many factors affect heart disease, diets low in saturated fat and cholesterol may reduce the risk of this disease."[3]

FOOD TECHNOLOGY

America's food supply has radically changed over the years. These changes, which have swept the food marketing system, are rooted in widespread social changes and scientific advances. The agricultural and food processing industries have developed various chemicals to increase and preserve the food supply. However, critics voice

FOR FURTHER FOCUS

GLOSSARY OF TERMS FOR CURRENT LABELS

To improve communication between producers and consumers, all producers must use the standard wording supplied by the U.S. Food and Drug Administration (FDA). Whether these terms are used in the Nutrition Facts box or elsewhere as part of the manufacturer's product description, all producers must use the commonly accepted terms. The following is a sampling of these terms.

Nutrition Facts Box
Daily Values
Daily values (DVs) are reference values that relate the nutrition information to a total daily diet of 2000 kcal, which is appropriate for most women and teenage girls as well as for some sedentary men. The footnote indicates the daily values for a 2500-kcal diet, which meets the needs of most men, teenage boys, and active women. To help consumers determine how a food fits into a healthy diet, the following nutrients, in the order given, must be listed as %DV:

- Total fat
- Saturated fat
- Trans fat
- Cholesterol
- Sodium
- Total carbohydrate
- Dietary fiber
- Vitamins A and C
- Calcium and iron

Other vitamins and minerals may be listed if the manufacturers choose to do so, but this is not required.

Daily Reference Value
As part of the DVs listed, the daily reference values are a set of dietary standards for the following nine nutrients: total fat; saturated fat; trans fat; cholesterol; total carbohydrate; dietary fiber; protein; potassium; and sodium. The daily reference values do not appear on the label, because they are part of a food's DV.

Reference Daily Intake
As part of the DVs listed, the Reference Daily Intakes (RDIs) are a set of dietary standards for essential vitamins, minerals, and protein. RDIs are based on the actual Recommended Dietary Allowances (RDAs), when available, or the Adequate Intake values. The term *RDI* replaces the old term *US RDA*, which was developed by food manufacturers as an estimate that was based on previous RDAs. RDIs do not appear on the label, because they are part of a food's DV.

Descriptive Terms on Products
The FDA has specifically defined many terms. Manufacturers must follow these definitions if they use these terms on their product. The following are examples:

- *Fat free:* Less than 0.5 g of fat per serving.
- *Low cholesterol:* 20 mg of cholesterol or less per serving and per 100 g; 2 g saturated fat or less per serving. Any label claim about low cholesterol is prohibited for all foods that contain more than 2 g of saturated fat per serving.
- *Light* or *Lite:* At least a one-third reduction in kilocalories. If fat contributes 50% or more of total kilocalories, fat content must be reduced by 50% compared with the reference food.
- *Less sodium:* At least a 25% reduction; 140 mg or less per reference amount per serving.
- *High:* 20% or more of the DV per serving.
- *Reduced saturated fat:* At least 25% less saturated fat than an appropriate reference food.
- *Lean:* Applied to meat, poultry, and seafood; less than 10 g of fat, 4 g of saturated fat, and 95 mg of cholesterol per serving.
- *Extra lean:* Applied to meat, poultry, and seafood; less than 5 g of fat, 2 g of saturated fat, and 95 mg of cholesterol per serving.

For more information, see "How to Understand and Use the Nutrition Facts Label" on the FDA Web site at www.fda.gov/Food/ResourcesForYou/Consumers/NFLPM/ucm274593.htm.

Health Claims
The FDA guidelines indicate that any health claim on a label must be supported by substantial scientific evidence. The following claims meet this test:

- Low sodium and the prevention of hypertension
- Calcium and vitamin D and the prevention of osteoporosis
- Low dietary fat and a reduced risk of cancer
- Low dietary cholesterol and saturated fat and a reduced risk of coronary heart disease
- Fiber-containing grain products, fruits, and vegetables and a reduced risk of cancer
- Grain products and fruits and vegetables that contain fiber, especially soluble fiber, and the prevention of coronary heart disease
- Fruits and vegetables that are rich in vitamins A or C and a lowered risk of cancer
- Folate and the prevention of neural tube defects
- Soy protein and a reduced risk of coronary heart disease
- Stanols/sterols and a reduced risk of coronary heart disease

For more information, refer to "Health Claims Meeting Significant Scientific Agreement" on the FDA Web site at www.fda.gov/Food/LabelingNutrition/LabelClaims/HealthClaimsMeetingSignificantScientificAgreementSSA/default.htm.

concerns about how these changes have affected food safety and the overall environment. Such concerns are usually focused on pesticide use and food additives.

Agricultural Pesticides

Reasons for Use

Large American agricultural corporations as well as individual farmers use a number of chemicals to improve their crop yields. These materials have made possible the advances in food production that are necessary to feed a growing population. For example, farmers use certain chemicals to control a wide variety of destructive insects that reduce crop yield (Figure 13-3).

Problems

Concerns and confusion continue regarding the use and effects of such chemicals. The four general areas of concern are as follows: (1) pesticide residues on foods; (2) the gradual leaching of the chemicals into groundwater and surrounding wells; (3) the increased exposure of farm workers to these strong chemicals; and (4) the increased amount of chemicals necessary as insects develop tolerance. Over time, the use of these chemicals has created a pesticide dilemma, and there is currently no clear answer regarding what to do in the face of conflicting interests. Thousands of pesticides are in use, and assessing the

risks of specific pesticides is an important but complicated task.

Alternative Agriculture

An increasing number of concerned farmers, with help from soil scientists, are turning away from heavy pesticide use toward alternative agricultural methods.

Organic Farming. Organic plant foods are grown without synthetic pesticides, fertilizers, sewage sludge, genetically modified organisms, or ionizing radiation. Organic meat, poultry, eggs, and dairy products are from animals that have been raised without antibiotics or growth hormones. In October 2002, the USDA enacted a set of nationally recognized standards to identify certified organic food. For a food to carry the USDA Organic Seal (Figure 13-4), the farm and processing plant where the food was grown and packaged must have undergone government inspections and met the strict USDA organic standards (see the For Further Focus box, "Organic Food Standards").[4] All foods that are produced organically are not required to use the organic label; it is a voluntary program. However, companies that are using the label on their food without certification face a large fine. Sales of organic foods are rapidly growing, and an increasing number of farmers—especially in California, which is the major supplier of U.S. fruits and vegetables—are using organic farming.

Certified organic foods are not recognized as being more safe or more nutritious than conventionally produced foods.[5] Organic farmers can still use natural pesticides and fertilizers; therefore, they are not producing pesticide-free foods. Other common points of confusion are with the use of the following terms: *natural, hormone free,* and *free range.* These terms are not synonymous with *organic.* Truthful terms about the production of a food can appear on the food label, but they do not mean that the product is organic. The term *natural* may be used on products that contain no artificial ingredients (e.g., coloring, chemical preservatives) and if the product and its ingredients are not more than minimally processed. The Food Safety and Inspection Service of the USDA does not approve use of the terms *hormone free* or *antibiotic free.*

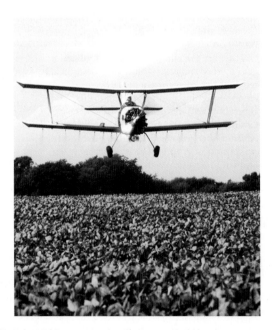

Figure 13-3 A farmer applies insecticide to a corn crop. (Courtesy Ken Hammond, Agricultural Research Service, U.S. Department of Agriculture, Washington, DC.)

organic farming the use of farming methods that employ natural means of pest control and that meet the standards set by the National Organic Program of the U.S. Department of Agriculture; organic foods are grown or produced without the use of synthetic pesticides or fertilizers, sewage sludge, genetically modified organisms, or ionizing radiation.

FOR FURTHER FOCUS

ORGANIC FOOD STANDARDS

The National Organic Program, which is a constituent of the U.S. Department of Agriculture (USDA), was established to ensure standards for organic foods. In response to the growing market, the National Organic Program has set strict standards for the growth, production, and labeling of organic foods. Although many methods prohibited by the organic standards (e.g., irradiation, genetic modification) are deemed safe by the USDA, these methods of farming have been banned in certified organic foods because of public concern.

Organic foods have four labeling categories with specific guidelines for each, as follows:

1. *100% organic:* Products that carry this label must be made or produced exclusively with certified organic ingredients, and they must have passed a government inspection. These products may use the USDA Organic Seal on their labels and advertisements.

2. *Organic:* Products labeled as organic must contain 95% to 100% organic ingredients and also must have passed a government inspection. The National Organic Program must approve all other ingredients for use as nonagricultural substances or as products not commercially available in organic form. These products may also use the USDA Organic Seal with the percentage of organic ingredients listed.

3. *70% organic ingredients:* Products made with at least 70% certified organic ingredients may state on the product label "made with organic ingredients" and list up to three ingredients or food groups. These foods also must meet the National Organic Program guidelines for growth or production without synthetic pesticides, fertilizers, sewage sludge, bioengineering, or ionizing radiation. The USDA Organic Seal may not be displayed on these products or used in any advertising.

4. *Less than 70% organic ingredients:* Foods made with less than 70% certified organic ingredients may not use the USDA Organic Seal or make any organic claims on the front panel of the package. They can list the specific organic ingredients on the side panel of the package.

All food products made with at least 70% organic ingredients must also supply the name and address of the government-approved certifying agent on the product.

For more information about the USDA organic standards, visit the National Organic Program Web site at www.ams.usda.gov/AMSv1.0/nop; call the National Organic Program at 202-720-3252; or write to USDA-AMS-National Organic Program, 1400 Independence Avenue, SW, Room 2646-South, Stop 0268, Washington, DC 20250.

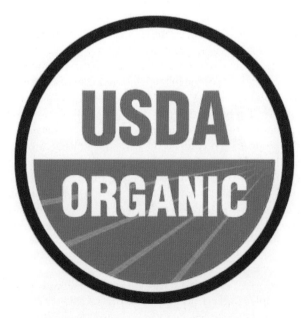

Figure 13-4 Official U.S. Department of Agriculture organic seal, which is available at www.ams.usda.gov/AMSv1.0/nop. (Courtesy the National Organic Program, Agricultural Marketing Service, U.S. Department of Agriculture, Washington, DC.)

Instead, the phrases *raised without added hormones* and *raised without added antibiotics* are allowed, provided that the producer is able to supply an affidavit that attests to the production practices that are used to support the claim. One important note about the use of hormones is that they are approved for use only in beef cattle and lamb production. Therefore, any such claim on a poultry product would be allowed only if it were immediately followed by this statement: "Federal regulations prohibit the use of hormones in poultry."

Organic farming is safer for the soil, the water, the agricultural workers, and the birds. Unfortunately, compared with conventional farming, organic farming is less efficient. Without synthetic pesticides and fertilizers, crops are smaller and require more land. As a result, the products are more expensive.

Biotechnology. Plant physiologists are developing strains of genetically modified (GM) foods that reduce the need for toxic pesticides and herbicides. Genetic manipulation in various forms has been used to improve crops for thousands of years, but most U.S. consumers are unaware of the extent to which these foods have entered the marketplace. In the United States, 93% of soybean crop acreage and a steadily increasing percentage of corn

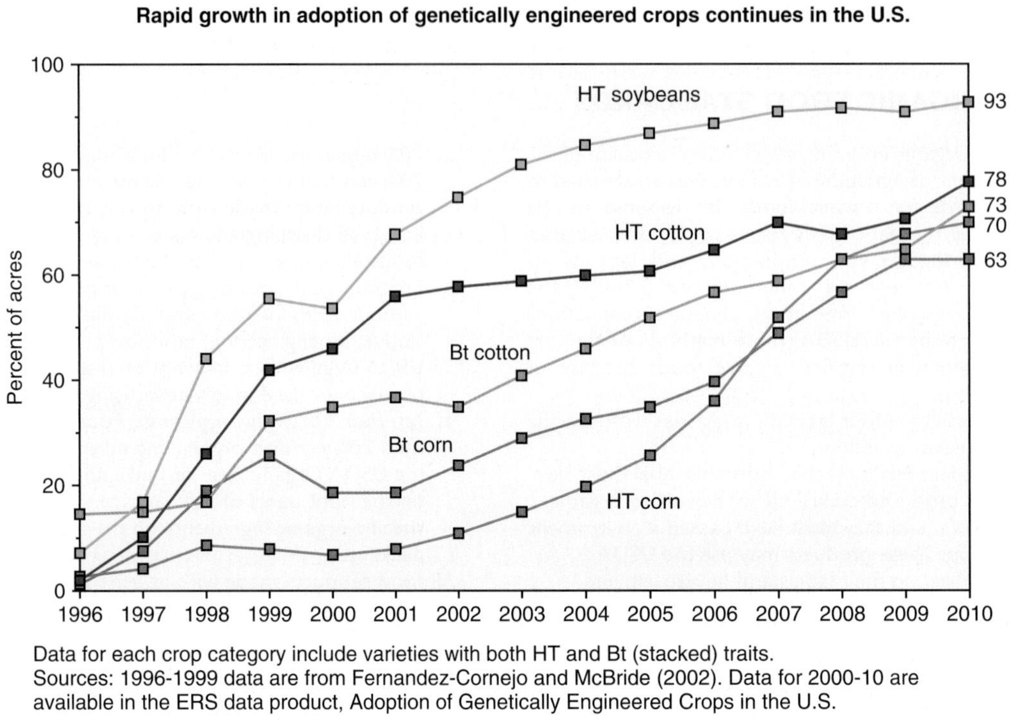

Rapid growth in adoption of genetically engineered crops continues in the U.S.

Data for each crop category include varieties with both HT and Bt (stacked) traits.
Sources: 1996-1999 data are from Fernandez-Cornejo and McBride (2002). Data for 2000-10 are available in the ERS data product, Adoption of Genetically Engineered Crops in the U.S.

Figure 13-5 Adoption of genetically engineered crops continues to grow rapidly in the United States. (Reprinted from the U.S. Department of Agriculture, Economic Research Service. *Adoption of genetically engineered crops in the U.S.,* 2010, U.S. Department of Agriculture: Washington, DC; 2010) Bt - *Bacillus thuringiensis bacterium* HT - *herbicide tolerant.*

crops are GM herbicide-tolerant varieties[6] (Figure 13-5). Most people in the United States have consumed some form of GM foods at some point, such as seedless oranges or watermelons. An example of biotechnology in today's agriculture is the use of GM corn that expresses a specific protein that ultimately serves as an insecticide. Approved genetic modifications are currently used to protect against virus infections and insects on tomatoes, potatoes, squash, papayas, and other crops. GM crops are extensively tested for their composition, safety, and environmental effects. The National Institutes of Health, the Animal Plant Health Inspection Service of the USDA, the FDA, and the Environmental Protection Agency are all involved in the strict regulation of GM foods in commercial use, which are the most heavily regulated new foods.

The benefits of biotechnology are not limited to the producer. Technology is advancing to the point of engineering food to increase its quality, safety, and nutritional value.[7] Plants are produced with increased antioxidants and improved fatty acid and amino acid profiles, all of which are beneficial to the consumer and which may have positive effects on human nutrition worldwide. More than 50 biotechnology crop products are approved for commercialization in the United States (Figure 13-6).

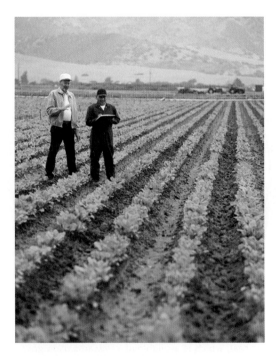

Figure 13-6 A geneticist and technician evaluate sugar beet breeding in California. (Courtesy Scott Bauer, Agricultural Research Service, U.S. Department of Agriculture, Washington, DC.)

Such forms of agriculture remain controversial around the world because of many unknown factors regarding the long-term effects on the environment and overall human health. Current testing procedures are unable to determine potential problems from long-term use, such as carcinogenicity or neurotoxicity. Research that was completed with soybeans revealed that wild-type and GM soybean varieties had exactly the same allergenicity; thus, genetic modification did not increase the likelihood of allergies in this crop.[8] This type of research will be important for all types of GM crops to ensure safety and improve consumer acceptability.

Irradiation. Irradiation can kill bacteria and parasites that are on food after harvest. Irradiation helps to prevent food-borne illness caused by *Escherichia coli, Salmonella, Campylobacter, Listeria, Cyclospora, Shigella,* and *Salmonella.*[9] Three different methods of irradiation are used, all of which are approved by the World Health Organization, the Centers for Disease Control and Prevention, the USDA, and the FDA. The use of irradiation is not a new science; wheat flour and white potatoes were approved for irradiation during the early 1960s. In addition to reducing or eliminating disease-causing germs, irradiation can be used to increase the shelf life of produce. Foods that are irradiated have unaltered nutritional value; they are not radioactive, they have no harmful substances introduced as a result of irradiation, but they may taste slightly different.[9] A variety of foods have been approved for irradiation in the United States, including meat, poultry, grains, some seafood, fruits, vegetables, herbs, and spices. The FDA requires that all irradiated foods be appropriately labeled with either the radura symbol for irradiation (Figure 13-7) or with a written description that states that the food has been exposed to irradiation.

Consumer rejection in the United States and around the world is mainly the result of altered taste and a fear of the unknown long-term effects of irradiation on human health. Irradiation does introduce a slight increase in trans fatty acid content in meats,[10] which is a known health risk. The U.S. government continues to support the use and safety of such foods; however, without consumer acceptance, companies that are using such procedures have limited success.

Food Additives

The use of food additives (i.e., chemicals that are intentionally added to foods to prevent spoilage and extend shelf life) is not new to the food industry, either. Table 13-1 lists examples of food additives. The two most common additives are sugar and salt, although consumers often do not recognize these basic ingredients as food additives. Some additives have been used for centuries as preservatives, especially salt in cured meats. The phrase *generally recognized as safe* is used to define additives that have been used in foods and that do not require FDA approval.

Over the past few decades, the number and variety of food additives in the food supply have increased; the current variety of food market items would be impossible without them. Scientific advances have created processed food products, and the changing society has created a market demand. The expanding population, a larger workforce, and more complex family life have increased the desire for more variety and convenience in foods as well as better safety and quality. Food additives help to achieve these needs, and they serve many other purposes, such as the following:

- They enrich foods with added nutrients.
- They produce uniform qualities (e.g., color, flavor, aroma, texture, general appearance).
- They standardize many functional factors (e.g., thickening, stabilization [i.e., keeping parts from separating]).
- They preserve foods by preventing oxidation.
- They control acidity or alkalinity to improve flavor and texture of the cooked product.

A number of micronutrients and antioxidants are used as additives in processed foods not for their ability to increase nutrient content but rather for their technical effects either during processing or in the final product.

FOOD-BORNE DISEASE

Prevalence

Many disease-bearing organisms inhabit the environment and can contaminate food and water. Much has been learned during the past decade about the pathogens that commonly contaminate food and water and about ways to prevent food-borne illness outbreaks. However, lapses in control still occur, and these can result in high

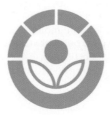

Figure 13-7 Radura symbol of irradiation. (Courtesy the Food Safety and Inspection Service, U.S. Department of Agriculture, Washington, DC.)

TABLE 13-1 **EXAMPLES OF FOOD ADDITIVES**

The following summary lists the types of common food ingredients, why they are used, and some examples of the names that can be found on product labels that refer to them. Some additives are used for more than one purpose.

Types of Ingredients	What They Do	Examples of Uses	Names Found on Product Labels
Preservatives	Prevent food spoilage from bacteria, molds, fungi, or yeast (antimicrobials); slow or prevent changes in color, flavor, or texture and delay rancidity (antioxidants); maintain freshness	Fruit sauces and jellies, beverages, baked goods, cured meats, oils and margarines, cereals, dressings, snack foods, fruits, and vegetables	Ascorbic acid, citric acid, sodium benzoate, calcium propionate, sodium erythorbate, sodium nitrite, calcium sorbate, potassium sorbate, BHA, BHT, EDTA, tocopherols (vitamin E)
Sweeteners	Add sweetness with or without the extra calories	Beverages, baked goods, confections, table-top sugar, substitutes, many processed foods	Sucrose (sugar), glucose, fructose, sorbitol, mannitol, corn syrup, high fructose corn syrup, saccharin, aspartame, sucralose, acesulfame potassium (acesulfame-K), neotame
Color additives	Offset color loss due to exposure to light, air, temperature extremes, moisture and storage conditions; correct natural variations in color; enhance colors that occur naturally; provide color to colorless and "fun" foods	Many processed foods, (candies, snack foods margarine, cheese, soft drinks, jams and jellies, gelatins, pudding and pie fillings)	FD&C Blue Nos. 1 and 2, FD&C Green No. 3, FD&C Red Nos. 3 and 40, FD&C Yellow Nos. 5 and 6, Orange B, Citrus Red No. 2, annatto extract, beta-carotene, grape skin extract, cochineal extract or carmine, paprika oleoresin, caramel color, fruit and vegetable juices, saffron (Note: Exempt color additives are not required to be declared by name on labels but may be declared simply as colorings or color added)
Flavors and spices	Add specific flavors (natural and synthetic)	Pudding and pie fillings, gelatin dessert mixes, cake mixes, salad dressings, candies, soft drinks, ice cream, BBQ sauce	Natural flavoring, artificial flavor, and spices
Flavor enhancers	Enhance flavors already present in foods (without providing their own separate flavor)	Many processed foods	Monosodium glutamate (MSG), hydrolyzed soy protein, autolyzed yeast extract, disodium guanylate or inosinate
Fat replacers (and components of formulations that are used to replace fats)	Provide expected texture and a creamy "mouth-feel" in reduced-fat foods	Baked goods, dressings, frozen desserts, confections, cake and dessert mixes, dairy products	Olestra, cellulose gel, carrageenan, polydextrose, modified food starch, microparticulated egg white protein, guar gum, xanthan gum, whey protein concentrate
Nutrients	Replace vitamins and minerals lost in processing (enrichment), add nutrients that may be lacking in the diet (fortification)	Flour, breads, cereals, rice, macaroni, margarine, salt, milk, fruit beverages, energy bars, instant breakfast drinks	Thiamine hydrochloride, riboflavin (vitamin B_2), niacin, niacinamide, folate or folic acid, beta carotene, potassium iodide, iron or ferrous sulfate, alpha tocopherols, ascorbic acid, vitamin D, amino acids (L-tryptophan, L-lysine, L-leucine, L-methionine)
Emulsifiers	Allow smooth mixing of ingredients, prevent separation Keep emulsified products stable, reduce stickiness, control crystallization, keep ingredients dispersed, and to help products dissolve more easily	Salad dressings, peanut butter, chocolate, margarine, frozen desserts	Soy lecithin, mono- and diglycerides, egg yolks, polysorbates, sorbitan monostearate

TABLE 13-1   **EXAMPLES OF FOOD ADDITIVES—cont'd**

Types of Ingredients	What They Do	Examples of Uses	Names Found on Product Labels
Stabilizers, thickeners, binders, and texturizers	Produce uniform texture, improve "mouth-feel"	Frozen desserts, dairy products, cakes, pudding and gelatin mixes, dressings, jams and jellies, sauces	Gelatin, pectin, guar gum, carrageenan, xanthan gum, whey
pH control agents and acidulants	Control acidity and alkalinity, prevent spoilage	Beverages, frozen desserts, chocolate, low-acid canned foods, baking powder	Lactic acid, citric acid, ammonium hydroxide, sodium carbonate
Leavening agents	Promote rising of baked goods	Breads and other baked goods	Baking soda, monocalcium phosphate, calcium carbonate
Anti-caking agents	Keep powdered foods free-flowing, prevent moisture absorption	Salt, baking powder, confectioner's sugar	Calcium silicate, iron ammonium citrate, silicon dioxide
Humectants	Retain moisture	Shredded coconut, marshmallows, soft candies, confections	Glycerin, sorbitol
Yeast nutrients	Promote growth of yeast	Breads and other baked goods	Calcium sulfate, ammonium phosphate
Dough strengtheners and conditioners	Produce more stable dough	Breads and other baked goods	Ammonium sulfate, azodicarbonamide, L-cysteine
Firming agents	Maintain crispness and firmness	Processed fruits and vegetables	Calcium chloride, calcium lactate
Enzyme preparations	Modify proteins, polysaccharides and fats	Cheese, dairy products, meat	Enzymes, lactase, papain, rennet, chymosin
Gases	Serve as propellant, aerate, or create carbonation	Oil cooking spray, whipped cream, carbonated beverages	Carbon dioxide, nitrous oxide

Reprinted from the International Food Information Council and the U.S. Food and Drug Administration. *Food ingredients and colors, 2010* (website): www.fda.gov/Food/FoodIngredientsPackaging/ucm094211.htm#types. Accessed December 2010.

incidences of illness and death as well as economic burden. The estimated annual incidence of food-borne illness has been on the decline for most pathogens during recent years[11] (Figure 13-8). Microbiologic diseases—both bacterial and viral—represent the majority of these outbreaks nationwide, with a large range of costs associated with each type of infection. *Salmonella, Campylobacter, Shigella,* and *Cryptosporidium* are the most common infections seen during home and community outbreaks.

Food Sanitation

Buying and Storing Food

The control of food-borne disease focuses on strict sanitation measures and rigid personal hygiene. First, the food itself should be of good quality and not defective or diseased. Second, dry or cold storage should protect it from deterioration or decay, which is especially important for products such as refrigerated convenience foods; this is the fastest growing segment of the convenience food market, and it is potentially the most dangerous, because these foods are not sterile. These vacuum-packaged or modified-atmosphere chilled food products are only minimally processed and not sterilized, and they are at risk of temperature abuse. Home refrigerator temperatures should be held at 40° F or lower. At temperatures of more than 45° F, any precooked or leftover foods are potential reservoirs for bacteria that survive cooking and that can then recontaminate cooked food. Food safety depends on the following critical actions[12] (Figure 13-9):

- *Clean:* Wash hands and surfaces often.
- *Separate:* Do not cross-contaminate.
- *Cook:* Cook to proper temperatures.
- *Chill:* Refrigerate promptly.

All food preparation areas must be scrupulously clean, and foods must be washed or cleaned well. Cooking procedures and temperatures must be followed as directed. All utensils, dishes, and anything else that comes in contact with food must be clean. Leftover food should be stored and reheated appropriately or discarded (Table 13-2). Food does not need to be cooled to room

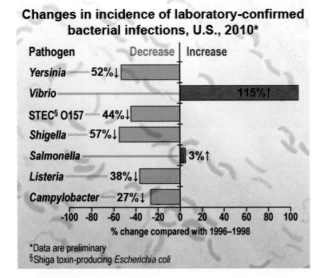

Figure 13-8 Changes in the incidence of laboratory-confirmed bacterial infections, United States, 2010. (From the Centers for Disease Control and Prevention. *Incidence of foodborne illness, 2010* (website): www.cdc.gov/Features/dsFoodbornelllness. Accessed February 2012.)

Figure 13-9 The Partnership for Food Safety Education developed the "Fight BAC!" (i.e., bacteria) campaign to prevent food-borne illness. Campaign graphics are available at www.fightbac.org. (Courtesy Partnership for Food Safety Education, Washington, DC.)

temperature before refrigerating; this practice allows food to sit in a temperature range that is perfect for bacterial growth. Leftovers should be refrigerated within 2 hours. Garbage must be contained and disposed of in a sanitary manner. Safe methods of food handling, cooking, and storage are simple and mostly common sense; however, they often are neglected, and this may lead to food-borne illness.

Food safety publications for all types of foods and populations can be found at the Food Safety and Inspection Service Web site at www.fsis.usda.gov.

Preparing and Serving Food

All people who handle food—especially those who work in public food services—should follow strict measures to prevent contamination. For example, washing hands properly and wearing clean clothing, gloves, and aprons are imperative. Basic rules of hygiene should apply to all people who are handling food, whether they work in food processing and packaging plants, process and package foods in markets, or prepare and serve food in restaurants. In addition, people with infectious diseases should have limited access to direct food handling.

The following are the minimal internal temperatures to be reached when cooking various foods:

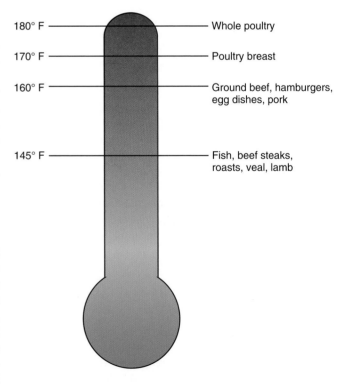

The Hazard Analysis & Critical Control Point (HACCP) food safety system focuses on preventing food-borne illness by identifying critical points and eliminating

TABLE 13-2 **COLD STORAGE**

Product	Refrigerator (40° F)	Freezer (0° F)
Eggs		
Fresh, in shell	3 to 5 weeks	Do not freeze
Raw yolks and whites	2 to 4 days	1 year
Hard cooked	1 week	Does not freeze well
Liquid Pasteurized Eggs, Egg Substitutes		
Opened	3 days	Does not freeze well
Unopened	10 days	1 year
Mayonnaise, Commercial		
Refrigerate after opening	2 months	Do not freeze
Frozen Dinners and Entrees		
Keep frozen until ready to heat	—	3 to 4 months
Deli and Vacuum-Packed Products		
Store-prepared (or homemade) egg, chicken, ham, tuna, and macaroni salads	3 to 5 days	Does not freeze well
Hot Dogs and Luncheon Meats		
Hot Dogs		
Opened package	1 week	1 to 2 months
Unopened package	2 weeks	1 to 2 months
Luncheon Meat		
Opened package	3 to 5 days	1 to 2 months
Unopened package	2 weeks	1 to 2 months
Bacon and Sausage		
Bacon	7 days	1 month
Sausage, raw—from chicken, turkey, pork, beef	1 to 2 days	1 to 2 months
Smoked breakfast links, patties	7 days	1 to 2 months
Hard sausage—pepperoni, jerky sticks	2 to 3 weeks	1 to 2 months
Summer Sausage Labeled "Keep Refrigerated"		
Opened	3 weeks	1 to 2 months
Unopened	3 months	1 to 2 months
Corned Beef		
Corned beef, in pouch with pickling juices	5 to 7 days	Drained, 1 month
Ham, Canned, Labeled "Keep Refrigerated"		
Opened	3 to 5 days	1 to 2 months
Unopened	6 to 9 months	Do not freeze
Ham, Fully Cooked		
Vacuum sealed at plant, undated, unopened	2 weeks	1 to 2 months
Vacuum sealed at plant, dated, unopened	"Use-By" date on package	1 to 2 months
Whole	7 days	1 to 2 months
Half	3 to 5 days	1 to 2 months
Slices	3 to 4 days	1 to 2 months
Hamburger, Ground and Stew Meat		
Hamburger and stew meat	1 to 2 days	3 to 4 months
Ground turkey, veal, pork, lamb, and mixtures of them	1 to 2 days	3 to 4 months
Fresh Beef, Veal, Lamb, and Pork		
Steaks	3 to 5 days	6 to 12 months
Chops	3 to 5 days	4 to 6 months
Roasts	3 to 5 days	4 to 12 months
Variety meats—tongue, liver, heart, kidneys, chitterlings	1 to 2 days	3 to 4 months
Prestuffed, uncooked pork chops, lamb chops, or chicken breasts stuffed with dressing	1 day	Does not freeze well
Soups and stews, vegetable or meat added	3 to 4 days	2 to 3 months

Continued

TABLE 13-2 **COLD STORAGE**—cont'd

Product	Refrigerator (40° F)	Freezer (0° F)
Fresh Poultry		
Chicken or turkey, whole	1 to 2 days	1 year
Chicken or turkey, pieces	1 to 2 days	9 months
Giblets	1 to 2 days	3 to 4 months
Cooked Meat and Poultry Leftovers		
Cooked meat and meat casseroles	3 to 4 days	2 to 3 months
Gravy and meat broth	1 to 2 days	2 to 3 months
Fried chicken	3 to 4 days	4 months
Cooked poultry casseroles	3 to 4 days	4 to 6 months
Poultry pieces, plain	3 to 4 days	4 months
Poultry pieces in broth, gravy	1 to 2 days	6 months
Chicken nuggets, patties	1 to 2 days	1 to 3 months
Other Cooked Leftovers		
Pizza, cooked	3 to 4 days	1 to 2 months
Stuffing, cooked	3 to 4 days	1 month

Reprinted from the Food Safety and Inspection Service. *Safe food handling: basics for handling food safely* (website): www.fsis.usda.gov/Fact_Sheets/Basics_for_Handling_Food_Safely/index.asp. Accessed December 2010.

hazards. Many organizations, including the USDA and the FDA, use the HACCP standards. The USDA has developed specific standards for a variety of food products. For more information about HACCP, visit www.fda.gov/Food/FoodSafety/HazardAnalysisCriticalControlPointsHACCP/default.htm.

Food Contamination

Food-borne illness usually presents itself with flu-like symptoms, but it can advance to a lethal illness. Not all bacteria found in foods are harmful, and some are even beneficial (e.g., the bacteria in yogurt). Bacteria that are harmful to people are referred to as *pathogens.* Certain subgroups of the population are at higher risk for the development of food-borne illness as a result of age and physical condition. Groups with the highest risks are young children, pregnant women, elderly individuals, and people with compromised immune systems.

Food-borne illness generally results from the ingestion of bacteria, viruses, or parasites. Illness that results from bacteria is caused by either an infection or by toxins that are produced by the bacteria.

Bacterial Food Infections

Bacterial food infections result from eating food that is contaminated by large colonies of different types of bacteria. Specific diseases result from specific bacteria (e.g., salmonellosis, shigellosis, listeriosis).

Salmonellosis. Salmonellosis is caused by *Salmonella,* a bacterium that was named for the American veterinarian pathologist Daniel Salmon (1850-1914), who first

isolated and identified the species that commonly cause food-borne infections: *Salmonella typhi* and *Salmonella paratyphi.* Approximately 40,000 cases of salmonellosis are reported in the United States each year, although thousands of other cases likely go unreported.[13] These organisms readily grow in common foods such as milk, custard, egg dishes, salad dressing, and sandwich fillings. Seafood from polluted waters—especially shellfish such as oysters and clams—may also be a source of infection. The unsanitary handling of foods and utensils can spread the bacteria. Resulting cases of gastroenteritis may vary from mild to severe diarrhea. Immunization, pasteurization, and sanitary regulations that involve community water and food supplies as well as food handlers help to control such outbreaks. Because the incubation and multiplication of the bacteria take time after the food is eaten, symptoms of food infection develop relatively slowly (i.e., up to 48 hours later). Symptoms include diarrhea, fever, vomiting, and abdominal cramps. The illness usually lasts 4 to 7 days, with most affected individuals recovering completely. Severe dehydration from diarrhea and vomiting may require intravenous fluids.

Shigellosis. Shigellosis is caused by the bacteria *Shigella,* which was named for the Japanese physician Kiyoshi Shiga (1870-1957), who first discovered a main species of the organism, *Shigella dysenteriae,* during a dysentery epidemic in Japan in 1898. Approximately 14,000 cases are reported annually, but because many cases are not diagnosed, the Centers for Disease Control and Prevention estimates that the actual number of cases may be as much as 20 times higher.[14] Shigellosis is usually confined to the large intestine; it may vary from a mild, transient intestinal disturbance in adults to fatal dysentery in young children. The bacteria grow easily in foods, especially milk, which is a common vehicle of transmission to infants and children. The boiling of water or the pasteurization of milk kills the organisms, but the food or milk may easily be reinfected through unsanitary handling. The disease is spread similarly to how salmonella is transmitted: by feces, fingers, flies and by foods such as milk and articles that are handled by unsanitary carriers. Shigellosis, similar to salmonellosis, is more common during the summer, and it most often occurs in young children.[14] Symptoms appear within 4 to 7 days and include cramps, diarrhea, fever, vomiting, and blood or mucus in the stool.

Listeriosis. Listeriosis is caused by the bacteria *Listeria,* which was named for the English surgeon Baron Joseph Lister (1827-1912), who first applied knowledge of bacterial infection to the principles of antiseptic surgery in a benchmark 1867 publication that led to "clean" operations and the development of modern surgery. However, only within the past 30 years has knowledge of bacteria's role as a direct cause of food-borne illness increased and the major species to cause human illness, *Listeria monocytogenes,* been identified. Before 1981, *Listeria* was thought to be an organism of animal disease that was transmitted to people only by direct contact with infected animals. However, this organism occurs widely in the environment and in high-risk individuals, such as elderly people, pregnant women, infants, and patients with suppressed immune systems. It can produce a rare but often fatal illness with severe symptoms such as diarrhea, flu-like fever and headache, pneumonia, sepsis, meningitis, and endocarditis. Approximately one third of all listeriosis cases occur in pregnant women.[15] Food-borne disease has been traced to a variety of foods, including soft cheese, poultry, seafood, raw milk, refrigerated raw liquid whole eggs, and meat products (e.g., pâté).

Escherichia Coli. Escherichia coli was discovered by Theodor Escherich (1857-1911), a German pediatrician and bacteriologist who discovered the rod-shaped bacteria in 1885. It was not recognized as a human pathogen until 1982. There are many types of *E. coli,* and not all types are harmful to humans. In fact, some strains are part of the healthy gut flora that survive in the intestines and produce a valuable supply of vitamin K. The most common form of *E. coli* that results in about 70,000 cases of illness in North America per year is the Shiga toxin-producing strain O157:H7. This strain is most dangerous to young children and elderly adults (see the Drug-Nutrient Interaction box, "Drug Resistant *Escherichia coli* and the Food Supply"). Most cases involve diarrhea, stomach cramps, and low-grade fevers that start within 3 to 4 days after

ingestion and that usually resolve within 5 to 7 days. About 5% to 10% of individuals infected with *E. coli* will develop hemolytic uremic syndrome, which is a potentially lethal condition. *E. coli* is most often spread through fecal contamination (e.g., contaminated foods, not properly washing hands after changing diapers), undercooked meat, and unpasteurized foods (e.g., milk, apple cider, soft cheeses).[16]

Vibrio. Filippo Pacini (1812-1883) first isolated microorganisms that he called "vibrions" from cholera patients in 1854. This particular bacterial infection has been on the rise in the United States for the past decade[17] (see Figure 13-8). It is a salt-requiring organism that inhabits the salt-water coastal regions of North America, and it is usually ingested by humans via contaminated seafood. Immunocompromised individuals are most susceptible to *Vibrio* infection. Thoroughly cooking seafood—especially shellfish such as oysters—reduces the risk of infection.

Bacterial Food Poisoning

Food poisoning is caused by the ingestion of bacterial toxins that have been produced in food as a result of the growth of specific kinds of bacteria before the food is eaten. The powerful toxin is directly ingested, so symptoms of food poisoning develop rapidly. Two types of bacterial food poisoning, staphylococcal and clostridial, are most commonly responsible.

Staphylococcal Food Poisoning. Staphylococcal food poisoning was named for the causative organism, which is mainly *Staphylococcus aureus,* a round bacteria that forms masses of cells. *S. aureus* poisoning is the most common form of bacterial food poisoning in the United States. Powerful preformed toxins in the contaminated food rapidly produce illness (i.e., 1 to 6 hours after ingestion). The symptoms appear suddenly, and they include severe cramping and abdominal pain with nausea, vomiting, and diarrhea, usually accompanied by sweating, headache, fever, and sometimes prostration and shock. However, recovery is fairly rapid, and symptoms subside within 24 to 48 hours[18] (see the Clinical Applications box, "Case Study: A Community Food Poisoning Incident"). The amount of toxin ingested and the susceptibility of the individual eating it determine the degree of severity. The source of the contamination is usually a staphylococcal

---

hemolytic uremic syndrome a condition that results most often from infection with *Escherichia coli* and that presents with a breaking up of red blood cells (i.e., hemolysis) and kidney failure.

DRUG-NUTRIENT INTERACTION

DRUG RESISTANT *ESCHERICHIA COLI* AND THE FOOD SUPPLY

The agricultural use of antimicrobial drugs is suspected in the development of drug-resistant bacterial strains that are transmitted to humans via the food supply.[1] Drug-resistant strains of *Escherichia coli* bacteria are highly prevalent in the retail meat and poultry supplies. Resistance to first-line antibiotics by these bacteria represents a major cause of illness, death, and increased health care costs. Researchers have found that drug-resistant *E. coli* infections in humans were more closely related to the strains of bacteria found in chickens than to those found in the gut flora of humans, which suggests that drug-resistant *E. coli* strains are likely transmitted to humans via poultry that is carrying the infection.[1]

In 2006, the United States experienced an outbreak of *E. coli* infection that was traced to commercially grown spinach. This prompted a nationwide recall of bagged spinach and of products that had been made with the contaminated spinach. Upon investigation, the U.S. Food and Drug Administration found several environmental risk factors, including proximity to waterways that were exposed to cattle and wildlife feces.[2]

Although the washing of the spinach would not have prevented the *E. coli* outbreak, the U.S. Food and Drug Administration recommends the employment of safe food-handling practices among all consumers to prevent contamination from many causes.[2] Populations that are at risk for infection with drug-resistant strains of bacteria include children, elderly adults, and those who are immunocompromised. In health care settings, proper food safety practices are especially important. Drug-resistant strains of bacteria necessitate the long-term use of strong antibiotics. Nausea, vomiting, and diarrhea are common with antibiotic use as a result of the destruction of the natural gut flora. Some antibiotics like ciprofloxacin (Cipro) can bind to calcium, magnesium, iron, and zinc, thereby interfering with their absorption. Thus, the long-term use of this antibiotic can result in poor bioavailability of these minerals.[3]

Kelli Boi

1. Johnson JR, Sannes MR, Croy C, et al. Antimicrobial drug-resistant Escherichia coli from humans and poultry products, Minnesota and Wisconsin, 2002-2004. *Emerg Infect Dis.* 2007;13(6):838-846.
2. U.S. Department of Health and Human Services. *FDA finalizes report on 2006 spinach outbreak.* 2007 [cited December 2011; Available from: www.fda.gov/NewsEvents/Newsroom/PressAnnouncements/2007/ucm108873.htm.
3. Pronsky Z. *Food-medication interactions.* 15th ed. Birchrunville, Penn: Food-Medication Interactions; 2008.

infection on the hand of a worker preparing the food. This infection is often minor and considered harmless, or it may even be unnoticed by the food handler. Foods that are particularly effective carriers of staphylococci and their toxins include custard or cream-filled bakery goods, processed meats, ham, tongue, cheese, ice cream, potato salad, sauces, chicken and ham salads, and combination dishes such as spaghetti and casseroles. The toxin causes no change in the normal appearance, odor, or taste of the food, so the victim has no warning. A careful food history helps to determine the source of the poisoning, and portions of the food are obtained for examination, if possible. Few bacteria may be found, because heating kills the organisms but does not destroy the toxins that have been produced.

Clostridial Food Poisoning. Clostridial food poisoning was named for the spore-forming, rod-shaped bacteria, mainly *Clostridium perfringens* and *Clostridium botulinum*, which can also form powerful toxins in infected foods.

C. perfringens spores are widespread in the environment, including soil, water, dust, refuse, and many other places. This organism multiplies in cooked meat and meat dishes, and it develops its toxin in foods that are held at warm or room temperatures for extended periods. A number of outbreaks from food eaten in restaurants,

college dining rooms, and school cafeterias have been reported. In most cases, cooked meat is improperly prepared or refrigerated. Control depends on the careful preparation and adequate cooking of meats, prompt service, and immediate refrigeration at sufficiently low temperatures.

The bacteria *C. botulinum* causes a far more serious and often fatal food poisoning, *botulism,* which results from the ingestion of food that contains its powerful toxin. Depending on the dose of toxin taken and the individual response, symptoms usually appear within 12 to 72 hours and, in severe cases, can result in death.[19] Mortality rates are high. Nausea, vomiting, weakness, and dizziness are the initial symptoms. The toxin progressively irritates motor nerve cells and blocks the transmission of neural impulses at the nerve terminals, thereby causing a gradual paralysis. Sudden respiratory paralysis with airway obstruction is the major cause of death. *C. botulinum* spores are widespread in soil throughout the world and may be carried on harvested food to the canning process. Like all *Clostridia,* this species is anaerobic or nearly so. The relatively air-free can and canning

---

anaerobic a microorganism that can live and grow in an oxygen-free environment.

CLINICAL APPLICATIONS

CASE STUDY: A COMMUNITY FOOD POISONING INCIDENT

John and Eva Wesson agreed that their lodge dinner had been the best they had ever had, especially the dessert: custard-filled cream puffs, John's favorite. He had eaten two of them, despite Eva's protests; maybe that was why he began to feel ill shortly after they arrived home. Eva's stomach felt a little upset, too, so they both took some antacid pills, thinking that their "stomachaches" were from eating more rich food than they were accustomed to eating. They went to bed early.

However, by 11:00 PM, Eva woke up alarmed. John was vomiting, and he had diarrhea and increasingly severe stomach cramps. He complained of a headache, and his pajamas were wet with sweat. He had a fever and appeared to be in shock. Eva began to have similar pains and symptoms, although they were not as severe as John's pains.

One of their friends who had also been at the lodge dinner telephoned; she and her husband had the same symptoms.

By now, John was prostrate and unable to move. Eva immediately called 911, and they were both taken to the hospital. After treatment in the emergency department for shock, followed by observational care and rest the following day, John's symptoms had subsided, and he was allowed to go home. The physician advised John and Eva to eat lightly for a few days and to get more rest. He said that he would investigate the cause in the meantime. During the next few days, John and Eva learned that almost all their friends who had been at the lodge dinner had had an experience that was similar to their own.

The physician contacted the public health department to report the incident. His was one of several similar calls, a public health officer said, and the department was already investigating.

The following week, the public health officer returned the physician's call to report his findings. The cream puffs that the lodge restaurant had served that evening had been purchased from a local bakery. At the bakery, health officials had located a worker with an infected cut on his little finger—"a small thing," the worker said. He could not understand what all the fuss was about.

The health officials also located the delivery truck driver, who had started out at midmorning to make his rounds and to take the cream puffs to the lodge. When they questioned the driver, they learned that the delivery truck had broken down during his afternoon deliveries, before he had reached the lodge. The driver said that he had been irritated by a 3-hour wait at the garage while the truck was being fixed, but he still got the order to the lodge restaurant in time for the dinner.

At the lodge, the chef said that everyone was so busy with the dinner that, when the cream puffs finally arrived, no one had time to give them much notice. They had decided not to put the cream puffs in the refrigerator because they were about to be served.

When John and Eva's physician called them afterward to report the story, John and Eva decided that they would not eat at the lodge restaurant again. Besides, by then, John had lost his taste for cream puffs.

Questions for Analysis
1. Why is the control of the community's food supply an important responsibility of the health department?
2. Which disease agents may be carried by food or water?
3. What agent caused John and Eva's illness? Was this a food infection or a food poisoning? Why?
4. While the investigation was occurring and before John and Eva learned the real cause of their illness, John thought it must have been caused by "those things farmers and food processors put into food these days." What substances did John mean? Give some examples.
5. Why are these materials used for growing and processing food?
6. What are some ways in which food is protected from its point of production to the table? How can food be preserved for later use?
7. Which agency controls food safety and quality? How does it do so?

---

temperatures (i.e., $\geq 27°$ C [$80°$ F]) provide good conditions for toxin production. The development of high standards in the commercial canning industry has eliminated this source of botulism, but cases still result each year, mainly from the ingestion of home-canned foods. Because boiling for 10 minutes destroys the toxin and not the spore, all home-canned food—no matter how well preserved it is considered to be—should be boiled for at least 10 minutes before it is eaten. Within the United States, Alaska and Washington have the highest incidence of botulism, with Alaska having more cases as a result of native customs of eating uncooked or partially cooked meat that has been fermented, dried, or frozen.

Table 13-3 summarizes examples of common food contamination.

Viruses

Illnesses that are produced by the viral contamination of food are few compared with those produced by bacterial sources. These include upper respiratory infections (e.g., colds, influenza) and viral infectious hepatitis. Explosive epidemics of infectious hepatitis have occurred in schools, towns, and other communities after the fecal contamination of water, milk, or food. Contaminated shellfish from polluted waters have also caused several outbreaks. Again, the stringent control of community water and food

TABLE 13-3 EXAMPLES OF FOOD-BORNE DISEASE

Organism	Common Name of Illness	Onset Time After Ingesting	Signs and Symptoms	Duration	Food Sources
Bacillus cereus	*B. cereus* food poisoning	10 to 16 hours	Abdominal cramps, watery diarrhea, nausea	24 to 48 hours	Meats, stews, gravies, vanilla sauce
Campylobacter jejuni	Campylobacteriosis	2 to 5 days	Diarrhea, cramps, fever, and vomiting; diarrhea may be bloody	2 to 10 days	Raw and undercooked poultry, unpasteurized milk, contaminated water
Clostridium botulinum	Botulism	12 to 72 hours	Vomiting, diarrhea, blurred vision, double vision, difficulty swallowing, muscle weakness; can result in respiratory failure and death	Variable	Improperly canned foods, especially home-canned vegetables; fermented fish, baked potatoes in aluminum foil, bottled garlic
Cryptosporidium	Intestinal cryptosporidiosis	2 to 10 days	Diarrhea (usually watery), stomach cramps, upset stomach, slight fever	May be remitting and relapsing over weeks to months	Uncooked food or food contaminated by an ill food handler after cooking, contaminated drinking water
Cyclospora cayetanensis	Cyclosporiasis	1 to 14 days, usually at least 1 week	Diarrhea (usually watery), loss of appetite, substantial loss of weight, stomach cramps, nausea, vomiting, fatigue	May be remitting and relapsing over weeks to months	Various types of fresh produce (imported berries, lettuce, basil)
Escherichia coli producing toxin	*E. coli* infection	1 to 3 days	Watery diarrhea, abdominal cramps, some vomiting	3 to 7 or more days	Water or food contaminated with human feces
Escherichia coli O157:H7	Hemorrhagic colitis or *E. coli* O157:H7 infection	1 to 8 days	Severe (often bloody) diarrhea, abdominal pain and vomiting; usually little or no fever is present; more common among children 4 years old or younger; can lead to kidney failure	5 to 10 days	Undercooked beef (especially hamburger), unpasteurized milk and juice, raw fruits and vegetables (e.g., sprouts), contaminated water
Hepatitis A	Hepatitis	28 days average (15 to 50 days)	Diarrhea, dark urine, jaundice, flu-like symptoms (i.e., fever, headache, nausea, abdominal pain)	Variable, usually 2 weeks to 3 months	Raw produce, contaminated drinking water, uncooked foods and cooked foods that are not reheated after contact with an infected food handler, shellfish from contaminated waters

Organism	Common Name of Illness	Onset Time After Ingesting	Signs and Symptoms	Duration	Food Sources
Listeria monocytogenes	Listeriosis	9 to 48 hours for gastrointestinal symptoms, 2 to 6 weeks for invasive disease	Fever, muscle aches, and nausea or diarrhea; pregnant women may have a mild flu-like illness, and infection can lead to premature delivery or stillbirth; elderly or immunocompromised patients may develop bacteremia or meningitis	Variable	Unpasteurized milk, soft cheeses made with unpasteurized milk, ready-to-eat deli meats
Noroviruses	Variously called viral gastroenteritis, winter diarrhea, acute nonbacterial gastroenteritis, food poisoning, and food infection	12 to 48 hours	Nausea, vomiting, abdominal cramping, diarrhea, fever, headache; diarrhea is more prevalent among adults, vomiting is more common among children	12 to 60 hours	Raw produce, contaminated drinking water, uncooked foods and cooked foods that are not reheated after contact with an infected food handler, shellfish from contaminated waters
Salmonella	Salmonellosis	6 to 48 hours	Diarrhea, fever, abdominal cramps, vomiting	4 to 7 days	Eggs, poultry, meat, unpasteurized milk or juice, cheese, contaminated raw fruits and vegetables
Shigella	Shigellosis or bacillary dysentery	4 to 7 days	Abdominal cramps, fever, diarrhea; stools may contain blood and mucus	24 to 48 hours	Raw produce, contaminated drinking water, uncooked foods and cooked foods that are not reheated after contact with an infected food handler
Staphylococcus aureus	Staphylococcal food poisoning	1 to 6 hours	Sudden onset of severe nausea and vomiting, abdominal cramps; diarrhea and fever may be present	24 to 48 hours	Unrefrigerated or improperly refrigerated meats, potato, and egg salads; cream pastries
Vibrio parahaemolyticus	V. parahaemolyticus infection	4 to 96 hours	Watery (occasionally bloody) diarrhea, abdominal cramps, nausea, vomiting, fever	2 to 5 days	Undercooked or raw seafood, such as shellfish
Vibrio vulnificus	V. vulnificus infection	1 to 7 days	Vomiting, diarrhea, abdominal pain, blood-borne infection, fever, bleeding within the skin, ulcers that require surgical removal; can be fatal to persons with liver disease or weakened immune systems	2 to 8 days	Undercooked or raw seafood, such as shellfish (especially oysters)

Reprinted from the U.S. Department of Health and Human Services and the U.S. Food and Drug Administration. *What you need to know about foodborne illness-causing organisms in the U.S.* (website): www.fda.gov/Food/ResourcesForYou/Consumers/ucm103263.htm. Accessed December 2010.

supplies as well as the personal hygiene and sanitary practices of food handlers are essential for the prevention of disease.

Parasites

The following two types of worms are of serious concern in relation to food: (1) roundworms, such as the *trichina (Trichinella spiralis)* worm found in pork; and (2) flatworms, such as the common tapeworms found in beef and pork. The following control measures are essential: (1) laws controlling hog and cattle food sources and pastures to prevent the transmission of the parasites to the meat produced for market; and (2) the avoidance of rare beef and undercooked pork as an added personal precaution.

Environmental Food Contaminants

Lead. Heavy metals such as lead may contaminate food and water as well as the air and environmental objects. Although lead poisoning in the United States has dramatically declined since the removal of lead from gasoline, it continues to plague certain subgroups of the population (see the Cultural Considerations box, "The Continued Burden of Lead Poisoning"). The average blood lead level among children between the ages of 1 and 5 years in the United States is 1.5 µg/dL.[20] Children are especially vulnerable to lead poisoning, particularly those of poor families who live in older homes or impoverished areas with peeling lead paint.[21] Eliminating high blood lead levels in children, which are defined as those of 10 µg/dL or greater, is one of the *Healthy People 2020* goals.[20]

Of all sources of lead, lead paint (which was banned in the United States in 1978) is the most problematic source of contamination for children. An estimated 37.1 million homes in the United States have lead in their paint surfaces.[22] Children who live in these homes face lead exposure as a result of breathing airborne particles of paint dust created by disturbed or deteriorating walls or by abrasive paint removal before remodeling. The amount of lead-containing dust on the floor of a home is significantly associated with the blood lead level in children.[21] Drinking water may be an important source of lead in high-risk households with water that comes through lead service pipes or plumbing joints that have been sealed with lead solder. Current Environmental Protection Agency rules for public drinking water, however, have lowered the controlled lead exposure levels even further. Children with elevated blood lead levels have lower intellectual performance compared with similar children who do not suffer from lead toxicity.[23] Studies have also found this same high-risk population group to be deficient in

iron; this condition can increase lead absorption four- to five-fold, it has a similar deleterious effect on neurology, and it can thus further complicate lead toxicity.[24]

Natural Toxins. Toxins that are produced by plants or microorganisms also contaminate the food and water supply. Mercury, which is found naturally in the environment in addition to being a by-product of human production, is converted to methyl mercury by bacteria. Methyl mercury is a toxin that contaminates large bodies of water and the fish within that water. This contamination can pass through the food chain to people who regularly consume large fatty fish. Aflatoxin, which is another natural toxin, is produced by fungi. It may contaminate foods such as peanuts, tree nuts, corn, and animal feed.

Other food contaminants and pollutants that may pose a risk to human health come from a variety of sources (e.g., factories, sewage, fertilizers) but end up leaching out into the ground, thereby contaminating food production areas and the water supply.

FOOD NEEDS AND COSTS

Hunger and Malnutrition

Worldwide Malnutrition

Hunger and even famine and death exist in many countries of the world today. Lack of sanitation, cultural inequality, overpopulation, and economic and political structures that do not appropriately use resources are all factors that may contribute to malnutrition. Chronic food or nutrient shortages within a population perpetuate the cycle of malnutrition, in which undernourished pregnant women give birth to low birth weight infants. These infants are then more susceptible to infant death or growth retardation during childhood. When high nutrient needs throughout childhood and adolescence are not met, the incidence of malnourished or growth-stunted adults with shorter life expectancies and reduced work capacities continues to rise. Figure 13-10 illustrates the two drastically different outcomes that occur depending

---

hepatitis the inflammation of the liver cells; symptoms of acute hepatitis (i.e., of less than 6 months' duration) include flu-like symptoms, muscle and joint aches, fever, feeling sick or vomiting, diarrhea, headache, dark urine, and yellowing of the eyes and skin; symptoms of chronic hepatitis (i.e., of more than 6 months' duration) include jaundice, abdominal swelling and sensitivity, low-grade fever, and fluid retention (i.e., ascites).

CULTURAL CONSIDERATIONS

THE CONTINUED BURDEN OF LEAD POISONING

Exposure to lead continues to be a problem in the United States. One of the *Healthy People 2020* goals is to eliminate blood lead levels (BLLs) of 10 µg/dL or greater in children. Although BLLs are declining, much work still needs to be done to reach the 2020 goal.

Among all age groups, children between the ages of 1 and 5 years have the highest risk for elevated BLLs. Among ethnic groups, non-Hispanic blacks have the highest occurrence rates. Following are the percentages of children between the ages of 1 and 5 years with elevated BLLs of 10 µg/dL or more[1]:

- All children between the ages of 1 and 5 years: 1.4%
- Non-Hispanic black children: 3.4%
- Mexican-American children: 1.2%
- Non-Hispanic white children: 1.2%

The accumulation of lead in the blood results in oxidative stress and interferes with the normal physiologic functions of calcium, zinc, and iron. Prolonged elevated lead in the body can cause anemia, kidney damage, seizures, encephalopathy, and eventually paralysis.[2]

The Centers for Disease Control and Prevention set the critical blood lead level for children at 10 µg/dL; however, there is evidence that neurologic damage may occur at lower levels of approximately 7.2 µg/dL.[3]

The figure here depicts the BLLs of children by ethnicity for the last three survey periods. Note the successful decrease in severely affected children over time and the disparity of minority groups with elevated blood lead levels.

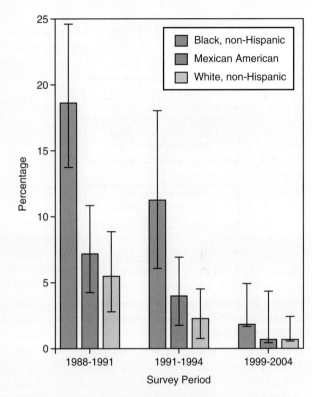

Percentage of children between the ages of 1 and 5 years with blood lead levels of 10 µg/dL or more by race or ethnicity and survey period according to the National Health and Nutrition Examination Surveys that took place in the United States from 1988 to 1991, 1991 to 1994, and 1999 to 2004. 95% confidence interval. (Data from Jones RL, Homa DM, Meyer PA, et al. Trends in blood lead levels and blood lead testing among US children aged 1 to 5 years, 1988-2004. *Pediatrics* 2009;123(3):e376-e385.)

1. Jones RL, Homa DM, Meyer PA, et al. Trends in blood lead levels and blood lead testing among US children aged 1 to 5 years, 1988-2004. *Pediatrics.* 2009;123(3):e376-e385.
2. Centers for Disease Control and Prevention and National Center for Environmental Health. *Fourth National Report on Human Exposure to Environmental Chemicals.* Centers for Disease Control and Prevention: Atlanta; 2009.
3. Jusko TA, Henderson CR, Lanphear BP, et al. Blood lead concentrations < 10 microg/dL and child intelligence at 6 years of age. *Environ Health Perspect.* 2008;116(2):243-248.

on whether a child has access to education, financial needs, and health care. Malnutrition may result from total kilocalorie deficiency or single-nutrient deficiencies. The most common deficiencies in the world today are iron-deficiency anemia, protein-energy malnutrition, vitamin-A deficiency, and iodine deficiency. Figure 13-11 shows the complicated interaction of the many factors that lead to malnutrition.

The United Nations Committee on World Food Security was formed to address the 842 million people worldwide who do not have enough food to meet their basic nutritional requirements. The long-term goals of this committee are to eliminate world hunger and to reduce the number of undernourished people by half by 2015.[25] The plan is composed of several commitments that are focused on stabilizing the social, economic, and

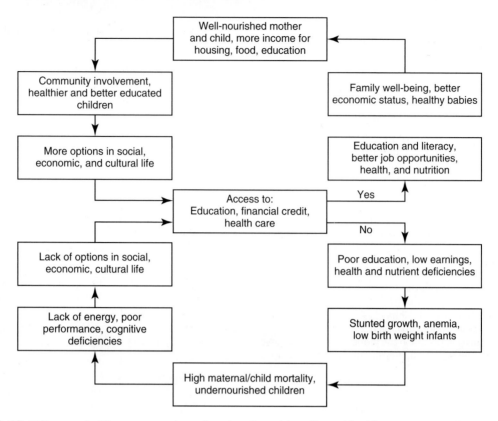

Figure 13-10 Differences in life outcomes when education, financial credit, and health care are accessible. (Adapted from Struble MB, Aomari LL. Position of the American Dietetic Association: addressing world hunger, malnutrition, and food insecurity. *J Am Diet Assoc.* 2003;103(8):1046-1057.)

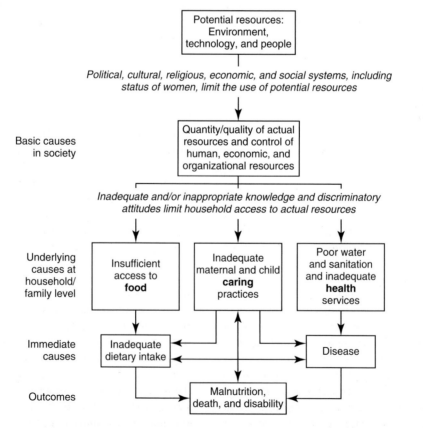

Figure 13-11 Multiple causes of malnutrition. (Adapted from Struble MB, Aomari LL. Position of the American Dietetic Association: addressing world hunger, malnutrition, and food insecurity. *J Am Diet Assoc.* 2003;103(8):1046-1057.)

environmental production and distribution of nutritionally adequate food. The committee is responsible for monitoring, evaluating, and consulting on the international food security situation with follow-up reports. Information and updates about the progress of this committee can be found at www.fao.org/monitoringprogress/index_en.html.

Malnutrition in America

Hunger does not stop at the U.S. border. In the United States, which is one of the wealthiest countries on earth, hunger and malnutrition among the poor persist. More than 49.1 million individuals (i.e., 17.1 million households) in the United States have food insecurity, which is defined as "limited or uncertain availability of nutritionally adequate and safe foods or limited or uncertain ability to acquire acceptable foods in socially acceptable ways."[26] Individuals who are at the highest risk for food insecurity within the United States are individuals who live below the income-to-poverty ratio, households with children that are headed by a single woman, African Americans, Hispanics, and households in central city areas.[26] At both the government and personal levels of any society, food availability and use involve money and politics. Various factors are implicated, such as land management practices, water distribution, food production and distribution policies, and food assistance programs for individuals and families in need.

Food Assistance Programs

In situations of economic stress and natural disasters, individuals and families require financial help. Many people in the United States experience hunger every day. Dietitians, nurses, and other health care providers may need to discuss available food assistance programs and make appropriate referrals.

Commodity Supplemental Food Program

Under the Commodity Supplemental Food Program (CSFP), the USDA purchases food items that are good sources of nutrients but that are often lacking in the diets of the target population (i.e., low-income pregnant and breast-feeding women, other new mothers up to 1 year postpartum, infants, children who are younger than 5 years old, and older people who are at least 60 years old). The USDA then distributes the food to state agencies and tribal organizations. From there, the food is dispersed to local agencies for public allocation. Local agencies (e.g., departments of health, social services, education, or agriculture) are responsible for evaluating eligibility, providing nutrition education, and dispersing food. This

program is not currently available in every state. The most recent report noted that an average of 467,000 people participate in the CSFP services each month.[27] Information about CSFP can be found at www.fns.usda.gov/fdd/programs/csfp/.

Supplemental Nutrition Assistance Program (SNAP)

SNAP, which was formerly known as the food stamp program, began during the late depression years of the 1930s and was expanded during the 1960s and 1970s. This program has helped many poor people to purchase needed food; the majority of the individuals that are served are children and elderly adults. The USDA estimated that 40.3 million people participated in SNAP services in the United States each month during 2010 at an annual cost of $64.7 trillion.[28] With this program, electronic benefits transfer cards are issued to the primary care provider of the household. These cards are used in a way that is similar to a debit card in approved retail stores to supplement the household's food needs for 1 month. Households must have a monthly income that is below the program's eligible poverty limit to qualify. SNAP is in operation in all 50 states, the District of Columbia, Guam, and the U.S. Virgin Islands, and it is administered at the local level. More information about this program can be found at the USDA's Food and Nutrition Service Web site at www.fns.usda.gov/snap.

Special Supplemental Food Program for Women, Infants, and Children

The Special Supplemental Food Program for Women, Infants, and Children (WIC) provides nutrition supplementation, education, and counseling in addition to referrals for health care and social services to women who are pregnant, postpartum, or breast-feeding and to their infants and children who are younger than 5 years old. WIC has established criteria for participation, and each applicant must be income eligible and determined to be at nutritional risk. The food packages provided through WIC meet the *Dietary Guidelines for Americans* and promote the consumption of fruits, vegetables, and whole grains. The average monthly food cost per participant as reported for fiscal year 2010 was $41.55.[29] Participants are provided with vouchers that are exchanged for foods such as milk, eggs, cheese, juice, fortified cereals, fruits, and vegetables at participating retailers. These foods supplement the diet with rich sources of protein, iron, and certain vitamins to help reduce risk factors such as poor growth patterns, low birth weight, prematurity, preeclampsia, miscarriage, and anemia.

WIC was established in 1972, and it currently has more than 9 million participants. WIC offices are established in every state, the District of Columbia, Guam, Puerto Rico, American Samoa, and the U.S. Virgin Islands. Approximately half of all participants are children between the ages of 1 and 5 years, and non-Hispanic Caucasians make up the largest race and ethnic percentage of those served.[30] More information can be found at www.fns.usda.gov/wic/default.htm.

School Meals Programs

There are several programs available to assist low-income children with receiving healthy food while at school. Current programs in the United States include the National School Lunch, Fresh Fruit and Vegetable, School Breakfast, and Special Milk programs. The National School Lunch program includes subprograms for low-income children that provide nutritionally balanced meals and snacks after school and during the summer months, when school is not in session. The USDA offsets the costs of the program by donating large quantities of a variety of foods to public schools. Children eat for free or at reduced rates, and these meals often comprise their main food intake for the day. The meals provided must fulfill approximately one third of a child's Recommended Dietary Allowance for protein, vitamin A, vitamin C, iron, calcium, and calories, and it must meet the *Dietary Guidelines for Americans,* which call for diets that are lower in total fat and that contain more fruits, vegetables, and whole grains.[31] The Special Milk Program provides milk to children who do not have access to the other meal programs. More information about School Meals programs can be found at www.fns.usda.gov/cnd.

Nutrition Services Incentive Program

The Nutrition Services Incentive Program, which was formerly known as the Nutrition Program for the Elderly, is operated through the U.S. Department of Health and Human Services Administration on Aging.

This program provides cash or commodities from the USDA for the delivery of nutritious meals to the elderly. Regardless of income, all people who are older than 60 years old can eat hot lunches at a community center under the Congregate Meals Program; if they are ill or disabled, they can receive meals at home by using the services of the Home-Delivered Meals Program. The act specifies that economically and socially needy people be given priority. Both programs accept voluntary contributions for meals. More information can be found at www.fns.usda.gov/fdd/programs/nsip.

Food Buying and Handling Practices

For many American families, the problem is spending their limited food dollars wisely. Even on a low-cost plan for food purchasing, an average family of four can expect to spend approximately $645 to $758 per month on food alone.[32] Shopping for food can be complicated, especially when each item in a supermarket's overabundant supply shouts, "Buy me!" Food marketing is big business, and producers compete for prize placement and shelf space. A large supermarket stocks many thousands of different food items. A single food item may be marketed a dozen different ways at as many different prices. In diet counseling, clients and families typically express their greatest need as help with buying food. The following wise shopping and handling practices help with the provision of healthy foods as well as with controlling food costs.

Planning Ahead

Use sales circulars in newspapers, plan general menus, and keep a checklist of basic pantry supplies. Make a list ahead of time according to the location of items in a regularly used grocery store. Such planning controls impulse buying and reduces extra trips.

Buying Wisely

Understanding packaging, carefully reading labels, and watching for sale items helps to improve purchasing power. Only buy in quantity if it results in real savings and if the food can be adequately stored or used. Be cautious when selecting so-called "convenience foods"; the time saved may not be worth the added cost. For fresh foods, try alternative food sources such as farmers' markets, consumer cooperatives, and gardens.

Storing Food Safely

Control food waste and prevent illness caused by food spoilage or contamination. Conserve food by storing items in accordance with their nature and use. Use dry storage, covered containers, and correct-temperature refrigeration as needed. Keep opened and partly used food items at the front of the shelf for timely use. Avoid waste by preparing only the amount needed. Use leftovers in creative ways.

Cooking Food Well

Use cooking processes that retain maximal food value and that maintain food safety. Cooking vegetables for shorter periods (e.g., stir frying, steaming) and with as little water as possible helps to retain their vitamin and mineral nutritive quality. Prepare food with imagination and good sense. Give zest and appeal to dishes with a variety of seasonings, combinations, and serving arrangements. No matter how much they know about nutrition and health, people usually eat because they are hungry and because the food looks and tastes good, not necessarily because it is healthy.

SUMMARY

- Common public concerns about the safety of the community food supply center on the use of chemicals such as pesticides and food additives. These substances have produced an abundant food supply, but they have also raised concerns, and they require close monitoring.
- The FDA is the main government agency that was established to maintain the control of the food supply. It conducts activities related to areas such as food safety, food labeling, food standards, consumer education, and research.
- Numerous organisms such as bacteria, viruses, and parasites that can contaminate food may cause food-borne disease. Rigorous public health measures control the sanitation of food handling areas and the personal hygiene of food handlers. The same standards should apply to home food handling preparation and storage.
- Families that are under economic stress may benefit from counseling about financial assistance. Various U.S. food assistance programs help families in need, and referrals can be made to appropriate agencies. Families may also need assistance with the buying and use of food.

CRITICAL THINKING QUESTIONS

1. What is the basis of concern about food additives and pesticide residues?
2. What are some ways that agriculture is changing to reduce the use of pesticides and their danger to workers as well as to protect the land?
3. Describe the ways that various organisms may contaminate food. What standards of food preparation and handling should be used to keep food safe?
4. Kaycee is a single mother with two children. She is working part time making minimum wage. During the school year, her children receive free breakfasts and lunches at school. However, she is concerned for her children's nutritional well-being during the summer months. For what assistance may Kaycee and her children qualify? What suggestions would you make to help establish a well-balanced diet for this family?
5. According to the food buying and handling practices described in this chapter, evaluate your own habits. Describe potential hazardous points for food-borne illness contamination, and discuss ways to improve your food-buying practices.

CHAPTER CHALLENGE QUESTIONS

True-False

Write the correct statement for each statement that is false.

1. *True or False:* U.S. surveys reveal little or no real malnutrition in the population.
2. *True or False:* The politics of a region or country is not involved in the nutritional status of the people.
3. *True or False:* The number of new processed food items that use food additives has declined in recent years because of public pressure and concern.
4. *True or False:* The use of pesticides on farm crops and food additives in processed foods is controlled by the USDA and the FDA.
5. *True or False:* Food poisoning is always caused by the viral contamination of food.
6. *True or False:* The Commodity Supplemental Food Program buys agricultural food surpluses to support market prices of food and then distributes these goods to needy people.
7. *True or False:* The Nutrition Services Incentive Program provides group meals for all people who are older than 60 years old, regardless of their income.

Multiple Choice

1. Food additives are used in processed food items to do which of the following? *(Circle all that apply.)*
   a. To preserve food and lengthen its market life
   b. To enrich food with added nutrients
   c. To improve flavor, texture, and appearance
   d. To enhance or improve some physical property of the food

2. The use of food additives in food products is controlled by the
   a. U.S. Public Health Service.
   b. USDA.
   c. FDA.
   d. Federal Trade Commission.

3. The National School Lunch program provides free or reduced-price lunches to children in need that provide approximately one third of a child's Recommended Dietary Allowance for protein, vitamin A, vitamin C, iron, calcium, and calories and meet the
   a. MyPlate.gov guidelines.
   b. *Dietary Guidelines for Americans.*
   c. Academy of Nutrition and Dietetics guidelines.
   d. American Diabetic Association guidelines.

⊖volve Please refer to the Students' Resource section of this text's Evolve Web site for additional study resources.

REFERENCES

1. Philipson T. Government perspective: food labeling. *Am J Clin Nutr.* 2005;82(1 Suppl):262S-264S.
2. U.S. Department of Health and Human Services. *How to understand and use the nutrition facts label* (Website): www.fda.gov/Food/ResourcesForYou/Consumers/NFLPM/ucm274593.htm. Accessed December 2010.
3. Office of Nutrition, Labeling, and Dietary Supplements; Center For Food Safety and Applied Nutrition. *Food labeling guide.* College Park, Md: U.S. Food and Drug Administration; 2008.
4. U.S. Department of Agriculture. *National organic program* (Website): http://www.ams.usda.gov/AMSv1.0/ams.fetchTemplateData.do?template=TemplateA&navID=NationalOrganicProgram&leftNav=NationalOrganicProgram&page=NOPNationalOrganicProgramHome&acct=AMSPW. Accessed December 2010.
5. Søltoft M, Nielsen J, Holst Laursen K, et al. Effects of organic and conventional growth systems on the content of flavonoids in onions and phenolic acids in carrots and potatoes. *J Agric Food Chem.* 2010;58(19):10323-10329.
6. U.S. Department of Agriculture, Economic Research Service. *Adoption of genetically engineered crops in the U.S..* Washington, DC: U.S. Department of Agriculture; 2010.
7. Bruhn C, Earl R. Position of the American Dietetic Association: agricultural and food biotechnology. *J Am Diet Assoc.* 2006;106(2):285-293.
8. Hoff M, Son DY, Gubesch M, et al. Serum testing of genetically modified soybeans with special emphasis on potential allergenicity of the heterologous protein CP4 EPSPS. *Mol Nutr Food Res.* 2007;51(8):946-955.
9. Centers For Disease Control and Prevention; National Center For Zoonotic, Vector-Borne, and Enteric Diseases. *Irradiation of food* (Website): www.cdc.gov/nczved/divisions/dfbmd/diseases/irradiation_food/. Accessed October 17, 2011.
10. Fan X, Kays SE. Formation of trans fatty acids in ground beef and frankfurters due to irradiation. *J Food Sci.* 2009;74(2):C79-C84.
11. Centers For Disease Control and Prevention. Preliminary foodnet data on the incidence of infection with pathogens transmitted commonly through food–10 states, 2008. *MMWR Morb Mortal Wkly Rep.* 2009;58(13):333-337.
12. Food Safety Inspection Service, U.S. Department of Agriculture. *Basics for handling food safely* (Website): www.fsis.usda.gov/fact_sheets/basics_for_handling_food_safely/index.asp. Accessed December 2010.
13. Centers For Disease Control and Prevention; National Center For Zoonotic, Vector-Borne, and Enteric Diseases. *Salmonellosis* (Website): www.cdc.gov/nczved/divisions/dfbmd/diseases/salmonellosis/. Accessed December 2010.
14. Centers For Disease Control and Prevention; National Center For Zoonotic, Vector-Borne, and Enteric Diseases. *Shigellosis* (Website): www.cdc.gov/nczved/divisions/dfbmd/diseases/shigellosis/. Accessed December 2010.
15. Centers For Disease Control and Prevention; National Center For Zoonotic, Vector-Borne, and Enteric Diseases. *Listeriosis* (Website): www.cdc.gov/listeria/index.html. Accessed December 2010.
16. Centers For Disease Control and Prevention; National Center For Zoonotic, Vector-Borne, and Enteric Diseases. *Escherichia Coli O157:H7* (Website): www.cdc.gov/nczved/divisions/dfbmd/diseases/ecoli_o157h7/. Accessed December 2010.
17. Centers For Disease Control and Prevention. *Incidence of foodborne illness* (Website): www.cdc.gov/features/dsfoodborneillness. Accessed December 2010.
18. Centers For Disease Control and Prevention; National Center For Zoonotic, Vector-Borne, and Enteric Diseases. *Staphylococcal food poisoning* (Website): www.cdc.gov/nczved/divisions/dfbmd/diseases/staphylococcal/. Accessed December 2010.
19. Centers For Disease Control and Prevention; National Center For Zoonotic, Vector-Borne, and Enteric Diseases. *Botulism* (Website): www.cdc.gov/nczved/divisions/dfbmd/diseases/botulism/. Accessed December 2010.
20. U.S. Department of Health and Human Services. *Healthy people 2020.* Washington, DC: U.S. Government Printing Office; 2010.

21. Dixon SL, Gaitens JM, Jacobs DE, et al. Exposure of U.S. children to residential dust lead, 1999-2004: ii. the contribution of lead-contaminated dust to children's blood lead levels. *Environ Health Perspect*. 2009;117(3): 468-474.

22. Stout II DM, Bradham KD, Egeghy PP, et al. American Healthy Homes Survey: a national study of residential pesticides measured from floor wipes. *Environ Sci Technol*. 2009;43(12):4294-4300.

23. Jusko TA, Henderson TA, Lanphear BP, et al. Blood lead concentrations < 10 microg/dl and child intelligence at 6 years of age. *Environ Health Perspect*. 2008;116(2): 243-248.

24. Wright RO, Tsaih SW, Schwartz J, et al. Association between iron deficiency and blood lead level in a longitudinal analysis of children followed in an urban primary care clinic. *J Pediatr*. 2003;142(1):9-14.

25. Skoet J, Stamoulis K. *The state of food insecurity in the world: 2006*. Rome: Food and Agriculture Organization of The United Nations; 2006.

26. Holben DH. Position of the American Dietetic Association: food insecurity in the United States. *J Am Diet Assoc*. 2010; 110(9):1368-1377.

27. U.S. Department of Agriculture Food and Nutrition Service. *Commodity supplemental food program* (Website): www.fns.usda.gov/fdd/programs/csfp/pfs-csfp.pdf. Accessed December 2010.

28. U.S. Department of Agriculture Food and Nutrition Service. *Program data: supplemental nutrition assistance program* (Website): www.fns.usda.gov/pd/snapmain.htm. Accessed December 2010.

29. U.S. Department of Agriculture Food and Nutrition Service. *Program data: WIC program* (Website): www.fns.usda.gov/pd/wicmain.htm. Accessed December 2010.

30. Connor P, Bartlett S, Mendelson M, et al. *WIC participant and program characteristics 2008*. Alexandria, Va: U.S. Department of Agriculture; 2010.

31. U.S. Department of Agriculture, U.S. Department of Health and Human Services. *Dietary guidelines for americans, 2010*. Washington, DC: U.S. Government Printing Office; 2010.

32. Center For Nutrition Policy and Promotion, U.S. Department of Agriculture. *Official USDA food plans: cost of food at home at four levels, U.S. average,* October 2010. Alexandria, Va: U.S. Department of Agriculture; 2010.

FURTHER READING AND RESOURCES

Explore these Web sites for current information and regulations regarding food safety, food-borne illness, and food labeling standards.

Centers for Disease Control and Prevention. Foodborne illness in the United States: www.cdc.gov/foodborneburden/

U.S. Department of Agriculture: Agricultural Marketing Service, The National Organic Program. www.ams.usda.gov/AMSv1.0/nop

U.S. Department of Agriculture. Food and nutrition services: nutrition assistance programs: www.fns.usda.gov

U.S. Food and Drug Administration: Food labeling and nutrition. www.fda.gov/Food/LabelingNutrition/default.htm

U.S. Food and Drug Administration: Food safety. www.fda.gov/food/foodsafety/default.htm

U.S. Department of Agriculture. Food Safety and Inspection Service food safety publications: www.fsis.usda.gov/fact_sheets/index.asp

U.S. Department of Agriculture: National Institute of Food and Agriculture. www.csrees.usda.gov

United States Regulatory Agencies Unified Biotechnology Web site. usbiotechreg.nbii.gov/

Holben DH. Position of the American Dietetic Association: food insecurity in the United States. *J Am Diet Assoc*. 2010;110(9):1368-1377.
The Academy of Nutrition and Dietetics (formerly known as the American Dietetic Association) addresses the issues of food insecurity and malnutrition in the United States and the interventions that are needed to eliminate such disparity. The role of the dietitian in such programs is also discussed.

CHAPTER 14

Food Habits and Cultural Patterns

Why do people eat what they eat? Food is necessary to sustain life and health, but people eat certain foods for many reasons other than good health and nutrition, although these are important factors. As stated in Chapter 13, the broader food environment from which we have to choose is often influenced by factors such as politics and poverty, which limit personal control and choice.

A variety of connotations are attached to food. All food habits are intimately related to people's entire way of life: their values, beliefs, and situations. However, sometimes these food patterns change over time with more exposure to other cultural patterns.

SOCIAL, PSYCHOLOGIC, AND ECONOMIC INFLUENCES ON FOOD HABITS

Social Influences

Social Structure

Human group behavior reveals many activities, processes, and structures that comprise social life. In any society, social groups are largely formed by factors such as economic status, education, residence, occupation, and family. Values and habits differ among groups. Subgroups also develop on the basis of region, religion, age, gender, social class, health issues, special interests, ethnic backgrounds, politics, and other common concerns such as group affiliations.

Food and Social Factors

Food is a symbol of acceptance, warmth, and friendliness in social relationships. People tend to accept food or food advice readily from friends, acquaintances, and people that they view as trusted authorities. These influences are especially strong in family relationships. Food habits that are closely associated with family sentiments stay with people throughout their lives. During adulthood, certain foods may trigger a flood of childhood memories and are valued for reasons apart from any nutritional importance.

Psychologic Influences

Understanding Diet Patterns

Understanding dietary patterns begins with the recognition of the psychologic influences that are involved. Food is a basic enjoyment—and necessity—of life. Social relationships may affect individual behavior as it relates to dietary patterns. Many of these psychologic factors are rooted in childhood experiences. For example, when a child is hurt or disappointed, parents may offer a cookie or a piece of candy to distract the child. Then, when adults feel hurt, they turn to similar sweets to help them feel good again. Certain foods, especially sweets and other pleasurable tastes, stimulate "feel good" body chemicals in the brain called *endorphins* that give a mild "high" that may help ease pain.

Food and Psychosocial Development

From infancy to old age, emotional maturity grows along with physical development. At each stage of human growth, food habits are part of both physical and psychosocial development. For example, a 2-year-old toddler who is taking his first steps toward eventual independence from his parents may learn to control his parents through food by becoming a picky eater or by refusing to eat at mealtimes. Psychologists believe that another normal developmental factor is involved; this is called *food neophobia*, which is the fear of unfamiliar foods. This universal trait may be an instinct from the evolutionary past that protected children from eating harmful foods when they were just becoming independent from their mothers.

Marketing and Environmental Influences

Food habits are also manipulated by television, radio, magazines, and other media messages. Influences from peers, convenience items, marketing at the local grocery store, and many other factors of persuasion may dictate the decision-making process for food choices throughout life. Advertising strategies that make use of cartoon characters on food packages that are marketed toward children negatively influence children's eating patterns by increasing the intake of high-energy, nutrient-poor "junk foods."[1] A recent study that compared the nutritional quality of the food endorsed on American television with that of nutrition guidelines found a drastic imbalance in advertising for the very food components that the dietary guidelines warn against overconsumption of (i.e., saturated fat, cholesterol, and sodium).[2]

Marketing trends and media also share a strong influence with regard to what a culture views as beautiful. In the United States, a very thin figure is heavily valued, and such influences may sway food choices.

Economic Influences

Family Income and Food Habits

Many American families live under socioeconomic pressures, especially during periods of recession and inflation. The problems of middle-income families differ in relative terms, but low-income families—especially those in poverty situations—suffer extreme needs. These families may lack adequate housing and have little or no access to educational opportunities. As a result, they are poorly prepared for jobs and often only make a day-to-day living at low-paying work, or they may be unemployed. Approximately 14.3% of Americans live with an income that is below the federal poverty level, with the highest burden on African-American and Hispanic families.[3]

The cost of a healthy diet composed of whole grains, lean meats, fruits, vegetables, and low-fat dairy is difficult to achieve for some families that are living at or below the federal poverty line. Thus, it is not surprising that people with low incomes bear the greater burden of unnecessary illness and malnutrition. Some organizations have suggested an additional taxation of selected foods with little or no nutritional quality in an attempt to subsidize healthy choices such as fruits and vegetables.[4]

CULTURAL DEVELOPMENT OF FOOD HABITS

Food habits, like any other form of human behavior, do not develop in a vacuum. They grow from many personal, cultural, social, economic, and psychologic influences. For each person, these factors are interwoven.

Strength of Personal Culture

Culture involves much more than the major and historic aspects of a person's communal life (e.g., language, religion, politics, technology); it also develops from all of the habits of everyday living and family relationships, such as preparing and serving food. In a gradual process of conscious and unconscious learning, cultural values, attitudes, habits, and practices become a deep part of individual lives. Although part of this heritage may be revised or rejected as adults, people are ultimately responsible for shaping their own lives and passing traditions on to the following generations. Americans have a broad range of food habits that have been influenced by a world of cultural diversity.

food neophobia the fear of new food.

Food in a Culture

Food habits are among the oldest and most deeply rooted aspects of many cultures. Food availability, economics, and personal food meanings and beliefs are the primary factors of influence. An individual's cultural background largely determines what is eaten as well as when and how it is eaten, but much variation exists. All types of customs, whether rational or irrational and beneficial or injurious, are found in every part of the world. Many foods take on symbolic meanings related to major life experiences (e.g., birth, death, religion, politics, general social organization). From ancient times, ceremonies and religious rites involving food have surrounded certain events and seasons. Food gathering, preparing, and serving have followed specific customs, many of which remain intact today.

Traditional Cultural Food Patterns

The United States has long been considered a "melting pot" of ethnic and racial groups. In more recent years, however, this image no longer seems appropriate. America's diversity has come to be recognized and even celebrated as a basis for its national strength. This recognition is particularly demonstrated by the diversity of America's cultural food patterns. Pockets of ethnic groups in which native lifestyles are somewhat retained are apparent in many American cities.

Many different cultural food patterns are part of American family and community life. These patterns have contributed special dishes or modes of cooking to American eating habits. In turn, many of these cultural food habits have been Americanized. Older members of the family use traditional foods more regularly, with younger members of the family using them mainly on special occasions or holidays. Nevertheless, traditional foods have strong meanings and bind families and cultural communities in close fellowship. A few representative cultural food patterns are briefly reviewed in this chapter. Individual tastes and geographic patterns may vary, but food patterns are connected with culture and have a strong influence on how people eat.

Religious Dietary Laws

The dietary practices within Christianity (e.g., Catholic, Protestant, and Eastern Orthodox churches), Judaism, Hinduism, Buddhism, and Islam fluctuate in accordance with each follower's independent understanding and interpretation of what constitutes a healthy and proper diet. Such dietary laws may apply to what, how, and when specific foods are allowed or avoided. Some dietary laws are applicable at all times (e.g., no pork at any time for Islamic followers), whereas other laws apply only during religious ceremonies (e.g., during Lent for Roman Catholics). Following are examples of two such religions and their dietary laws.

Jewish

Basic Food Pattern. All Jewish festivals are religious in nature and have historic significance, but the observance of Jewish food laws differs among the three basic groups within Judaism: (1) orthodox, with strict observance; (2) conservative, with less strict observance; and (3) reform, with less ceremonial emphasis and minimal general use. The basic body of dietary laws is called the *Rules of Kashrut.* Foods that are selected and prepared in accordance with these rules are called *kosher,* from the Hebrew word meaning "fit, proper." These laws originally had special ritual significance. Current Jewish dietary laws apply this significance to laws that govern the slaughter, preparation, and serving of meat; the combining of meat and milk; and the use of fish and eggs. The following are various Jewish food restrictions:

- *Meat:* Appropriate meats should come from animals that chew their cud and that have cloven hooves. Pork and birds of prey are avoided at all times. All forms of meat are rigidly cleansed of blood.
- *Meat and milk:* Meat and milk products are both part of the kosher Jewish diet; however, they are not to be eaten at the same meal or prepared with the use of the same dishes. Orthodox homes maintain two sets of regular dishes: one for serving meat and the other for meals that contain dairy products. An additional two sets of dishes are maintained especially for use during Passover.
- *Fish:* Only fish with fins and scales are allowed. These may be eaten with either meat or dairy meals. Shellfish and crustaceans are avoided.
- *Eggs:* No egg with a blood spot may be eaten. Eggs may be used with either meat or dairy meals.

Representative Foods and Influence of Festivals. Many traditional Jewish foods relate to festivals of the Jewish calendar that commemorate significant events in Jewish history. Special Sabbath foods are often used. A few representative foods, mostly of Eastern European influence, include the following:

- *Bagels:* doughnut-shaped hard yeast rolls
- *Blintzes:* thin, filled, rolled pancakes
- *Borscht (borsch):* a soup of meat stock, beaten egg or sour cream, beets, cabbage, or spinach that is served hot or cold
- *Challah:* a Sabbath loaf of white bread that is shaped as a twist or coil and that is used at the beginning

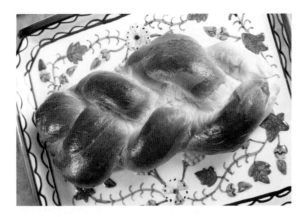

Figure 14-1 Challah, which is a traditional Jewish bread. (Copyright JupiterImages Corp.)

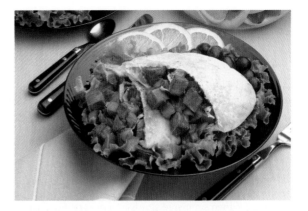

Figure 14-2 Traditional Muslim pita bread stuffed with sandwich fillings. (Copyright JupiterImages Corp.)

of the meal after the Kiddush, which is the blessing over the wine (Figure 14-1)

- *Gefüllte (gefilte) fish:* from a German word meaning "stuffed fish," this is usually the first course of the Sabbath evening meal; it is made of chopped and seasoned fish filets that are stuffed back into the skin or rolled into balls
- *Kasha:* buckwheat groats (hulled kernels) that are used as a cooked cereal or as a potato substitute with gravy
- *Knishes:* pastries that are filled with ground meat or cheese
- *Lox:* smoked and salted salmon
- *Matzo:* flat, unleavened bread
- *Strudel:* a thin pastry that is filled with fruit and nuts, rolled, and baked

Muslim

Basic Food Pattern. Muslim dietary laws are based on the restriction or prohibition of some foods and the promotion of others, and they are derived from the Islamic teachings found in the Koran. The laws are binding and must be followed at all times, even during pregnancy, hospitalization, and travel. These laws are also binding for visitors in the host Muslim country. Almost all foods are permitted unless specifically conditioned or prohibited as follows:

- *Milk products:* permitted at all times
- *Fruits and vegetables:* permitted except if fermented or poisonous
- *Breads and cereals:* permitted unless contaminated or harmful
- *Meats:* seafood (including fish, shellfish, eels, and sea animals) and land animals (except swine) are permitted; pork is strictly prohibited. Muslims typically eat kosher meats, because the blood of the

animal is not to be eaten. Halal meat is the equivalent of kosher meat.

- *Alcohol:* strictly prohibited

All food combinations are consumed as long as no prohibited items are included. Milk and meat may be eaten together, which is in contrast with Jewish kosher laws. The Koran mentions certain foods as being of special value, including figs, olives, dates, honey, milk, and buttermilk. Foods that are prohibited by the Muslim dietary laws may be eaten when no other sources of food are available.

Representative Foods. Following are a number of favorite foods and dishes that can be used as appetizers, main dishes, snacks, or salads:

- *Bulgur (or burghel):* partially cooked and dried cracked wheat that is available in a coarse grind as a base for pilaf or in a fine grind for use in tabouli and kibbeh
- *Falafel:* a "fast food" that is made from a seasoned paste of ground, soaked beans that is formed into shapes and fried
- *Fatayeh:* a snack or appetizer that is similar to a small pizza, with toppings of cheese, meat, or spinach
- *Kibbeh:* a meat dish that is made of cracked wheat shell filled with small pieces of lamb and fried in oil
- *Pilaf:* sautéed and seasoned bulgur or rice that is steamed in a bouillon, sometimes with poultry, meat, or shellfish
- *Pita:* a flat circular bread that is torn or cut into pieces and stuffed with sandwich fillings (Figure 14-2) or used as a scoop for a dip such as *hummus,* which is made from chickpeas
- *Tabouli:* a salad made from soaked bulgur that has been combined with chopped tomatoes, parsley,

CULTURAL CONSIDERATIONS

ID AL-FITR: THE POST-RAMADAN FESTIVAL

At the conclusion of Ramadan, Islam's holy month of prayer and fasting, wealthy merchants and princes in Muslim countries traditionally hold public feasts for the needy. This is known as the Festival of Id al-Fitr.

Over the years, many delicacies have been served to symbolize the joy of returning from fasting and the heightened sense of unity, brotherhood, and charity that the fasting experience has brought to the people. Among the foods served are chicken or veal sautéed with eggplant and onions and then simmered slowly in pomegranate juice and spiced with turmeric and cardamom seeds. The highlight of

the meal is usually *kharuf mahshi,* which is a whole lamb (i.e., a symbol of sacrifice) that is stuffed with a rich dressing made of dried fruits, cracked wheat, pine nuts, almonds, and onions and seasoned with ginger and coriander. The stuffed lamb is baked in hot ashes for many hours so that it is tender enough to be pulled apart and eaten with the fingers.

At the conclusion of the meal, rich pastries and candies are served; these may be flavored with spices or flower petals. Some of the sweets are taken home and savored for as long as possible as a reminder of the festival.

---

mint, and green onion and then mixed with olive oil and lemon juice

Influence of Festivals. The fourth pillar of Islam as commanded by the Koran is fasting. Among the Muslim people, a 30-day period of daylight fasting is required during Ramadan, which is the ninth month of the Islamic lunar calendar. Ramadan was chosen for the sacred fast because that was when Mohammed received the first of the revelations that were subsequently compiled to form the Koran, and it is also the month when Mohammed's followers first drove their enemies from Mecca in 624 AD. During the month of Ramadan, Muslims all over the world observe daily fasting by taking no food or drink from dawn until sunset. However, nights are often spent at special feasts. First, an appetizer such as dates or a fruit drink is served, and then followed by the family's "evening breakfast," which is called the *iftar*. At the end of Ramadan, a traditional feast that lasts up to 3 days concludes the observance. Special dishes that include delicacies such as thin pancakes dipped in powdered sugar, savory buns, and dried fruits mark this occasion (see the Cultural Considerations box, "Id al-Fitr: The Post-Ramadan Festival").

All Muslims, regardless of medical condition, observe the fast of Ramadan. Individuals with diabetes, who are on certain medications, or who are pregnant or breast-feeding may have complications during this time. Health care professionals must be sensitive to such religious practices when counseling patients.

Spanish and Native American Influences

Mexican

The food habits of the early Spanish settlers and Native American nations form the basis of the current food patterns among people of Mexican heritage who live in the

United States, chiefly in the South and Southwest. The following three foods are basic to this pattern: dried beans, chili peppers, and corn. Variations and additions may be found in different places or among those of different income levels. Relatively small amounts of meat are used, and eggs are occasionally eaten. Fruit (e.g., mango, papaya) is consumed in varying amounts, depending on availability and price. For centuries, corn has been the basic grain used for bread in the form of tortillas, which are flat cakes that are baked on a hot surface or griddle. Wheat is also used when making tortillas, and rice and oats are added cereals. Coffee is a popular beverage. Major seasonings are chili peppers, onions, and garlic; the basic fat is lard.

Puerto Rican

The Puerto Rican people share a common heritage with many Hispanic Caribbean countries, so many of their food patterns are similar[5] (Figure 14-3). However, Puerto Ricans add tropical fruits and vegetables, many of which are available in their neighborhood markets in the United States. *Viandas,* which are starchy vegetables and fruits such as plantains and green bananas, are popular foods (Figure 14-4). Two other basic foods are rice and beans. Milk, meat, yellow and green vegetables, and other fruits are used in limited quantities, but dried codfish is a staple. Coffee also is a well-liked beverage among Puerto Ricans, and the traditional cooking fat is lard.

Native American

The Native American population of Indian and Alaska Natives is composed of more than 500 federally

---

Ramadan the ninth month of the Muslim year, which is a period of daily fasting from sunrise to sunset.

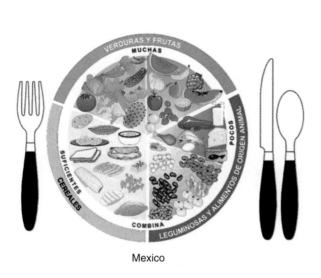

Mexico

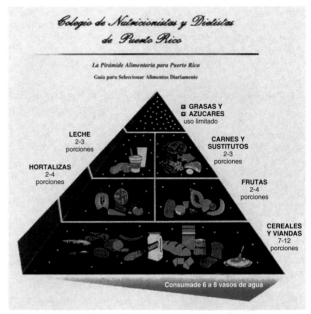

Puerto Rico

Figure 14-3 National food guides for Mexico and Puerto Rico. (Reprinted from Painter J, Rah JH, Lee YK. Comparison of international food guide pictorial representations. *J Am Diet Assoc.* 2002; 102:483-489, with permission from the Academy of Nutrition and Dietetics.)

recognized diverse groups that live on reservations, in small rural communities, and in metropolitan cities. Despite their individual diversity, the various groups share a spiritual attachment to the land and a determination to retain their culture. Food has great religious and social significance in these groups. Serving food is an integral part of celebrations, ceremonies, and everyday hospitality. Foods may be prepared and used in different ways from region to region. Variation reflects what can be grown locally, harvested, or hunted on the land or fished from its rivers; it also reflects what is available in food markets.

Among the American Indian groups of the Southwest United States, the food pattern of the Navajo people—whose reservation extends over a 25,000-mi^2 area at the junction of New Mexico, Arizona, and Utah—is one example. The Navajos learned farming from the early Pueblo people, and they established corn and other crops as staples. They later learned herding from the Spaniards, which made sheep and goats available for food and wool. Some families also raise chickens, pigs, and cattle. Today, American Indian food habits combine traditional dietary staples (e.g., corn/maize, beans, squash) with modern food products from available supermarkets and fast-food restaurants (Figure 14-5). Meat (e.g., fresh mutton [Figure 14-6], beef, pork, chicken, smoked or processed meat) is eaten daily. Other staples include bread (tortillas or fry bread, blue cornbread, and cornmeal mush), beverages

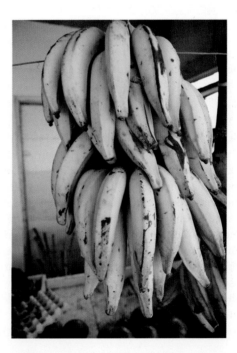

Figure 14-4 A plantain, which is a popular fruit in Puerto Rico. (Copyright JupiterImages Corp.)

Dairy Group
1 cup low-fat, skim, or acidophilus milk
1 cup low- or non-fat yogurt
1-1/2 ounces natural cheese (or 2 ounces processed), low- or non-fat preferred

*Breast milk for babies, goat's milk, bone soup, fish head soup, or canned salmon with bones

Vegetable Group
1 cup raw leafy greens
1/2 cup other vegetables, cooked or raw
3/4 cup vegetable juice, green beans, squash, kale, broccoli, or zucchini

*Sprouts or new shoots, wild mushrooms, nopalitos, wild onion, amaranth leaves (wild spinach), fresh or dried squash, lambsquarter (kappa), wild mustard, peeled stems, purslane or jicama

Bread Group
1 6-inch corn tortilla
1 7-1/2-inch flour tortilla**
4-6 crackers**
1 slice bread**
1/2 hamburger bun**
1/2 cup cooked cereal**
1 ounce ready-to-eat cereal**
1/2 cup rice or pasta (cooked)**

*Indian biscuits (bannock bread), popcorn, Indian wheat or psyllium (plantago), barley, wild oats, wild rice, amaranth and mesquite flour, popped amaranth seeds, wild peas, or corn (fresh, frozen or cooked)

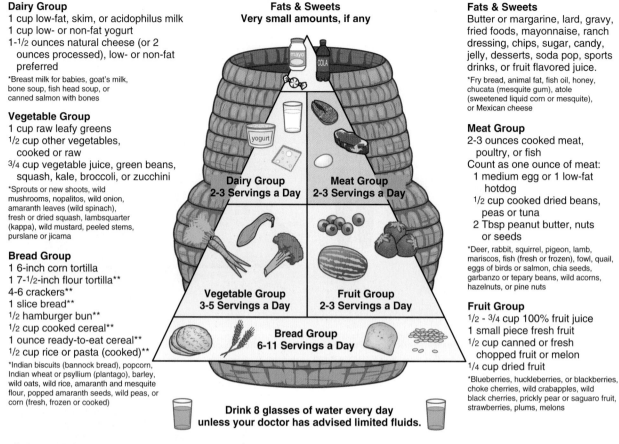

Fats & Sweets
Very small amounts, if any

Dairy Group
2-3 Servings a Day

Meat Group
2-3 Servings a Day

Vegetable Group
3-5 Servings a Day

Fruit Group
2-3 Servings a Day

Bread Group
6-11 Servings a Day

Drink 8 glasses of water every day
unless your doctor has advised limited fluids.

Fats & Sweets
Butter or margarine, lard, gravy, fried foods, mayonnaise, ranch dressing, chips, sugar, candy, jelly, desserts, soda pop, sports drinks, or fruit flavored juice.

*Fry bread, animal fat, fish oil, honey, chucata (mesquite gum), atole (sweetened liquid corn or mesquite), or Mexican cheese

Meat Group
2-3 ounces cooked meat, poultry, or fish
Count as one ounce of meat:
1 medium egg or 1 low-fat hotdog
1/2 cup cooked dried beans, peas or tuna
2 Tbsp peanut butter, nuts or seeds

*Deer, rabbit, squirrel, pigeon, lamb, mariscos, fish (fresh or frozen), fowl, quail, eggs of birds or salmon, chia seeds, garbanzo or tepary beans, wild acorns, hazelnuts, or pine nuts

Fruit Group
1/2 - 3/4 cup 100% fruit juice
1 small piece fresh fruit
1/2 cup canned or fresh chopped fruit or melon
1/4 cup dried fruit

*Blueberries, huckleberries, or blackberries, choke cherries, wild crabapples, wild black cherries, prickly pear or saguaro fruit, strawberries, plums, melons

Figure 14-5 Southern Arizona American Indian Food Guide: Choices for a Healthy Life. *Traditional foods. **Whole grain products recommended. (Osterkamp LK, Longstaff L. Development of a dietary teaching tool for American Indians and Alaskan Natives in Southern Arizona. *Nutr Educ Behav.* 2004;36:272-274.)

(coffee, soft drinks, and other fruit-flavored sweet drinks), eggs, vegetables (corn, potatoes, green beans, and tomatoes), and some fresh or canned fruit. Frying is a common method of food preparation, and lard and shortening are the traditional cooking fats. However, health concerns are growing as a result of the increased use of modern convenience or snack foods that are high in fat, sugar, calories, and sodium, especially among children and teenagers (see the Cultural Considerations box, "Acculturation to an American Diet").

Other Native American tribes in the United States have their own heritages and distinct dietary habits relative to customs and the regions in which they live.

Influences of the Southern United States

African Americans

African-American populations, especially in the Southern states, have contributed a rich heritage to American

food patterns, particularly to Southern cooking as a whole. Similar to their moving music styles (e.g., spirituals, blues, gospel, jazz), the food patterns of Southern African Americans developed through a creative ability to turn staples at hand into memorable food. Although regional differences occur, as with any basic food pattern, the representative use of foods from basic food groups is evident as follows:

- *Breads and cereals:* Traditional breads include hot breads such as biscuits, spoonbread (a soufflé-like dish of cornmeal with beaten eggs), cornmeal muffins, and skillet cornbread. Cooked cereals such as cornmeal mush, hominy grits (ground corn), and oatmeal are also commonly used.
- *Eggs and dairy products:* Eggs and some cheese but little milk are used, probably because of the greater prevalence of lactose intolerance among African Americans.
- *Vegetables:* Leafy greens such as turnip greens, collard greens, mustard greens, and spinach are

CULTURAL CONSIDERATIONS

ACCULTURATION TO AN AMERICAN DIET

Immigration from one part of the world to another is usually accompanied by changes with regard to dietary intake, lifestyle, and disease risk to match the new culture; this phenomenon is referred to as *acculturation*. Several studies have evaluated the changes that occur over time, specifically with Hispanic-Latino immigrants, because this population encompasses the fastest-growing ethnic group in the United States. One such large-scale review of the literature evaluated the relationship between ethnicity, acculturation, and overall diet quality among Latinos who were living in the United States. Researchers noted that Latinos who exhibited more acculturation consistently scored worse in overall diet quality by eating less fruit, rice, and beans and by consuming more sugar and sugar-sweetened beverages than their less acculturated counterparts.[1] Acculturation has been linked to the development of chronic diseases such as diabetes. A separate study that evaluated the diets of Latinos with diabetes showed that, as more acculturation takes place for the immigrants in their new environment, their diets include less dietary fiber and more saturated fat, both of which are contraindicated.[2]

One of the most notable negative effects of acculturation seems to be with the Native American and Alaska Native populations. According to the Centers for Disease Control and Prevention, the prevalence of obesity, diabetes, and cardiovascular disease among Native American and Alaska Natives is higher than that of any other major racial or ethnic group in the United States[3] (see figure). Researchers believe that the increase in disease risk is directly associated

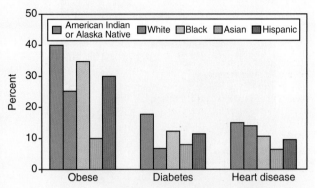

The prevalence of obesity, diabetes, and heart disease by ethnicity. From Barnes PM, Adams PF, Powell-Griner E. Health characteristics of the American Indian or Alaska Native adult population: United States, 2004-2008. *Natl Health Stat Report.* 2010;(20):1-22.

with dietary and lifestyle adaptations to the typical American diet and to a more sedentary lifestyle.

For more information about acculturation, see the references listed for this box and the article entitled "Dietary acculturation and the nutrition transition" by Satia, which is referenced in the Further Reading and Resources section at the end of this chapter.

1. Ayala GX, Baquero B, Klinger S. A systematic review of the relationship between acculturation and diet among Latinos in the United States: implications for future research. *J Am Diet Assoc.* 2008;108(8):1330-1344.
2. Mainous AG 3rd, Diaz VA, Geesey ME. Acculturation and healthy lifestyle among Latinos with diabetes. *Ann Fam Med.* 2008;6(2): 131-137.
3. Barnes PM, Adams PF, Powell-Griner E. Health characteristics of the American Indian or Alaska Native adult population: United States, 2004-2008. *Natl Health Stat Report.* 2010;(20):1-22.

frequently used and are usually cooked with bacon or salt pork. Cabbage is boiled or chopped raw and served with a salad dressing (e.g., coleslaw). Other vegetables that are used include okra (coated with cornmeal and fried), sweet potatoes (baked whole or sliced and "candied" with added sugar), green beans, tomatoes, potatoes, corn, butter beans, and dried beans such as black-eyed peas and red or pinto beans cooked with smoked ham hocks and served over rice. Black-eyed peas served over rice comprise a dish called "hoppin' John" that is traditionally served on New Year's Day to bring good luck for the new year.

- *Fruits:* Commonly eaten fruits include apples, peaches, berries, oranges, bananas, and fruit juices.

- *Meat:* Pork is a common meat, and this includes fresh cuts of ribs, sausage, and smoked ham. Some beef is eaten, and it is mainly ground for meat loaf or hamburgers. Poultry is frequently consumed, mainly as fried chicken and baked holiday turkey. Organ meats such as liver, heart, intestines (chitterlings), and poultry giblets (i.e., gizzard and heart) are consumed. Fish, including catfish and some flounder, and shellfish (e.g., crab and shrimp) are eaten when available. Frying is a common method of cooking; lard, shortening, and vegetable oils are the traditionally used fats.

- *Desserts:* Favorites include pies (e.g., pecan, sweet potato, pumpkin), deep-dish peach or berry

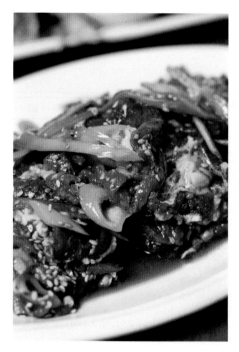

Figure 14-6 Mutton, which is the meat of sheep or goats. (Copyright JupiterImages Corp.)

cobblers, cakes (e.g., coconut, chocolate), and bread pudding.

- *Beverages:* Coffee, apple cider, fruit juices, lemonade, iced sweet tea, carbonated soft drinks, and buttermilk (which is a more easily tolerated, cultured form of milk) are consumed.

French Americans

The Cajun people, who are concentrated in the southwestern coastal waterways of southern Louisiana, have contributed a unique cuisine and food pattern to America's rich and varied fare. This pattern continues to provide a unique model for the rapidly expanding forms of American ethnic food. The Cajuns are descendants of the early French colonists of Acadia, which is a peninsula on the eastern coast of Canada that is now known as Nova Scotia. During the pre-Revolutionary wars between France and Britain, both countries contended for the area of Acadia. However, after Britain finally won control of Canada, the fear of an Acadian revolt led to a forcible deportation of the French colonists in 1755. After a long and difficult journey down the Atlantic coast and then westward along the Gulf of Mexico, a group of the impoverished Acadians finally settled along the bayou country of what is now Louisiana. To support themselves, they developed their unique food pattern from the seafood at hand and from what they could grow and harvest. Over time, Cajuns blended their own French culinary background with the Creole cooking that they found in their new homeland around New Orleans.

The unique Cajun food pattern of the Southern United States represents an ethnic blending of cultures that made use of the basic foods available in the area. Cajun foods are strong flavored and spicy, with the abundant seafood as a base and usually cooked as a stew and served over rice. The well-known hot chili sauce Tabasco, which is made from crushed and fermented red chili peppers blended with spices and vinegar, is still made by generations of a Cajun family on Avery Island on the coastal waterway of southern Louisiana. The most popular shellfish native to the region is the crawfish, which is now grown commercially in the fertile rice paddies of the bayou areas. Catfish, red snapper, shrimp, blue crab, and oysters are some of the other popular seafoods that are used. Popular vegetables include onions, bell peppers, okra, parsley, shallots, and tomatoes; seasonings include cayenne (red) pepper, Tabasco sauce, crushed black pepper, white pepper, bay leaves, thyme, and filé powder. Some typical Cajun dishes include seafood or chicken gumbo, jambalaya, red beans and rice, blackened catfish or red snapper, barbecued shrimp, breaded catfish with Creole sauce, and boiled crawfish. Breads and starches include French bread, hushpuppies (fried balls of a cornbread mixture), cornbread muffins, cush-cush (cornmeal mush cooked with milk), grits (ground white corn), rice, and yams. Desserts include ambrosia (freshly peeled orange segments and orange juice with sliced bananas and freshly grated coconut), sweet potato pie, pecan pie, berry pie, bread pudding, and pecan pralines.

Cajun a group of people with an enduring tradition whose French-Catholic ancestors established permanent communities in the southern Louisiana coastal waterways after being expelled from Acadia (now Nova Scotia, Canada) by the reigning English during the late eighteenth century; they developed a unique food pattern from a blend of native French influence and the Creole cooking that was found in the new land.

filé powder a substance that is made from ground sassafras leaves; it seasons and thickens the dish into which it is put.

jambalaya a dish of Creole origin that combines rice, chicken, ham, pork, sausage, broth, vegetables, and seasonings.

DRUG-NUTRIENT INTERACTION

THE FRENCH PARADOX: RED WINE AND HEART DISEASE

French cuisine is very rich, and it is high in saturated fat. Although the relationship between saturated fat intake and the risk of heart disease has been well established, cardiovascular disease risk among the French remains low; this concept is known as the *French paradox*. The suspected reason for this paradox is the high consumption of red wine. Red wine contains antioxidant compounds known as *polyphenols* that may be responsible for improved cardiovascular function. Although research supports that there are antioxidant benefits with moderate red wine consumption,

more studies are needed before recommendations can be formulated.[1]

Alcohol provides calories, and it can be considered a component of the diet as well as a drug substance. Excessive alcohol consumption can alter the absorption and metabolism of essential nutrients, thereby leading to malnutrition. Vitamin and mineral deficiencies often accompany chronic alcohol abuse, particularly of the B vitamins thiamine and folate.

1. Covas MI, Gambert P, Fitó M, de la Torre R. Wine and oxidative stress: up-to-date evidence of the effects of moderate wine consumption on oxidative damage in humans. *Atherosclerosis.* 2010;208(2):297-304.

Wine is a typical drink for people with French heritage, but this is true more so in France than the United States; however, wine is considered a staple for drinking and cooking (see the Drug-Nutrient Interaction box, "The French Paradox: Red Wine and Heart Disease").

Asian Food Patterns

Chinese

Chinese cooks believe that refrigeration diminishes natural flavors, so they select the freshest foods possible, hold them for the shortest time possible, and cook them quickly at a high temperature in a *wok* (a basic round-bottom pan) with small amounts of fat and liquid. The wok allows heat to be controlled with a quick stir-frying method that preserves natural flavor, color, and texture. Vegetables that are cooked just before serving are still crisp and flavorful when served. Meat is used in small amounts in combined dishes more so than as a single main entree. Little milk is used, but eggs and soybean products (e.g., tofu) add other sources of protein. Foods that have been dried, salted, pickled, spiced, candied, or canned may be added as garnishes or relishes to mask some flavors or textures or to enhance others. Fruits are usually eaten fresh, and rice is the staple grain that is used at most meals. The traditional beverage is unsweetened green tea. Seasonings include soy sauce, ginger, almonds, and sesame seeds. Peanut oil is the main cooking fat. Figure 14-7 illustrates the pictorial food guides for China, Japan, and Korea.

Japanese

In some ways, Japanese food patterns are similar to those of the Chinese. Rice is the basic grain served at meals, soy sauce is used for seasoning, and tea is the main beverage. The Japanese diet contains more seafood, especially in the form of sushi, than the Chinese diet does. Many varieties of fish and shellfish are used. The term *sushi* does not necessarily mean raw fish; some sushi is prepared with only vegetables or with cooked fish. Vegetables are usually steamed, and pickled vegetables are also used. Fresh fruit is eaten in season, and a tray of fruit is a regular course at main meals. The overall Japanese diet is high in sodium content and low in milk products because of the high prevalence of lactose intolerance among these individuals.

Southeast Asian

Since 1971, in the wake of the Vietnam War, more than 340,000 Southeast Asians have come to the United States as refugees. The largest groups of refugees are Vietnamese, but others have come from the adjacent war-torn countries of Laos and Cambodia. Refugees mainly settled in California, with other groups found in Florida, Texas, Illinois, and Pennsylvania. As a whole, their food patterns are similar and have an effect on American diet and agriculture. Asian grocery stores throughout the country stock many traditional Asian food items. Rice (both long grain and glutinous) forms the basis of the Indonesian food pattern and is eaten at most meals. The Vietnamese usually eat their rice plain in a separate rice bowl and not mixed with other foods, whereas other Southeast Asians may eat rice in mixed dishes.

Soups are also commonly used at meals. Many fresh fruits and vegetables are eaten along with fresh herbs and other seasonings such as chives, spring onions, chili peppers, ginger root, coriander, turmeric, and fish sauce. Many kinds of seafood (i.e., fish and shellfish) are included in the diet, as well as chicken, duck, and pork. Red meat is usually eaten only once or twice per month and in small

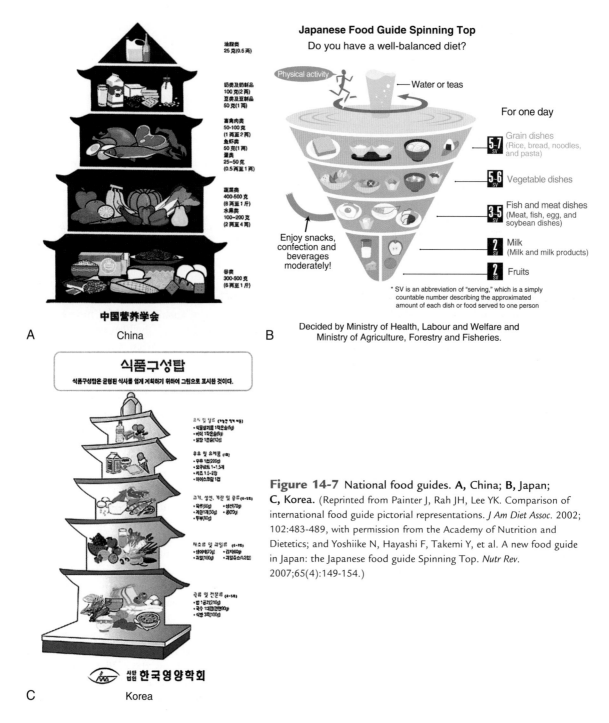

Figure 14-7 National food guides. **A,** China; **B,** Japan; **C, Korea.** (Reprinted from Painter J, Rah JH, Lee YK. Comparison of international food guide pictorial representations. *J Am Diet Assoc.* 2002; 102:483-489, with permission from the Academy of Nutrition and Dietetics; and Yoshiike N, Hayashi F, Takemi Y, et al. A new food guide in Japan: the Japanese food guide Spinning Top. *Nutr Rev.* 2007;65(4):149-154.)

quantities. Stir-frying in a wok with a small amount of lard or peanut oil is a common method of cooking. A variety of vegetables and seasonings are used, with small amounts of seafood or meat added. In a traditional Asian diet, nuts and legumes are the primary sources of protein.

Since coming to the United States, Vietnamese individuals have made some dietary changes that reflect American influence. These changes include the use of more eggs,

beef, pork, candy and other sweet snacks, bread, fast foods, soft drinks, butter, margarine, and coffee.

Mediterranean Influences

Italian

The sharing of food is an important part of Italian life. Meals are associated with warmth and fellowship, and special occasions are shared with families and friends. Bread and pasta are the basic ingredients of most meals. Milk, which is seldom used alone, is typically mixed with coffee in equal portions. Cheese is a favorite food, with many popular varieties available. Meats, poultry, and fish are used in many ways, and the varied Italian sausages and cold cuts are famous worldwide. Vegetables are used alone, in mixed main dishes, or in soups, sauces, and salads. Seasonings include herbs and spices, garlic, wine, olive oil, tomato puree, and salted pork. Main dishes are prepared by initially browning vegetables and seasonings in olive oil; adding meat or fish; covering with such liquids as wine, broth, or tomato sauce; and simmering slowly on low heat for several hours. Fresh fruit is often eaten as dessert or as a snack.

Greek

Everyday meals are simple, but Greek holiday meals are occasions for serving many delicacies. Bread is always the center of every meal, with other foods considered accompaniments. Milk is seldom used as a beverage but instead served in the cultured form of yogurt. Cheese is a favorite food, especially *feta,* which is a white cheese that is made from sheep's milk and preserved in brine. Lamb is the preferred meat, but others, especially fish, also are eaten. Eggs are sometimes a main dish, but they are never a breakfast food. Many vegetables are used, often as a main entree, and they are cooked with broth, tomato sauce, onions, olive oil, and parsley. A typical salad of thinly sliced raw vegetables and feta cheese, dressed with olive oil and vinegar, is often served with meals; the traditional Greek salad also is a favorite at many American restaurants. Rice is a main grain in many dishes. Fruit is an everyday dessert, but rich pastries such as *baklava* are served on special occasions. Figure 14-8 illustrates the Mediterranean Diet Pyramid.

See Appendix F for more information about the traditional foods of various cultures.

CHANGES IN AMERICAN FOOD HABITS

Personal Food Choices

Basic Determinants

As has been demonstrated, universal factors that determine personal food choices arise from physical, social, and psychologic needs. Box 14-1 lists some of these factors. Changing personal eating patterns is difficult enough; helping clients and patients to make needed changes for positive health reasons is even more

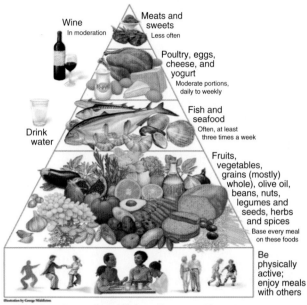

Figure 14-8 Mediterranean Diet Pyramid. (Copyright 2009, Oldways Preservation & Exchange Trust, Boston, Mass [www.oldwayspt.org/mediterranean-diet-pyramid]).

difficult. Such teaching requires a culturally sensitive and flexible understanding of the complex factors that are involved.

Factors That Influence Change

Ethnic patterns and regional cultural habits are strong influences that establish food habits early in life. However, shifts within a society result in changes in food consumption patterns for better or worse. Some examples include the following[6]:

- *Socioeconomic environment:* Increases or decreases in income will have direct effects on the food purchasing power of families. Other societal factors that drive food choices include urbanization, women in employment, and consumer attitudes toward healthy food.
- *Technology:* Expansion in the fields of science and technology increases the number and variety of food items available as well as the shelf-life of food.
- *Access to food:* Grocery store and farmers' market locations and fast-food availability affect the food choices of different individuals.
- *Vision:* America's expanding mass media, especially television, stimulates many options for new items

and changes expectations and desires. A landmark study published in the *New England Journal of Medicine* reported that "marketing strongly influences children's food preferences, requests, and consumption"; this fact has not necessarily benefited modern youth.[7] Authorities argue that the Federal Trade Commission has the obligation to protect children from the deceptive marketing of unhealthy foods, because children are not able to comprehend the intent of persuasive commercial marketing.[8]

Changing American Food Patterns

The stereotype of the all-American family of two parents and two children eating three meals a day with no snacks in between is no longer the norm. Far-reaching changes have occurred with regard to Americans' ways of living and, subsequently, their food habits.

Household Dynamics

American households are changing in nature. A growing proportion of households involve groups of unrelated people living together. The number of women in the workforce continues to increase rapidly, and this trend is not restricted to any social, economic, or ethnic group. Women of all racial and ethnic groups hold half of all management and professional positions in the U.S. labor market. The U.S. Department of Labor reports that women increased their labor force participation from 43% to 54.4% between 1970 and 2009.[9] Working parents increasingly rely on food items and cooking methods that save time, space, and labor.

With Whom and Where We Eat

Family meals, as they have been known, have changed. Breakfasts and lunches are seldom eaten in a family setting. Although research shows that frequent family meals are positively associated with improved dietary quality and beneficial developmental assets and that they are inversely related to high-risk behaviors among adolescents (e.g., substance abuse), family mealtime as a group is on the decline.[10,11] In addition, more Americans eat away from home at a higher frequency than in years past and choose foods that are higher in fat, lower in fiber, and lower in overall quality.[12,13]

How Often and How Much We Eat

Americans' habits have also changed with regard to when they eat. Mid-morning and mid-afternoon breaks at work usually involve food or beverages; evening television snacks and midnight refrigerator raids are common. Americans are increasing the number of times a day that they eat to as many as 11 "eating occasions"; this pattern has recently been termed *grazing*. This shift is not necessarily bad, depending on the nature of the periodic snacking or grazing. In fact, studies indicate that frequent small meals are better for the body than three larger meals per day, especially when healthy snacking and grazing contribute to needed nutrient and energy intake (see the For Further Focus box, "Snacking: An All-American Food Habit").

Growing portion sizes are a concerning trend in typical American meals and snacks. Portion sizes and energy consumption, especially from restaurants and prepackaged foods, have been getting larger since the 1970s.[14] Despite many reports about the "portion distortion" issues in American eating patterns, serving sizes remain unnecessarily large, and most consumers continue to eat and drink relative to the amount of food and beverage served instead of relative to their actual hunger and

FOR FURTHER FOCUS

SNACKING: AN ALL-AMERICAN FOOD HABIT

The snack market in the United States continues to grow. Consumer spending for all foods has increased, with a large portion of the increase being spent on snacks: mainly salty snacks, cookies, and crackers. Other popular snacks include soft drinks, candies, gum, fresh fruit, bakery items, milk, and chips.

Snacking is said to "ruin your appetite," and perhaps the consumption of excess soft drinks does, but is snacking altogether bad? Not necessarily. Surveys have shown a direct association between more complete nutrition and an increase in snacking. Those who snack more show higher

nutrient percentages in the "adequate" range of the Dietary Reference Intake standards. Many people snack on foods that are not empty calories but rather that are essential contributions to total nutritional adequacy (e.g., fruit, cheese, eggs, bread, crackers).

Snacking—or grazing, as some people do, which involves more frequent nibbling—is clearly a significant component of food behavior. Rather than rule against the practice, dietitians should promote snack foods that enhance nutritional well-being.

---

energy needs.[15-17] The Academy of Nutrition and Dietetic's (previously known as the American Dietetic Association) position paper entitled *Total Diet Approach* emphasizes the importance of portion control as a part of an overall healthy eating style.[18]

Fast Foods

Most Americans have eaten in a fast-food restaurant at least once. From McDonald's modest beginning in 1955 in Des Plaines, Ill, the fast-food business has grown into a multibillion-dollar enterprise that is now present around the world and that is a household name. An article in the *Journal of the American Dietetic Association* compared portion sizes of selected foods from the year they were introduced with the sizes that are commonly found today. For example, in 1954, a regular order of French fries from Burger King was 2.6 oz. Today, a medium order of Burger King fries averages 4.1 oz. Similarly, in 1955, the only size of fries that McDonald's had to offer was a 2.4-oz portion. Today, the McDonald's portions range from small (2.4 oz) to large (6.0 oz) (the Supersize 7.1-oz serving was discontinued in 2004 after the release of the documentary *Super Size Me*).[16] Such sizes dwarf the standard serving sizes on the U.S. Department of Agriculture's MyPlate food guide. According to MyPlate, a standard serving of soda is 12 fl oz. However, the average size of a soda served at a fast-food outlet is 23 fl oz.[19] Some researchers believe that the expanding portion sizes in America's most popular restaurants are closely linked with America's expanding weight problem. The U.S. Department of Health and Human Services created an interesting Portion Distortion Quiz that depicts serving size changes over the past 20 years (hp2010.nhlbihin.net/portion/index.htm).

Tempting advertisements often lure consumers into ordering more food than they need. Deals such as "two

for one" and "value meals" could be a great bargain, but they supply more food than is necessary for one person. In today's fast-food market, a variety of options are available outside of the customary hamburger and fries. Many fast-food chains offer grilled or baked chicken, turkey, or fish; fresh deli sandwiches with vegetables; side orders of salads or steamed vegetables; soup; and frozen yogurt. A well-balanced meal can be selected at almost any restaurant, provided that the consumer is selecting the healthier choice. As with foods from any ethnic or cultural background, "all foods fit in moderation."

Health and Fitness

Americans' interest in health and fitness has affected food buying in several ways, with more evidence of nutrition awareness, weight concerns, and interest in gourmet or specialty foods. New lines of low-fat, fat-free, sugar-free, high-protein, and similar foods are available. Prepackaged meals ready to eat on the go are available in most markets.

Economical Buying

Many Americans are making diet changes to save money, and no-frills grocery stores are becoming more and more popular across the country. With a warehouse-type store, the cost of overhead is significantly reduced, and store owners can pass that savings on to consumers. Many Americans also are members of bulk-food chains such as Costco and Sam's Club. Buying in bulk (i.e., economy size or family size) can save money, but only if the quantity can be efficiently used; no savings is incurred if the food is not properly stored or not eaten before it goes bad. Grocery stores also provide cost-per-unit pricing on the shelves to make comparing the prices of similar foods in different-sized containers or packages easier for the consumer.

SUMMARY

- All people grow up and live in a social setting. Each person inherits a culture and a particular social structure, complete with its food habits and attitudes about eating.
- The effects on health that are associated with major social and economic shifts should be understood—as well as the current social forces, including cultural, religious, and psychological—to help people make dietary changes that will benefit their health.
- Food patterns of Americans are changing. People who live fast-paced, complex lives increasingly rely on new forms of convenience food. More women are working, household dynamics are changing, and meal patterns are evolving.
- Eating away from the home and at fast-food restaurants continues to increase in popularity, along with excess energy intake and oversized portions.
- Authorities encourage people to be conscientious about serving sizes relative to their need and to make choices that include a healthy variety of low-energy-density fruits and vegetables.

CRITICAL THINKING QUESTIONS

1. What is the meaning of culture? How does it affect food patterns?
2. This chapter outlines the dietary laws of two religious groups. With what other dietary laws are you familiar? Use the Internet for references, and compare the dietary practices of another religious group with the ones that are given in the text. Could any practices be problematic for children, elderly adults, or sick individuals?
3. What social and psychologic factors influence food habits? Give examples of personal meanings related to food.
4. What are current trends in American food habits? Discuss their implications for nutrition and health.

CHAPTER CHALLENGE QUESTIONS

True-False

Write the correct statement for each statement that is false.

1. *True or False:* The structure of American social classes is largely determined by occupation, income, education, and residence.
2. *True or False:* Lifestyles and eating habits are modified in response to changes in society's values.
3. *True or False:* From the time of birth, eating is a social act that is built on social relationships.
4. *True or False:* Very few differences exist among various cultural eating and food patterns that would influence how a health care professional would counsel a patient.

Multiple Choice

1. A healthy body requires
   a. specific foods to control specific functions.
   b. certain food combinations to achieve specific physiologic effects.
   c. natural foods to prevent disease.
   d. specific nutrients from a variety of foods to perform specific body functions.

2. Food habits in a given culture are largely based on which of the following? *(Circle all that apply.)*
   a. Food availability
   b. Genetic differences in food tastes
   c. Food economics, market practices, and food distribution
   d. Symbolic meanings that are attached to certain foods

3. In the Jewish food pattern, the word *kosher* refers to food prepared by which of the following methods? *(Circle all that apply.)*
   a. The ritual slaughter of allowed animals for maximal blood drainage
   b. Avoidance of the combination of meat and milk in the same meal
   c. The use of special seasoning to avoid the use of salt
   d. The use of special cooking of food combinations to ensure purity and digestibility

4. The basic grain used in the Mexican food pattern is
   a. rice.
   b. corn.
   c. wheat.
   d. oat.

5. Stir-frying is a basic cooking method that is used in the food pattern of
a. Mexican individuals.
b. Jewish individuals.
c. Chinese individuals.
d. Greek individuals.

---

evolve Please refer to the Students' Resource section of this text's Evolve Web site for additional study resources.

REFERENCES

1. Roberto CA, Baik J, Harris JL, Brownell KD. Influence of licensed characters on children's taste and snack preferences. *Pediatrics*. 2010;126(1):88-93.
2. Mink M, Evans A, Moore CG, et al. Nutritional imbalance endorsed by televised food advertisements. *J Am Diet Assoc*. 2010;110(6):904-910.
3. DeNavas-Walt C, Proctor BD, Smith JC. *Income, poverty, and health insurance coverage in the United States: 2009, U.S. Census Bureau, current population reports*. Washington, DC: U.S. Government Printing Office; 2010.
4. Powell LM, Han E, Chaloupka FJ. Economic contextual factors, food consumption, and obesity among U.S. adolescents. *J Nutr*. 2010;140(6):1175-1180.
5. Painter J, Rah JH, Lee YK. Comparison of international food guide pictorial representations. *J Am Diet Assoc*. 2002;102(4):483-489.
6. Kearney J. Food consumption trends and drivers. *Philos Trans R Soc Lond B Biol Sci*. 2010;365(1554):2793-2807.
7. Nestle M. Food marketing and childhood obesity–a matter of policy. *N Engl J Med*. 2006;354(24):2527-2529.
8. Pomeranz JL. Television food marketing to children revisited: the Federal Trade Commission has the constitutional and statutory authority to regulate. *J Law Med Ethics*. 2010;38(1):98-116.
9. Solis HL, Hall K. *Women in the labor force: a databook*. Washintong, DC: U.S. Department of Labor and U.S. Bureau of Labor Statistics; 2010.
10. Eisenberg ME, Neumark-Sztainer D, Fulkerson JA, Story M. Family meals and substance use: is there a long-term protective association? *J Adolesc Health*. 2008;43(2):151-156.
11. Eisenberg ME, Olson RE, Neumark-Sztainer D, et al. Correlations between family meals and psychosocial well-being among adolescents. *Arch Pediatr Adolesc Med*. 2004;158(8):792-796.
12. Beydoun MA, Powell LM, Wang Y. Reduced away-from-home food expenditure and better nutrition knowledge and belief can improve quality of dietary intake among US adults. *Public Health Nutr*. 2009;12(3):369-381.
13. Briefel RR, Johnson CL. Secular trends in dietary intake in the United States. *Annu Rev Nutr*. 2004;24:401-431.
14. Ello-Martin JA, Ledikwe JH, Rolls BJ. The influence of food portion size and energy density on energy intake: implications for weight management. *Am J Clin Nutr*. 2005;82(1 Suppl):236S-241S.
15. Schwartz J, Byrd-Bredbenner C. Portion distortion: typical portion sizes selected by young adults. *J Am Diet Assoc*. 2006;106(9):1412-1418.
16. Young LR, Nestle M. Portion sizes and obesity: responses of fast-food companies. *J Public Health Policy*. 2007;28(2):238-248.
17. Burger KS, Kern M, Coleman KJ. Characteristics of self-selected portion size in young adults. *J Am Diet Assoc*. 2007;107(4):611-618.
18. Nitzke S, Freeland-Graves J. Position of the American Dietetic Association: total diet approach to communicating food and nutrition information. *J Am Diet Assoc*. 2007;107(7):1224-1232.
19. Young LR, Nestle M. Expanding portion sizes in the US marketplace: implications for nutrition counseling. *J Am Diet Assoc*. 2003;103(2):231-234.

FURTHER READING AND RESOURCES

Kearney J. Food consumption trends and drivers. *Philos Trans R Soc Lond B Biol Sci*. 2010;365(1554):2793-2807.
The author explores worldwide trends in food consumption patterns and the correlation to drivers such as economics, trade policies, consumer attitudes, marketing, availability, etc.

Satia JA. Dietary acculturation and the nutrition transition: an overview. *Appl Physiol Nutr Metab*. 2010;35(2):219-223.
This article explores dietary acculturation by immigrants— the process of adopting the dietary practices of a new culture— in the United States and the major forces that drive the nutritional transitions. The author takes an important look at the overall relevance and provides suggestions for future research.

CHAPTER 15

Weight Management

KEY CONCEPTS

- Underlying causes of obesity include a host of various genetic, environmental, and psychologic factors.
- Short-term food patterns or fads often stem from food misinformation that appeals to some human psychologic need; however, these fads do not necessarily meet physiologic needs.

- Realistic weight management focuses on individual needs and health promotion, including meal pattern planning and regular physical activity.
- Severe underweight carries physiologic and psychologic risk to the body.

---

urrently, 34.2% of adults in the United States are overweight, 33.8% are obese, and 5.7% are extremely obese.[1] This epidemic—which results in large part from poor diet, physical inactivity, and genetics—is not limited to adults. The National Center for Health Statistics reported that 16.9% of children and adolescents between the ages of 2 and 19 years are also obese.[2] Weight-loss diets are abundant and do not lack in variety with regard to the philosophy of the methods used to shed unwanted pounds. The use of these diets seems to increase daily, with new diet books constantly appearing in the public press. Despite this obsession with weight and the big-business industry of weight loss products and diets, Americans continue to grow in undesirable directions (Figure 15-1). This chapter examines the problem of weight management and seeks a more positive and realistic health model that recognizes personal needs and sound weight goals.

OBESITY AND WEIGHT CONTROL

Body Weight and Body Fat

Definitions

Obesity develops from many interwoven factors—including personal, physical, psychologic, and genetic—and is difficult to define. As used in the traditional medical sense, *obesity* is a clinical term for excess body fat, and it is generally used to describe people who are at least 20% above a desired weight for height. The terms *overweight* and *obesity* are often used interchangeably, but they technically have different meanings. *Overweight* denotes a body weight that is above a population weight-for-height standard; however, the word *obesity* is a more specific term that refers to the degree of fatness (i.e., the relative excess amount of fat in the total body composition). Over the past five decades, the percentage of obese adults (i.e., those with a body mass index [BMI] of 30 or greater) between the ages of 20 and 74 years has increased from 13.4% of the population to 34%.[1] The relative prevalence of overweight and obese adults in America is of epidemic proportions. Box 15-1 provides the classifications of BMI.

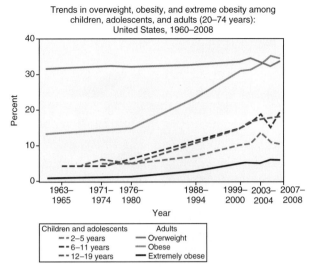

Figure 15-1 Overweight and obesity, by age: United States, 1960-2008. Estimates for adults are age adjusted. For adults: overweight, including obese, is defined as a body mass index (BMI) of 25 or greater; overweight but not obese as a BMI of 25 or more but less than 30; and obese as a BMI of 30 or more. For children: overweight is defined as a BMI at or above the sex- and age- specific 95th percentile BMI cut points from the 2000 CDC Growth Charts: United States. Obese is not defined for children. (Reprinted from Ogden CL, Carroll MD. *Prevalence of overweight, obesity, and extreme obesity among adults: United States, trends 1976-1980 through 2007-2008, Division of Health and Nutrition Examination Surveys.* Atlanta: National Center for Health Statistics; 2010. Ogden CL, Carroll MD. *Prevalence of obesity among children and adolescents: United States, trends 1963-1965 through 2007-2008, Division of Health and Nutrition Examination Surveys.* Atlanta: National Center for Health Statistics; 2010.

BMI can be tracked from childhood to adulthood with the Centers for Disease Control and Prevention growth charts (see Chapter 11). BMI is a reliable method of predicting the relative risk of becoming an overweight adult on the basis of the presence or absence of excess weight at various times throughout childhood. Children and adolescents who are overweight or obese during their school years are significantly more likely to continue to suffer from obesity as they age.[3,4]

Every person is different, and normal weight ranges in healthy people vary. Until recently, the important factor of age for setting a reasonable body weight for adults had been overlooked. With advancing age, body weight usually increases until approximately the age of 50 years for men and the age of 70 years for women, and then it declines.

The exclusive use of BMI to define obesity has undergone criticism because it does not measure body fat per se but rather total body weight relative to height. This

BOX 15-1   BODY MASS INDEX CLASSIFICATIONS

BODY MASS INDEX RANGE (kg/m²)	CLASSIFICATION
18.5 to 24.9	Normal
25 to 29.9	Overweight
30 to 35	Obese
> 35	Clinically or extremely obese

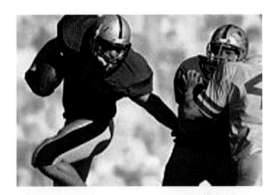

Figure 15-2 According to standard height/weight charts, some football players would be considered overweight. These charts should be used with discretion when assessing weight for individuals with more lean body mass (muscle) than the typical person.

method classifies some individuals as obese when they do not have excess body fat. For example, a football player in peak condition can be extremely "overweight" according to standard height/weight charts. In other words, he can weigh considerably more than the average man of the same height, but much more of his weight is lean muscle mass rather than excess fat (Figure 15-2). Thus, for individuals with more muscle mass than the average person, BMI may not be the most ideal means of assessing risks associated with weight. However, for the vast majority of the population, BMI is an appropriate tool and it is closely associated with health risks stemming from excess body fat.

Body Composition

BMI is closely related to body fat percentages (Figure 15-3). Because BMI is much easier to assess than body composition, it is recommended as the standard for

body composition the relative sizes of the four body compartments that make up the total body: lean body mass (muscle mass), fat, water, and bone.

body mass index (BMI) the body weight in kilograms divided by the square of the height in meters (i.e., kg/m²).

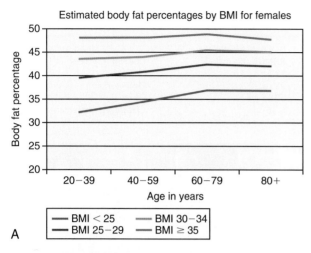

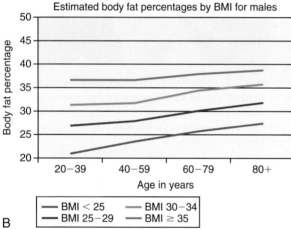

A

B

Figure 15-3 Body fat percentage as it correlates with body mass index (BMI) (A, females: B, males). (Adapted from Li C, Ford ES, Zhao G, et al. Estimates of body composition with dual-energy x-ray absorptiometry in adults. *Am J Clin Nutr.* 2009;90(6):1457-1465.)

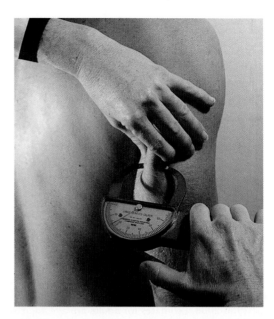

Figure 15-4 Assessment tools include skinfold calipers, which measure the relative amount of subcutaneous fat tissue at various body sites. (Reprinted from Mahan LK, Escott-Stump S. *Krause's food & nutrition therapy.* 12th ed. Philadelphia: Saunders; 2008.)

assessing health relative to weight. However, body composition assessment provides an additional measure of overall health and fitness. Health professionals can measure body fatness with the use of a variety of methods:

- *Body fat calipers* measure the width of skin folds at precise body sites, because most of the body fat is deposited in layers just under the skin. These measures are then used in specific formulas to calculate an estimated body fat composition (Figure 15-4). Calipers are an easy, portable, inexpensive, and noninvasive way to measure body fat. However, the reliability of the test depends on the skill of the technician, which can vary greatly.
- *Hydrostatic weighing,* which is a more precise method, is often used in athletic programs and research studies. Hydrostatic weighing requires the

complete submersion of an individual in water. The person must exhale as much air as possible and then stay underwater for a few seconds for an accurate reading to be obtained. Although this method is more accurate, it is not easy, portable, or inexpensive, and many patients are not willing or able to perform the test.

- *Bioelectrical impedance analysis* is an easy, portable, inexpensive, and noninvasive body composition measurement tool. One type, a foot-to-foot analyzer, requires that the person stand on a modified scale with bare feet while an unnoticeable electrical current travels through his or her body (Figure 15-5). The analyzer determines the individual's body fat percentage on the basis of gender, age, height, weight, total body water, and the rate at which the electrical current travels. Fat impedes the current; therefore, a lower total body fat composition results in a faster travel time of the electrical current. Such analyzers have both a standard adult setting and an athletic setting. Although this method does not require any special skill on either the client's part or the technician's part, discrepancies in some people have been noted between total body fat percentages as measured by bioelectrical impedance versus dual-energy x-ray absorptiometry.[5] Bioelectrical impedance machines that use a

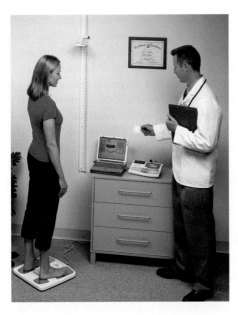

Figure 15-5 Tanita bioelectrical impedance body composition measurement tool. (Courtesy Tanita Corp., Arlington Heights, Ill.)

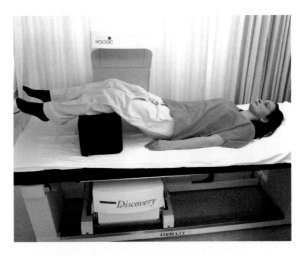

Figure 15-6 Dual-energy x-ray absorptiometry. (Courtesy University of Utah, Division of Nutrition, Salt Lake City, Utah.)

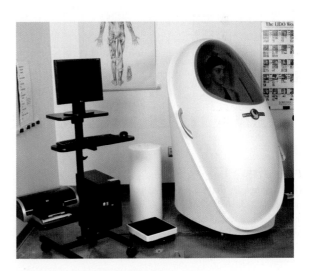

Figure 15-7 The BOD POD uses air displacement technology to measure body composition. (Courtesy Life Measurements, Inc., Concord, Calif.)

multiple-frequency bioelectrical impedance analysis with eight-point tactile electrodes have the least error and the highest correspondence to reference amounts of body fat.[6,7]

- *Dual energy x-ray absorptiometry,* which is a more accurate way to assess body composition (including bone density and body fat) uses radiation to distinguish bone, muscle, water, and fat density[8] (Figure 15-6). Although this method is less intimidating than hydrostatic weighing for some people, it is substantially more expensive.
- *Air displacement plethysmography* with the use of the BOD POD (Life Measurement, Inc, Concord, Calif), may prove to be a reliable method of assessing body composition that does not rely on technical expertise or radiation (Figure 15-7). However, it is also expensive and not easily portable. The BOD POD calculates the percentage of body fat using weight, body volume, thoracic lung volume, and body density. Current studies indicate that the BOD POD is a reliable measurement tool for most subgroups of the population, but discrepancies may arise when measuring children, athletes, and elderly individuals.[9-11] However, it does offer a reliable means of assessing body fat percentage in overweight and obese populations, whereas other methods are often not as reliable.[12]

A body fat content within the range of 21% to 25.8% of total body weight (i.e., a BMI of less than 25 kg/m^2) is

associated with the lowest risk of chronic disease for men between the ages of 20 and 79 years. For women, the ideal range is somewhat higher: 32.2% to 36.9%.[13] Body fat percentage ranges that are associated with fitness are slightly lower than those associated with BMI and chronic disease prevention. The American College of Sports Medicine classifies men as having "above average" and "well above average" fitness levels when their body fat percentages are between 7% and 15.8%, for 20- to 29-year-old men and when they are between 14.5% and 22%, for women of the same age group (Figure 15-8).[14] Health risks associated with too little or too much body fat rise

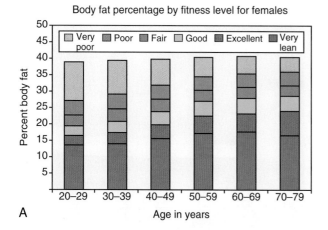

Body fat percentage by fitness level for females

A   Age in years

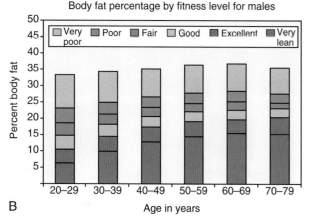

Body fat percentage by fitness level for males

B   Age in years

Figure 15-8 Body fat percentage by fitness level (A, females; B, males). (Adapted from the American College of Sports Medicine. *ACSM's health-related physical fitness assessment manual.* 3rd ed. Baltimore, Md: American College of Sports Medicine; 2010.)

as the percentage of body fat exceeds or falls below these ranges.

Measures of Weight Maintenance Goals

Standard Height/Weight Tables

Height/weight tables are general population guides and should be regarded only as such. Individual needs must be considered. One of the standard tables that is used in the United States is the Metropolitan Life Insurance Company's ideal weight-for-height chart. These charts are based on life expectancy information gathered since the 1930s from the company's population of life insurance policyholders. Many people have questioned how well these tables represent the total current population,

because the data are based on such a select group of individuals (most of whom were Caucasian, middle- to upper-class men for the first few decades of data gathering) and may not consider the wide variety of individuals who are found within a diverse community.

More recent height/weight tables rely on BMI calculations and are based on the National Research Council data for weight and health, the current *Dietary Guidelines for Americans,* and recent medical studies. These guidelines directly relate height and weight ranges to relative risks for chronic diseases (Table 15-1). Within each age group, obesity is significantly associated with higher all-cause mortality rates.[15-17]

Healthy Weight Range

Following are general calculations that make use of the Hamwi method for determining healthy or ideal weight goals:

- *Men:* 106 lb for the first 5 feet, then add or subtract 6 lb for each inch above or below 5 feet, respectively. A range is then taken by adding and subtracting 10% to account for small and large body frames.
- *Women:* 100 lb for the first 5 feet, then add or subtract 5 lb for each inch above or below 5 feet, respectively. A range is then taken by adding and subtracting 10% to account for small and large body frames.

For example, a 5-foot, 6-inch woman would have an ideal body weight range of 100 lb + (6 in × 5 lb) = 130 ± 10%. Therefore, her ideal body weight range is 117 to 143 lb.

As with BMI, this calculation does not account for acceptable changes that are associated with age (i.e., a loss of stature and slight increases in weight) or for individuals with very high muscle mass. A person's ideal weight may give him or her a ballpark figure for a healthy weight goal. Three important considerations must be taken into account when relying on ideal body weight calculations: frame size, variation, essentiality of body fat.

Body Frame. Height (in centimeters) divided by wrist circumference (in centimeters) provides an estimate of body frame size. For an accurate measurement, the patient's arm should be flexed at the elbow with the palm facing up and the hand relaxed. With a flexible measuring tape, measure the wrist circumference at the joint distal

Hamwi method   a formula for estimating the ideal body weight on the basis of gender and height.

TABLE 15-1 **BODY MASS INDEX TABLE**

$$\text{Body mass index} = \frac{\text{Weight (kg)}}{\text{Height (m)}^2} \quad \text{or} \quad \frac{\text{Weight (lb)} \times 703}{\text{Height (in)}^2}$$

Body Mass Index	HEALTHY WEIGHT						OVERWEIGHT					OBESE										EXTREMELY OBESE					
	19	20	21	22	23	24	25	26	27	28	29	30	31	32	33	34	35	36	37	38	39	40	41	42	43	44	45
HEIGHT	BODY WEIGHT (POUNDS)																										
4'10"	91	96	100	105	110	115	119	124	129	134	138	143	148	153	158	162	167	172	177	181	186	191	196	201	205	210	215
4'11"	94	99	104	109	114	119	124	128	133	138	143	148	153	158	163	168	173	178	183	188	193	198	203	208	212	217	222
5'	97	102	107	112	118	123	128	133	138	143	148	153	158	163	168	174	179	184	189	194	199	204	209	215	220	225	230
5'1"	100	106	111	116	122	127	132	137	143	148	153	158	164	169	174	180	185	190	195	201	206	211	217	222	227	232	238
5'2"	104	109	115	120	126	131	136	142	147	153	158	164	169	175	180	186	191	196	202	207	213	218	224	229	235	240	246
5'3"	107	113	118	124	130	135	141	146	152	158	163	169	175	180	186	191	197	203	208	214	220	225	231	237	242	248	254
5'4"	110	116	122	128	134	140	145	151	157	163	169	174	180	186	192	197	204	209	215	221	227	232	238	244	250	256	262
5'5"	114	120	126	132	138	144	150	156	162	168	174	180	186	192	198	204	210	216	222	228	234	240	246	252	258	264	270
5'6"	118	124	130	136	142	148	155	161	167	173	179	186	192	198	204	210	216	223	229	235	241	247	253	260	266	272	278
5'7"	121	127	134	140	146	153	159	166	172	178	185	191	198	204	211	217	223	230	236	242	249	255	261	268	274	280	287
5'8"	125	131	138	144	151	158	164	171	177	184	190	197	203	210	216	223	230	236	243	249	256	262	269	276	282	289	295
5'9"	128	135	142	149	155	162	169	176	182	189	196	203	209	216	223	230	236	243	250	257	263	270	277	284	291	297	304
5'10"	132	139	146	153	160	167	174	181	188	195	202	209	216	222	229	236	243	250	257	264	271	278	285	292	299	306	313
5'11"	135	143	150	157	165	172	179	186	193	200	208	215	222	229	236	243	250	257	265	272	279	286	293	301	308	315	322
6'	140	147	154	162	169	177	184	191	199	206	213	221	228	235	242	250	258	265	272	279	287	294	302	309	316	324	331
6'1"	144	151	159	166	174	182	189	197	204	212	219	227	235	242	250	257	265	272	280	288	295	302	310	318	325	333	340
6'2"	148	155	163	171	179	186	194	202	210	218	225	233	241	249	256	264	272	280	287	295	303	311	319	326	334	342	350
6'3"	152	160	168	176	184	192	200	208	216	224	232	240	249	256	264	272	279	287	295	303	311	319	327	335	343	351	359

Locate the height of interest in the leftmost column, and then read across the row for that height to the weight of interest. Follow the column of the weight up to the top row that lists the body mass index (BMI). A BMI of 18.5 to 24.9 is in the healthy weight range; a BMI of 25 to 29.9 is in the overweight range; and a BMI of 30 or more is the obese range. Modified from the National Institutes of Health; National Heart, Lung, and Blood Institute. *Evidence report of clinical guidelines on the identification, evaluation, and treatment of overweight and obesity in adults.* Bethesda, Md: National Institutes of Health; 1998.

(i.e., toward the hand) to the styloid process (i.e., the bony wrist protrusion). Individuals with a small frame size would have an ideal body weight at the lower end of their ideal body weight range and vice versa for individuals with a large frame size. The following example indicates the standards for body frame size, which are useful for interpreting ideal body weight:

Height: 5 ft, 4 in = 64 in × 2.54 cm/in = 162.56 cm

Wrist circumference = 15.4 cm

162.56/15.4 = 10.56 = Medium frame

FRAME SIZE	MALE RATIO	FEMALE RATIO
Small	> 10.4	> 10.9
Medium	10.4 to 9.6	10.9 to 9.9
Large	< 9.6	< 9.9

Individual Variation. Ideal weight varies with time and circumstance throughout the life span. A person's ideal weight depends on many factors, including gender, age, body shape, metabolic rate, genetics, and physical activity. Specific individual situations govern needs.

Necessity of Body Fat. Some body fat is essential for survival. Every cell membrane in the body has fat molecules within it. Fat is used for insulation, temperature regulation, the cushioning of vital organs, and many other functions. The estimated essential body fat level (i.e., the minimum amount required for health) is approximately 5% for men and 12% for women.[18] It should be noted that these are minimum amounts of body fat and not optimal levels. Hormonal regulation of the reproductive system is negatively affected by inadequate body fat and severe caloric restriction in women. Some women who drop below the critical body fat percentage experience amenorrhea because of a decrease in hormone levels.[19]

Obesity and Health

Weight Extremes

Clinically severe or significant obesity is a health hazard in itself and creates other medical problems by placing strain on all body systems. Both extremes of weight—fatness and thinness—pose health problems.

Overweight and Health Problems

Obesity increases the risk of related conditions such as hypertension, type 2 diabetes, heart disease, arthritis, and certain types of cancer.[20-23] Weight loss can reduce elevated blood glucose levels and blood pressure in obese people.[24,25] In turn, these improvements reduce risks related to heart disease.

Causes of Obesity

Basic Energy Balance

How does a person become overweight? Although some people have congenital obesity, a major contributor to obesity in Americans is physical inactivity. In fact, one study found that a simple and well-defined walking program can help to reduce total body weight, percentage of body fat, and BMI among overweight people even without any noticeable changes in dietary intake.[26] Regular exercise has a significant effect on increasing lean body mass and reducing the risk of the chronic diseases associated with obesity.

The overall energy imbalance (i.e., more energy intake from food and drink than energy output through physical activity and basal metabolic needs) is the primary cause of excess weight. Excess intake is stored in the body as fat. Approximately 3500 kcal is stored in each 1 lb (0.45 kg) of body fat (Box 15-2). A minor daily imbalance in which energy intake exceeds output by a mere 100 kcal can result in a significant weight gain in 1 year, as follows:

100 kcal/day × 365 days/year = 36,500 extra kcal/year

36,500 kcal ÷ 3500 kcal/lb = 10.4 lb/year (4.7 kg)

However, some overweight people only eat moderate amounts of food, and some people of average weight eat much more but never seem to gain unwanted pounds. Because many individual differences exist, more factors

---

BOX 15-2   KILOCALORIE ADJUSTMENT NECESSARY FOR WEIGHT LOSS

To lose 454 g (1 lb) per week there needs to be a 500 kcal energy deficit per day.

Basis of estimation:
1 lb body fat = 454 g
1 g pure fat = 9 kcal
1 g body fat = 7.7 kcal (differences due to water in fat cells)
454 g × 7.7 kcal/g = 3496 kcal/454 g body fat (or ≈ 3500 kcal)
500 kcal energy deficit × 7 days = 3500 kcal = 454 g body fat = 1 lb

---

amenorrhea the absence of a menstrual period in a woman of reproductive age.

clinically severe or significant obesity a body mass index of 40 or more or a body mass index of 35 to 39 with at least one obesity-related disorder; also referred to as *extreme obesity* and *morbid obesity*.

than energy balance are involved in maintaining a healthy weight.

Hormonal Control

Leptin. A research group at Rockefeller University first reported to have found the "obesity gene" in an overweight strain of laboratory mice. Soon thereafter, these researchers located the human equivalent of the same gene.[27] This gene encodes for a hormone that is released primarily from adipose tissue and that is believed to play a role in determining a person's set point for fat storage. The researchers named the hormone *leptin* from the Greek word *leptos,* meaning "thin or slender." Leptin production was first understood to control satiety in people by serving as a negative feedback mechanism against the overconsumption of total energy. Plasma leptin levels rise after weight gain and drop after weight loss.[28,29] At one point, scientists thought that obese individuals were resistant to leptin's negative feedback because the hormone did not cross the blood-brain barrier. However, studies indicate that leptin is also produced in the brain and influenced by the amount of adiposity and gender.[30] With the discovery of leptin production in the brain, the theory of leptin resistance has been refuted as a primary cause of obesity. Some individuals have been identified as having severe early-onset obesity and to lack the leptin receptor, thereby receiving no negative feedback regarding energy intake.[31] Even so, such incidence was found in only 3% of individuals with early-onset obesity. The exact role that leptin plays in the neurobiology of human obesity remains unclear but is being extensively researched.

Ghrelin. The counterpart to leptin is the enteric peptide ghrelin. Ghrelin is an appetite stimulant that is secreted from the stomach to activate the appetite-regulating network. When administered peripherally, ghrelin increases appetite and promotes adiposity.[32] Such a discovery has led to investigations of the use of a ghrelin antagonist to fight obesity.[33] Many questions remain unanswered about the roles of leptin and ghrelin and with regard to how some individuals do not respond to fluctuations of these substances in their plasma levels.

Genetic and Family Factors

Genetic inheritance probably influences a person's chances of obesity more than any other factor. Family food patterns provide an environment that allows this genetic trait to present itself.

Genetic Control. The predisposition for obesity is highly associated with genetics, thereby making certain people highly susceptible to becoming obese in an environment that allows for such a genetic expression (see the Cultural Considerations box, "Genetics and the Predisposition for Obesity").[34-36] Genetic regulation may control the amount of body fat that an individual has the potential to carry. A person then eats to regain or lose whatever amount of fat the body is naturally set or programmed for in accordance with the weight below or above this internally regulated set point. Thus, people who have lost body fat below their programmed level will eat to regain to their genetic set point when food is again available. Similarly, people with lower programmed fat levels who have gained excess body fat will lose weight when they resume their regular food intake. This is not to say that a person has no control over his or her own body weight: the genetic influence is the predisposing factor but not the determining factor. The daily life, environment, and habits that a person chooses influence the expression of this genetic trait (Figure 15-9). In one thorough review of environmental and genetic influences on obesity, the author states that, "although we might say that obesity has a large genetic component to it, this doesn't mean that the obese have somehow miraculously deposited enormous quantities of body fat without eating too much food, or expending too little energy, or doing both."[37]

Family Reinforcement. An individual's genetic predisposition for increased body fat is reinforced by inappropriate family food patterns. Studies show that that the greatest risk for obesity is a history of being overweight.[4,36] In addition to genetic influence, families also exert social pressure and teach children habits and attitudes toward food. Thus, the development of healthy eating habits during the childhood and teenage years with fat- and calorie-controlled cooking and family mealtimes is highly encouraged to establish balanced food patterns.[38]

Physiologic Factors. The amount of body fat that a person carries is related to the number and size of fat cells in the body. Critical periods for becoming obese occur during early growth periods, when cells are multiplying rapidly during childhood and adolescence. After the body has added extra fat cells for more fuel storage, these cells remain and can store varying amounts of fat. Basal metabolic rate, physical activity, and lean muscle mass are major physiologic factors for determining individual fat storage. Women store more fat during pregnancy and after menopause in response to hormonal changes.

---

early-onset obesity a genetically associated obesity that occurs during early childhood.

appetite-regulating network a hormonally controlled system of appetite stimulation and suppression.

CULTURAL CONSIDERATIONS

GENETICS AND THE PREDISPOSITION FOR OBESITY

When comparing the prevalence of obesity among various racial and ethnic groups in the United States, researchers have found a significant differences with regard to the risk for obesity in women (see graph below).[1] Few differences are seen among different racial and ethnic groups of men. According to the National Center for Health Statistics, the female prevalence of adolescent and adult obesity per racial and ethnic group is as follows:

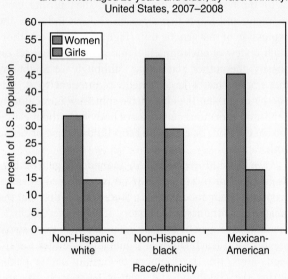

Prevalence of obesity among girls aged 12–19 and women aged 20 years and older, by race/ethnicity: United States, 2007–2008

An even more dramatic trend noted throughout the National Center for Health Statistics data for the past few decades is the significant increase in obesity in both genders. Summarized below are the findings from these surveys, which include all racial and ethnic groups. The numbers show the prevalence of obesity in both genders among adults who are 20 years old and older as percentages of the population[1,2]:

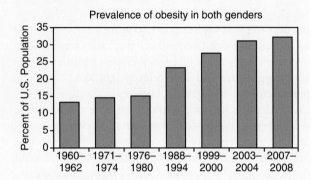

Prevalence of obesity in both genders

Although genetics does play a role in the prevalence of and predisposition for obesity, such influences cannot explain such an increase in obesity among the entire population.

1. Flegal KM, Carroll MD, Ogden CL, Curtin LR. Prevalence and trends in obesity among US adults, 1999-2008. *JAMA.* 2010;303(3):235-241.
2. National Center for Health Statistics. *Health, United States, 2006, with chartbook on trends in the health of Americans,* Hyattsville, Md: U.S. Government Printing Office; 2006.

Psychologic Factors. Work, family, and social environments may cultivate emotional stress, which many people respond to by eating for comfort. Societal pressures to maintain the cultural "ideal" thin body type contribute to the strain of constant dieting, which in turn can perpetuate the chronic dieters' dilemma of yo-yo dieting (i.e., weight loss followed by weight gain) and cause reductions in metabolic rate and lean body mass.

Other Environmental Factors. Many environmental factors add to the ever-increasing problem of obesity in the United States. The following are only a few: an increase in energy-dense food availability, fast and convenient foods, an increase in portion sizes, a decrease in food preparation time and skills, a decrease in physical activity, an increase in screen time (e.g., television, computer, video games), and the decreased physical requirements of

household chores (e.g., domestic appliances such as washing machines, vacuum cleaners, and dishwashers; central heating).

Individual Differences and Extreme Practices

Individual Energy Balance Levels

Several factors influence a person's energy balance. Estimating energy requirements is a useful starting point for practitioners to assess an individual's calorie needs.

Energy Out. Factors such as the basal metabolic rate (BMR), body size, lean body mass, age, gender, and physical activity influence the total daily calorie expenditure. Some people have more genetic-based metabolic

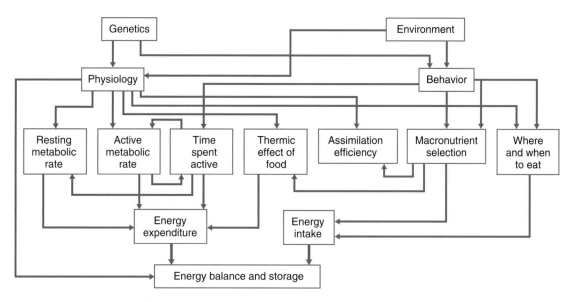

Figure 15-9 The major causal links among genetics, environmental effects, physiology, behavior, and energy balance. (Reprinted from Speakman JR. Obesity: the integrated roles of environment and genetics. *J Nutr.* 2004;134[8 Suppl]:2090S-2105S.)

efficiency (i.e., the ability to "burn" energy more readily than others do).

Energy In. When calculating a person's energy intake, Nutrition Facts labels and dietary analysis software indicate only an estimated value. Reported food values represent the averages of many samples of that type of food. Thus, determining the exact amount of kcals consumed by a person throughout the day is difficult.

Extreme Practices

Desperate attempts to lose weight may drive people to extreme measures, which sometimes worsen health risks.

Fad Diets. A constant array of diet books and weight loss supplements that promise to "melt the fat away" continue to flood the American market (Table 15-2). These books and supplements usually sell briefly and then fade away, largely because their quick fixes do not work. Such a complex problem has no simple answers. Most of the fad diets fail on the following two counts:

1. *Scientific inaccuracies and misinformation:* Fad diets and supplements are often nutritionally inadequate and based on false claims.
2. *Failure to address the necessity of changing long-term habits and behaviors:* People are often set up for failure regarding the maintenance of a healthy weight once it is achieved. The basic behavioral problem involved in changing food and exercise habits for life—thereby developing a new lifestyle—is unrecognized.

With some diets, the degree of energy restriction is impossible to maintain long-term. Many fad dieters find themselves caught in a vicious cycle of chronic dieting syndrome and its harmful physical and psychologic effects.

Fasting. The drastic fasting approach takes many forms, from literal fasting to the use of very-low-calorie diets (e.g., 800 kcal or less per day). Possible effects of a semistarvation diet include acidosis, low blood pressure, electrolyte imbalance, a loss of lean muscle mass, and decreased BMR. Such programs cannot be maintained for the long term without deleterious effects on health. The regaining of body fat mass is often overshot after a semistarvation diet; in other words, when the individual resumes normal eating, he or she gains back more fat mass than he or she had to begin with.[39]

Specific Macronutrient Restrictions. Avoiding any food group or macronutrient (i.e., carbohydrates, fats, or proteins) as a means for weight loss is unfounded. Such diets that are extremely low fat or extremely low in carbohydrates are too restrictive to maintain for extended periods, and they also carry health risks.

chronic dieting syndrome a cyclic pattern of weight loss by dieting followed by rapid weight gain; this abnormal psychophysiologic food pattern becomes chronic, changing a person's natural body metabolism and relative body composition to the abnormal state of a *metabolically obese* person of normal weight.

TABLE 15-2 COMPARISON OF SELECT COMMON DIETS

Diet	Philosophy	Foods to Eat	Foods to Avoid	Diet Composition (Average for 3 Days)	Recommended Supplements	Health Claims Scientifically Proven?	Practicality	Lose and Maintain Weight?
Atkins*	Eating too many carbohydrates causes obesity and other health problems; ketosis leads to decreased hunger; carbohydrates prevent your body from burning fat	Meat, fish, poultry, eggs, cheese, high-fiber vegetables, butter, oil, nuts, seeds	Carbohydrates, specifically bread, pasta, most fruits and high-carbohydrate vegetables, milk, alcohol	Protein: 27% Carbohydrates: 5% Fat: 68% (saturated, 26%)	Atkins supplement that includes chromium picolinate, carnitine, coenzyme Q10	No long-term validated studies published	Limited food choices; difficult to eat in restaurants, because only plain protein sources and limited vegetables and salads allowed	Yes, but initial weight loss is mostly water; does not promote a positive attitude toward food groups; difficult to maintain for the long term because the diet restricts food choices
Eat Right 4 Your Type†	Blood type determines the way your body absorbs nutrients and dictates the diet and exercise plan that will suit you best	*Type O:* meat, seafood, fruits, vegetables *Type A:* fruits, vegetables, beans, most seafood, grains *Type B:* meat, beans, fruits, vegetables, seafood, low-fat dairy *Type AB:* seafood, dairy, fruits, vegetables	*Type O:* wheat, beans *Type A:* meat, dairy, wheat *Type B:* chicken, wheat, lentils *Type AB:* meat	Not applicable (diet varies according to blood type, ancestry, and so on)	Depends on your blood type and overall health, which includes immune, skin, digestive, bone, joint, circulation, mental, and hormonal health as well as concurrent medications	No; theories and long-term results not validated	Not applicable (diet varies according to blood type, ancestry, and so on)	Possibly, if caloric intake is less than energy output
Protein Power‡	Eating carbohydrates releases insulin in large quantities, which contributes to obesity and other health problems	Meat, fish, poultry, eggs, cheese, low-carbohydrate vegetables, butter, oil, salad dressings, alcohol in moderation	Foods high in carbohydrates	Protein: 26% Carbohydrates: 16% Fat: 54% (saturated, 18%) Alcohol: 4%	Multivitamin and mineral supplement	No long-term validated studies published	Not practical for the long term; rigid rules	Yes, by caloric restriction; limited food choices are not practical for the long term
The South Beach Diet§	Switching to the "right" carbohydrates stops insulin resistance, reduces cravings, and causes weight loss	Seafood, chicken breast, lean meat, low-fat cheese, nut oils, most vegetables, low-fat dairy; later, most whole grains and beans	Fatty meats, full-fat cheese, refined grains, sweets, juice, potatoes	Phase 1: Protein: 34% Carbohydrates: 14.8% Fat: 50%	Multivitamins and omega-3 fatty acids; Metamucil recommended during phase 1	Evidence does exist to link the avoidance of saturated fats with the reduced risk of heart disease	First phase is more difficult; later phases are mostly healthy foods and more practical	Yes, although initial weight loss is mostly water; sustained weight loss through reduced calorie intake

Diet								
Sugar Busters‖	Sugar is toxic to the body and causes the release of insulin, which promotes fat storage	Foods high in protein and fat; low glycemic index foods; olive oil, canola oil, and alcohol in moderation	Protein: 27% Carbohydrates: 52% Fat: 21% (saturated, 4%)	None	Potatoes, white rice, corn, carrots, beets, white bread, all refined white flour products	No long-term validated studies published	Eliminates many carbohydrate foods; discourages eating fruit with meals	Yes, by caloric restriction; limited food choices are not practical for the long term
Stillman¶	High-protein foods burn body fat; if carbohydrates are consumed, the body stores fat instead of burning it	Lean meats, skinless poultry, lean fish and seafood, eggs, cottage cheese, skim milk, cheeses	Protein: 64% Carbohydrates: 3% Fat: 33% (saturated, 13%)	Multivitamin and mineral supplement	All foods high in carbohydrates: bread, pasta, fruit, vegetables, fats, oils, dairy products, alcohol	No long-term validated studies published	Extreme limitations with regard to food choices; very little variety	Yes, but loss is mostly water; maintenance is based on strict calorie counting; very limited food choices are not practical for the long term
Zone 1-2-3 Program**	Eating the right combination of foods leads to a metabolic state at which the body functions at peak performance and stabilizes hormonal communication, thereby leading to decreased hunger, increased weight loss, increased energy, and increased control of cellular inflammation	Protein, fat, and carbohydrates in exact proportions only (40/30/30); alcohol in moderation	Protein: 34% Carbohydrates: 36% Fat: 29% (saturated, 9%) Alcohol: 1%	200 IU of vitamin E	Fruit (some types), saturated fats	No; theories and long-term results not validated	Food must be eaten in required proportions of protein, fat, and carbohydrates; menus are plain and unappealing; vegetable portions are very large; difficult to calculate portions	Yes, by caloric restriction; could result in weight maintenance if carefully followed; diet is rigid and difficult to maintain

*Atkins RC. Dr. Atkins' new diet revolution. New York: Avon Books; 1999.
†D'Adamo PJ, Whitney C. Eat right 4 your type. New York: Riverhead Books; 2002.
‡Eades MR, Eades MD. Protein power. New York: Bantam Books; 1996.
§Agatston A. The South Beach diet. Emmaus, Pa: Rodale Inc; 2003.
‖Steward HL, Bethea M, Andrews S, Balart LA. Sugar busters. New York: Ballantine Books; 1998.
¶Stillman IM, Baker SS. The doctor's quick weight loss diet. New York: Dell; 1967.
**Sears B. The zone. New York: HarperCollins; 1995.
Modified from St Jeor ST, Howard BV, Prewitt TE, et al. Nutrition Committee of the Council on Nutrition, Physical Activity, and Metabolism of the American Heart Association: Dietary protein and weight reduction: a statement for healthcare professionals from the Nutrition Committee of the Council on Nutrition, Physical Activity, and Metabolism of the American Heart Association. Circulation. 2001;104(15):1869-1874.

Clothing and Body Wraps. Special "sauna suits" and body wrapping have been claimed to help weight loss in certain body areas or to reduce cellulite tissue. Some people endure mummy-like body wrapping in an attempt to reduce body size. However, the resulting small weight loss is caused only by temporary water loss. Fat mass cannot be melted away without using the stored energy (i.e., burning the calories) in the adipocytes.

Drugs. Diuretics and exogenous hormones should never be used to alter body weight or lean tissue mass without strict medical indication and supervision. Various amphetamine compounds were once popular for the medical treatment of obesity, but they are no longer used because of their dangerous health consequences. Common over-the-counter drugs have included phenylpropylamine (Accu-trim, Dexatrim), which is a stimulant that is similar to amphetamine; and ephedra, which is currently banned in the United States. In addition, there are many herbs that claim weight-loss benefits. The U.S. Food and Drug Administration (FDA) keeps an updated list of contaminated and potentially dangerous over-the-counter drugs and supplements on its Web site at www.fda.gov/Drugs/ResourcesForYou/Consumers/default.htm.

A pair of related weight loss drugs—fenfluramine and phentermine—were prescribed to be used together in the popular "fen-phen" combination for weight loss. Shortly thereafter, physicians found that one in eight patients who were using fen-phen developed valvular regurgitation, which is a sometimes fatal condition.[40] The FDA, with the support of the medical community, quickly removed these drugs from the market in 1997. Likewise, in 2010, the FDA withdrew sibutramine (Meridia) from the U.S. market as a result of an increased risk of heart attack and stroke with its use. Sibutramine was another weight-loss medication that worked by increasing the heart rate and thus increasing energy expenditure. Although the pursuit of pharmacotherapy for the treatment of obesity is intense, few safe options are currently available.

Drugs that are used to treat obesity generally work in one of the following four ways:

1. Reducing energy intake by suppressing the appetite
2. Increasing energy expenditure by stimulating the BMR
3. Reducing the absorption of food in the gut
4. Altering lipogenesis and lipolysis

The FDA approved orlistat (Alli, Xenical) for the treatment of clinically significant obesity in 1999. Orlistat inhibits dietary fat absorption. Orlistat has been successful with weight loss, but reports indicate that maximal benefits occur only when it is combined with lifestyle changes that induce a negative energy balance.[41,42] As with many medications, unpleasant side effects are associated with this medication, including diarrhea, gas, and abdominal pain (see the Drug-Nutrient Interaction box, "Orlistat: An Over-The-Counter Weight-Loss Aid".

Surgery. Surgical techniques are usually reserved for the medical treatment of clinically severe obesity among patients who have not had success with other methods of long-term weight loss. Studies show that weight-loss surgery provides significant and sustained weight loss and a reduced relative risk of death as a result of a decrease in several conditions and comorbid diseases associated with obesity.[43,44] Although surgery historically has been the most successful method of permanent weight loss among patients with severe obesity, it is not without risks and complications.

Two types of surgical procedures are performed for weight loss: gastric restriction (i.e., making the stomach smaller) and combination procedures (i.e., making the stomach smaller and inducing malabsorption). Gastric restriction involves the creation of a small stomach pouch that is designed to reduce the space available for food in the stomach, thereby limiting appetite and eating (Figure 15-10, A and B). Adjustable gastric bands can be placed by laparoscopic surgery, and the band is subcutaneously adjusted as needed with the use of a small port. Malabsorptive procedures rearrange the small intestine to decrease the length and efficiency of the gut for nutrient absorption (Figure 15-10, C, D, and E).[45] Weight-loss surgeries require a skilled team of specialists, nutrition care, careful patient selection, and continuous follow-up in partnership with the patient and his or her family. The inherent risks of surgery and postsurgical malnutrition are critical issues that should be thoroughly addressed with the patient.

A more limited type of cosmetic surgery developed during the 1980s is a form of local fat removal, lipectomy, which is commonly called *liposuction*. Lipectomy removes fat deposits under the skin in places of cosmetic concern, such as the hips and thighs. A thin tube is inserted

---

adipocytes fat cells.

negative energy balance what occurs when more total energy is expended than consumed.

lipectomy the surgical removal of subcutaneous fat by suction through a tube that is inserted into a surface incision or by the removal of larger amounts of subcutaneous fat through a major surgical incision.

DRUG-NUTRIENT INTERACTION

ORLISTAT: AN OVER-THE-COUNTER WEIGHT-LOSS AID

In February 2007, the U.S. Food and Drug Administration approved the drug orlistat (Alli) as an over-the-counter weight-loss aid for overweight adults. When combined with a low-fat diet, the drug can be an effective adjunct to a weight-loss program. Orlistat works by inhibiting the absorption of fat in the intestine by up to 30%, thereby reducing the caloric impact of food.[1]

However, as a result of its mechanism of action, orlistat also inhibits the absorption of fat-soluble vitamins. A multivitamin taken at least 2 hours before or after a dose of orlistat is recommended to prevent the suboptimal absorption of vitamins A, D, E, and K. Even with vitamin supplementation, vitamin D and E absorption may be significantly decreased.[2]

In addition, orlistat can cause uncomfortable gastrointestinal side effects such as flatulence and loose stools. Eating large amounts of fat can increase these side effects, whereas fiber supplements that contain psyllium may help to reduce them.[3]

Orlistat is not approved for use by children who are younger than 18 years old, and it is contraindicated for people with absorptive disorders (e.g., pancreatitis, gall bladder disorders) and for those who are not overweight. Because this drug is now available over the counter, patients may take orlistat irresponsibly. It is important for clinicians to inquire about all medications and nutritional supplements that their patients are taking so that they may accurately advise these individuals about potential interactions and negative health consequences.

Kelli Boi

1. Halpern A, Mancini MC. Treatment of obesity: an update on anti-obesity medications. *Obes Rev.* 2003;4(1):25-42.
2. Filippatos TD, Derdemezis CS, Gazi IF, et al. Orlistat-associated adverse effects and drug interactions: a critical review. *Drug Saf.* 2008;31(1):53-65.
3. Cavaliere H, Floriano I, Medeiros-Neto G. Gastrointestinal side effects of orlistat may be prevented by concomitant prescription of natural fibers (psyllium mucilloid). *Int J Obes Relat Metab Disord.* 2001;25(7):1095-1099.

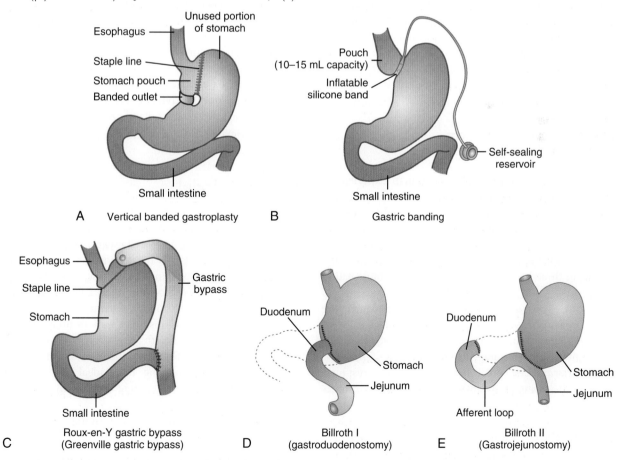

Figure 15-10 Surgical procedures for the treatment of clinically severe obesity (**A-E**). (Reprinted from Mahan LK, Escott-Stump S. *Krause's food & nutrition therapy.* 12th ed. Philadelphia: Saunders; 2008.)

through a small incision in the skin, and the desired amount of fat is suctioned away. This procedure can be quite painful, however, and it carries risks such as infection, large disfiguring skin depressions, and blood clots that can lead to dangerous circulatory problems or even kidney failure. Any surgical procedure carries risk and may cause other problems and side effects.

A SOUND WEIGHT-MANAGEMENT PROGRAM

Essential Characteristics

There are no shortcuts to successful weight control or weight loss. Weight loss requires hard work and strong individual motivation. Weight management requires a personalized program that focuses on changing lifestyle factors such as food and exercise behaviors. Choices that build a healthy mental and physical state with ample positive social support are desirable. The most recent position paper by the Academy of Nutrition and Dietetics regarding weight management makes note of the following: "A healthful lifestyle requires significant planning, proficiency in making appropriate choices and estimating portion sizes, and diligence in monitoring energy intake and activity, all of which take time to develop and maintain."[46]

Behavior Modification

Basic Principles

Food behavior is rooted in many human experiences. Behavior-oriented therapies are designed to help change patterns that contribute to excessive weight and that can help empower individuals to plan constructive actions to meet personal health goals. This behavioral approach must begin with a detailed examination of the following three basic aspects of each undesirable eating behavior:

1. *Cues or antecedents:* What stimulates the behavior?
2. *Response:* What happens during the eating or sedentary behavior after the cue?
3. *Consequences:* What happens after the response to the eating or sedentary behavior that reinforces it?

Basic Strategies and Actions

A program of personal behavior modification for weight management is directed toward the following: (1) the control of eating behavior (e.g., a food diary that includes when, where, why, how, and how much); (2) the promotion of physical activity to increase energy output; and (3) emotional, social, and psychologic health. Three progressive actions follow for the planning of individual strategies.

Defining Problem Behavior. Specifically define the problem behavior and the desired behavior outcome. This process clearly establishes goals and contributing objectives.

Recording and Analyzing Baseline Behavior. Record eating and exercise behavior, and carefully analyze it in terms of physical setting and people involved. What types of patterns emerge? How often do these patterns occur? What conditions seem to trigger desirable and undesirable behaviors? What consequent events seem to maintain the habits (e.g., time, place, people, social responses, hunger before and after, emotional mood, other factors)?

Planning a Behavior Management Strategy. Set up controls of the external environment that involve the situational forces related to each of the three behavior areas involved: (1) what occurs before the behavior; (2) the response to the behavior; and (3) the results of the behavior. The goal is to break the identified links to old and undesirable behaviors and to recondition them to the desired new eating and exercise behaviors. The Clinical Applications box entitled "Breaking Old Links: Strategies for Changing Food Behavior" provides a few examples of reconditioning personal food and exercise habits to more positive behaviors.

Dietary Principles

The central dietary approach in a weight-management program that may achieve a degree of lasting success must be based on the following five characteristics:

1. *Realistic goals:* Goals must be realistic in terms of overall weight loss and rate of loss, averaging $\frac{1}{2}$ to 1 lb per week (or no more than 2 lb per week for clinically severely obese patients). Even minor amounts of weight loss (i.e., 10% of body weight) can reduce the health risks that are associated with obesity.[46] Therefore, patients do not need to focus on achieving their ideal body weight but rather a relative weight loss on the basis of current weight.
2. *Negative energy balance:* The most important factor that affects weight loss is the establishment of a negative energy balance with a reduction of 500 to 1000 kcal/day.[46] The negative energy balance should

CLINICAL APPLICATIONS

BREAKING OLD LINKS: STRATEGIES FOR CHANGING FOOD BEHAVIOR

Old habits die hard. They are never easy to change, but the effort is worthwhile in the case of undesirable eating behaviors that contribute to excess body fat and that are thus harmful to health. Following are some behavioral suggestions.

1. Deal with Behavioral Cues
Minimize as many cues for the problem behavior as possible. Minimize situations that are associated with problem foods, put temptation out of reach, and make the problem behavior as difficult as possible to perform. Freeze leftovers, remove problem food items from the kitchen or store them in hard-to-reach places, and take a route home other than by the familiar bakery or candy shop.

Suppress the cues that cannot be entirely eliminated. Control social situations that maintain the behavior, reward the alternate desired behavior, have a trusted person monitor your eating patterns, reduce stress, minimize contact with excessive food, use smaller plates to make smaller food portions appear larger, and make use of positive nonfood "treat" activities (e.g., physical activity).

Strengthen cues for desirable behaviors. Follow the MyPlate guidelines and the *Dietary Guidelines for Americans* for appropriate food choices and amounts. Use food behavior aids (e.g., records, a diary or journal). Distribute appropriate foods among meal and snack patterns. Make desirable food behavior as attractive and as enjoyable as possible.

2. Deal with Actual Food Behavior in Response to Cues
Slow the pace of eating. Take one bite at a time, and place the utensil on the plate between bites. Chew each bite slowly. Sip a beverage. Consciously plan conversation with meal companions for between bites. Visualize eating in slow motion. Enhance the social aspect of eating.

Savor the food. Eat slowly, and sense the taste, smell, and texture of the food. Develop and practice these sensory feelings to the extent that they can be described and brought to mind afterward. Look for food seasonings and combinations that will enhance this process and bring to mind positive feelings about the food experience.

3. Deal with the Follow-up Behavior
Decelerate the problem behavior. Slow down its frequency, and respond neutrally when it occurs rather than with negative talk or thoughts. Give social reinforcement to the decreasing number of times that the problem behavior occurs. Acknowledge the ultimate consequences of the undesirable behavior in the development of health problems.

Accelerate the desired behavior. Update the progress records or personal journal daily. Respond positively to all desired behavior, and provide material reinforcement for positive behavior. Provide social reinforcement by enlisting the help of close friends or family for constructive efforts to modify behavior.

Such a program requires effort, motivation, and work. Continuously evaluate progress toward desired behavior while maintaining a realistic goal, and then plan individual or group maintenance and support activities during an extended follow-up period.

---

be achieved through a combination of reduced energy in and increased energy out.

3. *Nutritional adequacy:* The diet must be nutritionally adequate. Consuming less food requires conscious choices of nutrient-dense foods. In addition, the ratio of macronutrients should have an appropriate balance that is based on a wide variety of food sources.

4. *Cultural appeal:* The food plan must be similar enough to an individual's cultural eating patterns to form the basis for a permanent alteration of eating habits.

5. *Energy readjustment to maintain weight:* When the desired weight level is reached, the kilocalorie level is adjusted in accordance with maintenance needs.

Basic Energy Balance Components

The two sides of energy balance are energy intake in the form of food and drink and energy output in the form of metabolic work and physical activity. For successful weight reduction, both components must be addressed.

Energy Input: Food Behaviors

Clinicians should not assign arbitrary serving sizes and numbers of servings without knowledge of the patient's actual eating patterns. Food diaries are helpful for establishing what the patient's normal food choices are, the amounts typically eaten, and the distribution of meals throughout the day. From this baseline information, clinicians can help to identify minor changes to start with, such as eating smaller portions, replacing soda with water, and encouraging patients to eat slowly to savor the food's taste and to improve satiety.[46,47] Whole foods should be emphasized and processed foods minimized. Ideally, meals should be evenly distributed throughout the day. The use of fat, sugar, salt, and fiber should be quantified and modified, if necessary, to meet the *Dietary Guidelines for Americans, 2010.* Table 15-3 provides suggested servings of the food groups and subgroups to meet recommended nutrient intakes. These guides can serve as a focal point for sound nutrition education. Some additional suggestions are provided in the Clinical Applications box, "Practical Suggestions for Changing Food Behaviors."

Energy Output: Exercise Behaviors

Energy output in physical activity must be increased relative to normal activity. For someone who has no planned physical activity, a regular daily exercise schedule that starts with simple walking for approximately a half hour each day and building up to a brisk pace is a great way to begin. Some form of aerobic exercise (e.g., swimming, running, biking) or resistance exercise should be added (see the For Further Focus box, "Benefits of Aerobic Exercise in Weight Management"). An exercise class may be helpful to maintain motivation. Encourage patients to experiment with various activities until they find one that they enjoy and that they feel they can maintain for the long term. Following are current recommendations by the *Dietary Guidelines for Americans, 2010,* regarding exercise and weight maintenance or weight loss[48]:

- Prevent or reduce overweight and obesity through improved eating and physical activity behaviors.
- Increase physical activity and reduce time spent in sedentary behaviors.

Specific physical activity recommendations are discussed in greater detail in Chapter 16.

Principles of a Sound Food Plan

A careful diet history (see Chapter 17) can be the basis for a sound personalized food plan and should involve the principles of energy and nutrition balance, distribution balance and portion control, a food guide, and a preventive approach.

Energy Balance

Under normal circumstances, when energy expenditure is greater than energy intake, weight loss occurs. Because 1 lb of fat is equal to approximately 3500 kcal, an energy deficit of 500 kcal/day results in a weight loss of about 1 lb per week; a deficit of 250 kcal equals a ½-lb weight loss per week (see Box 15-2). All people who are pursuing weight loss should determine their current total energy needs as a basis for diet planning (Box 15-3). Modifications to energy intake and energy output can then be adjusted to produce a negative energy balance. As discussed throughout this text, individual energy needs vary greatly. Therefore, assuming that all people on a weight-loss program should limit caloric intake to 1400 kcal/day (or any other prefabricated amount) is not appropriate. For a person who normally consumes 2000 kcal/day, the ideal scenario is a deficit of approximately 500 kcal/day. The total of those 500 kcal should not all come from diet. Reducing calorie intake by 25% (2000 × 25% = 500 kcal) would undoubtedly leave a person hungry and constantly thinking about food. Instead, the weight-loss program could include a 250-kcal reduction in energy intake and a 250-kcal increase in energy expenditure for a total deficit of 500 kcal (see the Clinical Applications box, "Case Study: John's Energy Balance and Weight-Management Plan.")

Nutrient Balance

Basic energy nutrients are outlined in the diet to achieve the following nutrient balance:

- *Carbohydrate:* Approximately 45% to 65% of the total kilocalories, with emphasis on complex forms such as starch with fiber and a limit on simple sugars
- *Protein:* Approximately 10% to 35% of the total kilocalories, with emphasis on lean foods and small portions

---

BOX 15-3 **ESTIMATION OF ADULT ENERGY NEEDS**

Mifflin-St. Jeor Equation
Men:
Total Energy Expenditure (kcal/day) = (Weight [kg] × 10 + Height [cm] × 6.25 − Age × 5 − 5) × Physical activity coefficient

Women:
Total Energy Expenditure (kcal/day) = (Weight [kg] × 10 + Height [cm] × 6.25 − Age × 5 − 161) × Physical activity coefficient

Physical Activity Coefficient:
1.200 = Sedentary (little or no exercise)
1.375 = Lightly active (light exercise or sports 1 to 3 days per week)
1.550 = Moderately active (moderate exercise or sports 3 to 5 days per week)
1.725 = Very active (hard exercise or sports 6 to 7 days per week)
1.900 = Extra active (very hard exercise or sports and physical job)

TABLE 15-3   **U.S. DEPARTMENT OF AGRICULTURE FOOD PATTERNS**

For each food group or subgroup,[a] recommended average daily intake amounts[b] at all calorie levels. Recommended intakes from vegetable and protein foods subgroups are per week. For more information and tools for application, go to MyPlate.gov.

Calorie level of pattern[c]	1,000	1,200	1,400	1,600	1,800	2,000	2,200	2,400	2,600	2,800	3,000	3,200
Fruits	1 c	1 c	1½ c	1½ c	1½ c	2 c	2 c	2 c	2 c	2½ c	2½ c	2½ c
Vegetables[d]	1 c	1½ c	1½ c	2 c	2½ c	2½ c	3 c	3 c	3½ c	3½ c	4 c	4 c
Dark-green vegetables	½ c/wk	1 c/wk	1 c/wk	1½ c/wk	1½ c/wk	1½ c/wk	2 c/wk	2 c/wk	2½ c/wk	2½ c/wk	2½ c/wk	2½ c/wk
Red and orange vegetables	2½ c/wk	3 c/wk	3 c/wk	4 c/wk	5½ c/wk	5½ c/wk	6 c/wk	6 c/wk	7 c/wk	7 c/wk	7½ c/wk	7½ c/wk
Beans and peas (legumes)	½ c/wk	½ c/wk	½ c/wk	1 c/wk	1½ c/wk	1½ c/wk	2 c/wk	2 c/wk	2½ c/wk	2½ c/wk	3 c/wk	3 c/wk
Starchy vegetables	2 c/wk	3½ c/wk	3½ c/wk	4 c/wk	5 c/wk	5 c/wk	6 c/wk	6 c/wk	7 c/wk	7 c/wk	8 c/wk	8 c/wk
Other vegetables	1½ c/wk	2½ c/wk	2½ c/wk	3½ c/wk	4 c/wk	4 c/wk	5 c/wk	5 c/wk	5½ c/wk	5½ c/wk	7 c/wk	7 c/wk
Grains[e]	3 oz-eq	4 oz-eq	5 oz-eq	5 oz-eq	6 oz-eq	6 oz-eq	7 oz-eq	8 oz-eq	9 oz-eq	10 oz-eq	10 oz-eq	10 oz-eq
Whole grains	1½ oz-eq	2 oz-eq	2½ oz-eq	3 oz-eq	3 oz-eq	3 oz-eq	3½ oz-eq	4 oz-eq	4½ oz-eq	5 oz-eq	5 oz-eq	5 oz-eq
Enriched grains	1½ oz-eq	2 oz-eq	2½ oz-eq	2 oz-eq	3 oz-eq	3 oz-eq	3½ oz-eq	4 oz-eq	4½ oz-eq	5 oz-eq	5 oz-eq	5 oz-eq
Protein foods[d]	2 oz-eq	3 oz-eq	4 oz-eq	5 oz-eq	5 oz-eq	5½ oz-eq	6 oz-eq	6½ oz-eq	6½ oz-eq	7 oz-eq	7 oz-eq	7 oz-eq
Seafood	3 oz/wk	5 oz/wk	6 oz/wk	8 oz/wk	8 oz/wk	8 oz/wk	9 oz/wk	10 oz/wk	10 oz/wk	11 oz/wk	11 oz/wk	11 oz/wk
Meat, poultry, eggs	10 oz/wk	14 oz/wk	19 oz/wk	24 oz/wk	24 oz/wk	26 oz/wk	29 oz/wk	31 oz/wk	31 oz/wk	34 oz/wk	34 oz/wk	34 oz/wk
Nuts, seeds, soy products	1 oz/wk	2 oz/wk	3 oz/wk	4 oz/wk	4 oz/wk	4 oz/wk	4 oz/wk	5 oz/wk	5 oz/wk	5 oz/wk	5 oz/wk	5 oz/wk
Dairy[f]	2 c	2½ c	2½ c	3 c	3 c	3 c	3 c	3 c	3 c	3 c	3 c	3 c
Oils[g]	15 g	17 g	17 g	22 g	24 g	27 g	29 g	31 g	34 g	36 g	44 g	51 g
Maximum SoFAS[h] **limit, calories (% of calories)**	137 (14%)	121 (10%)	121 (9%)	121 (8%)	161 (9%)	258 (13%)	266 (12%)	330 (14%)	362 (14%)	395 (14%)	459 (15%)	596 (19%)

[a]All foods are assumed to be in nutrient-dense forms, lean or low-fat and prepared without added fats, sugars, or salt. Solid fats and added sugars may be included up to the daily maximum limit identified in the table. Food items in each group and subgroup are:

Fruits	All fresh, frozen, canned, and dried fruits and fruit juices: for example, oranges and orange juice, apples and apple juice, bananas, grapes, melons, berries, raisins.
Vegetables	
■ Dark-green vegetables	All fresh, frozen, and canned dark-green leafy vegetables and broccoli, cooked or raw: for example, broccoli; spinach; romaine; collard, turnip, and mustard greens.
■ Red and orange vegetables	All fresh, frozen, and canned red and orange vegetables, cooked or raw: for example, tomatoes, red peppers, carrots, sweet potatoes, winter squash, and pumpkin.
■ Beans and peas (legumes)	All cooked beans and peas: for example, kidney beans, lentils, chickpeas, and pinto beans. Does not include green beans or green peas. (See additional comment under protein foods group.)
■ Starchy vegetables	All fresh, frozen, and canned starchy vegetables: for example, white potatoes, corn, green peas.
■ Other vegetables	All fresh, frozen, and canned other vegetables, cooked or raw: for example, iceberg lettuce, green beans, and onions.
Grains	
■ Whole grains	All whole-grain products and whole grains used as ingredients: for example, whole-wheat bread, whole-grain cereals and crackers, oatmeal, and brown rice.
■ Enriched grains	All enriched refined-grain products and enriched refined grains used as ingredients: for example, white breads, enriched grain cereals and crackers, enriched pasta, white rice.
Protein foods	All meat, poultry, seafood, eggs, nuts, seeds, and processed soy products. Meat and poultry should be lean or low-fat and nuts should be unsalted. Beans and peas are considered part of this group as well as the vegetable group, but should be counted in one group only.
Dairy	All milks, including lactose-free and lactose-reduced products and fortified soy beverages, yogurts, frozen yogurts, dairy desserts, and cheeses. Most choices should be fat-free or low-fat. Cream, sour cream, and cream cheese are not included because of their low calcium content.

[b]Food group amounts are shown in cup (c) or ounce-equivalents (oz-eq). Oils are shown in grams (g). Quantity equivalents for each food group are:
- Grains, 1 ounce-equivalent is: 1 one-ounce slice bread; 1 ounce uncooked pasta or rice; ½ cup cooked rice, pasta, or cereal; 1 tortilla (6″ diameter); 1 pancake (5″ diameter); 1 ounce ready-to-eat cereal (about 1 cup cereal flakes).
- Vegetables and fruits, 1 cup-equivalent is: 1 cup raw or cooked vegetable or fruit; ½ cup dried vegetable or fruit; 1 cup vegetable or fruit juice; 2 cups leafy salad greens.
- Protein foods, 1 ounce-equivalent is: 1 ounce lean meat, poultry, seafood; 1 egg; 1 Tbsp peanut butter; ½ ounce nuts or seeds. Also, ¼ cup cooked beans or peas may be counted as 1 ounce-equivalent.
- Dairy, 1 cup equivalent is: 1 cup milk, fortified soy beverage, or yogurt; 1½ ounces natural cheese (e.g., cheddar); 2 ounces of processed cheese (e.g., American).

[c]See the Dietary Guidelines for Americans, 2010 for estimated calorie needs per day by age, gender, and physical activity level. Food intake patterns at 1,000, 1,200, and 1,400 calories meet the nutritional needs of children ages 2 to 8 years. Patterns from 1,600 to 3,200 calories meet the nutritional needs of children ages 9 years and older and adults. If a child aged 4 to 8 years needs more calories and, therefore, is following a pattern at 1,600 calories or more, the recommended amount from the dairy group can be 2½ cups per day. Children aged 9 years and older and adults should not use the 1,000, 1,200, or 1,400 calorie patterns.

[d]Whole-grain and protein foods subgroup amounts are shown in this table as weekly amounts, because it would be difficult for consumers to select foods from all subgroups daily.

[e]Whole-grain subgroup amounts shown in this table are minimums. More whole grains up to all of the grains recommended may be selected, with offsetting decreases in the amounts of enriched refined grains.

[f]The amount of dairy foods in the 1,200 and 1,400 calorie patterns have increased to reflect new Recommended Dietary Allowances for calcium that are higher than previous recommendations for children aged 4 to 8 years.

[g]Oils and soft margarines include vegetable, nut, and fish oils and soft vegetable oil table spreads that have no *trans* fats.

[h]SoFAS are calories from solid fats and added sugars. The limit for SoFAS is the remaining amount of calories in each food group after selecting the specified amounts in each food group in nutrient-dense forms (forms that are fat-free or low-fat and with no added sugars). The number of SoFAS is lower in the 1,200, 1,400, and 1,600 calorie patterns than in the 1,000 calorie pattern. The nutrient goals for the 1,200 to 1,600 calorie patterns are higher and require that more calories be used for nutrient-dense foods from the food groups.

U.S. Department of Agriculture and U.S. Department of Health and Human Services, *Dietary Guidelines for Americans*, 2010. Washington, DC: U.S. Government Printing Office; 2010.

CLINICAL APPLICATIONS

PRACTICAL SUGGESTIONS FOR CHANGING FOOD BEHAVIORS

Goals

Be realistic. Do not set your goals too high. Adapt your rate of loss to equal ½ lb to 2 lb per week.

Kilocalories

Do not be an obsessive calorie counter. Instead, become familiar with food exchanges in your diet list, learn the general values of some of your home-prepared meals, and then modify recipes or make occasional substitutes.

Plateaus

Anticipate plateaus; they happen to everyone. As the body adjusts to a new energy balance, lean-to-fat body mass ratio, and metabolic rate, weight loss rates can slow down. Increase exercise during these periods to help get started again.

Binges

Do not be discouraged if you binge. Individuals who have previously struggled with binge eating behavior may have an occasional setback. Try to keep these binges infrequent and, when possible, plan ahead for special occasions. Adjust the following day's diet or the remainder of the same day accordingly. Changing binge eating behavior is not easy. The assistance of a psychologic and nutritional expert may be helpful.

Special Diet Foods

Purchasing special low-calorie foods is not necessary. Learn to read labels carefully. Most special diet foods are expensive foods that are not much lower in kilocalories than regular foods. All foods can fit into a diet plan, with moderation. The amount of kilocalories and fat should be chosen within the context of the overall diet.

Home Meals

Try to avoid making a separate menu for yourself (or another person on a weight-loss program). Adapt your needs to the family meal, and then adjust the seasonings or method of preparation to involve fewer kilocalories, especially by reducing or omitting fat.

Eating Away From Home

Watch your portions. When you are a guest, limit extras such as sauces and dressings, and trim your meat well. In restaurants, select singly prepared items rather than combination dishes. Avoid items with heavy sauces or fat seasonings as well as fried foods. Select fruit or sherbet for dessert rather than pastries.

Appetite Control

Avoid dependence on appetite-depressant medications, which typically are only crutches. Try nibbling on food items from the free food list, or save other meal items, such as fruit or bread exchanges, for use between meals.

Meal Pattern

Eat three or more meals a day. If snacks between meals help you, then plan part of your day's allowance to account for them. The point is to spread your daily energy allowance throughout the day. Avoid the common pattern of no breakfast, little or no lunch, and a huge dinner.

FOR FURTHER FOCUS

BENEFITS OF AEROBIC EXERCISE IN WEIGHT MANAGEMENT

The goal of weight management is to reduce excess body fat and, in most cases, build lean body mass (muscle). However, both tissues may be lost when a person tries to reach a weight goal merely by reducing food intake.

Optimal body composition can be achieved by combining food restriction with aerobic exercise. Aerobic exercise consists of activities sustained long enough to draw on the body's fat reserve for fuel while oxygen intake is increased (thus the term *aerobic*). Lean body tissue burns fats in the presence of oxygen. Therefore aerobic activity is best suited for achieving the ideal balance of high lean body mass and low fatty tissue in the body.

The benefits of aerobic exercise to an overweight person in a weight management program include the following:

- Suppressed appetite
- Reduced total body fat
- Higher BMR
- Increased circulatory and respiratory function
- Increased energy expenditure
- Retention of tissue protein and building of lean body mass levels

Some individuals complain about the slow rate of weight loss, difficulty in controlling appetite, and consistent "flabbiness" despite continuing diet management. These individuals may welcome the suggestion of aerobic activity to help manage weight loss. Suggestions include a brisk daily walk, jumping rope, swimming, bicycling, jogging, running, aerobic or spinning classes, or another activity that increases the heart rate enough to have an aerobic effect and can be maintained for 20 to 30 minutes. Carefully note the physical stress this activity may place on individuals who have not exercised for some time or who have medical problems related to exertion. These individuals should have a medical checkup before beginning such a program on their own or joining a local gym or other community fitness center.

CLINICAL APPLICATIONS

CASE STUDY: JOHN'S ENERGY BALANCE AND WEIGHT-MANAGEMENT PLAN

John is a 21-year-old college student who leads a more or less sedentary life because of his classes and studying. He is interested in wrestling, however, and he wants to make the university team. To do so, he must lose some excess weight.

John begins to look carefully at his energy balance. He weighs 180 lb, and is 5 feet, 8 inches tall. John's average food intake is approximately 3000 kcal/day. He wants to lose weight in a healthy, long-term way by adjusting his energy balance.

Questions for Analysis
1. What are John's present daily total energy needs in kilocalories according to the Mifflin-St. Jeor equation?
2. How does this total energy need compare with his food energy intake?
3. To lose approximately 1 lb per week, how much should John reduce the caloric value of his daily diet?
4. In addition to reducing his dietary kilocalories, what else could John do to help create a negative energy balance and improve his body condition?

- *Fat:* 15% to 25% of the total kilocalories, with emphasis on minimal animal and trans fats, adequate essential fatty acids from plant foods, and alternate nonfat seasonings
- The food plan should meet the recommendations of the *Dietary Guidelines for Americans, 2010* (see Figure 1-4).

Distribution Balance and Portion Control

Spreading food fairly evenly throughout the day with four to five meals or snacks is advised.[46] Hunger usually peaks every 4 to 5 hours. If an individual has certain "problem times" of the day, planning simple snacks for those periods helps to maintain balance. Long periods without refueling can result in low blood sugar and subsequent periods of overeating, usually of whatever can be found at the time, which is often "junk foods" with empty calories from vending machines. Balanced meals require the foresight of planning and preparation.

Inappropriately large portion sizes continue to contribute to the energy intake imbalance for many Americans. Portion sizes and portion control are important factors in a sound food plan. Please see Chapter 14 for a discussion of portion control.

Food Guide

The Academy of Nutrition and Dietetics publishes the "Choose Your Foods: Weight Management" food exchange list (available from www.eatright.org) that follows the general *Dietary Guidelines for Americans.* This basic food exchange system is a good general reference guide for comparative food values and portions, variety in food choices, and basic meal planning. Table 15-3 provides examples of food plans that meet nutrient needs at 12 different calorie levels. A simple plan also can be outlined by using the food groups of the MyPlate guidelines (see Figure 1-3).

Preventive Approach

The most positive work with weight management is aimed at prevention. Current trends indicate that the U.S. population of children and adolescents continues to gain excess weight, and these overweight children are becoming obese adults. Major culprits in this health epidemic are inappropriate eating patterns and inadequate physical inactivity. Support for young parents and children before obesity develops can help to prevent many problems later in adulthood. This support and guidance should include early nutrition counseling and education, which can help to build positive health habits, especially in the forms of positive eating behaviors and increased exercise through active play and physical activities for the entire family. Many programs for young children—such as Head Start, school lunch programs, and the Special Supplemental nutrition Program for Women, Infants and Children (WIC) program (see Chapter 13)—address obesity issues through education and prevention for both parents and children.

FOOD MISINFORMATION AND FADS

A fad is any popular fashion or pursuit that is embraced with fervor. Food fads are scientifically unsubstantiated beliefs about certain foods that may persist for a short time in a given community or society. The word *fallacy* means "a deceptive, misleading, or false notion or belief." Food fallacies are false or misleading beliefs that underlie food fads. The jargon term *quack* is a shortened form of *quicksalver,* a term that was invented centuries ago by the Dutch to describe the pseudophysician or pseudoprofessor who sold worthless salves, magic elixirs, and cure-all tonics. He proclaimed his wares in a patter that skeptical people compared with the quacking of a duck. In medicine, nutrition, and allied health fields, a quack is a fraudulent pretender who claims to have skill, knowledge, or qualifications that he or she does not truly possess. The motive for such quackery is usually money, and the quack uses a hoax to feed on the physical and emotional needs of his or her victims.

Unscientific statements about food often mislead consumers and contribute to poor food habits. False information may come from folklore or fraud. Food choices should be based on sound scientific knowledge from responsible authorities; misinformation should be recognized as such.

Food Fads

Types of Claims

Food faddists make exaggerated claims about certain types of food. These claims generally fall into the following four basic groups:

1. *Food cures:* Certain foods cure specific conditions.
2. *Harmful foods:* Certain foods are harmful and should be omitted from the diet.
3. *Food combinations:* Special food combinations restore health and are effective for reducing weight.
4. *Natural foods:* Only "natural" foods can meet body needs and prevent disease. The term *natural* may be used on unprocessed or minimally processed products that contain no artificial ingredients, coloring ingredients, or chemical preservatives. Some people consider all processed foods unhealthy, including those that are enriched or fortified.

Erroneous Claims

Claims that are simply erroneous require careful examination. On the surface, they seem to be simple statements about food and health. However, further observation reveals that they focus on a food itself and not on the specific nutrients that are in the food, which are the actual physiologic agents of life and health. Some individuals may be allergic to specific foods and obviously should avoid them. In addition, certain foods may supply relatively large amounts of individual nutrients and therefore are good sources of those nutrients. However, the nutrients—and not the whole foods themselves—have specific functions in the body. Each nutrient is found in a wide variety of different foods. Remember that people require specific nutrients and not necessarily specific foods.

Dangers

Why should health care workers be concerned about food fads and their effect on food habits? What harm do food fads cause? Food fads generally involve four possible negative effects.

Danger to Health. Responsibility for one's health is fundamental. Self-diagnosis and self-treatment can be dangerous, however, especially when such action follows questionable sources. By following such a course, people with real illness may fail to seek appropriate medical care. Many ill and anxious people have been misled by fraudulent claims of cures and have postponed proven effective therapy.

Cost. Some foods and supplements used by faddists are harmless, but many are expensive. Money spent for useless items is wasted. When dollars are scarce, a family may neglect to buy foods that fill basic needs in an attempt to purchase a "miracle cure."

Lack of Sound Knowledge. Misinformation hinders the development of individuals and society and ignores scientific progress. The perpetuation of certain superstitions can counteract sound teaching about health.

Distrust of the Food Market. America's food environment is changing. People should be watchful, but a blanket rejection of all modern food production is unwarranted. People must develop intelligent concerns and rational approaches to meet their nutrition needs.

What Is the Answer?

What can be done to counter food habits that are associated with food fads, misinformation, or even outright deception? Helpful instruction is based on personal conviction, practice, and enthusiasm. The following approaches to positive teaching can then be used.

Using Reliable Sources

Sound background knowledge is essential and should include the following:

1. Knowing the product being pushed and the people or company behind it
2. Knowing how human physiology and biochemistry work
3. Knowing the scientific method of problem solving (e.g., collect the facts, identify the problem, determine a reasonable solution or action, carry it out, and evaluate the results)

Sound community resources include the following:

- Extension educators work in the community through state and county Extension Service offices and direct highly successful community nutrition activities, such as their Expanded Food and Nutrition Education Program. These specialists develop many food and nutrition guides, especially for those with limited education or who speak English as a second language. Information about the program can be found at www.csrees.usda.gov/nea/food/efnep/efnep.html.

- The FDA and U.S. Department of Agriculture (USDA) produce many educational materials related to food and nutrition (see Chapter 13). Requests for these mostly free materials can be directed to FDA and USDA agency offices.
- "Cultural and Ethnic Food and Nutrition Education Materials: A Resource List for Educators" is provided by the USDA at www.nal.usda.gov/fnic/pubs/bibs/gen/ethnic.html.
- Public health nutritionists located in county and state public health offices and as part of special programs (e.g., WIC) can provide information. WIC state agencies are listed at www.fns.usda.gov/wic/Contacts/statealpha.htm.
- Registered dietitians in local medical care centers and those who serve hospitalized patients, outpatient clinics, and others in private practice also are valuable resources. The Academy of Nutrition and Dietetics nationwide nutrition network can be accessed at www.eatright.org/programs/rdfinder/.

Recognizing Human Needs

Consider the emotional needs that food and food rituals help to fulfill. These needs are a part of life, and they should be used in a positive way in nutrition teaching. Even if a person is using food as an emotional crutch, the emotional need is still real. Never take away crutches without offering a better and wiser form of support. Food and all the associations that go along with it compose a basic enjoyment of life. Maintaining a balance between food as entertainment and food as fuel is the challenge of identifying what human needs are being met by certain foods. The establishment of a healthy diet must consider all such human needs; it may involve specialized help, such as that provided by behavioral therapists.

Remaining Alert to Teaching Opportunities

Use any opportunity that arises to present sound nutrition and health information, whether formally or informally. Learn about the available resources described previously. Develop communication skills, avoid monotony, and use a well-disciplined imagination.

Thinking Scientifically

Even very young children can be taught to use the problem-solving approach to everyday situations. Children are naturally curious. With their eternal

---

BOX 15-4 THE FOOD AND NUTRITION SCIENCE ALLIANCE'S 10 RED FLAGS OF JUNK SCIENCE

1. Recommendations that promise a quick fix
2. Dire warnings of danger from a single product or regimen
3. Claims that sound too good to be true
4. Simplistic conclusions drawn from a complex study
5. Recommendations based on a single study
6. Dramatic statements that are refuted by reputable scientific organizations
7. Lists of "good" and "bad" foods
8. Recommendations made to help sell a product
9. Recommendations based on studies published without peer review
10. Recommendations from studies that ignore differences among individuals or groups

Reprinted from the Food and Nutrition Science Alliance (FANSA): *10 red flags of junk science,* Chicago: Food and Nutrition Science Alliance; 1995.

---

questioning—"Why?"—they often seek evidence to support the statements that they hear. Three basic questions help with the evaluation of claims in any situation: (1) "What do you mean?"; (2) "How do you know?"; and (3) "What is your evidence?"

The Food and Nutrition Science Alliance is a partnership of seven professional scientific societies that have joined together to disseminate sound nutrition information. This organization issued a list of 10 red flags to help guide consumers toward making educated decisions about nutrition and health issues (Box 15-4). This list is an excellent guide when evaluating reports and claims about various diets, supplements, and other nutrition-related fads.

Knowing Responsible Authorities

The FDA is legally responsible for controlling the quality and safety of food and drug products marketed in the United States. However, this is a tremendous task that requires public help. Other government, professional, and private organizations can provide additional resources (see the Further Reading and Resources list at the end of the chapter).

UNDERWEIGHT

General Causes and Treatment

Extremes in underweight—just as in overweight—can pose health problems. Although general malnutrition and excessive thinness is a less-common problem in the U.S. population than overweight, it does occur, and it is usually associated with poor living conditions or long-term disease. A person who is more than 10% below the average weight for height and age is considered underweight; someone who is 20% or more below the average weight has cause for significant health concerns. Physiologic and psychologic effects may occur, especially among young children. Their resistance to infection is lowered, their general health is poor, and their strength is reduced.

Causes

Underweight is associated with conditions that cause general malnutrition, including the following:

- *Wasting disease:* long-term disease with chronic infection and fever that raise the BMR
- *Poor food intake:* diminished food intake that results from psychologic factors that cause a person to refuse to eat, loss of appetite, or personal poverty and limited available food supply
- *Malabsorption:* poor nutrient absorption that results from chronic diarrhea, a diseased gastrointestinal tract, the excessive use of laxatives, or drug-nutrient interactions
- *Hormonal imbalance:* hyperthyroidism or a variety of other hormonal imbalances that increase the caloric needs of the body
- *Energy imbalance:* condition that results from greatly increased physical activity without a corresponding increase in food or a lack of available food supply
- *Poor living situation:* an unhealthy home environment that results in irregular and inadequate meals, where eating is considered unimportant, and where an indifferent attitude toward food exists

Dietary Treatment

Special nutrition care to rebuild body tissues and to regain health is necessary for underweight and undernourished patients. Food plans should be adapted to each person's unique situation, whether it involves his or her personal needs, living situation, economic needs, or any underlying disease. The dietary goal, in accordance with each person's tolerance, is to increase energy and nutrient intake, with adherence to the following needs:

- *High-caloric diet:* above the standard requirement for that individual
- *High protein:* to rebuild tissues
- *High carbohydrate:* to provide the primary energy source in an easily digested form
- *Moderate fat:* to provide essential fatty acids and add energy without exceeding tolerance limits

- *Good sources of vitamins and minerals:* provided by a variety of nutrient-dense foods and dietary supplements when individual deficiencies require them

A variety of foods attractively served may help to revive the appetite and increase the desire to eat more. Nourishing meals and snacks should be spread throughout the day and should include favorite foods often. A basic aim is to help build good food habits so that improved nutritional status and weight can be maintained. Residents in long-term care facilities are especially vulnerable to weight-loss problems, and they have special needs (see the Clinical Applications box, "Problems of Weight Loss among Older Adults in Long-Term Care Facilities"). In addition, several medications that are often prescribed to elderly individuals may result in anorexia or weight loss. This rehabilitation process requires creative counseling for the patient and the family along with practical guides and support. In some cases, tube feeding or intravenous feeding (e.g., total parenteral nutrition) may be necessary (see Chapter 22).

Ideal weight gain includes both lean and fat tissue. To gain muscle, physical exercise must be part of the treatment. Resistance training increases lean tissue and, in turn, boosts appetite. A variety of weight-lifting and strength-training programs can be designed, depending on the desires of the individual, and they should be encouraged as an important part of healthy weight gain.

Disordered Eating

To discuss disordered or abnormal eating, we must first define "normal eating". Normal eating is when an individual is capable of the following:

- Eating when he or she is hungry and stopping when full
- Demonstrating moderate restraint with regard to food selection
- Recognizing that overeating and undereating are sometimes acceptable and trusting his or her body to establish a balance
- Having the ability to be flexible with his or her eating schedule

Disordered eating is defined as any eating pattern that is not normal, and it can include a variety of subclinical problems. Disordered eating can range from an insurmountable fear of eating fat to an inability to eat in public. Family and personal tensions as well as social pressures for thinness may result in serious body image disturbances and eating problems that push the disordered

PROBLEMS OF WEIGHT LOSS AMONG OLDER ADULTS IN LONG-TERM CARE FACILITIES

The American population of adults who are 65 years old and older is rapidly increasing. The most rapid population increase over the next decade will be among those who are older than 85 years old, and many of these elderly people will require long-term care in nursing homes.

One of the problems that is encountered among elderly residents is low body weight and rapid unintentional weight loss. These conditions can become serious health problems, and they are a sensitive indicator of malnutrition that can contribute to illness and death. Because weight loss is such a strong predictor of morbidity and mortality in clinical settings, early and continuing observation to assess needs is important, especially in relation to factors that contribute to weight loss.

In general, weight loss in this population can be caused by the following: (1) the physical effects of the metabolic changes of aging; (2) the physical effects of disease; or (3) certain factors that alter the amount and type of food eaten. Physical disease (e.g., cancer) can cause extreme weight loss as a result of metabolic abnormalities, taste changes, loss of appetite, nausea, and vomiting. Other diseases that affect weight include gastrointestinal problems; uncontrolled diabetes; cardiovascular disorders (e.g., congestive heart failure); pulmonary disease; infection; and alcoholism. Psychologic factors or psychiatric disorders may also contribute to malnutrition and weight loss from depression, memory loss, disorientation, apathy, and appetite disturbance. Some altered mental states may be caused by nutritional deficiencies (e.g., low levels of folate and B-complex vitamins) as well as by protein energy malnutrition. These conditions can be corrected with specific nutritional support.

The following additional physiologic, psychologic, and social factors may influence food intake and body weight and thus contribute to malnutrition among elderly people:

- *Body composition changes:* Height and body weight gradually decline as people age. Body weight usually peaks between the ages of 34 and 54 years in men and 55 and 75 years in women, and it decreases thereafter. Body fat losses are generally not significant. One cause of weight loss is a decline in body water, which is caused in part by the weakening of the normal thirst mechanism. Therefore, a feeling of thirst cannot be relied upon to secure adequate water intake, so water must frequently be offered and encouraged. More constant attention to fluid intake also helps with the common problem of xerostomia (i.e., dry mouth) in older adults. Xerostomia results from inadequate salivary secretions, which makes eating difficult, thereby contributing to malnutrition. Lean body mass also declines with age, and this results in a lower basal metabolic rate and decreased physical activity and energy requirements. Thus, any possible increase in physical activity and the use of nutrient-dense foods are encouraged.
- *Taste changes:* The regeneration of taste bud cells slows with age, but the extent and effect on food intake vary widely. The sense of smell also declines with age and may negatively affect taste. The

increased use of appropriate seasoning and flavoring in food preparation is needed.
- *Dentition:* About half of Americans have lost some or all of their teeth by the age of 65 years. Many have dentures, but chewing problems are often present. Nursing home residents frequently report chewing, biting, and swallowing problems that interfere with eating and adequate food intake. The assessment of specific needs and dental care solutions helps to correct eating problems.
- *Gastrointestinal problems:* Delayed gastric emptying may contribute to distention and lack of appetite. A decrease in gastric secretions, including hydrochloric acid, may hinder the absorption of vitamin B_{12}, folate, and iron, thereby contributing to anemia and a loss of appetite. Constipation is a common complaint that often leads to laxative abuse and that results in interference with nutrient absorption. An increase in dietary fiber, liquids, and physical activity can help to provide a more natural approach to establishing normal bowel movements.
- *Drug-nutrient interactions:* Elderly people often take a number of prescribed and over-the-counter drugs, some of which are the direct cause of anorexia, nausea, and vomiting. Other drugs are indirect causes in that they induce nutrient malabsorption; this leads to deficiencies that in turn cause anorexia and weight loss. Drug therapy for elderly patients should involve constant medical, nutrition, and nursing attention to ensure appropriate use.
- *Functional disabilities:* Eating problems can prevent or alter the capacity of elderly people to take in sufficient food. These problems may vary from more difficult functional disabilities that interfere with putting food into the mouth and swallowing (e.g., problems that often require a trained therapist) to dependence on feeding assistance that can be provided by sensitive nursing care.
- *Social problems:* Socioeconomic problems are often involved in the care of the elderly. A specially trained geriatric social worker can help to secure possible sources of financial assistance. A sense of social isolation can also lead to decreased food intake. Family support, sensitive contact with nursing home staff and residents, and as much involvement as possible in group activities are necessary.

Health care workers in geriatric settings need continuing education and sensitization to the potential dangers of low body weight and weight loss among their patients. Older individuals with acute and chronic illnesses and functional disabilities are at the greatest risk for nutrition-related problems. These people require continual nutrition assessment and the monitoring of their body weight. Some of the restrictions of "special diets" should be relaxed or discontinued when the risk of malnutrition is evident, with the goal of increasing nutrient intake and making eating as enjoyable as possible.

eating behavior to the point of becoming clinical eating disorders. The three most common eating disorders are anorexia nervosa, bulimia nervosa, and binge eating disorder (Box 15-5).

The most recent position paper from the Academy of Nutrition and Dietetics regarding eating disorders states that eating disorders are "medical illnesses with diagnostic criteria based on psychological, behavioral, and physiologic characteristics."[49] Mortality rates from eating disorders are significant compared with other psychologic diseases: 4.0% for anorexia nervosa, 3.9% for bulimia nervosa, and 5.2% for eating disorders not otherwise specified.[50] Eating disorders are secretive in nature; therefore, establishing a true estimate of population prevalence is difficult. However, research indicates that eating disorders occur less frequently among males than females and that homosexual and bisexual males are at higher risk than their heterosexual counterparts.[51]

Anorexia Nervosa

The estimated lifetime prevalence of anorexia nervosa is 0.9% in women and 0.3% in men.[52] This complex psychologic disorder results in self-imposed starvation. In addition to the diagnostic criteria provided in Box 15-5, Table 15-4 outlines the clinical signs that are associated with both anorexia nervosa and bulimia nervosa.

Risk factors for anorexia nervosa include the following[49]:

- Genetic predisposition
- Dieting behavior
- High level of exercise
- Body dysmorphic disorder
- Obsessive-compulsive disorder
- Acculturation
- Perfectionism
- Negative self-evaluation

All forms of eating disorders require an interdisciplinary team for treatment success. Nutrition therapy goals that are specific to anorexia nervosa are focused on restoring a healthy weight and normalizing eating patterns.

Bulimia Nervosa

The estimated lifetime prevalence of bulimia nervosa is 1.5% in women and 0.5% in men.[52] Bulimia is an eating disorder that involves repeated episodes of binge eating followed by one or more compensatory mechanisms to rid the body of excess calories. Compensatory mechanisms include self-induced vomiting, laxative abuse, strict dieting or fasting, and excessive exercise. What a binge consists of will vary among patients, but it generally involves the consumption of excessive quantities of food during a short period of time. Oral and dental problems from the purging behavior may involve oral mucosal irritation, decreased salivary secretions (xerostomia), and irreversible tooth enamel erosion. Table 15-4 provides other clinical signs of bulimia nervosa.

Individuals with bulimia nervosa often go unnoticed and undiagnosed compared with individuals with anorexia nervosa. Their body weights are generally within a normal range, but they may fluctuate. Risk factors for bulimia nervosa include the following[49]:

- Negative self-evaluation
- Parental influences such as comments about weight
- Parental obesity
- Childhood obesity
- High use of escape-avoidance coping
- Low perceived social support
- "All or none" perceptions about eating
- Impulsive personality

Nutrition therapy goals for patients with bulimia nervosa are focused on eliminating episodes of binging and purging.

Binge Eating Disorder

The estimated lifetime prevalence of binge eating disorder is 3.5% for women and 2.0% for men.[52] This eating disorder includes binging episodes without compensatory behaviors. This reactive type of eating often follows stress or anxiety as an emotional eating pattern to soothe or

anorexia nervosa an extreme psychophysiologic aversion to food that results in life-threatening weight loss; a psychiatric eating disorder that results from a morbid fear of fatness in which a person's distorted body image is reflected as fat when the body is malnourished and extremely thin as a result of self-starvation.

bulimia nervosa a psychiatric eating disorder related to a person's fear of fatness in which cycles of gorging on large quantities of food are followed by compensatory mechanisms (e.g., self-induced vomiting, the use of diuretics and laxatives) to maintain a "normal" body weight.

binge-eating disorder a psychiatric eating disorder that is characterized by the occurrence of binge eating episodes at least twice a week for a 6-month period.

eating disorders not otherwise specified subthreshold disordered eating that is not consistent with the diagnostic criteria for bulimia nervosa or anorexia nervosa (e.g., binge eating disorder)

body dysmorphic disorder an obsession with a perceived defect of the body.

BOX 15-5   AMERICAN PSYCHIATRIC ASSOCIATION DIAGNOSTIC CRITERIA

Anorexia Nervosa

A. Refusal to maintain body weight at or above a minimally normal weight for age and height (e.g., weight loss that leads to the maintenance of body weight of less than 85% of that expected or failure to make expected weight gain during period of growth that leads to body weight of less than 85% of that expected)

B. Intense fear of gaining weight or becoming fat even though underweight

C. Disturbance in the way in which one's body weight or shape is experienced; undue influence of body weight or shape on self-evaluation or denial of the seriousness of the current low body weight

D. In postmenarchal women, amenorrhea (i.e., the absence of at least three consecutive menstrual cycles)

   1. *Restricting type:* During the current episode of anorexia nervosa, the person has not regularly engaged in binge eating or purging behavior

   2. *Binge eating/purging type:* During the current episode of anorexia nervosa, the person has regularly engaged in binge eating and purging behavior

Bulimia Nervosa

A. Recurrent episodes of binge eating that are characterized by both of the following:

   1. Eating, during a discrete period of time (e.g., within any 2-hour period), an amount of food that is larger than most people would eat during a similar period of time and under similar circumstances

   2. A sense of a lack of control regarding eating during the episode (e.g., a feeling that one cannot stop eating or control what or how much one is eating)

B. Recurrent inappropriate compensatory behavior to prevent weight gain, such as self-induced vomiting; the misuse of laxatives, diuretics, enemas, or other medications; fasting; or excessive exercise

C. The binge eating and inappropriate compensatory behaviors both occur, on average, at least twice a week for 3 months

D. Self-evaluation is unduly influenced by body shape and weight

E. The disturbance does not occur exclusively during episodes of anorexia nervosa

   1. *Purging type:* During the current episode of bulimia nervosa, the person has regularly engaged in self-induced vomiting or the misuse of laxatives, diuretics, or enemas

   2. *Nonpurging type:* During the current episode of bulimia nervosa, the person has used other inappropriate compensatory behaviors (e.g., fasting, excessive exercise) but has not regularly engaged in self-induced vomiting or the misuse of laxatives, diuretics, or enemas

Eating Disorder Not Otherwise Specified

This category is for disorders of eating that do not meet the criteria for any specific eating disorder. For example:

A. For females, all of the criteria for anorexia nervosa are met except that the individual has regular menses

B. All of the criteria for anorexia nervosa are met except that, despite significant weight loss, the individual's current weight is within the normal range

C. All of the criteria for bulimia nervosa are met except that the binge eating and inappropriate compensatory mechanisms occur at a frequency of less than twice a week or for a duration of less than 3 months

D. The regular use of inappropriate compensatory behavior by an individual of normal body weight after eating small amounts of food

E. Repeatedly chewing and spitting out (but not swallowing) large amounts of food

Binge Eating Disorder

A. Recurrent episodes of binge eating that are characterized by the following:

   1. Eating a larger amount of food than normal during a short period of time (e.g., within any 2-hour period)

   2. Lack of control over eating during the binge episode (i.e., the feeling that one cannot stop eating)

B. Binge eating episodes are associated with three or more of the following:

   1. Eating until feeling uncomfortably full

   2. Eating large amounts of food when not physically hungry

   3. Eating much more rapidly than normal

   4. Eating alone because you are embarrassed by how much you are eating

   5. Feeling disgusted, depressed, or guilty after overeating

C. Marked distress regarding binge eating is present

D. Binge eating occurs, on average, at least 2 days a week for 6 months

E. The binge eating is not associated with the regular use of inappropriate compensatory behavior (e.g., purging, excessive exercise) and does not occur exclusively during the course of bulimia nervosa or anorexia nervosa

Modified from the American Psychiatric Association. *Diagnostic and statistical manual of mental disorders.* 4th ed. text revision, Washington, DC: American Psychological Association Press; 2000.

TABLE 15-4 **NUTRITION-RELATED CLINICAL SIGNS COMMONLY ASSOCIATED WITH ANOREXIA NERVOSA AND BULIMIA NERVOSA**

Clinical Signs	Anorexia Nervosa	Bulimia Nervosa
Electrolyte abnormalities	Hypokalemia with refeeding syndrome; hypomagnesemia; hypophosphatemia	Hypokalemia accompanied by hypochloremic alkalosis; hypomagnesemia
Cardiovascular effects	Hypotension; irregular, slow pulse; orthostasis; sinus bradycardia	Cardiac arrhythmias; palpitations; weakness
Gastrointestinal effects	Abdominal pain; bloating; constipation; delayed gastric emptying; feeling of fullness; vomiting	Constipation; delayed gastric emptying; dysmotility; early satiety; esophagitis; flatulence; gastroesophageal reflux disease; gastrointestinal bleeding
Endocrine imbalances—reproductive, metabolic	Cold sensitivity; diuresis; fatigue; hypercholesterolemia; hypoglycemia; menstrual irregularities	Menstrual irregularities; rebound fluid retention with edema
Nutrient deficiencies	Protein–energy malnutrition; various micronutrient deficiencies	Variable
Skeletal and dental effects	Bone pain with exercise; osteopenia; osteoporosis	Dental caries; erosion of the surface of the teeth
Muscular effects	Wasting; weakness	Weakness
Weight status	Underweight state	Variable
Cognitive status	Poor concentration	Poor concentration
Growth status	Arrested growth and maturation	Typically not affected

American Dietetic Association. Position of the American Dietetic Association: nutrition in the treatment of anorexia nervosa, bulimia nervosa, and other eating disorders. *J Am Diet Assoc.* 2006;106(12):2073-2082.

relieve painful or tense feelings. The binges may be triggered by psychologic factors that involve the self and the body image. Patients with binge eating disorder are most often overweight or obese. Risk factors for binge eating disorder include the following[49]:

- Repeated exposure to negative comments about shape, weight, and eating
- Negative self-evaluation
- Perfectionism
- Childhood obesity
- Low self-esteem
- High levels of body concern
- High use of escape-avoidance coping
- Low levels of perceived social support

Nutrition therapy goals for patients with binge eating disorder are focused on eliminating binge episodes and often involve psychotherapy, behavioral weight-loss treatment, and psychopharmacology.

Treatment

These psychologic disorders require therapy from a team of skilled professionals, including physicians, psychologists, and dietitians. Even with the best of care, recovery is slow, and the word *cure* is seldom used. Many patients with eating disorders have persistent food and weight preoccupations throughout their lives.

Patients with eating disorders often have neurologic disturbances. These chemical disturbances were first thought of as the cause of disordered eating behavior. However, researchers have found that, when a normal weight and eating pattern are reestablished in the patient, the neurologic chemistry returns to normal. Therefore, one of the first issues to address for the treatment of an eating disorder is establishing a healthy weight in the patient. Psychologic therapy is more successful when neurologic disturbances are reduced. Next, the team of professionals must work together to restore eating habits and attitudes toward food, to optimize physical and mental health, and to restore intrapersonal and interpersonal problems. Continuing support groups that include friends, family, and health care professionals are critical for long-term treatment.

SUMMARY

- In the traditional medical model, obesity has been viewed as an illness and a health hazard, which is true in cases of clinically severe obesity. Newer approaches view moderate overweight differently, however, in terms of the important aspects of fatness, leanness, and body composition, and they propose a more person-centered positive health model.

- Planning a weight-management program for either an overweight or underweight person must involve the metabolic and energy needs of the individual. Personal food choices and habits as well as fatty tissue needs during different stages of the life cycle must be considered.

- Important aspects of such a weight-reduction program include changing food behaviors and increasing physical activity. A sound program is based on reduced energy intake for gradual weight loss and nutrient balance, with meals distributed throughout the day for energy needs. The ideal plan begins with prevention and stresses the formation of positive food habits during early childhood to prevent major problems later in life.

- Food fads and misinformation are increasingly popular within all facets of American society. Identifying harmful practices and providing accurate information are basic functions of the health care provider.

- Excessive thinness is a cause for health concern. Malnutrition may result in underweight individuals for a variety of medical and psychologic reasons.

- Eating disorders require professional team therapy that includes medical, psychologic, and nutrition care.

CRITICAL THINKING QUESTIONS

1. Why is the term *ideal weight* difficult to define? Explain some of the problems with determining this measure. What role does it play in weight management?
2. What does *set point* mean with regard to individual weight? How does it relate to diet and exercise in a personal weight-management program?
3. Describe the components of a positive health model for weight management. What are the basic principles of a sound food plan for such a program?
4. Describe two major eating disorders that are associated with a growing obsession with thinness. What are the contributing social and psychologic factors? What is the treatment?
5. How does chronic dieting syndrome relate to and contribute to the prevalence of disordered eating?

CHAPTER CHALLENGE QUESTIONS

True-False
Write the correct statement for each statement that is false.
1. *True or False:* The development of childhood obesity results exclusively from genetic inheritance.
2. *True or False:* Increasing the energy expended during physical activity is a means of weight reduction.
3. *True or False:* A certain percentage of stored fat in the body is necessary for life.
4. *True or False:* A reasonable weight-reduction diet for an adult involves an energy deficit of approximately 500 kcal per day, depending on individual size and need.
5. *True or False:* A weight-reduction diet should not include between-meal snacks.
6. *True or False:* Food fads usually are long lasting and seldom change.

Multiple Choice

1. Overweight is a direct risk factor for which of the following conditions? *(Circle all that apply.)*
   a. Cancer
   b. Type 2 diabetes mellitus
   c. Arthritis
   d. Hypertension

2. A 500-kcal deficit in the daily energy expenditure of an obese person enables him or her to lose weight at approximately which of the following rates?
   a. 1 lb per week
   b. 2 lb per week
   c. 3 lb per week
   d. 4 lb per week

3. An individual who has repeated episodes of binging and purging, who expresses severe self-criticism, and who is often depressed may have which of the following conditions?
   a. Anorexia nervosa
   b. Bulimia nervosa
   c. Compulsive overeating
   d. None of the above

⊖volve **Please refer to the Students' Resource section of this text's Evolve Web site for additional study resources.**

REFERENCES

1. Ogden CL, Carroll MD. *Prevalence of overweight, obesity, and extreme obesity among adults: United States, trends 1976-1980 through 2007-2008, Division of Health and Nutrition Examination Surveys*. Atlanta: National Center for Health Statistics; 2010.
2. Ogden CL, Carroll MD. *Prevalence of obesity among children and adolescents: United States, trends 1963-1965 through 2007-2008, Division of Health and Nutrition Examination Surveys*. Atlanta: National Center for Health Statistics; 2010.
3. The NS, Suchindran C, North KE, et al. Association of adolescent obesity with risk of severe obesity in adulthood. *JAMA*. 2010;304(18):2042-2047.
4. Nader PR, O'Brien M, Houts R, et al; National Institute of Child Health and Human Development Early Child Care Research Network. Identifying risk for obesity in early childhood. *Pediatrics*. 2006;118(3):e594-e601.
5. Demura S, Sato S, Kitabayashi T. Estimation accuracy of percent total body fat and percent segmental fat measured by single-frequency bioelectrical impedance analysis with 8 electrodes: the effect of difference in adiposity. *J Sports Med Phys Fitness*. 2005;45(1):68-76.
6. Demura S, Sato S, Kitabayashi T. Percentage of total body fat as estimated by three automatic bioelectrical impedance analyzers. *J Physiol Anthropol Appl Human Sci*. 2004;23(3):93-99.
7. Kriemler S, Puder J, Zahner L, et al. Cross-validation of bioelectrical impedance analysis for the assessment of body composition in a representative sample of 6- to 13-year-old children. *Eur J Clin Nutr*. 2009;63(5):619-626.
8. Wang Z, Heymsfield SB, Chen Z, et al. Estimation of percentage body fat by dual-energy x-ray absorptiometry: evaluation by in vivo human elemental composition. *Phys Med Biol*. 2010;55(9):2619-2635.
9. Ittenbach RF, Buison AM, Stallings VA, Zemel BS. Statistical validation of air-displacement plethysmography for body composition assessment in children. *Ann Hum Biol*. 2006;33(2):187-201.
10. Silva AM, Minderico CS, Teixeira PJ, et al. Body fat measurement in adolescent athletes: multicompartment molecular model comparison. *Eur J Clin Nutr*. 2006;60(8):955-964.
11. Bertoli S, Battezzati A, Testolin G, Bedogni G. Evaluation of air-displacement plethysmography and bioelectrical impedance analysis vs dual-energy x-ray absorptiometry for the assessment of fat-free mass in elderly subjects. *Eur J Clin Nutr*. 2008;62(11):1282-1286.
12. Ginde SR, Geliebter A, Rubiano F, et al. Air displacement plethysmography: validation in overweight and obese subjects. *Obes Res*. 2005;13(7):1232-1237.
13. Li C, Ford ES, Zhao G, et al. Estimates of body composition with dual-energy x-ray absorptiometry in adults. *Am J Clin Nutr*. 2009;90(6):1457-1465.
14. American College of Sports Medicine. *ACSM's health-related physical fitness assessment manual*. 3rd ed. Baltimore, Md: American College of Sports Medicine; 2010.
15. Ringback Weitoft G, Eliasson M, Rosen M. Underweight, overweight and obesity as risk factors for mortality and hospitalization. *Scand J Public Health*. 2008;36(2):169-176.
16. Nejat EJ, Polotsky AJ, Pal L. Predictors of chronic disease at midlife and beyond–the health risks of obesity. *Maturitas*. 2010;65(2):106-111.
17. Zajacova A, Dowd JB, Burgard SA. Overweight adults may have the lowest mortality–do they have the best health? *Am J Epidemiol*. 2011;173(4):430-437.
18. Heymsfield S, Lohman T, Wang Z-M, Going S. *Human body composition*. 2nd ed. Champaign, Ill: Human Kinetics; 2005.
19. Miller KK, Grinspoon S, Gleysteen S, et al. Preservation of neuroendocrine control of reproductive function despite severe undernutrition. *J Clin Endocrinol Metab*. 2004;89(9):4434-4438.
20. Wannamethee SG, Shaper AG, Walker M. Overweight and obesity and weight change in middle aged men: impact on cardiovascular disease and diabetes. *J Epidemiol Community Health*. 2005;59(2):134-139.

21. Houston DK, Nicklas BJ, Zizza CA. Weighty concerns: the growing prevalence of obesity among older adults. *J Am Diet Assoc.* 2009;109(11):1886-1895.

22. Good D, Morse SA, Ventura HO, Reisin E. Obesity, hypertension, and the heart. *J Cardiometab Syndr.* 2008;3(3):168-172.

23. Probst-Hensch NM. Chronic age-related diseases share risk factors: do they share pathophysiological mechanisms and why does that matter? *Swiss Med Wkly.* 2010;140:w13072.

24. Tejada T, Fornoni A, Lenz O, Materson BJ. Nonpharmacologic therapy for hypertension: does it really work? *Curr Cardiol Rep.* 2006;8(6):418-424.

25. Shapiro JR, Stout AL, Musante GJ. "Structure-size me": weight and health changes in a four week residential program. *Eat Behav.* 2006;7(3):229-234.

26. Schneider PL, Bassett DR Jr, Thompson DL, et al. Effects of a 10,000 steps per day goal in overweight adults. *Am J Health Promot.* 2006;21(2):85-89.

27. Zhang Y, Proenca R, Maffei M, et al. Positional cloning of the mouse obese gene and its human homologue. *Nature.* 1994;372(6505):425-432.

28. Kerksick CM, Wismann-Bunn J, Fogt D, et al. Changes in weight loss, body composition and cardiovascular disease risk after altering macronutrient distributions during a regular exercise program in obese women. *Nutr J.* 2010;9:59.

29. Eikelis N, Esler M. The neurobiology of human obesity. *Exp Physiol.* 2005;90(5):673-682.

30. Eikelis N, Wiesner G, Lambert G, Esler M. Brain leptin resistance in human obesity revisited. *Regul Pept.* 2007;139(1-3):45-51.

31. Farooqi IS, Wangensteen T, Collins S, et al. Clinical and molecular genetic spectrum of congenital deficiency of the leptin receptor. *N Engl J Med.* 2007;356(3):237-247.

32. Gil-Campos M, Aguilera CM, Cañete R, Gil A. Ghrelin: a hormone regulating food intake and energy homeostasis. *Br J Nutr.* 2006;96(2):201-226.

33. Kiewiet RM, van Aken MO, van der Weerd K, et al. Effects of acute administration of acylated and unacylated ghrelin on glucose and insulin concentrations in morbidly obese subjects without overt diabetes. *Eur J Endocrinol* 2009;161(4):567-573.

34. Blakemore AI, Froguel P. Is obesity our genetic legacy? *J Clin Endocrinol Metab.* 2008;93(11 Suppl 1):S51-S56.

35. Hinney A, Vogel CI, Hebebrand J. From monogenic to polygenic obesity: recent advances. *Eur Child Adolesc Psychiatry.* 2010;19(3):297-310.

36. Bouchard C. Childhood obesity: are genetic differences involved? *Am J Clin Nutr.* 2009;89(5):1494S-1501S.

37. Speakman JR. Obesity: the integrated roles of environment and genetics. *J Nutr.* 2004;134(8 Suppl):2090S-2105S.

38. American Dietetic Association. Position of the American Dietetic Association: individual-, family-, school-, and community-based interventions for pediatric overweight. *J Am Diet Assoc.* 2006;106(6):925-945.

39. Hall KD. Computational model of in vivo human energy metabolism during semistarvation and refeeding. *Am J Physiol Endocrinol Metab.* 2006;291(1):E23-E37.

40. Sachdev M, Miller WC, Ryan T, Jollis JG. Effect of fenfluramine-derivative diet pills on cardiac valves: a meta-analysis of observational studies. *Am Heart J.* 2002;144(6):1065-1073.

41. O'Meara S, Riemsma R, Shirran L, et al. A systematic review of the clinical effectiveness of orlistat used for the management of obesity. *Obes Rev.* 2004;5(1):51-68.

42. Schnee DM, Zaiken K, McCloskey WW. An update on the pharmacological treatment of obesity. *Curr Med Res Opin.* 2006;22(8):1463-1474.

43. Perry CD, Hutter MM, Smith DB, et al. Survival and changes in comorbidities after bariatric surgery. *Ann Surg.* 2008;247(1):21-27.

44. Christou NV. Impact of obesity and bariatric surgery on survival. *World J Surg.* 2009;33(10):2022-2027.

45. Kelly JJ, Shikora S, Jones DB, et al. Best practice updates for surgical care in weight loss surgery. *Obesity (Silver Spring).* 2009;17(5):863-870.

46. Seagle HM, Strain GW, Makris A, et al. Position of the American Dietetic Association: weight management. *J Am Diet Assoc.* 2009;109(2):330-346.

47. Kokkinos A, le Roux CW, Alexiadou K, et al. Eating slowly increases the postprandial response of the anorexigenic gut hormones, peptide YY and glucagon-like peptide-1. *J Clin Endocrinol Metab.* 2010;95(1):333-337.

48. U.S. Department of Agriculture, U.S. Department of Health and Human Services. *Dietary Guidelines for Americans, 2010.* Washington, DC: U.S. Government Printing Office; 2010.

49. American Dietetic Association. Position of the American Dietetic Association: Nutrition intervention in the treatment of anorexia nervosa, bulimia nervosa, and other eating disorders. *J Am Diet Assoc.* 2006;106(12):2073-2082.

50. Crow SJ, Peterson CB, Swanson SA, et al. Increased mortality in bulimia nervosa and other eating disorders. *Am J Psychiatry.* 2009;166(12):1342-1346.

51. Austin SB, Ziyadeh NJ, Corliss HL, et al. Sexual orientation disparities in purging and binge eating from early to late adolescence. *J Adolesc Health.* 2009;45(3):238-245.

52. Hudson JI, Hiripi E, Pope HG Jr, Kessler RC. The prevalence and correlates of eating disorders in the National Comorbidity Survey Replication. *Biol Psychiatry.* 2007;61(3):348-358.

FURTHER READING AND RESOURCES

Academy of Nutrition and Dietetics: Healthy Weight. www.eatright.org/Public/content.aspx?id=6843

Centers for Disease Control and Prevention: Healthy Weight. www.cdc.gov/healthyweight/index.html

Intuitive Eating. www.intuitiveeating.org

Nutrition.gov. www.nutrition.gov; click on "Weight Management"

Office of the Surgeon General. Obesity. www.surgeongeneral.gov/topics/obesity/

Sim LA, McAlpine DE, Grothe KB, et al. Identification and treatment of eating disorders in the primary care setting. *Mayo Clin Proc.* 2010;85(8):746-751.

CHAPTER 16

Nutrition and Physical Fitness

KEY CONCEPTS

- Regular physical activity is an important part of a healthy lifestyle, and it relies on healthy muscle structure.
- Different levels of physical activity draw on a variety of body fuel sources.

- Sedentary lifestyles are a contributing factor to poor health.
- A healthy personal exercise program combines both strengthening and aerobic activities.

This chapter demonstrates that balanced nutrition and physical fitness are essential interrelated parts of an overall healthy lifestyle. Both reduce risks associated with chronic diseases, and both are important therapies for the treatment of chronic conditions. Health care workers should provide their patients with sound guidelines for nutrition and physical fitness while setting good examples.

PHYSICAL ACTIVITY RECOMMENDATIONS AND BENEFITS

Guidelines and Recommendations

Technology is rapidly reducing the requirement for physical activity as part of everyday life. Many modern conveniences (e.g., moving sidewalks, escalators) are contributing to sedentary lifestyles and the overall health issues that accompany them. Approximately 39% of American adults do not engage in any form of leisure-time physical activity on a regular basis, and only 31% of adults participate in 30 minutes of moderate physical activity five or more times per week, which is the minimum recommendation.[1]

Increased participation in regular physical activity is a national health goal. The U.S. Department of Health and Human Services has set nutrition and physical fitness goals for Americans—among many other health-related goals—in its *Healthy People 2020* report.[2] The 2020 targets for participation in physical activity are listed in Box 16-1. In addition to the goals of *Healthy People 2020*, the *Physical Activity Guidelines for Americans*, the *Dietary*

Guidelines for Americans, the MyPlate guidelines, and the Dietary Reference Intakes all address the need to participate in physical activity on a regular basis.

Physical activity differs from exercise according to the following definition[3]:

- *Physical activity*: bodily movement produced by the contraction of skeletal muscles that substantially increases energy expenditure above the basal level
- *Exercise*: a subcategory of physical activity that is planned, structured, repetitive, and with the purpose of improving or maintaining one or more component of physical fitness

The *Physical Activity Guidelines for Americans* are based on the following three components[3]:

- *Intensity*: how hard a person works to do the activity
  - Moderate intensity is equivalent in effort to brisk walking.
  - Vigorous intensity is equivalent in effort to running or jogging.
- *Frequency*: how often a person performs aerobic activity
- *Duration*: how long a person performs an activity during any one session

BOX 16-1 *HEALTHY PEOPLE 2020* PHYSICAL ACTIVITY OBJECTIVES

- Reduce the proportion of adults who engage in no leisure-time physical activity. Target: 32.6%.
- Increase the proportion of adults who meet current federal physical activity guidelines for aerobic physical activity and for muscle-strengthening activity.
  - Increase the proportion of adults who engage in aerobic physical activity of at least moderate intensity for at least 150 minutes per week, 75 minutes per week of vigorous-intensity exercise, or an equivalent combination. Target: 47.9%.
  - Increase the proportion of adults who engage in aerobic physical activity of at least moderate intensity for more than 300 minutes per week, more than 150 minutes per week of vigorous-intensity exercise, or an equivalent combination. Target: 31.3%.
  - Increase the proportion of adults who perform muscle-strengthening activities on 2 or more days of the week. Target: 24.1%.
  - Increase the proportion of adults who meet the objectives for aerobic physical activity and muscle-strengthening activity. Target: 20.1%.
- Increase the proportion of adolescents who meet current federal physical activity guidelines for aerobic physical activity and for muscle-strengthening activity.
  - Aerobic physical activity. Target: 20.2%.
  - Muscle-strengthening activity. Target not yet set.
  - Aerobic physical activity and muscle-strengthening activity. Target not yet set.

From the U.S. Department of Health and Human Services. *Healthy People 2020*. Washington, DC: U.S. Government Printing Office; 2010.

The *Physical Activity Guidelines for Americans* are as follows[3]:

- *Children and adolescents:* Children and adolescents should engage in 60 minutes or more of physical activity each day.
  - *Aerobic:* Most of the 60 or more minutes per day should be either moderate- or vigorous-intensity aerobic physical activity and should include vigorous-intensity physical activity at least 3 days a week.
  - *Muscle strengthening:* As part of their 60 or more minutes of daily physical activity, children and adolescents should include muscle-strengthening physical activity on at least 3 days of the week.
  - *Bone strengthening:* As part of their 60 or more minutes of daily physical activity, children and adolescents should include bone-strengthening physical activity on at least 3 days of the week.
- *Adults:* Adults should avoid inactivity. Some physical activity is better than none, and adults who participate in any amount of physical activity gain some health benefits. (Note that the following recommendations for adults are given as minutes per week.)
  - For substantial health benefits, adults should perform at least 150 minutes a week of moderate-intensity aerobic physical activity, 75 minutes a week of vigorous-intensity aerobic physical activity, or an equivalent combination of moderate- and vigorous-intensity aerobic activity. Aerobic activity should be performed in episodes of at least 10 minutes and should preferably be spread throughout the week.
  - For additional and more extensive health benefits, adults should increase their aerobic physical activity to 300 minutes a week of moderate-intensity aerobic activity, 150 minutes a week of vigorous-intensity aerobic physical activity, or an equivalent combination of moderate- and vigorous-intensity activity. Additional health benefits are gained by engaging in physical activity beyond this amount.
  - Adults should also perform moderate- or high-intensity muscle-strengthening activities that involve all major muscle groups on 2 or more days a week, because these activities provide additional health benefits.
- *Older adults:* The guidelines given for adults also apply to older adults. In addition, the following guidelines are just for older adults:
  - When older adults cannot perform 150 minutes of moderate-intensity aerobic activity a week because of chronic conditions, they should be as physically active as their abilities and conditions allow.
  - Older adults should do exercises that maintain or improve balance if they are at risk of falling.
  - Older adults should determine their level of effort for physical activity relative to their level of fitness.
  - Older adults with chronic conditions should understand whether and how their conditions affect their ability to perform regular physical activity safely.

Figure 16-1 suggests guidelines for how to incorporate recommended activities into daily life.

Health Benefits

With a personalized program that has been designed to meet individual needs, all people can develop healthy lifestyles. The longer that people follow some form of regular exercise routine, the more committed they become. Water aerobics, walking, and other low-impact workouts are becoming more and more popular in health clubs and have enabled more people to participate (e.g., those who cannot lift heavy weights or participate in "go for the burn" aerobics). Several of these new gym members

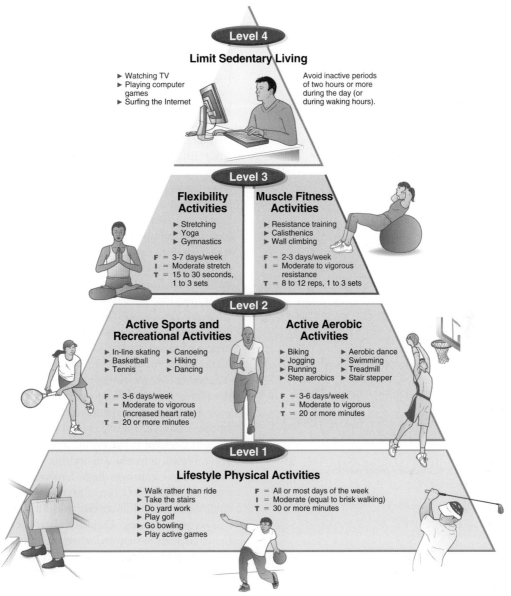

Figure 16-1 Physical activity pyramid. (Modified from Corbin RB, Lindsey R. *Fitness for life*. 5th ed. Champaign, Ill: Human Kinetics; 2005.) F - frequency, I - intensity, T - time.

are older adults who have health problems that may improve with moderate exercise. Regular exercise helps with the management of health, reduces the risk of chronic disease, promotes independence, and increases quality of life (Box 16-2).

For most people, physical activity should not pose any problem or hazard. The Physical Activity Readiness Questionnaire has been designed to identify the small number

of adults for whom physical activity may be inappropriate or those who should have medical advice regarding the type of activity that is most suitable for them (Figure 16-2). All practitioners in the health care field should be well informed with regard to their scope of practice for exercise recommendations and prescriptions. This chapter discusses general recommendations. Much like dietetics, in which the registered dietitian is recognized as the

BOX 16-2 **HEALTH BENEFITS ASSOCIATED WITH REGULAR PHYSICAL ACTIVITY**

Children and Adolescents
Strong Evidence
- Improved cardiorespiratory and muscular fitness
- Improved bone health
- Improved cardiovascular and metabolic health biomarkers
- Favorable body composition

Moderate Evidence
- Reduced symptoms of depression

Adults and Older Adults
Strong Evidence
- Lower risk of early death
- Lower risk of coronary heart disease
- Lower risk of stroke
- Lower risk of high blood pressure
- Lower risk of adverse blood lipid profile
- Lower risk of type 2 diabetes
- Lower risk of metabolic syndrome
- Lower risk of colon cancer
- Lower risk of breast cancer
- Prevention of weight gain
- Weight loss, particularly when combined with reduced calorie intake
- Improved cardiorespiratory and muscular fitness
- Prevention of falls
- Reduced depression
- Better cognitive function (for older adults)

Moderate to Strong Evidence
- Better functional health (for older adults)
- Reduced abdominal obesity

Moderate Evidence
- Lower risk of hip fracture
- Lower risk of lung cancer
- Lower risk of endometrial cancer
- Weight maintenance after weight loss
- Increased bone density
- Improved sleep quality

Note: The Advisory Committee rated the evidence of health benefits of physical activity as strong, moderate, or weak. To do so, the Committee considered the type, number, and quality of studies available, as well as consistency of findings across studies that addressed each outcome. The Committee also considered evidence for causality and dose response in assigning the strength-of-evidence rating.
U.S. Department of Health and Human Services. *2008 Physical Activity Guidelines for Americans.* Washington, D.C.: U.S. Department of Health and Human Services; 2008.

nutrition expert, exercise scientists, physiologists, and certified personal trainers are the experts in exercise.

The sense of fitness that exercise creates helps people to feel good physically, emotionally, and psychologically. However, in addition to this general sense of well-being, exercise (especially aerobic exercise) has special benefits for people with certain health problems.[4,5]

Coronary Heart Disease

Exercise reduces the risk for heart disease in several ways, including improved heart function, blood cholesterol levels, and oxygen transport.

Heart Muscle Function. The heart is a four-chambered organ that is approximately the size of an adult fist. Exercise—especially aerobic conditioning—strengthens the heart muscle, thereby enabling it to pump more blood per beat (i.e., stroke volume). A heart that has been strengthened by exercise has an increased aerobic capacity; in other words, the heart can pump more blood per minute without an undue increase in the heart rate. Therefore, exercises that rely primarily on the aerobic oxygen system for energy (e.g., walking, jogging, workouts on cardiopulmonary exercise machines) improve heart function.

Blood Lipid Levels. A recent large-scale meta-analysis concluded that progressive resistance training programs improved blood lipid profiles by significantly lowering the total cholesterol level, the low-density lipoprotein level, the total cholesterol to high-density lipoprotein ratio, and the triglyceride level.[6] Improvements in high-density lipoprotein cholesterol levels are associated with increases in fat-free mass (i.e., muscle mass) in both men and women. Because exercise is the means for which muscle mass is accumulated, physical activity that specifically increases muscle mass improves high-density lipoprotein levels.[7] Both exercise effects (i.e., improved heart function and cholesterol profile) lower the risks for diseased arteries.

Oxygen-Carrying Capacity. Exercise also enhances the circulatory system by increasing the oxygen-carrying capacity of the blood. As training continues, a person's efficiency of oxygen use and uptake (VO_2max) will improve.

Hypertension

Cardiovascular complications increase along with rising levels of blood pressure. According to the American Heart Association, approximately one in three adults in the United States has hypertension. People with stage 1

VO_2max the maximal uptake volume of oxygen during exercise; this is used to measure the intensity and duration of exercise that a person can perform.

hypertension chronically elevated blood pressure; systolic blood pressure is consistently 140 mm Hg or more or diastolic blood pressure is consistently 90 mm Hg or more.

Physical Activity Readiness
Questionnaire - PAR-Q
(revised 2002)

PAR-Q & YOU

(A Questionnaire for People Aged 15 to 69)

Regular physical activity is fun and healthy, and increasingly more people are starting to become more active every day. Being more active is very safe for most people. However, some people should check with their doctor before they start becoming much more physically active.

If you are planning to become much more physically active than you are now, start by answering the seven questions in the box below. If you are between the ages of 15 and 69, the PAR-Q will tell you if you should check with your doctor before you start. If you are over 69 years of age, and you are not used to being very active, check with your doctor.

Common sense is your best guide when you answer these questions. Please read the questions carefully and answer each one honestly: check YES or NO.

YES	NO	
☐	☐	**1. Has your doctor ever said that you have a heart condition <u>and</u> that you should only do physical activity recommended by a doctor?**
☐	☐	**2. Do you feel pain in your chest when you do physical activity?**
☐	☐	**3. In the past month, have you had chest pain when you were not doing physical activity?**
☐	☐	**4. Do you lose your balance because of dizziness or do you ever lose consciousness?**
☐	☐	**5. Do you have a bone or joint problem (for example, back, knee or hip) that could be made worse by a change in your physical activity?**
☐	☐	**6. Is your doctor currently prescribing drugs (for example, water pills) for your blood pressure or heart condition?**
☐	☐	**7. Do you know of <u>any other reason</u> why you should not do physical activity?**

If

you

answered

YES to one or more questions

Talk with your doctor by phone or in person BEFORE you start becoming much more physically active or BEFORE you have a fitness appraisal. Tell your doctor about the PAR-Q and which questions you answered YES.

- You may be able to do any activity you want — as long as you start slowly and build up gradually. Or, you may need to restrict your activities to those which are safe for you. Talk with your doctor about the kinds of activities you wish to participate in and follow his/her advice.
- Find out which community programs are safe and helpful for you.

NO to all questions

If you answered NO honestly to <u>all</u> PAR-Q questions, you can be reasonably sure that you can:

- start becoming much more physically active – begin slowly and build up gradually. This is the safest and easiest way to go.
- take part in a fitness appraisal – this is an excellent way to determine your basic fitness so that you can plan the best way for you to live actively. It is also highly recommended that you have your blood pressure evaluated. If your reading is over 144/94, talk with your doctor before you start becoming much more physically active.

DELAY BECOMING MUCH MORE ACTIVE:
- if you are not feeling well because of a temporary illness such as a cold or a fever – wait until you feel better; or
- if you are or may be pregnant – talk to your doctor before you start becoming more active.

PLEASE NOTE: If your health changes so that you then answer YES to any of the above questions, tell your fitness or health professional. Ask whether you should change your physical activity plan.

<u>Informed Use of the PAR-Q</u>: The Canadian Society for Exercise Physiology, Health Canada, and their agents assume no liability for persons who undertake physical activity, and if in doubt after completing this questionnaire, consult your doctor prior to physical activity.

Figure 16-2 Physical Activity Readiness Questionnaire. (Courtesy Canadian Society for Exercise Physiology. Copyright 2002.)

hypertension (i.e., a systolic pressure of 140 to 159 mm Hg or a diastolic pressure of 90 to 104 mm Hg) represent the overwhelming majority of hypertensive individuals in the general population, and exercise has become one of the most effective nondrug treatments for this condition.[8] Even for people with higher levels of blood pressure, exercise has proven to be an important adjunct to drug therapy by offsetting adverse drug effects and lowering medication requirements.

Normal rises in blood pressure occur during both aerobic and resistance-type exercises, and both forms of exercise are beneficial for individuals with hypertension. However, exercisers with diagnosed hypertension should avoid excess exertion to prevent severe stress on the cardiovascular system. An example would be holding your breath during the exertion phase of the exercise, such as with the lifting of heavy weights.

Diabetes

Physically active lifestyles are especially beneficial for individuals with type 2 diabetes to improve overall health and to reduce the risk of the chronic complications associated with diabetes.[9] Exercise improves the action of a person's naturally produced insulin by increasing the sensitivity of insulin receptor sites. When managing type 1 diabetes mellitus, the type of exercise and when it is performed must be balanced with food and insulin injections to prevent reactions that are caused by drops in blood glucose[10] (see Chapter 20 for a more detailed discussion of diabetes).

Weight Management

Exercise is extremely beneficial for weight management in the following ways: (1) it helps to regulate appetite; (2) it increases the basal metabolic rate; (3) it reduces the genetic fat deposit set point level; and (4) it is critical for weight-loss maintenance. Together with a well-planned diet, physical exercise corrects the energy balance in favor of increased energy output (see Chapter 15). Fat is used efficiently as the primary fuel source during lower-intensity aerobic exercise such as walking, jogging, swimming, and light cycling (Table 16-1).

Bone Disease

Weight-bearing exercises (e.g., walking, running) help to strengthen bones by increasing osteoblast activity. The weight-bearing load increases calcium deposits in bone, thereby increasing bone density and reducing the risk for osteoporosis. The benefits of exercise on bone density are most notable during the peak bone growth periods of adolescents and young adults. However, excessive forms of training can have a rebound effect in which bone

TABLE 16-1 SOURCE OF ENERGY FOR VARYING EXERCISE INTENSITY

Exercise Intensity	Fuel Used by Muscle
< 30% VO$_2$max (easy walking)	Mainly muscle fat stores
40% to 60% VO$_2$max (jogging, brisk walking)	Fat and carbohydrate used evenly
75% VO$_2$max (running)	Mainly carbohydrate
> 80% VO$_2$max (sprinting)	Nearly 100% carbohydrate

VO$_2$max, Peak oxygen uptake.

density is lost as a result of overtraining, undernutrition, or both.

Mental Health

Exercise stimulates the production of brain opiates, which are substances called *endorphins*. These natural chemicals decrease pain and improve mood, which may include an exhilarating type of "high." Mental health benefits from physical activity are persistent throughout life. Recent studies that have evaluated the quality of life of both community-dwelling and institutionalized older adults found physical and mental health benefits among those who regularly participated in light physical activity.[11,12]

Types of Physical Activity

A variety of exercises in a person's fitness plan is best. A well-balanced exercise program incorporates resistance training, aerobic activities, flexibility and stretching exercises, and a variety of activities of daily living. A good fitness plan is a combination of different enjoyable activities that most effectively reduce the risk of several chronic diseases.

Activities of Daily Living

Many activities of daily living do not reach aerobic levels (e.g., walking to work or to the store, walking the dog, playing catch with children) but are enjoyable and should be incorporated into daily life. If the activity of choice is not enjoyable and appreciated, it will likely be discontinued and thus not result in any potential benefit. Many people question whether exercise is most beneficial during the morning or at night. Again, the bottom line is that it is best whenever one can commit to doing it. No significant differences occur in the overall outcome as

osteoblast cells that are responsible for the mineralization and formation of bone.

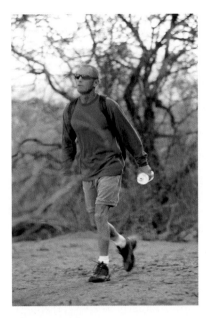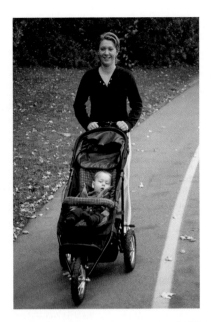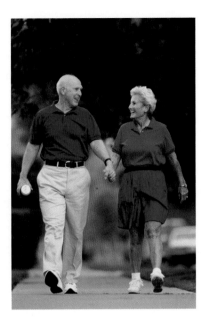

Figure 16-3 Aerobic walking is an exercise that can fit into almost anyone's lifestyle. (Left and center, copyright JupiterImages Corp. right, copyright PhotoDisc.)

long as exercise is incorporated into a daily routine and consistently maintained.

Resistance Training

Resistance training creates and maintains muscle and bone strength, which are physical traits that are necessary for health and an enhanced quality of life. An ideal resistance program should include 8 to 10 separate exercises (with 8 to 12 repetitions of each) that focus on all major muscle groups and that are performed 2 to 3 days per week for novice-level training. A more progressive model incorporates gradual load increases to stimulate muscle overload, more muscle specificity and variation, and a training regimen of 4 to 5 days per week.[13] For an individual whose primary goal is to gain strength and power, the repetitions should be of high intensity, with fewer than 6 repetitions before muscle fatigue occurs. For improved endurance, a lower weight should be used that will allow for at least 15 repetitions before muscle fatigue occurs.

Aerobic Exercise

Forms of exercise that can be sustained at a necessary level of intensity to provide aerobic benefits include activities such as swimming, running, jogging, bicycling, and aerobic dancing routines and similar workouts (Table 16-2). Perhaps the simplest and most popular form of stimulating exercise is walking. Figure 16-3 illustrates

TABLE 16-2   AEROBIC EXERCISES FOR PHYSICAL FITNESS

Type of Exercise	Aerobic Forms
Ball playing	Handball
	Racquetball
	Squash
Bicycling	Stationary
	Touring or mountain biking
Dancing	Aerobic routines
	Ballet
	Disco
Jumping rope	Brisk pace
Running or jogging	Brisk pace
Skating	Ice skating
	Roller skating
Skiing	Cross country
Swimming	Steady pace
Walking	Brisk pace

Maintained at an aerobic level for at least 30 minutes.

how aerobic walking can fit into almost anyone's lifestyle. If the pace is fast enough to elevate the pulse rate and if it is maintained for at least 20 minutes, then walking can be an excellent form of aerobic exercise. It is convenient, and it requires no equipment other than good walking shoes. Table 16-3 provides information about energy expenditure per pound of body weight per hour for various activities.

TABLE 16-3 APPROXIMATE ENERGY EXPENDITURE PER HOUR DURING VARIOUS ACTIVITIES

Activity	Kilocalories per Hour*
Sleeping	63
Lying or sitting, awake	70
Standing, relaxed	84
Rapid typing, sitting	105
Dressing and undressing	140
Walking slowly (24 min/mile)	210
Water aerobics	280
High-impact aerobics	490
Football, flag or touch	560
Walking quickly (12 min/mile)	560
Stair, treadmill	630
Swimming, vigorous effort	700
Running (8 min/mile)	875

*For an adult who weighs 70 kg (154 lb).

TABLE 16-4 TARGET ZONE HEART RATE ACCORDING TO AGE TO ACHIEVE AEROBIC PHYSICAL EFFECT OF EXERCISE

Age (Years)	MAXIMAL ATTAINABLE Heart Rate (Pulse = 220 − Age)	TARGET ZONE 70% Maximal Rate	85% Maximal Rate
20	200	140	170
25	195	136	166
30	190	133	161
35	185	129	157
40	180	126	153
45	175	122	149
50	170	119	144
55	165	115	140
60	160	112	136
65	155	108	132
70	150	105	127
75	145	101	124

Weight-Bearing Exercise

Both aerobic and resistance-type exercises may fit into this category as well. Weight-bearing exercises such as walking, jogging, aerobic dancing, and jumping rope are important for bone structure and strength. In each of these exercises, muscles are working against gravity. Bones will adapt to the environment, and the load put on them during weight-bearing exercises stimulates bones to become more dense.

Meeting Personal Needs

Health Status and Personal Gains

When planning a personal exercise program, first assess an individual's health status, present level of fitness, personal needs, and resources necessary for equipment or cost. Discussing an exercise program with a medical practitioner is always recommended, and getting medical clearance before beginning an exercise program is especially important for older persons and those with chronic diseases. Seeking advice and guidance from a certified personal trainer or an exercise physiologist will be of great benefit. There are many organizations that certify personal trainers, but some are more reputable than others. The American College of Sports Medicine is one of the leading authorities for certifying professionals as Health Fitness Specialists, Certified Personal Trainers, Clinical Exercise Specialists, and Registered Clinical Exercise Physiologists (visit www.acsm.org).

The exercise that is chosen should be something that is both enjoyable and of aerobic value. In addition, the individual should start slowly and build gradually to avoid burnout and injury. Moderation and regularity are the chief guides.

Achieving Aerobic Benefits

To build aerobic capacity, the level of exercise must raise the pulse rate to within 60% to 90% of an individual's maximal heart rate. An acceptable way to estimate the maximal heart rate is to subtract the person's age from 220. For aerobic benefits, 70% of maximal heart rate should then be maintained for approximately 20 minutes three to six times per week (Table 16-4). Resting pulse should be checked before starting the exercise period then again during and immediately afterward to monitor progress toward the target exercising heart rate and aerobic capacity. Heart rate monitors are a convenient way to monitor and keep track of the heart rate.

Exercise Preparation and Care

Whatever the choice of exercise, preparation and continuing care are important. It is not in the scope of this nutrition text to explore the details of various exercise programs. However, some very basic guidelines include warming up the muscles to prevent stress or injury and taking time to cool down after exercising. Do not go beyond tolerance limits; instead, listen to the body. Rest when tired, and stop when hurting. Contact a physician if symptoms do not subside. When more challenge is desired, gradually increase the exercise level by number of repetitions, weight intensity, or endurance—not all three at the same time.

DIETARY NEEDS DURING EXERCISE

Muscle Action and Fuel

Structure and Function

The synchronized action of millions of specialized cells that make up our skeletal muscle mass makes possible all forms of physical activity. A finely coordinated series of small bundles within the muscle fibers produces a smooth symphony of action through simultaneous and alternating contraction and relaxation. Muscular activity requires energy and oxygen.

Fuel Sources

The fuel sources required for energy are the basic energy nutrients: primarily carbohydrate (glucose and glycogen) and some fat. Protein is only used as an energy source when the other fuels are exhausted.

The relative use of stored fat for energy during exercise depends on the level of fitness of the person and the exercise intensity. Trained endurance athletes are more efficient at using fat for energy than are their untrained counterparts. However, the use of fat for energy declines as the exercise intensity increases above approximately 70% VO_2max, at which point the body becomes more reliant on the use of glucose for immediate energy. More sustained low-intensity exercises (i.e., 25% to 65% VO_2max) rely primarily on muscle fat stores for energy through the aerobic pathway.[14] As intensity increases, the source of energy gradually shifts to carbohydrates (see Table 16-1).

Oxygen

The most profound limit to exercise is the person's ability to deliver oxygen to his or her tissues and to then use that oxygen for energy production. This vital ability depends on the fitness of the pulmonary and cardiovascular systems. Fitness level—and thus oxygen and fuel use—is influenced by two major factors: (1) the fitness of the lungs, heart, and blood vessels; and (2) body composition.

Cardiovascular Fitness. Cardiovascular fitness is defined in terms of aerobic capacity, which depends on the body's ability to deliver and use oxygen in sufficient quantities to meet the demands of increasing levels of exercise. Oxygen uptake increases with exercise intensity until either the demand is met or the ability to supply it

is exceeded. The maximum rate at which the body can take in oxygen (i.e., aerobic capacity) is the VO_2max. This capacity determines the intensity and duration of exercise that a person can perform.

Body Composition. Body composition is a reflection of the four body compartments that make up the total body weight: lean body mass, fat, water, and bone (see Chapter 15). Lean body mass is more metabolically active (i.e., requires more fuel) than other body tissues such as adipose tissue. Thus, a person's fitness level is influenced by the amount of energy-demanding lean body mass relative to total fat mass.

Fluid and Energy Needs

Fluid

Dehydration limits performance and exercise capacity, especially in untrained individuals.[15,16] Its extent depends on the intensity and duration of the exercise, the surrounding temperature, the level of fitness, and the pre-exercise state of hydration. With continued exercise, the body temperature rises in response to heat that is released during energy production. To control this temperature rise, the body sends as much heat as possible to the skin, where it is released in sweat to evaporate on the skin. Over time—and especially in hot weather—this excessive sweating can lead to dehydration. To prevent dehydration, water must be frequently replaced. If dehydration continues, athletes may experience problems such as cramps, delirium, vomiting, hypothermia, or hyperthermia. By providing fluid replacement throughout periods of exercise, many of these problems can be prevented. Regular fluid intake should be planned for all types of athletes. Athletes who are engaged in longer and more demanding endurance events (i.e., more than 1 hour), especially in a warm environment, may benefit from an electrolyte and glucose sports drinks that has rapid gastric emptying and intestinal absorption times (see the For Further Focus box, "Hydrating With Water or a Sports Drink").[17]

Energy and Nutrient Stores

Exercise raises energy needs and helps regulate the appetite to meet this need. See Table 16-3 for some examples of the amount of kilocalories expended by general activities. For athletes as well as for other active individuals, proper diet choices are essential for daily energy needs,

---

aerobic capacity   a state in which oxygen is required to proceed; milliliters of oxygen consumed per kilogram of body weight per minute as influenced by body composition.

FOR FURTHER FOCUS

HYDRATING WITH WATER OR A SPORTS DRINK

Sports drinks began with a solution called *Gatorade,* a beverage that its developers named for their university's football team. They reasoned that, if they analyzed the sweat of their players, then they could replace the lost minerals and water in a drink that contained some flavoring, coloring, and sugars to make it acceptable; it would taste better and have more benefits than plain water. Although Gatorade proved beneficial for some athletes, most do not need it during general nonendurance exercise.

The ideal fluid to prevent dehydration depends on how demanding the exercise is and how long it lasts. For nonendurance exercise, physically fit athletes can maintain hydration with plain water. However, long-term endurance athletes need both water and fuel (i.e., carbohydrate), especially during hot weather. For athletes who are losing substantial amounts of water and sodium through sweat, electrolyte replacement is also an important consideration. Although it is rare, hyponatremia (i.e., a plasma sodium concentration of less than 135 mEq/L) can be fatal. The most common cause of hyponatremia among endurance athletes is excess sodium loss through sweat in combination with fluid replacement by plain water. Water dilutes the plasma sodium even more, thereby exacerbating the condition. Thus, sports drinks that contain sodium (0.5 to 0.7 g/L) and potassium (0.8 to 2.0 g/L) as well as carbohydrate are recommended for athletes during endurance events that last 2 hours or more.[1]

Other products that are entering the sports-drink market claim to have no added sugar but supply ample amounts of fructose and glucose from their fruit-juice bases. Fructose does not leave the stomach rapidly, and it is absorbed more slowly from the intestine compared with glucose, which often causes bloating or diarrhea. Another category of sports drinks on the market adds large amounts of vitamins and minerals to their solutions. These extra vitamins do not help an athlete's performance; on a hot day, a perspiring athlete could easily consume a megadose of vitamins after drinking four or five bottles of such a product.

As a general guide, it is worth the time to sort out the costs and claims made by sports drink manufacturers. These products are not for everyone. Furthermore, several functional foods (i.e., food components with physiologic actions) are marketed specifically to athletes as performance enhancers. Examples include the addition of citric acid, branched-chain amino acids, creatine, caffeine, carnitine, antioxidants, glutamine, and arginine to drinks or foods. Scientific evidence exists regarding the beneficial physiologic function of some of these components, but most do not yet have evidence with regard to efficacy.[2] Although sports drinks may meet the needs of athletes who are competing in physically demanding endurance events, they are not required by those who are participating in less-demanding sports activities. Water is the best solution for regular needs, and it costs far less.

1. Rodriguez NR, DiMarco NM, Langley S. Position of the American Dietetic Association, Dietitians of Canada, and the American College of Sports Medicine: nutrition and athletic performance. *J Am Diet Assoc.* 2009;109(3):509-527.
2. Aoi W, Naito Y, Yoshikawa T. Exercise and functional foods. *Nutr J.* 2006;5:15.

nutrient reserves, and winning performances. Without adequate energy during prolonged exercise, nutrient levels fall too low to sustain the body's continued demands. Fatigue follows, and exhaustion may result.

Energy and nutrient needs for most individuals who participate in physical activity are discussed later in this chapter under the "Macronutrient and Micronutrient Recommendations" heading. Specific dietary recomendations for meeting energy needs and maximizing nutrient stores for athletic performance during competition are discussed separately, because the needs of athletes are greater than what most people need for daily physical activity.

Macronutrient and Micronutrient Recommendations

Carbohydrate

Carbohydrate is the preferred fuel, and it is the critical energy source for an active person both before an exercise

period and during the recovery period. The complex carbohydrate forms sustain energy needs and supply added fiber, vitamins, and minerals. Carbohydrate fuels come from two sources: circulating blood glucose and glycogen stored in muscle and liver tissue. Complex carbohydrates (i.e., starches) are preferable to simple carbohydrates (i.e., monosaccharides and disaccharides). Starches break down gradually, help to maintain blood glucose levels more evenly (thus avoiding hypoglycemia), and maintain glycogen storage as a constant primary fuel.

During prolonged bouts of intense exercise, diets that are low in carbohydrate are less efficient for maintaining energy homeostasis.[18] A low-carbohydrate diet decreases the body's capacity for work, which intensifies over time. Physically active individuals on low-carbohydrate diets

hypoglycemia an abnormally low blood glucose level that may lead to muscle tremors, cold sweat, headache, and confusion.

are susceptible to fatigue, ketoacidosis, and dehydration. Conversely, a high-carbohydrate diet enhances muscle glycogen concentrations and exercise performance.[18] In addition, consuming small amounts of carbohydrates during exercise bouts improves whole-body carbohydrate oxidation and metabolic efficiency.[19,20] Therefore, eating foods with adequate carbohydrates before and during exercise helps to maintain the glucose concentrations that are necessary to exercise strenuously and delay fatigue.

Fat

Dietary recommendations for fat intake during physical activity do not vary from standard guidelines. In the presence of oxygen, fatty acids serve as a fuel source from stored fat tissue. No evidence supports improved physical performance with a dietary fat intake of more than 30% of the total daily energy intake. However, an extremely low fat intake can be dangerous if the diet is deficient in the essential fatty acids (i.e., linoleic and α-linolenic acids). A moderate level of fat is necessary in the diet for the absorption of fat-soluble vitamins and to ensure the adequate intake of the essential fatty acids.

Protein

Under normal circumstances, protein makes a relatively insignificant contribution to energy resources during exercise. Therefore, no more than the usual adult requirement (i.e., 0.8 g/kg body weight) is needed to meet the general protein needs of a healthy, physically active adult. For highly trained endurance and strength-trained athletes, the protein requirement may increase (see "Athletic Performance" later in this chapter). Protein requirements are influenced by sex, age, and intensity, duration, and type of exercise as well as by energy intake and carbohydrate availability.[17]

Vitamins and Minerals

Vitamins and minerals are not oxidized during the process of energy production. However, vitamins and minerals are essential as catalytic cofactors in enzyme reactions (see Chapters 7 and 8). Increased physical exertion during exercise or athletic training does not require a greater intake of vitamins and minerals beyond currently recommended intakes. A well-balanced diet supplies adequate amounts of vitamins and minerals, and exercise may improve the body's efficient use of them. Because athletes have an increased dietary need for energy, a larger kilocalorie intake from nutrient-dense foods would automatically boost their general intake of vitamins and minerals.

Multivitamin and mineral supplementation does not improve physical performance in healthy people who are eating well-balanced diets, and the potential side effects from megavitamin supplements are well known. However, therapeutic iron supplements may be necessary for some individuals who are experiencing iron-deficiency anemia (see the Drug-Nutrient Interaction box, "Iron Supplementation"). In addition, the special assessment of nutrient-energy status is needed for amenorrheic female athletes. Chronic negative energy balance is not uncommon among athletes such as gymnasts, ballet dancers, and runners, who may also suffer from disordered eating. Disordered eating patterns may involve low calcium intake, which can have serious consequences for bone development (see the Clinical Applications box, "The Female Athlete Triad: How Performance and Social Pressure Can Lead to Low Bone Mass").

ATHLETIC PERFORMANCE

General Training Diet

All individuals who regularly participate in physical activity must apply the general principles of exercise and energy balance that have been previously described. At what point does a person who regularly exercises become an athlete? It is often difficult to determine exactly when someone's nutrient needs require additional attention. From a nutrition standpoint, one of the main differences in an athlete's diet compared with that of the general public is that athletes require more fluid and energy to cover their needs during exercise. However, it is well accepted that physical activity, athletic performance, and exercise recovery are enhanced by optimal nutrition for everyone.[17]

Athletes who are involved in heavy training are more susceptible to immunosuppression because of the extreme demands that are placed on the body. A well-balanced diet with plenty of carbohydrates and protein from a variety of foods helps to prevent exercise-induced malnutrition and the risk for injury and infection.[21]

Total Energy

When exercise levels rise from mild or moderate amounts up to strenuous levels, caloric needs also rise to supply needed fuel. Exact energy needs vary depending on gender, body size, genetics, body composition, and the type of training involved. Adequate total energy intake allows athletes to maintain appropriate weight and body composition while maximizing performance.[17] Methods

---

amenorrheic the absence or abnormal cessation of the menses.

DRUG-NUTRIENT INTERACTION

IRON SUPPLEMENTATION

Iron plays an essential role in oxygen transport and energy metabolism, which are crucial during exercise. Injury, excessive losses in sweat, inadequate nutrient intake, periods of rapid growth, hemolysis, and menstrual losses all increase the risk for iron depletion in athletes. Iron deficiency—with or without anemia—can affect performance, so athletes should aim to meet the Dietary Reference Intakes for iron from the diet: 18 mg for women and 8 mg for men.[1] This can be accomplished by eating iron-rich foods such as red meat, legumes, dark green leafy vegetables, dried fruits, and fortified grains.

Research supports the importance of the periodic screening of athletes to monitor iron status before clinical symptoms of deficiency occur.[2,3] Groups that are at higher risk for low iron stores are females, adolescents, vegetarians, and long-distance runners.[1] The most common blood indices for iron status are as follows:

- *Hemoglobin:* a protein structure that contains iron that is needed for oxygen transport
- *Hematocrit:* the proportion of packed red blood cells with regard to total blood volume
- *Ferritin:* a protein that stores iron for later use

During periods of intense training, athletes may benefit from supplemental iron, particularly in the presence of iron-deficiency anemia.[2,3] When iron supplements are prescribed, the following precautions should be taken:

- Oral iron supplements provide nonheme iron. The absorption of nonheme iron is increased in the presence of vitamin C. Taking supplements with vitamin-C–rich foods will enhance absorption.
- Supplemental iron may cause heartburn, nausea, constipation, and abdominal pain.[4] Taking supplements with meals and drinking plenty of fluids can help to alleviate these symptoms.
- Iron and calcium compete for absorption. Avoid taking iron supplements with milk or other calcium-containing products.
- Other dietary components that inhibit iron absorption include polyphenols (found in tea and coffee), oxalic acid (found in spinach, chard, and berries), and phytates (found in whole grains and legumes).

At the initiation of a training program, individuals commonly experience a transient decrease in hemoglobin and serum ferritin as a result of increased plasma volume. This is sometimes referred to as "sports anemia," and it is not true iron deficiency.[1] Iron supplementation is not appropriate in these cases.

Kelli Boi

1. Rodriguez NR, DiMarco NM, Langley S. Position of the American Dietetic Association, Dietitians of Canada, and the American College of Sports Medicine: nutrition and athletic performance. *J Am Diet Assoc.* 2009;109(3):509-527.
2. Reinke S, Taylor WR, Duda GN, et al. Absolute and functional iron deficiency in professional athletes during training and recovery. *Int J Cardiol.* 2010 Dec 7 [Epub ahead of print].
3. McClung JP, Karl JP, Cable SJ, et al. Randomized, double-blind, placebo-controlled trial of iron supplementation in female soldiers during military training: effects on iron status, physical performance, and mood. *Am J Clin Nutr.* 2009;90(1):124-131.
4. Clark SF. Iron deficiency anemia: diagnosis and management. *Curr Opin Gastroenterol.* 2009;25(2):122-128.

for calculating basic energy needs are discussed in Chapter 6. Total energy needs should first be estimated with the use of the Dietary Reference Intakes, the Harris-Benedict equation, or the Mifflin-St. Jeor equation; energy requirements specific to the duration, frequency, and intensity of the exercise performed can then be added to those of basic needs.

Athletes' nutrient needs are best met by consuming a variety of foods to meet energy needs; these are represented by the MyPlate guidelines (Figure 1-3).

Carbohydrate

Athletes who are competing in prolonged endurance events should increase their energy intake from carbohydrates. General training needs are usually met with 6 to 7 g/kg body weight per day of carbohydrate. Endurance athletes have higher needs of 7 to 10 g/kg body weight per day.[17]

Fat

Dietary fat is needed to meet energy needs, to supply essential fatty acids, and to maintain weight. No performance benefit occurs from consuming a diet that is less than 20% or greater than 35% fat.

Protein

For highly trained endurance and strength-trained athletes, the protein requirement may increase to 1.2 to 1.7 g/kg/day.[17] Protein needs, even for highly trained athletes, can usually be met through the diet alone. For example, a 170-lb (77-kg) strength-training male athlete may have protein needs of 1.5 g/kg body weight: 77 kg × 1.5 g protein/kg = 115.5 grams of protein per day. The average daily protein intake by men and women who are 20 years old and older in the U.S. is 102 grams and 70 grams per day, respectively.[22] Thus, even for an athlete who is heavily building muscle mass, a slight increase of 13 grams of

CLINICAL APPLICATIONS

THE FEMALE ATHLETE TRIAD: HOW PERFORMANCE AND SOCIAL PRESSURE CAN LEAD TO LOW BONE MASS*

The female athlete triad consists of three health afflictions that are faced by women who are extremely physically active: (1) disordered eating; (2) menstrual disturbances and irregularities; and (3) osteopenia (low bone mass) or osteoporosis. Low bone mineral density (BMD) is often the final result of the triad, and it is the leading cause of stress fractures and injuries throughout the body, some of which may be irreversible. Ironically, many women who are in top physical form are the most likely to develop these three linked complications and health problems, because social and performance pressure may steer them toward extreme eating habits and exercise regimens. The dilemma that female athletes face today is how to maintain optimal physical performance while not provoking health risks.

Women who participate in competitive endurance sports (e.g., rowing, long-distance running) or who are judged partially on physical appearance (e.g., ice skating, diving, or dancing) are more likely to be preoccupied with their weight and to have self-image issues. Social and competitive pressure for a woman to be thin can contribute to her sense of imperfection. These demands can lead some women to develop disordered eating patterns that, in combination with strenuous exercise, result in low energy levels. This drop in energy will be followed by a drop in performance as the athlete loses focus and concentration and as she becomes fatigued. Some women develop psychologic eating disorders, such as bulimia nervosa (i.e., binge eating followed by forced vomiting, purging, or excessive laxative intake) or anorexia nervosa (i.e., refusal or inability to consume sufficient calories for daily requirements). These disorders may in turn progress to additional health problems, including depression, low self-esteem, seizures, cardiac arrhythmia, myocardial infarction, and other health complications. The seriousness of the eating disorder is linked to the amount of stress and concern that the woman feels about her body image in combination with the amount of emphasis put on her weight by herself, her trainers, and her coaches. Athletes often believe that leanness enhances performance, and some are willing to take health risks to satisfy their perfectionist needs and habits.

Poor caloric intake and disordered eating can cause menstrual irregularity. Amenorrhea is the suppression of menstrual cycles to three or fewer menses a year; primary amenorrhea is the repression of all menstrual cycles until the age of 16 years. This condition is often found in young female gymnasts who, in the most competitive circles, may strive to delay the onset of puberty to maintain their small, child-like physiques. Some women may have oligomenorrhea, which involves sporadic cycles that occur 3 to 9 times a year. The levels of estrogen and progesterone that regulate menses can be affected by metabolism, intensive exercise, dieting, or stress.

Several treatments are available for female athletes: hormone replacement therapy, increased caloric intake, decreased exercise, weight gain, and calcium supplements. Evidence suggests that raising estrogen and progesterone levels and increasing caloric intake are the most effective measures; however, a wide range of treatments are prescribed. Hormone therapy alone will not improve BMD. Education and further research are needed to determine the optimal course.

Bone density reaches its peak before the age of 30 years; therefore, young women must strive for dense bones during early adulthood to have healthy bone density later in life. If the density of the bones is diminished early, osteopenia occurs; if it is severe enough, this can be a sign of future osteoporosis. In active young women with inadequate diets and menstrual irregularities, cases of bone density that is 25% lower than normal have been reported. These thin bones increase the likelihood of stress fractures and injuries, and women are far more likely to incur such injuries than men.

However, some studies indicate that weight-bearing activities (e.g., gymnastics) seem to improve BMD and may help to prevent density decreases later in life. Yet the problem facing female athletes who eat improperly is that the rate of decline in BMD intensifies as menstrual cycles continue to be erratic. Weight-bearing sports will not overcome the tendency toward low BMD if diet and exercise levels are not carefully monitored. In today's weight-conscious society, the emphasis must not be on a perfect image, size, or body but rather on the perfect balance of health and training. The female athlete's skeletal integrity suffers as she resorts to drastic measures in her aspiration for an overly lean physical image.

The need to educate trainers, athletes, and health professionals about the consequences of neglected nutrition is imperative. Young female athletes must understand that depriving themselves of life's essential nutrients does significant bodily harm.

*With contributions from Meredith Catherine Williams.

---

protein per day over the average American intake would meet his needs. Furthermore, excess consumption from whole protein or amino acid supplements may put a taxing load on the kidneys as a result of excess nitrogen excretion.

Competition

Carbohydrate Loading

To prepare for an endurance event, athletes sometimes follow a dietary process called *carbohydrate* or *glycogen loading* (see the For Further Focus box, "Carbohydrate Loading for Endurance"). The current practice—which has been modified from earlier, more stressful plans—takes place the week before the event. The protocol includes a moderate and gradual tapering of exercise while increasing total carbohydrate intake in the diet (Table 16-5).

Pregame Meal

The ideal pregame meal depends on the tolerance of the athlete. It usually is a light meal that is eaten 3 to 4 hours before the event. This meal should be high in carbohydrates (approximately 200 to 300 g carbohydrate), low in fat and fiber, and moderate in protein; it should also provide sufficient fluid and be familiar to the athlete.[17] Fat and protein slow the rate of emptying in the stomach and thus should not be consumed in high quantities immediately before a workout or competition.

This schedule gives the body time to digest, absorb, and transform the meal into stored glycogen. Good food choices include pasta, bread, bagels, muffins, and cereal with nonfat milk. Box 16-3 outlines a sample pregame meal. Of most importance, however, is defining the pregame meal in accordance with what works well for the specific athlete.

Hydration Before, During, and After Exercise

Adequate hydration is an important consideration for athletes. Dehydration limits exercise capacity during endurance- and resistance-training activities. Fluid needs depend on the following: (1) the intensity and duration of the exercise; (2) the surrounding temperature, altitude, and humidity; (3) the individual's fitness level; and (4) the

pregame or pre-exercise state of hydration. The thirst mechanism cannot keep up with the loss of water that occurs during exercise; therefore, athletes are advised to make specific plans for fluid intake relative to individualized needs (Figure 16-4). In addition to water loss, which can be as much as 2.4 L/hr in extreme conditions, sweat also contains sodium and small amounts of other minerals (e.g., potassium, magnesium, chloride).

To maximize performance and to avoid the complications of dehydrations, athletes are advised to do the following:

Before exercise: Establish euhydration at least 4 hours before exercise by drinking 5 to 7 mL/kg body weight of water or a sports beverage. Void excess

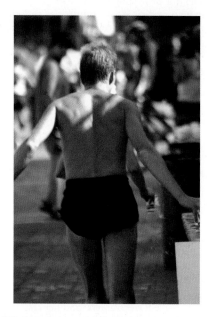

Figure 16-4 Frequent small drinks of cold water during extended exercise prevent dehydration.

TABLE 16-5 PRECOMPETITION PROGRAM FOR CARBOHYDRATE LOADING

Day	Exercise	Diet
1	90-minute period at 70% to 75% peak oxygen uptake	Mixed diet; 5 g of carbohydrate/kg body weight
2 and 3	Gradual tapering of time and intensity: < 40-minute period	Same as day 1
4 and 5	Continuation of tapering: < 20-minute period	Mixed diet; 10 g of carbohydrate/kg body weight
6	Complete rest	Same as days 4 and 5
7	Day of competition	High-carbohydrate pre-event meal

Modified from Coleman EJ. Carbohydrate and exercise. In Dunford M, editor. *Sports nutrition: a practice manual for professionals.* 4th ed. Chicago: The American Dietetic Association; 2006.

BOX 16-3 SAMPLE PREGAME MEAL

This sample pregame meal includes approximately 234 g of carbohydrates; it is high in complex carbohydrates and low in protein, fat, and fiber:

- 1½ cups cooked spaghetti (332 kcal, 65 g carbohydrate)
- ¾ cup tomato sauce (135 kcal, 20 g carbohydrate)
- 1 slice French bread, large (281 kcal, 55 g carbohydrate)
- 1 baked potato, large (278 kcal, 63 g carbohydrate)
- 1 cup apple juice (125 kcal, 31 g carbohydrate)

FOR FURTHER FOCUS

CARBOHYDRATE LOADING FOR ENDURANCE

Glycogen is the body storage form of carbohydrate in the liver and skeletal muscle that is designed to provide an immediate source of fuel and to protect blood glucose levels. Glycogen is restored with each day's food intake, but, during heavy exercise, normal glycogen stores are quickly exhausted. Without glucose available from oral intake or glycogen breakdown, not even stored fat can be used effectively as an energy source.

During the 1960s, trainers and coaches began to explore ways of avoiding this state of exhaustion in their athletes during endurance events. They reasoned that, if the athletes exercised heavily and ate a low-carbohydrate diet for 3 days to use the stored glycogen and then only exercised lightly and ate a high-carbohydrate diet for the next 3 days, their glycogen stores would become supersaturated, thereby

enabling them to perform at a higher level. When this practice was tested, the increase in glycogen stores in muscle and the athletes' performance was significantly improved compared with their previous work capacity.

This practice has become known as *carbohydrate* or *glycogen loading*, and it is specifically designed for endurance athletes. Glycogen loading is only effective when total energy intake is adequate as well. Athletes who consume low-calorie diets do not benefit from glycogen loading.[1]

Today, a less-stressful and modified process of tapered depletion is used to prevent possible injury to muscle tissue. This method can be used more often than the previously used schedule, and it is more productive in the long run. See Table 16-5 for the exercise and carbohydrate regimen.

1. Tarnopolsky MA, Zawada C, Richmond LB, et al. Gender differences in carbohydrate loading are related to energy intake. *J Appl Physiol.* 2001;91(1):225-230.

---

fluid before competition, and do not attempt hyperhydration.

During exercise: Drink during exercise to avoid excessive water loss, which is defined as a loss of more than 2% of body weight from water. The amount of fluid that is necessary to accomplish this will be highly individualized.

After exercise: Replace fluid loss after the completion of exercise by drinking 16 to 24 oz of fluid for every pound of body weight that is lost.[17]

A number of sports drinks with added sugar, electrolytes, and flavorings are available, but questions have been raised about their use or misuse (see the For Further Focus box, "Hydrating With Water or a Sport Drink"). Except for endurance events that last more than 1 hour, plain water usually is the rehydration fluid of choice. Electrolytes are replaced during the athlete's next meal. For events that last longer than 1 hour, beverages with 6% to 8% carbohydrate concentrations may be beneficial.

Energy During Exercise

For activities that last less than 1 hour, most athletes do not require dietary sources of energy during the exercise period. However, performance is enhanced during longer endurance events with the interval consumption of carbohydrates. The American College of Sports Medicine, the Academy of Nutrition and Dietetics, and the Dietitians of Canada recommend eating or drinking 0.7 g of carbohydrate per kg of body weight per hour (approximately 30 to 60 g/hr) during long events.[17] Consuming equal amounts of the preferred

food or drink every 15 to 20 minutes throughout the event is ideal compared with consuming the entire amount at once. Athletes should experiment with various forms of glucose before a competition to determine what is best tolerated. A large variety of sports drinks, gels, and other forms of carbohydrates are available from which athletes can choose. The food of choice should provide carbohydrates primarily from glucose, with little or no fat, protein, or fiber.

Energy After Exercise: Recovery

Proper nutrition is important to the athlete before and during exercise, and it also plays a major role in recovery after the event. Fluid and carbohydrate replacement beverages that are consumed immediately after a glycogen-depleting endurance event result in higher glycogen synthesis and muscle recovery than if replacement beverages are delayed for 2 hours or more.[17] Beverages with a 6% glucose concentration are adequate during this period, but higher concentrations may be consumed, depending on the tolerance of the athlete. For athletes who are taking only a short break in between events (e.g., triathletes), foods and beverages that are ingested should primarily contain simple carbohydrates. For athletes who will be recovering for longer periods of time, a replacement beverage that contains at least 1.2 g of carbohydrate per kg of body weight (taken over several hours) results in an increased rate of muscle glycogen recovery.[23] Muscle recovery is optimal after a strenuous workout, and protein intake during this time period is also beneficial.

Ergogenic Aids and Misinformation

Since ancient times, athletes have been seeking and experimenting with "magic" substances or treatments to gain a competitive edge. Nutritional supplements and ergogenic aids are highly prevalent in the sporting world among athletes, although very few of these substances have been proven to be effective for promoting performance, and several are questionable with regard to safety (see Evolve). Most of the marketed ergogenic aids do not work as they claim but are relatively harmless (see the Drug-Nutrient Interaction box, "Nutritional Ergogenic Supplements").

The use of androgens is of great concern; it is dangerous, and, in competitive sports, it is illegal. The use of steroids is widespread among athletes and bodybuilders, sometimes starting as early as high school or even junior high school. Steroids are synthetic sex hormones that have two actions: (1) anabolic (i.e., tissue growth) and (2) androgenic (i.e., masculinization). Athletes have been known to take steroids in megadoses of 10 to 30 times their normal body hormonal output to increase muscle

---

DRUG-NUTRIENT INTERACTION

NUTRITIONAL ERGOGENIC SUPPLEMENTS

Athletes and other individuals who are interested in improving their athletic performance often seek the help of ergogenic aids. Supplement manufacturers can make health claims about the effect of a substance on the structure or function of the body, but they are not required to demonstrate safety or efficacy. Therefore, a myriad of nutritional supplements are targeted to those who seek to enhance performance. The Academy of Nutrition and Dietetics, the Dietitians of Canada, and the American College of Sports Medicine have classified ergogenic aids into four categories on the basis of their efficacy and safety: (1) those that perform as claimed; (2) those that *may* perform as claimed; (3) those that do *not* perform as claimed; and (4) those that are dangerous, banned, or illegal.[1]

Those That Perform as Claimed

- *Creatine* is the most commonly used ergogenic aid. At moderate doses, it is considered safe, but high doses and creatine "loading" can cause a rapid increase in body mass that likely relate to increased water content in the muscle. Instances of gastrointestinal distress (e.g., cramping, diarrhea, nausea) may be associated with ingesting other substances along with creatine.[2]
- *Caffeine* was removed from the World Anti-Doping Agency's restricted list in 2004, but it is still a restricted substance for the National Collegiate Athletic Association. High-dose caffeine intake may cause gastrointestinal distress and could interfere with the ergogenic effects of creatine. There is conflicting evidence about caffeine's effect on glucose transport, with some studies showing impaired insulin-stimulated glucose uptake and others showing enhanced glucose uptake when carbohydrate is ingested with higher doses of caffeine.[2] Using caffeine-containing energy drinks can be ergolytic (i.e., performance impairing), especially in combination with other stimulants, alcohol, or other supplements.[1]

- *Alkalizing agents* such as sodium bicarbonate and sodium citrate may cause abdominal pain, nausea, cramps, and diarrhea. Excessive doses can cause severe metabolic acidosis.[2]
- *Protein and amino acid supplements* are as effective as food for promoting lean body mass, but supplements may contain banned ingredients that are not listed on the label. These supplements should be used with caution.

Those That May Perform as Claimed

- *Ribose, β-hydroxymethylbutyrate,* and *bovine colostrum* have all been studied for potential ergogenic benefits, and the research is inconclusive. Serious adverse effects have not been demonstrated in studies, but few studies investigating potential nutrient interactions have been conducted. More research is needed before safe recommendations can be made.[2]

Those That Do Not Perform as Claimed

- *Branched-chain amino acids* are essential amino acids that are oxidized in skeletal muscle. Exercise increases the oxidation of these substances in the muscle, but there is insufficient evidence that supplemental branched-chain amino acids will improve exercise performance. High doses may cause gastrointestinal distress and interfere with the absorption of other essential amino acids.[2]
- Other substances in this category include *carnitine, chromium picolinate, conjugated linoleic acid, medium-chain triglycerides,* and *pyruvate.* Research has not conclusively determined that these substances have any ergogenic benefit, and some may have adverse effects.[1]

Those That Are Dangerous, Banned, or Illegal

- A limited list of banned substances is found on Evolve.

Kelli Boi

---

1. Rodriguez NR, DiMarco NM, Langley S. Position of the American Dietetic Association, Dietitians of Canada, and the American College of Sports Medicine: nutrition and athletic performance. *J Am Diet Assoc.* 2009;109(3):509-527.
2. Bishop D. Dietary supplements and team-sport performance. *Sports Med.* 2010;40(12):995-1017.

size, strength, and performance. However, the physiologic side effects can be devastating, including such things as masculinization and gynecomastia; liver abnormalities such as dysfunction, tumor, and hepatitis; an increased risk of atherosclerosis; and the atrophy of the testicles and decreased sperm production. Psychologic effects vary from mood swings to depression and mania or hypomania.

Athletes and their coaches are particularly susceptible to claims and myths about foods and dietary supplements. All athletes, particularly those who are involved in highly competitive sports, constantly search for the competitive edge. Knowing this, manufacturers sometimes make distorted or false claims about their products. Health care providers should be familiar with common fads and myths that are circulating in the community.

Understanding these myths is important, and health care practitioners must know how to approach these individuals and what to recommend as effective alternatives.

ergogenic the tendency to increase work output; various substances that increase work or exercise capacity and output.

masculinization a condition marked by the attainment of male characteristics (e.g., facial hair) either physiologically as part of male maturation or pathologically by either sex.

gynecomastia the excessive development of the male mammary glands, frequently as a result of increased estrogen levels.

SUMMARY

- Many fine muscle fibers and cells, which are triggered by nerve endings, work together to make physical activity possible. Carbohydrate, mainly in the form of complex-carbohydrate foods or starches, is the primary fuel for energy to run this system.
- Carbohydrate metabolism yields circulating blood glucose and stored glycogen in muscles and the liver for fuel. Stored body fat supplies additional fuel as fatty acids, whereas protein provides insignificant energy for exercise. Vitamins and minerals are important parts of coenzymes for the process of energy production.
- Activities of daily living, aerobic exercise, and resistance training have many benefits that increase with practice. Excellent aerobic exercises include sustained fast walking, swimming, jogging, running,

and aerobic dancing or similar workouts. Resistance training increases muscle strength, which has a direct influence on metabolic rate and bone density.
- Exercise increases the need for energy and water. Water in small, frequent amounts is generally the best way to avoid dehydration. Electrolytes that are lost in sweat are replaced during the next meal. The macronutrient needs of athletes do not differ from those of the general population, except that more total calories and fluids are needed.
- During the week before an athletic event (especially an endurance event), athletes may practice carbohydrate loading to meet the energy demands of competition. However, pregame meals should contain small amounts of mainly complex carbohydrates, with little fat, protein, or fiber.

CRITICAL THINKING QUESTIONS

1. What is the primary role of each macronutrient (i.e., carbohydrates, fats, and protein) in terms of fuel for exercise?
2. Outline the nutrition and physical fitness principles that you would discuss with a client who is an athlete. Plan a diet for this person that meets his or her nutrient and energy needs.
3. Why is fluid balance vital during exercise periods? How are water and electrolyte balance achieved?

4. Describe the health benefits of exercise for a person with heart disease and for a person with hypertension. In addition, describe the benefits of exercise for an overweight person with type 2 diabetes.
5. Describe several factors to consider when planning a personal exercise program. Define the term *aerobic exercise,* and list the benefits of this type of exercise.

CHAPTER CHALLENGE QUESTIONS

True-False

Write the correct statement for each statement that is false.

1. *True or False:* Sports drinks that contain electrolytes and sugar are the best way to replace fluids that are lost during short bouts of exercise, such as a 30-minute jog.
2. *True or False:* Drinking water before and during an athletic event causes cramps and is not recommended, regardless of the endurance of the event.
3. *True or False:* Carbohydrate-containing sports drinks are best absorbed from the stomach when they have glucose concentrations of 6% to 8%.
4. *True or False:* Athletes need protein for extra energy.
5. *True or False:* Vitamins and minerals are burned for energy during workouts and training sessions.
6. *True or False:* Protein and fat do not contribute to glycogen stores.
7. *True or False:* Sweating is the main mechanism for dissipating body heat.
8. *True or False:* Aerobic exercise is of limited benefit for controlling heart disease and diabetes.
9. *True or False:* Walking can be an excellent form of aerobic exercise.

Multiple Choice

1. Which of the following activities is most likely to provide aerobic exercise?
   a. Golf
   b. Swimming
   c. Gardening
   d. Baseball

2. To develop aerobic capacity, an exercise should
   a. raise the pulse to 50% of the maximal heart rate.
   b. be maintained for alternating 10-minute periods.
   c. be practiced consistently every day.
   d. be practiced several times a week at an appropriate pulse rate for sustained periods.

3. Characteristics of a healthful exercise program should include which of the following? *(Circle all that apply.)*
   a. Enjoyable activities
   b. Ergogenic aids
   c. Regularity
   d. Going beyond tolerance limits

4. Exercise is beneficial for weight management because it serves which of the following purposes? *(Circle all that apply.)*
   a. Helps to regulate appetite
   b. Decreases the basal metabolic rate
   c. Reduces stress-related eating
   d. Increases the set point for fat deposition

5. Which of the following meals is the best choice for an athlete's pregame meal?
   a. Large grilled steak, fried potatoes, and ice cream
   b. Fried fish, vegetable salad with cream dressing, and fresh fruit
   c. Spaghetti with tomato sauce, French bread, and fruit
   d. Hamburger, french fries, and cola

⊖volve Please refer to the Students' Resource section of this text's Evolve Web site for additional study resources.

REFERENCES

1. U.S. Department of Health and Human Services. *Progress review: physical activity and fitness.* Washington, DC: U.S. Government Printing Office; 2008.
2. U.S. Department of Health and Human Services. *Healthy People 2020.* Washington, DC: U.S. Government Printing Office; 2010.
3. U.S. Department of Health and Human Services. *2008 physical activity guidelines for Americans.* Washington, DC: U.S. Department of Health and Human Services; 2008.
4. Kruk J. Physical activity and health. *Asian Pac J Cancer Prev.* 2009;10(5):721-728.
5. Martins RA, Veríssimo MT, Coelho e Silva MJ, et al. Effects of aerobic and strength-based training on metabolic health indicators in older adults. *Lipids Health Dis.* 2010;9:76.
6. Kelley GA, Kelley KS. Impact of progressive resistance training on lipids and lipoproteins in adults: a meta-analysis of randomized controlled trials. *Prev Med.* 2009; 48(1):9-19.
7. Schubert CM, Rogers NL, Remsberg KE, et al. Lipids, lipoproteins, lifestyle, adiposity and fat-free mass during middle age: the Fels Longitudinal Study. *Int J Obes (Lond).* 2006; 30(2):251-260.
8. Blumenthal JA, Babyak MA, Hinderliter A, et al. Effects of the DASH diet alone and in combination with exercise and weight loss on blood pressure and cardiovascular biomarkers in men and women with high blood pressure: the ENCORE study. *Arch Intern Med.* 2010;170(2):126-135.
9. Campbell HM, Khan N, Cone C, Raisch DW. Relationship between diet, exercise habits, and health status among patients with diabetes. *Res Social Adm Pharm.* 2011;7(2): 151-161.
10. Riddell M, Perkins BA. Exercise and glucose metabolism in persons with diabetes mellitus: perspectives on the role for continuous glucose monitoring. *J Diabetes Sci Technol.* 2009;3(4):914-923.

11. Salguero A, Martínez-García R, Molinero O, Márquez S. Physical activity, quality of life and symptoms of depression in community-dwelling and institutionalized older adults. *Arch Gerontol Geriatr.* 2011;53(2):152-157.

12. Buman MP, Hekler EB, Haskell WL, et al. Objective light-intensity physical activity associations with rated health in older adults. *Am J Epidemiol.* 2010;172(10):1155-1165.

13. American College of Sports Medicine. American College of Sports Medicine position stand. Progression models in resistance training for healthy adults. *Med Sci Sports Exerc.* 2009;41(3):687-708.

14. Horowitz JF, Klein S. Lipid metabolism during endurance exercise. *Am J Clin Nutr.* 2000;72(Suppl 2):558S-563S.

15. Merry TL, Ainslie PN, Cotter JD. Effects of aerobic fitness on hypohydration-induced physiological strain and exercise impairment. *Acta Physiol (Oxf).* 2010;198(2):179-190.

16. Casa DJ, Stearns RL, Lopez RM, et al. Influence of hydration on physiological function and performance during trail running in the heat. *J Athl Train.* 2010;45(2):147-156.

17. Rodriguez NR, DiMarco NM, Langley S. Position of the American Dietetic Association, Dietitians of Canada, and the American College of Sports Medicine: nutrition and athletic performance. *J Am Diet Assoc.* 2009;109(3): 509-527.

18. Green HJ, Ball-Burnett M, Jones S, Farrance B. Mechanical and metabolic responses with exercise and dietary carbohydrate manipulation. *Med Sci Sports Exerc.* 2007;39(1): 139-148.

19. Harger-Domitrovich SG, McClaughry AE, Gaskill SE, Ruby BC. Exogenous carbohydrate spares muscle glycogen in men and women during 10 h of exercise. *Med Sci Sports Exerc.* 2007;39(12):2171-2179.

20. Dumke CL, McBride JM, Nieman DC, et al. Effect of duration and exogenous carbohydrate on gross efficiency during cycling. *J Strength Cond Res.* 2007;21(4):1214-1219.

21. Gleeson M. Can nutrition limit exercise-induced immuno-depression? *Nutr Rev.* 2006;64(3):119-131.

22. Rhodes D, Clemens J, Goldman J, Moshfegh A. *What we eat in America, NHANES 2005-2006.* Washington, DC: U.S. Department of Agriculture; 2010.

23. Millard-Stafford M, Childers WL, Conger SA, et al. Recovery nutrition: timing and composition after endurance exercise. *Curr Sports Med Rep.* 2008;7(4):193-201.

FURTHER READING AND RESOURCES

Review the following Web sites for information, guidelines, research, and suggestions regarding exercise and physical fitness.

American College of Sports Medicine. www.acsm.org

Nancy Clark's Sports Nutrition Guidebook. www.nancyclarkrd.com

National Academies Press. www.nap.edu

National Coalition for Promoting Physical Activity. www.ncppa.org

National Institutes of Health, Office of Dietary Supplements. ods.od.nih.gov

The Surgeon General's Vision for a Healthy and Fit Nation. www.surgeongeneral.gov/library/obesityvision/obesityvision2010.pdf

Kruk J. Physical activity and health. *Asian Pac J Cancer Prev.* 2009;10(5):721-728.
This review of current scientific literature discusses the benefits of physical activity on several areas of health as well as the personal and societal cost of physical inactivity.

Rodriguez NR, DiMarco NM, Langley S. Position of the American Dietetic Association, Dietitians of Canada, and the American College of Sports Medicine: nutrition and athletic performance. *J Am Diet Assoc.* 2009;109(3): 509-527.

CHAPTER **17**

Nutrition Care

KEY CONCEPTS

- Valid health care is centered on the patient and his or her individual needs.
- Comprehensive health care is best provided by a team of health professionals and support staff.
- A personalized health care plan, evaluation, and follow-up care guide actions to promote healing and health.
- Drug-nutrient interactions can create significant medical complications.

People face acute illness or chronic disease and treatment in a variety of settings: the hospital, an extended-care facility, an outpatient clinic, and the home. Nutrition support is fundamental for the successful treatment of disease, and it is often the primary therapy. To meet individual needs, a broad knowledge of nutrition status, requirements, and ways of meeting the identified needs is essential. Each member of the health care team plays an important role in developing and maintaining a person-centered health care plan.

This chapter focuses on the comprehensive care of the patient's nutrition needs as provided by the registered dietitian. Nurses are intimately involved in the care process and often identify nutrition needs within the nursing diagnosis. An effective care plan involves all health care team members as well as the patient, the family, and the support system.

THE THERAPEUTIC PROCESS

Setting and Focus of Care

Health Care Setting

Modern hospitals are a marvel of medical technology, but medical advances sometimes bring confusion to patients, whose illnesses place them in the midst of a complex system of care. Various members of the medical staff come and go, and sometimes the day's schedule does not proceed as planned. Patients need personal advocates. Primary health care providers such as the nurse and the dietitian provide essential support and personalized care.

Person-Centered Care

Nutrition care must be based on individual needs and be person centered. Figure 17-1 demonstrates the nutrition care process model, with the person-centered approach defining the relationship between the patient and the dietetic professional. Needs must constantly be updated with the patient's status. Such personalized care demands great commitment from the health care team. Despite all of the methods, tools, and technologies described in this text and elsewhere, remember this basic fact: the therapeutic use of the self is the most healing tool that a person will ever use. This is a simple yet profound truth, because

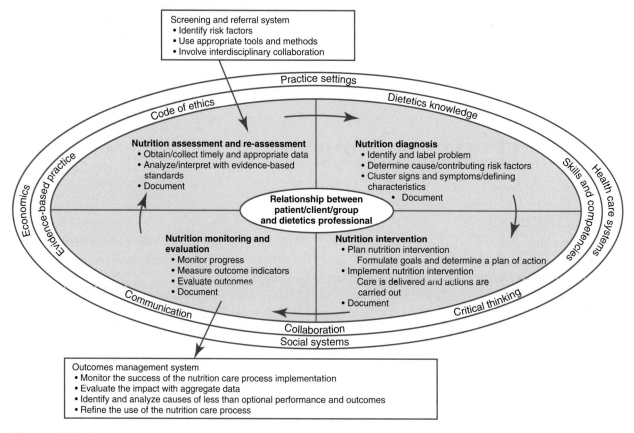

Figure 17-1 The nutrition care process model. (Reprinted from the Writing Group of the Nutrition Care Process/Standardized Language Committee. Nutrition care process and model part I: the 2008 update. *J Am Diet Assoc.* 2008;108(7):1113-1117.)

the human encounter is where health care workers bring themselves and their skills.

Health Care Team

In the area of nutrition care, the registered dietitian (RD) carries the major responsibility of medical nutrition therapy. Box 17-1 outlines the qualifications of an RD. Working closely with the physician, the dietitian determines individual nutrition therapy needs and a plan of care. Team support is essential throughout this process. Nurses are in a unique position to provide additional nutrition support by referring patients to the dietitian when necessary. Of all of the health care team members, nurses are in the closest continuous contact with patients and their families. Patients and caretakers with emotional and social support have a more positive experience with hospitalizations and overall medical care, regardless of clinical status.[1,2] Such a relationship is important to ensure the most beneficial health care approach. When developing this team relationship, all involved parties need each other's expertise for a successful outcome.

Physician and Support Staff

The health care team is headed by the physician and may include several other allied health professionals, depending on the needs of the patient. The team may include some or all of the following members: nurse, dietitian,

nursing diagnosis "[a] clinical judgment about individual, family, or community responses to actual or potential health problems/life processes. Nursing diagnoses provide the basis for selection of nursing interventions to achieve outcomes for which the nurse is accountable," as defined by the North American Nursing Diagnosis Association.

medical nutrition therapy a specific nutrition service and procedure that is used to treat an illness, injury, or condition; it involves an in-depth nutrition assessment of the patient, nutrition diagnosis, nutrition intervention (which includes diet therapy, counseling, and the use of specialized nutrition supplements), and nutrition monitoring and evaluation.

BOX 17-1 QUALIFICATIONS OF A REGISTERED DIETITIAN

What is a Registered Dietitian?

A registered dietitian (RD) is a food and nutrition expert who has met academic and professional requirements, including the following:

- Earned a bachelor's degree with course work approved by the Academy of Nutrition and Dietetics Commission on Accreditation for Dietetics Education; coursework typically includes food and nutrition sciences, food service systems management, business, economics, computer science, sociology, biochemistry, physiology, microbiology, and chemistry
- Completed an accredited, supervised practice program at a health care facility, community agency, or food service corporation
- Passed a national examination administered by the Commission on Dietetic Registration
- Completes continuing professional educational requirements to maintain registration

Approximately 50% of RDs hold advanced degrees. Some RDs also hold additional certifications in specialized areas of practice, such as pediatric or renal nutrition, nutrition support, and diabetes education.

How Is a Registered Dietitian Different From a Nutritionist?

- The "RD" credential is a legally protected title that can only be used by practitioners who are authorized by the Commission on Dietetic Registration of the Academy of Nutrition and Dietetics.
- Some RDs may call themselves "nutritionists," but not all nutritionists are registered dietitians. The definition and requirements for the term *nutritionist* vary. Some states have licensure laws that define the scope of practice for someone who is using the designation, but, in other states, virtually anyone can call himself or herself a "nutritionist," regardless of education or training.

To find out more about what services RDs provide and what the qualifications are for Dietetic Technician, Registered, please visit www.eatright.org.

Reprinted from the Academy of Nutrition and Dietetics: *RDs = nutrition experts* (website): www.eatright.org/HealthProfessionals/content.aspx?id=6856. Accessed February 2011.

physical therapist, occupational therapist, speech therapist, respiratory therapist, radiologist, physician assistant, kinesiotherapist, pharmacist, and social worker. The group must work together as a unit to best serve the patient's needs.

Roles of the Nurse and the Clinical Dietitian

The nurse and the dietitian form an important team for the provision of nutrition care. The dietitian determines nutrition needs, plans and manages nutrition therapy, evaluates the plan of care, and records results. Throughout this entire process, the nurse helps to develop, support, and carry out the plan of care. Successful care depends on the close teamwork of the dietitian and the nurse. The nursing process is a specific process by which nurses deliver care to patients and includes the following steps: assessment, diagnosis, outcome/planning, implementation, and evaluation. The nursing diagnosis is the nurse's clinical judgment about a client's response to actual or potential health conditions or needs.[3] A nursing diagnosis may include several issues that are nutrition related, such as diarrhea, malnutrition, failure to thrive, and fluid volume deficit. Although covering the nursing process is not within the scope of this text, an appreciation of the interconnected work of the nurse and the dietitian on the health care team is important.

A skilled nurse is well respected as the thread that ties all of the health care workers on a team together. Nurses are skilled multitaskers, and they carry a heavy load of the overall responsibilities in a clinical setting. When necessary, nurses may also serve as essential coordinators, advocates, interpreters, teachers, and counselors.

Coordinators and Advocates. Nurses work more closely with patients than do any other practitioners. They are best able to coordinate the patient's special services and treatments, and they can consult and refer as needed. Unfortunately, malnutrition is common in hospital settings. Many factors are involved in malnutrition (e.g., lack of appetite because of pain, medicine-induced anorexia, surgery, emotional and psychologic distress). However, sometimes patients have reduced food intake because of conflicts with medical procedures or appointments during mealtime. The nurse may be able to help resolve such conflicts by coordinating meal-delivery times with a consideration of the patient's scheduled procedures.

Interpreters. The nurse can help to reduce a patient's anxiety with the use of careful, brief, and easily understood explanations about various treatments and plans of care. This may include a basic reinforcement of special diet

kinesiotherapist a health care professional who treats the effects of disease, injury, and congenital disorders through the application of scientifically based exercise principles that have been adapted to enhance the strength, endurance, and mobility of individuals with functional limitations or for those patients who require extended physical conditioning.

nursing process the means by which nurses deliver care to patients; it includes the following steps: assessment, diagnosis, planning, implementation, and evaluation.

needs, the resulting food choices from menus, and illustrations of needs from foods on the tray. These activities may be difficult with uninterested patients, but efforts to understand such patient behaviors are important. A patient's psychologic and emotional status has a strong influence on his or her overall ability to deal with the medical problem at hand and to adhere to the treatment protocol. Patients who are discharged without a proper interpretation of their prognosis or plan of continued care may be noncompliant and experience unnecessary stress, confusion, medical complications, and hospital readmission.

Teachers and Counselors. Basic teaching and counseling skills are essential in nursing. Many opportunities exist during daily care for planned conversations about sound nutrition principles, which will reinforce the dietitian's work with the patient. Learning about the patient's nutrition needs should begin with hospital admission or initial contact, carry through the entire period of care, and continue in the home environment, with the support of community resources as needed.

PHASES OF THE CARE PROCESS

The Academy of Nutrition and Dietetics has developed a standardized Nutrition Care Process for RDs (see the Student Resources section on the Evolve Web site).[4] The Nutrition Care Process is defined as "a systematic problem-solving method that dietetics professionals use to critically think and make decisions to address nutrition-related problems and provide safe and effective quality nutrition care."[5] It is composed of the following four distinct and interrelated nutrition steps: (1) assessment; (2) diagnosis; (3) intervention; and (4) monitoring and evaluation. The Nutrition Care Process provides a consistent structure and framework for nutrition professionals to use to provide individualized care for patients. This process is used for patients, clients, and groups that have identified nutrition risk factors and that need assistance to achieve or maintain health goals.[5]

Nutrition Assessment

To assess nutrition status and provide person-centered care, as much information as possible about the patient's situation is collected. Family and medical history questionnaires are useful methods of gathering pertinent information on admission or during the initial office visit. Appropriate care considers the patient's nutrition status, food habits, and living situation as well as his or her needs, desires, and goals. The patient and his or her family are the primary sources of this information (Figure 17-2). Other sources include the patient's medical chart, oral or written communication with hospital staff, and related research. Data obtained during the nutrition assessment are organized into five categories. The table below gives examples of information that is gathered within each of the five categories.[6]

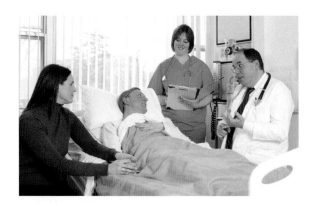

Figure 17-2 Interviewing a patient to plan personal care. (Copyright Photos.com.)

FOOD-/NUTRITION-RELATED HISTORY	ANTHROPOMETRIC MEASUREMENTS	BIOCHEMICAL DATA, MEDICAL TESTS, AND PROCEDURES	NUTRITION-FOCUSED PHYSICAL FINDINGS	CLIENT HISTORY
• Food and nutrient intake • Food and nutrient administration • Medication and herbal supplement use • Knowledge and beliefs • Availability of food and supplies • Physical activity	• Height • Weight • Body mass index • Waist circumference • Growth pattern indices and percentile ranks • Weight history	• Laboratory data • Results of tests and procedures	• Physical appearance • Muscle and fat wasting • Swallow function • Appetite • Affect	• Personal history • Medical, health, and family history • Treatment and complementary or alternative medicine use • Social history

Academy of Nutrition and Dietetics. *Nutrition Care Process SNAPshots* (website): www.eatright.org/HealthProfessionals/content.aspx?id=5902. (Step 1) Accessed February 2011.

CLINICAL APPLICATIONS

NUTRITION HISTORY: ACTIVITY-ASSOCIATED FOOD PATTERN OF A TYPICAL DAY

Name: _____ Date: _____

Height: _____ Weight (lb): _____ / (kg): _____ Body mass index: _____ Ideal weight: _____ Usual weight: _____

Referral:

Diagnosis:

Diet order:

Occupation:

Recreation, physical activity:

Present food intake:

Time/Location	Food (and Method of Preparation)	Serving Size	Tolerance/Comments
Breakfast			
Snack			
Lunch			
Snack			
Dinner			

Summary: Total servings of foods in each category:

Breads/grains: ____ Vegetables: ____ Fruits: ____ Dairy: ____ Meat: ____ Fat/sugar: ____

Dietary supplements and herbs:

Name of supplement: _____ Dose per day: _____

Food- and Nutrition-Related History

In most cases, the RD is responsible for evaluating the diet. Knowledge of the patient's basic eating habits may help to identify possible nutrition deficiencies. The Clinical Applications box entitled "Nutrition History: Activity-Associated Food Pattern of a Typical Day" shows an example of a general guide for gathering a nutrition history. Sometimes a more specific food history is obtained by using a 3-day food record; this involves the patient recording everything that is consumed, the food items that are used, and the amounts and methods of preparation for 3 full days. A more extended view of the diet may reveal additional information about food habits or problems as they relate to the individual's socioeconomic status, family, living situation, and general support system.

Clinicians should be aware that underreporting energy intake is quite common and that this may affect dietary assessment and recommendations.[7-10] A variety of methods are used to collect dietary intake, all of which have strengths and weaknesses (Table 17-1). Specific questioning about various supplements (e.g., vitamins, minerals, multivitamin/mineral combinations, herbs) is more likely to yield accurate answers and to provide insight into overall consumption. Patients often do not report supplement intake (see the Drug-Nutrient Interaction box, "Dietary Supplement Use and Safety"). Allergies and intolerances should be noted so that alternative recommendations meet nutrition needs without causing negative reactions.

Physical activity logs are similar to dietary intake logs in that all activity is recorded throughout the day in an effort to calculate energy expenditure. Like diet logs, physical activity questionnaires tend to be inaccurate relative to fitness in a portion of the population.[11] Thus, the overreporting or underreporting of energy expenditure is another important consideration when providing nutrition recommendations.

Anthropometric Measurements

Practice taking correct anthropometric measurements to avoid errors, and maintain proper equipment and

---

anthropometric measurements the physical measurements of the human body that are used for health assessment, including height, weight, skinfold thickness, and circumference (i.e., of the head, hip, waist, wrist, and mid-arm muscle).

TABLE 17-1 STRENGTHS AND LIMITATIONS OF TECHNIQUES USED TO MEASURE DIETARY INTAKE

Technique	Brief Description	Strengths	Limitations
24-hour food record	A trained interviewer asks the respondent to recall, in detail, all food and drink consumed during a period in the recent past	Requires less than 20 minutes to administer Inexpensive Easy to administer Can provide detailed information about the types of foods consumed Low respondent burden More objective than a dietary history Does not alter respondent's usual intake Useful in clinical settings Can be used to estimate the nutrient intake of certain groups	One recall rarely illustrates typical intake Underreporting and overreporting occur Depends on respondent's memory Omissions of sauces, dressings, and beverages can lead to low estimates of energy intake Data entry can be labor intensive
Food record or diary	The respondent records, at the time of consumption, the identities and amounts of all foods and beverages consumed for a period of time, usually ranging from 1 to 7 days	Does not rely on memory Can provide detailed intake data Can provide information about eating habits Multiple-day data are more representative of usual intake Reasonably valid for up to 5 days	Requires high degree of cooperation Subject must be literate Takes more time to obtain data Act of recording may alter usual intake Response burden can result in low response rates when used in large national surveys Analysis is labor intensive
Food frequency questionnaires	The respondent indicates how many times a day, week, month, or year that he or she usually consumes foods by using a questionnaire that consists of a list of approximately 150 foods or food groups that are important with regard to the intake of energy and nutrients	Can be self-administered Machine readable Modest demand on respondents Relatively inexpensive May be more representative of usual intake than a few days of diet records Design can be based on large population data	May not represent usual food or portion sizes chosen by respondent Intake data can be compromised when multiple foods are grouped within single listings Depends on the ability of the respondent to describe his or her diet
Diet history	The respondent is interviewed by a trained interviewer about the number of meals eaten per day; his or her appetite and food dislikes; the presence or absence of nausea and vomiting; the use of nutritional supplements and herbal products; cigarette smoking; and habits related to sleep, rest, work, and exercise	Assesses usual nutrient intake Can detect seasonal changes Data about all nutrients can be obtained Can correlate well with biochemical measures	Lengthy interview process Requires highly trained interviewers May overestimate nutrient intake Requires the cooperation of a respondent with the ability to recall his or her usual diet Difficult and expensive to code for group analysis

Modified from Lee RD, Neiman DC. *Nutrition assessment.* 4th ed. Boston: McGraw-Hill; 2007.

DRUG-NUTRIENT INTERACTION

DIETARY SUPPLEMENT USE AND SAFETY

In October 1994, the Dietary Supplement Health and Education Act (DSHEA) was passed by Congress. Since then, the dietary supplement industry has grown dramatically. Although the Act provides regulatory guidelines for safety, supplement manufacturers are not held to the same standards as drug companies with regard to demonstrating the safety and effectiveness of their products.[1]

Dietary supplements include vitamins, minerals, amino acids, fatty acids, herbs, botanicals, and other substances that have physiologic effects in the body.[1] As noted in the Drug-Nutrient Interaction boxes in previous chapters, vitamins and minerals can interact with one another and have detrimental effects on the body. Any substance that has a physiologic effect has the potential for nutrient and drug interactions that may cause harm. Nutrient intake from food compounded with high doses of micronutrients from supplements and from fortified foods and beverages can result in habitual intake above the Upper Tolerable Limit for many vitamins and minerals. This may manifest in gastrointestinal symptoms or overt signs of toxicity from specific nutrients.[2]

Supplement use has been monitored in research studies since the 1970s. In a recent National Health and Nutrition Examination Survey (NHANES), which took place from 2005 to 2008, dietary supplement use was reported by 50.9% of the adult population who were 20 years old and older.[3] In a study that researched alternative therapies in cancer patients, 73% of subjects were using some form of

dietary supplement; of those, 47% did not disclose supplement use to their medical providers.[4] Many patients do not feel that it is important to disclose dietary supplements because they are unaware of potential interactions with drugs or other therapies. When speaking with patients or clients, be objective about supplement use. Always encourage patients to discuss supplementation with a physician or pharmacist to avoid potential drug-nutrient interactions.

Kelli Boi

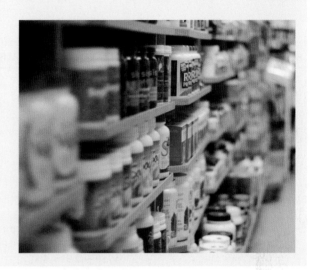

1. Hathcock J. Dietary supplements: how they are used and regulated. *J Nutr*. 2001;131(3s):1114S-1117S.
2. Carlsohn A, Cassel M, Linné K, Mayer F. How much is too much? A case report of nutritional supplement use of a high-performance athlete. *Br J Nutr*. 2011 Jan 25:1-5. [Epub ahead of print]
3. National Center for Health Statistics. *Health, United States, 2010: with special feature on death and dying*. Hyattsville, Md: U.S. Government Printing Office; 2011.
4. Rausch SM, Winegardner F, Kruk KM, et al. Complementary and alternative medicine: use and disclosure in radiation oncology community practice. *Support Care Cancer*. 2010;19(4):521-529.

careful technique. Height, weight, and body mass index are the most common anthropometric measurements that are used in clinical practice, and they provide basic nutrition risk parameters. Depending on the situation, body composition measurements and waist circumference may be taken as well.

Height. Use a fixed measuring stick against the wall, if possible, or use the moveable measuring rod on a platform clinic scale. Have the person stand as straight as possible, without shoes or a cap. Children who are younger than 2 years old should be measured while they are lying down with a stationary headboard and a movable footboard (Figure 17-3). Alternative measures for non-ambulatory patients provide estimates for people who are confined to a bed, who cannot stand up straight, or who have lower-body amputations (Box 17-2).

Weight and Body Mass Index. Weigh patients at consistent times (e.g., in the early morning after the bladder is emptied and before breakfast). If the patient is wearing the same clothing each time that he or she is weighed (e.g., an examination gown), a more consistent weight measurement will be obtained. Ask the patient about his or her usual body weight, and compare it with standard body mass index tables (see Chapter 15). Inquire about recent weight loss (e.g., how much over what period of time?). Rapid unintentional weight loss is significantly associated with increased health risks. Patients who have lost more than 5% body weight in 1 month or more than 10% body weight over any amount of time for unknown reasons should be referred to an RD for a thorough evaluation. Recent weight gain should be noted as well. Understanding the patient's

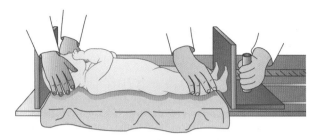

Figure 17-3 Measuring height in an infant. (Reprinted from Mahan LK, Escott-Stump S. *Krause's food & nutrition therapy.* 12th ed. Philadelphia: Saunders; 2008.)

general weight history over time (e.g., peaks and lows at what ages) will give a broad view of expected weight fluctuations.

The body mass index is calculated by using both weight and height measurements, and it is a helpful assessment tool throughout the life cycle (see Chapter 15).

Body Composition. The dietitian may measure various aspects of body size and composition to determine relative levels of fat compared with muscle. Several methods that are used to measure body composition are covered in Chapter 15. Some methods include a

---

BOX 17-2 ALTERNATIVE MEASURES FOR NONAMBULATORY PATIENTS

Total Arm Span
- With a flexible metric tape, measure the patient's full arm span from fingertip to fingertip across the front of the clavicles.
- For patients with limited movement in one arm, measure from the fingertip to the midpoint of the sternum on the dominant hand, and then double the measurement.

Knee HEIGHT[1,2]
- With the client's knees bent at a 90-degree angle, measure the left knee-to-floor height from the outside bony point just under the kneecap (i.e., the fibular head) and down to the floor surface.
- Use the following equations to calculate total body height from knee height:

AGE, GENDER, AND ETHNICITY	EQUATION	STANDARD ERROR FOR AN INDIVIDUAL
Black females		
>60 years old	$89.58 + (1.61 \times KH) - (0.17 \times A)$	3.83 cm
19 to 60 years old	$68.10 + (1.86 \times KH) - (0.06 \times A)$	3.80 cm
6 to 18 years old	$46.59 + (2.02 \times KH)$	4.39 cm
White females		
>60 years old	$82.21 + (1.85 \times KH) - (0.21 \times A)$	3.98 cm
19 to 60 years old	$70.25 + (1.87 \times KH) - (0.06 \times A)$	3.60 cm
6 to 18 years old	$43.21 + (2.15 \times KH)$	3.90 cm
Black males		
>60 years old	$79.69 + (1.85 \times KH) - (0.14 \times A)$	3.81 cm
19 to 60 years old	$73.42 + (1.79 \times KH)$	3.60 cm
6 to 18 years old	$39.60 + (2.18 \times KH)$	4.58 cm
White males		
>60 years old	$78.31 + (1.94 \times KH) - (0.14 \times A)$	3.74 cm
19 to 60 years old	$71.85 + (1.88 \times KH)$	3.97 cm
6 to 18 years old	$40.54 + (2.22 \times KH)$	4.21 cm

KH, knee height in cm; A, age in years.

Recumbent Bed Length
- Align the body so that the lower extremities, trunk, shoulders, and head are in a straight line.
- Mark on the bed sheet the position of the base of the heels and the top of the crown.
- Measure the distance with a tape measure.

Measurement While Lying in the Fetal Position
- Measure four segments of body while the person is lying on his or her side in a "fetal" position: heel (foot flexed) to knee, knee to hip, hip to shoulder, and shoulder to top of head.
- Add the segment measurements together.

1. Chumlea WC, Guo SS, Steinbaugh ML. Prediction of stature from knee height for black and white adults and children with application to mobility-impaired or handicapped persons. *J Am Diet Assoc.* 1994;94(12):1385-1388, 1391; quiz 1389-1390.
2. Chumlea WC, Guo SS, Wholihan K, et al. Stature prediction equations for elderly non-Hispanic white, non-Hispanic black, and Mexican-American persons developed from NHANES III data. *J Am Diet Assoc.* 1998;98(2):137-142.

skinfold thickness measurement with calipers, hydro-static weighing, bioelectrical impedance analysis, dual-energy x-ray absorptiometry, and the BOD POD body composition tracking system (Life Measurement, Inc., Concord, Calif).

Waist Circumference. Body mass index and body composition measurements indicate the risk for over-weight and obesity (i.e., body fatness), but they do not evaluate where excess fat is stored. The location of body fat is an important factor in nutrition assessment, because not all body fat is the same. An important study published in 2002 found that individuals who store body fat in the abdominal region have significantly more health risks than their counterparts of the same weight who store fat more in the hip and thigh regions.[12] The National Institutes of Health guidelines state that, for a lowered health risk, waist circumference should be less than 102 cm for men and less than 88 cm for women.[13] Waist circumference assessment is important for both overweight and normal-weight individuals, because it indicates the risk for chronic diseases (e.g., type 2 diabetes), even among individuals of normal weight.[14]

Biochemical Data, Medical Tests, and Procedures

Laboratory and radiographic tests help with the nutrition status assessment. Such reports generally are available in the patient's chart. Examples of biochemical tests pertinent to nutrition include the following:

- *Plasma proteins:* serum albumin and prealbumin
- *Liver enzymes:* evaluate liver function
- *Blood urea nitrogen and serum electrolytes:* evaluate renal function
- *Urinary urea nitrogen excretion:* estimate nitrogen balance
- *Creatinine height index:* evaluate protein tissue breakdown
- *Complete blood count:* evaluate for anemia
- *Fasting glucose:* evaluate for high or low blood glucose levels
- *Total lymphocyte count:* evaluate immune function

Depending on the patient, some medical tests or procedures may be warranted, such as the following:

Skeletal System Integrity. Several tests may be used, especially with older patients, to determine the status of bone integrity and possible osteoporosis. Some tests that are commonly used are x-rays, dual-energy x-ray absorptiometry, and full-body bone scanning.

Gastrointestinal Function. Medical procedures are also useful to evaluate function, disease, or malfunction along the gastrointestinal tract (e.g., gastric emptying time, peptic ulcer disease, inflammatory bowel disease).

Resting Metabolic Rate. Evaluating a patient's resting metabolic rate helps to establish total energy needs. Both direct and indirect measurement methods are discussed in Chapter 6.

The medical tests that are used for nutrition assessment are generally reliable for people of any age, but some conditions may interfere with test results and should be considered when evaluating laboratory values. For example, laboratory values may be affected by hydration status, the presence of chronic diseases, changes in organ function, and certain medications.

Nutrition-Focused Physical Findings

The careful observation of various areas of the patient's body may reveal signs of poor nutrition. Table 17-2 lists some clinical signs of nutrition status that should be kept in mind when providing general patient care.

Other members of the health care team (e.g., physician, nurse, physical therapist) may perform physical examinations that are useful for evaluating nutrition status.

Client History

The patient's personal history may provide critical information about his or her situation. Guided questioning helps clients to identify and remember elements of their histories that may be pertinent. As mentioned previously, dietary supplements such as herbs are often not mentioned unless they are specifically asked about. Other complementary and alternative medicine use should be identified during this stage. Many elements of a client's personal history can affect his or her current nutrition status and help to guide the plan of action; such elements include socioeconomic status, religion, culture, ethnicity, family interactions, living situation, education level, and employment status. Economic needs are paramount for many people in high-risk populations. Health care providers who are cognizant of the personal, cultural, and ethnic needs of their patients will be more effective when helping a patient plan for immediate and long-term nutrition needs.

Psychologic and emotional problems can weigh heavily on the overall outcome of a patient's prognosis and well-being. For example, geriatric patients in long-term health care facilities often suffer from depression and weight loss, which are confounding problems when individuals are already in poor health. Researchers have found that poor nutritional status and depression are associated, but they are not sure if depression is a cause or consequence of poor nutrition.[15,16] Thus, by inquiring about a patient's psychologic well-being during this step, perhaps some of the confounding factors can be alleviated.

TABLE 17-2 **SIGNS THAT SUGGEST NUTRIENT IMBALANCE**

Area of Concern	Possible Deficiency	Possible Excess
Hair		
Dull, dry, and brittle	Pro	
Easily plucked, with no pain	Pro	
Hair loss	Pro, Zn, biotin	Vit A
Flag sign (i.e., loss of hair pigment in strips around the head)	Pro, Cu	
Head and Neck		
Bulging fontanel (in infants)		Vit A
Headache		Vit A, D
Epistaxis (i.e., nosebleed)	Vit K	
Thyroid enlargement	Iodine	
Eyes		
Conjunctival and corneal xerosis (i.e., dryness)	Vit A	
Pale conjunctiva	Fe	
Blue sclerae	Fe	
Corneal vascularization	Vit B_2	
Mouth		
Cheilosis or angular stomatitis (i.e., lesions at the corners of the mouth)	Vit B_2	
Glossitis (i.e., red, sore tongue)	Niacin, folate, vit B_{12}, and other B vit	
Gingivitis (i.e., inflamed gums)	Vit C	
Hypogeusia or dysgeusia (i.e., poor sense of taste or distorted taste)	Zn	
Dental caries	Fluoride	
Mottling of teeth		Fluoride
Atrophy of papillae on tongue	Fe, B vit	
Skin		
Dry or scaly	Vit A, Zn, EFAs	Vit A
Follicular hyperkeratosis (resembles gooseflesh)	Vit A, EFAs, B vit	
Eczematous lesions	Zn	
Petechiae or ecchymoses	Vit C, K	
Nasolabial seborrhea (i.e., greasy, scaly areas between the nose and lip)	Niacin, vit B_{12}, B_6	
Darkening and peeling of skin in areas exposed to sun	Niacin	
Poor wound healing	Pro, Zn, vit C	
Nails		
Spoon shaped	Fe	
Brittle and fragile	Pro	
Heart		
Enlargement, tachycardia, or failure	Vit B_1	
Small heart	Energy	
Sudden failure or death	Se	
Arrhythmia	Mg, K, Se	
Hypertension	Ca, K	Na
Abdomen		
Hepatomegaly	Pro	Vit A
Ascites	Pro	
Musculoskeletal Extremities		
Muscle wasting (especially in the temporal area)	Energy	
Edema	Pro, vit B_1	
Calf tenderness	Vit B_1 or C, biotin, Se	
Beading of ribs or "rachitic rosary" in a child	Vit C, D	
Bone and joint tenderness	Vit C, D, Ca, P	
Knock knees, bowed legs, or fragile bones	Vit D, Ca, P, Cu	

TABLE 17-2 **SIGNS THAT SUGGEST NUTRIENT IMBALANCE—cont'd**

Area of Concern	Possible Deficiency	Possible Excess
Neurologic		
Paresthesias (i.e., pain and tingling or altered sensation in the extremities)	Vit B_1, B_6, B_{12}, biotin	
Weakness	Vit C, B_1, B_6, B_{12}, energy	
Ataxia and decreased position and vibratory senses	Vit B_1, B_{12}	
Tremor	Mg	
Decreased tendon reflexes	Vit B_1	
Confabulation or disorientation	Vit B_1, B_{12}	
Drowsiness and lethargy	Vit B_1	Vit A, D
Depression	Vit B_1, biotin, B_{12}	

Ca, Calcium; Cu, copper; EFAs, essential fatty acids; Fe, iron; K, potassium; Mg, magnesium; Na, sodium; P, phosphorus; Pro, protein; Se, selenium; Vit, vitamin(s); Zn, zinc.

At the conclusion of the gathering of nutrition assessment data, health care providers must distinguish relevant from irrelevant data, validate the data, and then determine whether there is a need to obtain additional information.

Nutrition Diagnosis

A nutrition diagnosis involves the "identification and labeling [of] an actual occurrence, risk of, or potential for developing a nutrition problem that dietetics professionals are responsible for treating independently."[5] A careful study of all information that has been gathered reveals basic patient needs. Other needs develop and guide the care plan as the hospitalization or consultation continues. Nutrition diagnoses are organized into the following three categories[6]:

INTAKE	CLINICAL	BEHAVIORAL AND ENVIRONMENTAL
• Too much or too little of a food or nutrient as compared with actual or estimated needs	• Nutrition problems that are related to medical or physical conditions	• Knowledge, attitudes, beliefs, physical environment, access to food, and food safety

Academy of Nutrition and Dietetics. *Nutrition Care Process SNAPshots* (website): www.eatright.org/HealthProfessionals/content. aspx?id=5902. (Step 2) Accessed February 2011.

Problem

After the careful assessment of nutrition indices, data is analyzed, and a nutrition diagnostic category is assigned. The nutrition diagnostic statement helps to identify nutrition problems, which may include nutrient deficiencies (e.g., evidence of iron-deficiency anemia) or underlying disease that requires a special modified diet (e.g., diabetes, liver disease). Such a diagnosis also "provides a link to setting realistic and measurable expected outcomes, selecting appropriate interventions, and tracking progress in attaining those expected outcomes."[5]

Etiology

The causes or contributing risk factors are identifiable factors that are directly leading to the stated problem. The Academy of Nutrition and Dietetics defines etiology as the "factors contributing to the existence of, or maintenance of pathophysiological, psychosocial, situational, developmental, cultural, and/or environmental problems."[5] Correctly identifying the cause is the only way to adequately design an intervention plan.

Signs and Symptoms

Signs and symptoms of nutrition problems are an accumulation of subjective and objective changes in the patient's health status that indicate a nutrition problem and that are the results of the identified etiology.

The nutrition diagnosis will change as the patient's nutrition needs change. The following is an example of a nutrition diagnosis statement:

Excessive caloric intake (*problem*) related to frequent consumption of large portions of high-fat meals (*etiology*) as evidenced by average daily intake of calories exceeding recommended amount by 500 kcal and 12-pound weight gain during the past 18 months (*signs*).[5]

Nutrition Intervention

After the assessment and diagnosis, health care providers should now be ready to plan and implement the most suitable nutrition intervention. Objectives of the written care plan give attention to personal needs and goals as well as to the identified requirements of medical care for the patient. Suitable and realistic actions then carry out

the personal care plan. Such activities ideally include family members and caretakers as well.

The nutrition intervention strategies are organized into four categories[6]:

FOOD AND NUTRIENT DELIVERY	NUTRITION EDUCATION	NUTRITION COUNSELING	COORDINATION OF NUTRITION CARE
• An individualized approach for food and nutrient provision • Includes meals and snacks, enteral and parenteral feeding, and supplements	• A formal process to instruct or train a patient in a skill • Imparts knowledge to help patients voluntarily manage or modify food choices and eating behaviors to maintain or improve health	• A supportive process that is characterized by a collaborative counselor–patient relationship • Sets priorities, establishes goals, and creates individualized action plans that acknowledge and foster responsibility for self-care to treat an existing condition • Promotes health	• Consultation with, referral to, or coordination of nutrition care with other health care providers, institutions, or agencies that can assist with the treatment or management of nutrition-related problems

Academy of Nutrition and Dietetics. *Nutrition Care Process SNAPshots* (website): www.eatright.org/HealthProfessionals/content.aspx?id=5902. (Step 3) Accessed February 2011.

Food and/or Nutrient Delivery

Personal Adaptation. Successful nutrition therapy can occur only when the diet is personalized (i.e., adapted to meet individual needs). This can be done best by planning with the patient and his or her family. The following four areas must be explored together:

1. *Personal needs:* What personal desires, concerns, goals, or life situation needs must be met?
2. *Disease:* How does the patient's disease or condition affect the body and its normal metabolic functions?
3. *Nutrition therapy:* Prioritize diagnoses on the basis of urgency, impact, and resources. How and why must the diet change to meet the needs created by the patient's particular disease or condition?
4. *Food plan:* How do these necessary nutritional modifications affect daily food choices? Write a nutrition prescription that is focused on the cause of the problem to meet these needs.

Mode of Feeding. The primary principle of diet therapy is based on a patient's normal nutrition requirements, and it is only modified as an individual's specific condition requires. Nutrition components of the oral diet may be modified in the following three ways:

1. *Energy:* The total energy value of the diet, expressed in kilocalories, may be increased or decreased.
2. *Nutrients:* One or more of the essential nutrients (i.e., protein, carbohydrate, fat, minerals, vitamins, and water) may be modified in amount or form.
3. *Texture:* The texture or seasoning of the diet may be modified (e.g., liquid and low-residue diets).

In the event that nutrient needs cannot be adequately satisfied through oral intake, other methods of nutrient delivery may be considered. When a patient's gastrointestinal tract is functioning but he or she cannot consume food orally, *enteral* feedings are an option. Enteral feedings are administered by a tube and make use of the digestion and absorption functions of the gastrointestinal tract at some point below the mouth. Feeding tubes are placed within the gastrointestinal tract at the point at which the patient is able to tolerate introduction of food or nutrients. The tube may pass through the nasal cavity down the esophagus to the stomach or small intestine for short-term feedings, or the tube may be surgically placed into the gastrointestinal tract for long-term enteral feedings. Details about when enteral feedings are used, tube placement, and types of formula will be discussed further in Chapter 22.

If patients are unable to tolerate any nutrient delivery into the gastrointestinal tract, health care providers may consider *parenteral* nutrition therapy. Parenteral

---

enteral a mode of feeding that makes use of the gastrointestinal tract through oral or tube feeding.

parenteral a mode of feeding that does not make use of the gastrointestinal tract but that instead provides nutrition support via the intravenous delivery of nutrient solutions.

nutrition therapy is administered intravenously and thus carries risks associated with its invasive nature. However, it is an effective way of meeting the nutrient needs of a patient whose gastrointestinal tract is not functioning. Chapter 22 will also cover parenteral nutrition therapy in greater detail.

Nutrition Education and Counseling

Communicating with a patient about his or her specific nutrition intervention plan is a critical step in the potential success of the treatment. Patients and families that understand the necessary changes to food or nutrient delivery methods are able to appreciate the benefit from such adjustments and are more likely to be compliant. Education may be a one-on-one experience with the dietitian, or it may occur in a group setting. Initial education and counseling interactions during inpatient stays can continue through outpatient appointments, when necessary.

Nutrition intervention plans are generally long-term lifestyle modifications that are meant to promote and improve health. Some patients will have more changes to make than others, and they will need continued nutrition counseling support to reach one goal at a time. Establishing a long-term plan to make such changes takes a commitment to education, counseling, and both professional and personal support. The plan of care will be modified over time as needed and in response to intervention.

Coordination of Nutrition Care

Several health care providers may be involved in a nutrition intervention plan. For example, enteral tube feedings will require the coordination of dietitians, nurses, the prescribing physician, and possibly the pharmacist. Interdisciplinary connections within health care make the coordination of nutrition care possible and more effective. In addition, family, friends, care providers, and other members of the patient's personal support group may be helpful during the coordination of the patient's care.

Nutrition Monitoring and Evaluation

Nutrition monitoring and evaluation identify patient outcomes relevant to the nutrition diagnosis and the intervention plan. This step measures progress toward the patient's goals. The three components of this process are as follows[4]:

1. Monitor progress.
2. Measure outcomes.
3. Evaluate outcomes.

Outcome measures that are used during this step are organized into the same categories as the nutrition assessment categories, excluding client history: food- and nutrition-related history outcomes; anthropometric measurement outcomes; biochemical data, medical tests, and procedure outcomes; and nutrition-focused physical finding outcomes.[6]

FOOD-/NUTRITION-RELATED HISTORY OUTCOMES	ANTHROPOMETRIC MEASUREMENT OUTCOMES	BIOCHEMICAL DATA, MEDICAL TESTS, AND PROCEDURE OUTCOMES	NUTRITION-FOCUSED PHYSICAL FINDING OUTCOMES
• Food and nutrient intake • Food and nutrient administration • Medication/herbal supplement use • Knowledge and beliefs • Availability of food and supplies • Physical activity, nutrition quality of life	• Height • Weight • Body mass index • Waist circumference • Growth pattern indices and percentile ranks • Weight history	• Lab data (e.g., electrolytes, glucose) and tests (e.g., gastric emptying time, resting metabolic rate)	• Physical appearance • Muscle and fat wasting • Swallow function • Appetite • Affect

Academy of Nutrition and Dietetics. *Nutrition Care Process SNAPshots* (website): www.eatright.org/HealthProfessionals/content.aspx?id=5902. (Step 4) Accessed February 2011.

Depending on the care plan, nutrition professionals will collect data that are pertinent to the outcome goals and then compare these data with the patient's previous status to assess progress. Efficacy of the care plan is assessed, and changes are made, if necessary. If changes are not necessary and the patient's goals have been satisfied, the dietitian may discharge the patient at this point.

DRUG INTERACTIONS

Many negative reactions can occur with polypharmacy, especially among elderly patients, who are also likely to take several dietary supplements and herbs. A total of 47% of the U.S. population takes at least one prescription drug per day, and 21% take three or more prescription drugs.[17] Patients may respond quite differently from one another, depending on normal dietary habits, the specific disease being treated, compliance, and other medications or supplements that are currently being taken.

Gathering information about all drug use is essential to the care process; this includes over-the-counter medications and prescribed drugs as well as alcohol and street drugs. The nurse should be particularly familiar with drug-food interactions, because he or she is most commonly administering both items to patients (Figure 17-4). However, all members of the health care team should be aware of potential drug-nutrient reactions and communicate regularly with the pharmacist.

Below is a brief description of the different types of drug-nutrient interactions. It is not within the scope of this textbook to extensively cover the many possible drug-nutrient interactions. There are Drug-Nutrient Interaction boxes throughout the text to highlight common interactions of interest within each chapter. Pocket guides such as *Food-Medication Interactions* (www.foodmedinteractions.com) are helpful for onsite reference.

Drug-Food Interactions

Interactions in which food increases or decreases the effect of a drug can adversely influence the health of a patient. Certain foods may affect the absorption, distribution, metabolism, or elimination of a drug, thereby altering the intended dose response (Table 17-3). The timing, size, and composition of meals relative to medication administration are all common causes of drug-food interactions. For example, a high-fat meal increases the absorption of some drugs that are lipophilic (i.e., "fat loving"), whereas a high-fiber meal may bind other drugs and reduce their absorption.

The interaction of grapefruit juice and several medications has been under critical evaluation during recent years. A substance called *furanocoumarin* in grapefruit juice can dramatically alter the bioavailability of certain drugs to a dangerous level.[18] The anticoagulation medication warfarin is a commonly prescribed drug for patients with heart disease, and it is also one of the most highly interactive medications with certain foods, specifically with those that are high in vitamin K.[19] Other examples of drug-food interactions would be as follows: (1) medications that interfere with the appetite as a result of changes in taste or smell sensations (e.g., amitriptyline, metronidazole); and (2) medications that stimulate the appetite (e.g., antihistamines, steroids). Over time, these alterations in appetite may affect nutritional status.[20]

Drug-Nutrient Interactions

Drug-nutrient interactions are primarily reactions that occur when medications are taken in combination with over-the-counter vitamin and mineral supplements (see the Clinical Applications box, "Case Study: Drug-Nutrient Interaction"). Unfortunately, the use of vitamin and mineral supplements is seldom reported to physicians or pharmacists by patients, and 49% of Americans who are older than 1 year old regularly use dietary supplements.[21] Patients should be asked what other medications they are taking, with specific questions asked about vitamin and mineral supplement use. Drug-nutrient interactions may result in the depletion of a nutrient, or the nutrient may induce a change in the rate of metabolism of the drug (see Table 17-3). The Cultural Considerations box entitled "Prescription Medication and Dietary Supplement Use" discusses the issue of nondisclosure among patients who are taking both dietary supplements and prescription medications.

Drug-Herb Interactions

Interactions that involve prescription drugs and herbs are the least well-defined drug interactions. St. John's wort

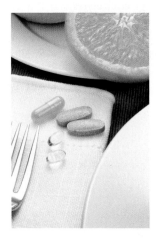

Figure 17-4 Many drugs, foods, and nutrients interact and cause medical problems. (Copyright Photos.com.)

polypharmacy the use of multiple medications by a patient.

TABLE 17-3 FOODS AND NUTRIENTS THAT AFFECT MEDICATIONS

Drug Class	Examples	Use	Food or Nutrient	Action	How to Avoid
Alcohol, particularly excessive use	Beer, wine, spirits	Lowers inhibitions, central nervous system depressant	Food	Slowed absorption	Consume alcohol with food or meals
Analgesics and nonsteroidal anti-inflammatory drugs	Salicylates (aspirin), ibuprofen (Motrin, Advil), naproxen (Anaprox, Aleve, Naprosyn), acetaminophen (Tylenol)	Pain and fever	Alcohol	Alcohol ingestion increases hepatotoxicity, liver damage, and stomach bleeding	Limit alcohol intake to 2 drinks per day for men and 1 drink per day for women
			Caffeine	Caffeine increases absorption and gastrointestinal side effects	Avoid excessive caffeine intake while taking these drugs
			Natural products that affect coagulation (e.g., garlic, gingko, ginger)	Natural anticoagulants counteract effects	Use caution when taking botanical supplements, including natural anticoagulants
Antibiotics	Ciprofloxacin (Cipro), penicillin	Infection	Dairy products	Decreased absorption	Interaction with foods is minimal Avoid eating dairy products 2 hours before and 6 hours after taking these medications
			Caffeine	Increased central nervous system stimulation	Limit caffeine-containing foods and beverages (e.g., chocolate, cola, tea, coffee)
			Fiber	Binds drug, thereby reducing absorption (only penicillin)	Do not take these drugs with high-fiber foods
Anticoagulant	Warfarin (Coumadin)	Blood clots	Vitamins K and E (supplements) may reduce efficacy	Reduced efficacy	Consistent intake of foods high in vitamin K (e.g., broccoli, spinach, kale, turnip greens, cauliflower, Brussels sprouts); avoid high doses of vitamin E (e.g., 400 IU)
			Alcohol and garlic	Increased anticoagulation	Avoid alcohol and supplements that contain garlic
Anticonvulsants	Phenobarbital, phenytoin	Seizures, epilepsy	Alcohol	Increased sedation	Avoid alcohol

Continued

TABLE 17-3 FOODS AND NUTRIENTS THAT AFFECT MEDICATIONS—cont'd

Drug Class	Examples	Use	Food or Nutrient	Action	How to Avoid
Antidepressants:		Depression, anxiety	Alcohol, caffeine[†]	Increased central nervous system effects of caffeine and alcohol or increased plasma drug levels	Avoid excessive alcohol and caffeine consumption with antidepressant drugs
Monoamine oxidase inhibitors	Phenelzine (Nardil), tranylcypromine (Parnate)		Foods and alcoholic beverages that contain tyramine	Rapid and potentially fatal increase in blood pressure	Avoid tyramine-containing foods*
Selective serotonin reuptake inhibitors	Sertraline (Zoloft), fluvoxamine (Luvox)		Grapefruit-related citrus	Potential for increased serum drug levels	Caution with grapefruit-related citrus
Selective serotonin norepinephrine reuptake inhibitors	Duloxetine (Cymbalta)		Caffeine	Increased serum drug levels when high doses used	Limit caffeine-containing foods and beverages (e.g., chocolate, cola, tea, coffee)
Tricyclic antidepressants	Amitriptyline (Elavil), clomipramine (Anafranil)		Fiber	Decreased drug effect	Avoid taking with high-fiber foods or supplements
			Grapefruit related citrus	Increased serum drug levels	Avoid grapefruit-related citrus fruits and juices
Antiemetics	Amitriptyline (Elavil), chlorpromazine (Thorazine), metoclopramide (Reglan)	Antidepressant, antipsychotic, antiemetic	Alcohol	Increased sedation	Avoid alcohol
Antihistamines	Fexofenadine (Allegra), loratadine (Claritin), cetirizine (Zyrtec), astemizole (Hismanal)	Allergies	Alcohol	Increased drowsiness and slowed mental and motor performance	Use caution when operating machinery or driving
Antihyperlipidemics (3-hydroxy-3-methylglutaryl coenzyme A reductase inhibitors), statins	Atorvastatin (Lipitor), lovastatin (Mevacor), pravastatin (Pravachol), simvastatin (Zocor)	High serum low-density lipoprotein cholesterol	Food and meals	Enhanced absorption	Lovastatin should be taken with the evening meal to enhance absorption
			Alcohol	Increased risk of liver damage	Avoid large amounts of alcohol
			Grapefruit-related citrus	Increased drug effect	Avoid grapefruit-related citrus juice and fruit
Antihypertensives	Angiotensin-converting enzyme inhibitors, angiotensin II receptor antagonists, β-blockers, verapamil	Hypertension	Natural licorice (Glycyrrhiza glabra)	Reduced effectiveness	Avoid consuming natural licorice
			Tyramine-rich foods		Avoid tyramine-containing foods*
			High-protein foods (e.g., eggs, meat, protein supplements)	Increased drug bioavailability and increased risk for adverse events	Take drugs separately from high-protein foods

Drug category	Drug	Condition	Food or substance	Effect	Recommendation
Antineoplastic drugs	Methotrexate	Cancer, psoriasis	Alcohol	Increased hepatotoxicity with chronic alcohol use	Avoid alcohol
			Dairy products	Decreased drug levels	Separate consumption of dairy products from that of drugs by 2 to 4 hours
Antiparkinson agents	Levodopa (Dopar, Larodopa)	Parkinson's disease	High-protein foods (e.g., eggs, meat, protein supplements), vitamin B_6	Decreased absorption	Spread protein intake equally across three to six meals per day to minimize reaction; avoid vitamin B_6 supplements or multivitamin supplement in doses of more than 10 mg
Antituberculotics	Isoniazid	Tuberculosis	Food	Reduced absorption with foods	Take on an empty stomach
			Alcohol	Increased hepatotoxicity and reduced isoniazid levels	Avoid alcohol
Antiulcer agents (histamine blockers)	Cimetidine (Tagamet)	Ulcers	Alcohol	Increased blood alcohol levels	Limit alcohol intake to 2 drinks per day for men and 1 drink per day for women
			Caffeine-containing foods and beverages	Reduced caffeine clearance	Limit caffeine intake
Bronchodilators	Theophylline (Slo-Bid, Theo-Dur)	Asthma, chronic bronchitis, emphysema	Caffeine	Increased stimulation of central nervous system	Avoid caffeine-containing foods and beverages (e.g., chocolate, cola, tea, coffee)
			Alcohol	Alcohol can increase nausea, vomiting, headache, and irritability	Avoid alcohol if taking theophylline medications
Corticosteroids	Prednisone (Pediapred, Prelone, Solu-Medrol), hydrocortisone	Inflammation and itching	Food	Stomach irritation	Take with food or milk to decrease stomach upset
Hypoglycemic agents	Sulfonylurea (Diabinese), metformin (Glucophage)	Diabetes	Alcohol	Severe nausea and vomiting	Avoid alcohol
			Fiber	Decreased drug absorption	Avoid taking with high-fiber foods or supplements

*Tyramine-containing foods include beer; red wine; American processed, cheddar, bleu, brie, mozzarella, and parmesan cheeses; yogurt and sour cream; beef and chicken liver; cured meats such as sausage and salami; game meats; caviar and dried fish; avocados, bananas, raisins, and broad (fava) beans; sauerkraut; yeast extracts; soy sauce and miso soup; ginseng; and caffeine-containing products (e.g., cola, chocolate, coffee, tea).

†These interact with most antidepressant medications. The central nervous system depressant effects of alcohol and the central nervous system stimulant effects of caffeine interfere with the therapeutic benefits of the antidepressant drugs. There are occasional interactions with the metabolism mechanisms (e.g., CYP enzyme inhibition), but many are not clinically significant, and the cytochrome P450 enzymes that are affected vary.

Data from Anderson J, Hart H. *Nutrient-drug interactions and food* (website): www.ext.colostate.edu/pubs/foodnut/09361.html. Accessed October 26, 2011; Hulisz D, Jakab J. *Food-drug interactions: which ones really matter?* (website): www.uspharmacist.com/content/t/bone_disorders,calcium/c/10374/. Accessed October 26, 2011; National Center for Biotechnology Information, US National Library of Medicine, National Institutes of Health. *PubMed Health* (website): www.ncbi.nlm.nih.gov/pubmedhealth/. Accessed February 2011; Pronsky ZM. *Food-medication interactions*. 15th ed. Birchrunville, Penn: Food-Medication Interactions; 2008; and Seden K, Dickinson L, Khoo S, Back D. Grapefruit-drug interactions. *Drugs* 2010;70(18):2373-2407.

CLINICAL APPLICATIONS

CASE STUDY: DRUG-NUTRIENT INTERACTION

Linda, a 24-year-old woman, reported to her doctor with symptoms that included fatigue; headaches; muscle, joint, and bone pain; dry, flaking skin; amenorrhea; hair loss; depression; nausea and vomiting; and weight loss. After a physical examination and laboratory work, Linda was determined to have liver damage. The only prescription medication that Linda takes is isotretinoin (Accutane) for acne. Isotretinoin is known as 13-*cis* retinoic acid, and it is a vitamin-A–related compound. She also reported taking several dietary supplements, including a multivitamin; a vitamin E supplement and a vitamin D supplement, each of which contains 500% of the Recommended Dietary

Allowance of its respective vitamin; an antioxidant liquid mix that contains β-carotene; and an occasional multimineral.

1. Could Linda's dietary supplement use have anything to do with her liver problems? Why?
2. What foods or nutrients should be avoided when taking isotretinoin?
3. What would you counsel Linda to do regarding her supplement and medication use?
4. Linda also mentions that she is trying to become pregnant. Would you recommend that she change anything with regard to her supplement or medication use?

CULTURAL CONSIDERATIONS

PRESCRIPTION MEDICATION AND DIETARY SUPPLEMENT USE

Prescription drug use and dietary supplement use are common in the United States[1]:

Ethnicity	Prescription Drug Use as a Percentage of the Population	Dietary Supplement Use Among Persons 20 Years Old and Older as a Percentage of the Population
White males	45.1%	48.7%
White females	56.3%	61.3%
Black males	37.1%	31.0%
Black females	45.7%	43.0%
Mexican males	28.4%	30.0%
Mexican females	38.2%	41.5%

Several studies have explored the issue of patients not reporting dietary supplement use to their health care providers. One study found that 69% of the participants who were using both prescription medications and herbal dietary supplements did not tell any of their conventional health

care providers about their herbal supplement use.[2] Another study looked specifically at the likelihood of disclosure on the basis of ethnicity and found significant variation among groups. When comparing disclosure rates among Asian, Hispanic, White, and Black supplement users, Asians and Hispanics were much less likely to inform their health care providers about their supplement use.[3] The same low rates of disclosure were true even for patients who were being treated for chronic conditions: only 51% of patients with one or more chronic disease who were currently taking prescription medications told their conventional health care providers about their dietary supplement use.[3]

It is evident that patients need more education about the importance of talking to their health care providers about the use of vitamin, mineral, and herbal supplements. Health care providers may need additional training to elicit information about dietary supplement use from their patients. It is helpful to understand the high use of supplements among certain ethnic groups in combination with the low reporting rates so that extra attention may be given to the matter when working with these patients.

1. National Center for Health Statistics. *Health, United States, 2010: with special feature on death and dying.* Hyattsville, Md: U.S. Government Printing Office; 2011.
2. Gardiner P, Graham RE, Legedza AT, et al. Factors associated with dietary supplement use among prescription medication users. *Arch Intern Med.* 2006;166(18):1968-1974.
3. Mehta DH, Gardiner PM, Phillips RS, McCarthy EP. Herbal and dietary supplement disclosure to health care providers by individuals with chronic conditions. *J Altern Complement Med.* 2008;14(10):1263-1269.

(*Hypericum perforatum*), which is one of the most commonly taken herbs (as an antidepressant), has been extensively studied for drug interactions. The exact mechanism by which St. John's wort interacts with medications varies. This herb is thought to have the most drug-herb interactions of the commonly used herbal products, some of

which are clinically severe. Medication groups that have documented adverse reactions when taken with St. John's wort include immunosuppressants; contraceptives; cardiovascular medications; anti-HIV drugs; anticancer drugs; anxiolytics; antidepressants; anticonvulsants; anesthetics; medications used to treat addicted patients (e.g., methadone); muscle relaxers; hypoglycemic, antimicrobic, and antimigraine medicines; and drugs that act on the gastrointestinal tract and the respiratory system.[22]

Other common herbs that are involved in drug interactions include papaya extract *(Carica papaya)*, devil's claw *(Harpagophytum procumbens)*, *Ginkgo biloba*, evening primrose *(Oenothera biennis)*, valerian *(Valeriana officinale)*, kelp *(Fucus vesiculosus)*, ginseng *(Panax ginseng)*, and ginger *(Zingiber officinale)*.[23] Many herbs also have clinically documented medicinal properties and should be evaluated on an individual basis to determine their appropriateness with the patient's current dietary habits and prescribed medications.

SUMMARY

- The basis for effective nutrition care begins with the patient's nutrition needs and must involve the patient and his or her family. Such person-centered care requires initial assessment and planning by the dietitian and continuous close teamwork among all team members who are providing primary care.
- The careful assessment of factors that influence nutrition status requires a broad foundation of pertinent information (e.g., physiologic, psychosocial, medical, personal). The patient's medical record is a basic means of communication among health care team members.

- Nutrition therapy is based on the personal and physical needs of the patient. Successful therapy requires a close working relationship among dietetic, medical, and nursing staff in the health care facility. The nurse is in a unique position to reinforce the nutrition principles of the diet with the patient and his or her family.
- Drug interactions with nutrients, foods, or other medications can present complications with patient care. Careful questioning to determine all prescription and over-the-counter supplements and medications that are being taken will help to guide the patient's education needs.

CRITICAL THINKING QUESTIONS

1. Identify and discuss the possible effects of various psychosocial factors on the outcome of nutrition therapy.
2. Describe commonly used measures for determining nutrition status in an outpatient setting and a long-term care facility. Include the following measurement tools: (1) anthropometric measures; (2) biochemical tests; (3) clinical observations; and (4) diet evaluation.
3. Describe the roles of the dietitian and the nurse with regard to the nutrition care plan. In what part of the care plan are nurses most closely involved? In what situation would a nurse refer a patient to the dietitian?
4. When questioning a patient about his diet history after cardiac bypass surgery, you determine that the patient is fond of spinach, kale, and broccoli. The patient reports eating at least two servings of these foods almost every day. Knowing that most patients who undergo a bypass take an anticoagulant medication after surgery, how would you counsel this patient?

CHAPTER CHALLENGE QUESTIONS

True-False
Write the correct statement for each statement that is false.
1. *True or False:* Nutrition care is based on the needs of individual patients.
2. *True or False:* Patients' housing situations have little relationship with their illnesses or continuing care.
3. *True or False:* History taking is an important skill when planning nutrition care.
4. *True or False:* After a diet treatment plan has been established, it should be continuously followed, without any changes.
5. *True or False:* The involvement of the patient's family in the diet therapy and teaching usually creates problems and is best avoided.
6. *True or False:* Patients' personal goals relate to their diet therapy and instruction.
7. *True or False:* Drug-nutrient interactions only create complications when the patient is taking dietary supplements; they do not occur with whole foods.

Multiple Choice

1. Which of the following personal details help to determine a patient's nutrition needs? *(Circle all that apply.)*
   a. Gastrointestinal function
   b. Blood protein level
   c. Skinfold thickness
   d. Symptoms of illness

2. A nutrition history should include which of the following items of nutrition information? *(Circle all that apply.)*
   a. General food habits
   b. Food-buying practices
   c. Cooking methods
   d. Food likes and dislikes

3. Knowledge of which of the following items is necessary for carrying out valid nutrition therapy for a hospitalized patient? *(Circle all that apply.)*
   a. The specific diet and its relation to the patient's disease
   b. Family member meal plans and restrictions
   c. The mode of the hospital's food service and the patient's need for any eating assistance devices
   d. The patient's response to the diet

⊖volve Please refer to the Students' Resource section of this text's Evolve Web site for additional study resources.

REFERENCES

1. Okkonen E, Vanhanen H. Family support, living alone, and subjective health of a patient in connection with a coronary artery bypass surgery. *Heart Lung.* 2006;35(4):234-244.
2. Stricker KH, Kimberger O, Schmidlin K, et al. Family satisfaction in the intensive care unit: what makes the difference? *Intensive Care Med.* 2009;35(12):2051-2059.
3. American Nurses Association. *The nursing process: a common thread amongst all nurses* (website): www.nursingworld.org/EspeciallyForYou/StudentNurses/Thenursingprocess.aspx. Accessed February 2011.
4. Writing Group of the Nutrition Care Process/Standardized Language Committee: Nutrition care process and model part I: the 2008 update. *J Am Diet Assoc.* 2008;108(7):1113-1117.
5. Lacey K, Pritchett E. Nutrition Care Process and Model: ADA adopts road map to quality care and outcomes management. *J Am Diet Assoc.* 2003;103(8):1061-1072.
6. Academy of Nutrition and Dietetics. *Nutrition care process SNAPshots* (website): www.eatright.org/HealthProfessionals/content.aspx?id=5902. Accessed February 2011.
7. Singh R, Martin BR, Hickey Y, et al. Comparison of self-reported, measured, metabolizable energy intake with total energy expenditure in overweight teens. *Am J Clin Nutr.* 2009;89(6):1744-1750.
8. Scagliusi FB, Ferrioli E, Pfrimer K, et al. Characteristics of women who frequently under report their energy intake: a doubly labelled water study. *Eur J Clin Nutr.* 2009;63(10):1192-1199.
9. Bothwell EK, Ayala GX, Conway TL, et al. Underreporting of food intake among Mexican/Mexican-American women: rates and correlates. *J Am Diet Assoc.* 2009;109(4):624-632.
10. Bailey RL, Mitchell DC, Miller C, Smiciklas-Wright H. Assessing the effect of underreporting energy intake on dietary patterns and weight status. *J Am Diet Assoc.* 2007;107(1):64-71.
11. Neilson HK, Robson PJ, Friedenreich CM, Csizmadi I. Estimating activity energy expenditure: how valid are physical activity questionnaires? *Am J Clin Nutr.* 2008;87(2):279-291.
12. Janssen I, Katzmarzyk PT, Ross R. Body mass index, waist circumference, and health risk: evidence in support of current National Institutes of Health guidelines. *Arch Intern Med.* 2002;162(18):2074-2079.
13. Clinical guidelines on the identification, evaluation, and treatment of overweight and obesity in adults–the evidence report. National Institutes of Health. *Obes Res.* 1998;6(Suppl 2):51S-209S.
14. Feller S, Boeing H, Pischon T. Body mass index, waist circumference, and the risk of type 2 diabetes mellitus: implications for routine clinical practice. *Dtsch Arztebl Int.* 2010;107(26):470-476.
15. Smoliner C, Norman K, Wagner KH, et al. Malnutrition and depression in the institutionalised elderly. *Br J Nutr.* 2009;102(11):1663-1667.
16. Grieger JA, Nowson CA, Ackland LM. Nutritional and functional status indicators in residents of a long-term care facility. *J Nutr Elder.* 2009;28(1):47-60.
17. National Center for Health Statistics. *Health, United States, 2010: with special feature on death and dying.* Hyattsville, Md: U.S. Government Printing Office; 2011.
18. Paine MF, Widmer WW, Hart HL, et al. A furanocoumarin-free grapefruit juice establishes furanocoumarins as the mediators of the grapefruit juice-felodipine interaction. *Am J Clin Nutr.* 2006;83(5):1097-1105.
19. Holbrook AM, Pereira JA, Labiris R, et al. Systematic overview of warfarin and its drug and food interactions. *Arch Intern Med.* 2005;165(10):1095-1106.
20. Genser D. Food and drug interaction: consequences for the nutrition/health status. *Ann Nutr Metab.* 2008;52(Suppl 1):29-32.
21. Bailey RL, Gahche JJ, Lentino CV, et al. Dietary supplement use in the United States, 2003-2006. *J Nutr.* 2011;141(2):261-266.
22. Borrelli F, Izzo AA. Herb-drug interactions with St John's wort (*Hypericum perforatum*): an update on clinical observations. *AAPS J.* 2009;11(4):710-727.
23. Sorensen JM. Herb-drug, food-drug, nutrient-drug, and drug-drug interactions: mechanisms involved and their medical implications. *J Altern Complement Med.* 2002;8(3):293-308.

FURTHER READING AND RESOURCES

American Society for Parenteral and Enteral Nutrition. www.nutritioncare.org

This association provides education, publications, conferences, and resources about clinical nutrition therapy for health care professionals. The association is made up of physicians, dietitians, nurses, pharmacists, scientists, and other allied health care professionals.

National Policy and Resource Center on Nutrition and Aging, Nutrition Screening and Assessment. Nutrition Screening Initiative and Mini Nutritional Assessment. www2.fiu.edu/~nutreldr/SubjectList/N/Nutrition_Screening_Assessment.htm

This site provides research, reports, resources, and additional Web links for nutrition assessment tools.

Gershwin ME, Borchers AT, Keen CL, et al. Public safety and dietary supplementation. *Ann N Y Acad Sci.* 2010;1190:104-117.

Writing Group of the Nutrition Care Process/Standardized Language Committee. Nutrition care process and model part I: the 2008 update. *J Am Diet Assoc.* 2008;108(7):1113-1117.

CHAPTER 18

Gastrointestinal and Accessory Organ Problems

KEY CONCEPTS

- Diseases of the gastrointestinal (GI) tract and its accessory organs interrupt the body's normal cycle of digestion, absorption, and metabolism.
- Food allergies result from sensitivity to certain proteins.

- Underlying genetic diseases may cause metabolic defects that block the body's ability to handle specific foods.

The body's highly organized and intricate system for handling food is often taken for granted. However, when something goes wrong with the system, the whole body is affected. The GI tract is a sensitive mirror, both directly and indirectly, of the individual human condition.

This chapter looks at the system that manages food and its nutrients. The digestive process requires a series of cascading events throughout the GI tract and the accessory organs: the pancreas, the liver, and the gallbladder. Nutrition therapy must be based on the functioning of this finely integrated network and on the person whose life it affects.

THE UPPER GASTROINTESTINAL TRACT

Major diseases that affect the GI tract are not limited to just the small or large intestine. The most affected areas are discussed in this chapter under the headings that state where their primary problems exist.

Problems of the Mouth

Dental Problems

Although the incidence of dental caries has declined somewhat during recent years, tooth decay still plagues children and adults. Some of the decline is associated with the increased use of fluoridated public water and toothpaste as well as better dental hygiene. Fluoride toothpastes are clearly effective for preventing dental caries at fluoride concentrations of 1000 ppm or more

in children and adolescents.[1] In elderly people, loss of teeth or ill-fitting dentures may cause problems with eating, decreased fruit and vegetable intake, and compromised overall nutrition. About half of the older adults in the United States have severe tooth loss, with 0 to 10 teeth remaining.[2,3] Sometimes a mechanical soft diet is helpful for individuals who are lacking teeth. For such a diet, all foods are soft cooked, and meats are ground and mixed with sauces or gravies so that less chewing is necessary.

Surgical Procedures

A fractured jaw and other surgeries that involve the mouth and neck poses obvious eating problems. Nutrients must be supplied, usually in the form of high-protein, high-caloric liquids. Table 18-1 provides an example of a simple milkshake, and other commercial formulas are also available (see Chapter 22). As healing progresses, soft

TABLE 18-1 **HIGH-PROTEIN, HIGH-KILOCALORIE FORMULA FOR LIQUID FEEDINGS**

Ingredient	Amount
Whole milk, 3.25% milk fat	1 cup
Egg substitute powder	0.35 oz or equivalent of 2 eggs
Ensure Plus	½ cup
Sugar, granulated	2 Tbsp
Ice cream, vanilla	½ cup
Vanilla flavoring	A few drops, as desired

Approximate food value: 23 g protein, 22 g fat, 80 g carbohydrate, and 618 kcal.
Prepackaged supplemental feedings are generally used instead of homemade liquid feedings.

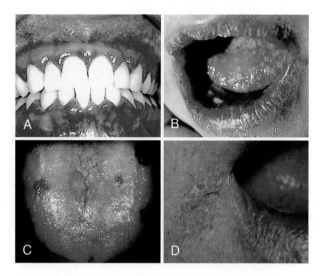

Figure 18-1 Tissue inflammation of the mouth. **A,** Gingivitis. **B,** Stomatitis. **C,** Glossitis. **D,** Cheilosis. (**A,** Reprinted from Murray PR, Rosenthal KS, Pfaller MA. *Medical microbiology.* 2nd ed. St. Louis: Mosby; 1994. **B,** Reprinted from Doughty DB, Broadwell-Jackson D. *Gastrointestinal disorders.* St. Louis: Mosby; 1993. **C,** Reprinted from Hoffbrand AV, Pettit JE, eds. *Sandoz atlas of clinical hematology.* London: Gower Medical; 1988. **D,** Reprinted from Lemmi FO, Lemmi CAE. *Physical assessment findings* [CD-ROM]. Philadelphia: Saunders; 2000.)

foods that require little chewing effort can be added, with the individual building to a full diet in accordance with his or her personal tolerance.

Oral Tissue Inflammation

Tissues of the mouth often reflect a person's general nutrition status. Malnutrition—especially severe states—causes the deterioration of the oral tissues, which results in local infection or injury that brings pain and difficulty with eating. The following conditions of the oral cavity may contribute to malnutrition:

- *Gingivitis:* inflammation of the gums that involves the mucous membrane and its supporting fibrous tissue that circles the base of the teeth (Figure 18-1, *A*)
- *Stomatitis:* inflammation of the oral mucous lining of the mouth (Figure 18-1, *B*)
- *Glossitis:* inflammation of the tongue (Figure 18-1, *C*)
- *Cheilosis:* a dry, scaling process at the corners of the mouth that affects the lips and the corner angles, thereby making opening the mouth to eat uncomfortable (Figure 18-1, *D*)

Mouth ulcers may develop from three infectious sources: (1) the herpes simplex virus, which causes mouth sores on the inside mucous lining of the cheeks and lips or on the external portion of the lips, where they are commonly called *cold sores* or *fever blisters;* (2) *Candida albicans,* which is a fungus that causes similar sores on the oral mucosa and results in a condition called *candidiasis* or *thrush;* and (3) hemolytic *Streptococcus,* which is a bacteria that causes the mucosal ulcers that are commonly called *canker sores.* Mouth ulcers are usually self-limiting and short lived. Other causes include simple toothbrush abrasions and allergies. Patients with an underlying illness such as cancer or HIV—both of which

lower the body's immune system—often have mouth ulcers. Chemotherapy and radiation treatment to the mouth destroy the fast-replicating cells and can result in painful mouth sores.

In these situations, eating may hurt; adequate nutrition should be considered in severe cases. Progressing from nutritionally dense liquids that are high in protein and calories to soft foods (e.g., usually nonacidic and bland to avoid irritation) is well tolerated. Extremes in temperature are avoided if they cause discomfort. Room-temperature soft or liquid foods are usually better accepted. For a person suffering from mouth pain, a mouthwash that contains a mild topical local anesthetic before meals helps to relieve the irritation that can be caused by eating.

Salivary Gland Problems

Disorders of the salivary glands in the mouth also affect eating and related nutrition status. Problems may arise from infection, such as the mumps virus that attacks the parotid gland (Figure 18-2). Other problems arise from mucous cysts (i.e., mucoceles) in obstructed salivary ducts, usually on the lower lip or the insides of the cheeks. Both excess salivation and inadequate salivation can interfere with eating and salivary gland function. Excess salivation is seen with numerous disorders that affect the

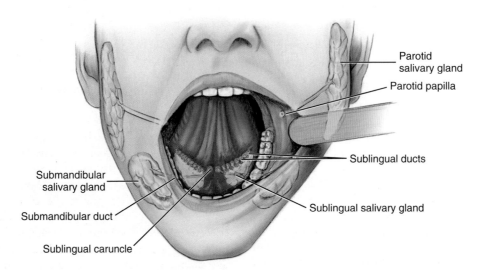

Figure 18-2 Location of the salivary glands. (Reprinted from Fehrenbach MJ, Herring SW. *Illustrated anatomy of the head and neck.* 3rd ed. Saunders: St. Louis; 2007.)

nervous system, local mouth infections, injuries, and drug reactions. Conversely, a dry mouth from a lack of salivation may be temporary and caused by fear, infection, or a drug reaction. Chronic dry mouth, which is called *xerostomia*, sometimes occurs in middle-aged and elderly adults, and it is often associated with rheumatoid arthritis or radiation therapy, or it may occur as a side effect from many drugs that are taken on a long-term basis. Xerostomia causes swallowing and speaking difficulties, taste interference, and tooth decay. More liquid food items such as beverages, soups, stews, juicy fruits, and gravies or sauces may facilitate the eating process. Extreme mouth dryness may be partially relieved by spraying an artificial saliva solution inside the mouth.

Swallowing Disorders

Swallowing is not as simple an act as it may seem. It involves highly integrated actions of the mouth, the pharynx, and the esophagus; in addition, after it has been started, swallowing is beyond voluntary control. Swallowing difficulty is a fairly common problem with a variety of causes. It may be only temporary (e.g., as a result of a piece of food lodged in the back of the throat), and the Heimlich maneuver may be appropriate first aid. However, dysphagia is a more chronic problem in some patients, and it is particularly common among patients with neurologic disorders such as Alzheimer's disease, Parkinson's disease, and stroke. Other common causes of dysphagia are head and neck cancer, tooth loss, xerostomia, and muscular weakness of the larynx.[4] To treat

mechanical soft diet a meal plan that consists of foods that have been chopped, blended, ground, or prepared with extra fluid to make chewing and swallowing easier.

parotid glands the largest of the three pairs of salivary glands; the parotid glands lie, one on each side, above the angle of the jaw and below and in front of the ear; they continually secrete saliva, which passes along the duct of the gland and into the mouth through an opening in the inner cheek that is level with the second upper molar tooth; normal saliva flow facilitates the chewing and swallowing of food and prevents problems that occur with a dry mouth.

xerostomia a dryness of the mouth from a lack of normal secretions.

pharynx the muscular membranous passage that extends from the mouth to the posterior nasal passages, the larynx, and the esophagus.

Heimlich maneuver a first-aid maneuver that is used to relieve a person who is choking from the blockage of the breathing passageway by a swallowed foreign object or food particle; to perform the maneuver, when standing behind the choking person, clasp the victim around the waist, place one fist just under the sternum (i.e., the breastbone), grasp the fist with the other hand, and then make a quick, hard, thrusting movement inward and upward to dislodge the object.

dysphagia difficulty swallowing.

dysphagia effectively, the problem must be identified as either a mechanical obstruction or a neuromuscular disorder, and it is usually diagnosed by a speech-language pathologist.

Subtle symptoms of dysphagia include an unexplained drop in food intake or repeated episodes of pneumonia related to aspiration. Patients with dysphagia have significantly longer hospital stays and compromised nutritional statuses compared with similar patients without dysphagia.[5,6] Watch for warning signs of dysphagia, and report them immediately. These signs may include the reluctance to eat certain food consistencies or any food at all, very slow chewing or eating, fatigue from eating, frequent throat clearing, complaints of food "sticking" in the throat, pockets of food held in the cheeks, painful swallowing, regurgitation, and coughing or choking during attempts to eat.

The problem usually is referred to a team of specialists that includes a physician, a nurse, a dietitian, and a speech-language pathologist. Thin liquids are the most difficult food form to swallow. Thus, the diet is adapted to individual needs in stages of thickened liquids and pureed foods. Pureed foods are generally the consistency of mashed potatoes or pudding. Regular table food can be pureed in a food processor to achieve the desired consistency. Several manufacturers produce pureed foods or food molds that are shaped like various meats or vegetables. Placing pureed food in a food mold to take the shape of the original food (e.g., corn on the cob, a chicken breast) enhances the appeal and appetite of patients who are faced with swallowing disorders, and it has been shown to improve overall nutrition intake.[7]

Problems of the Esophagus

Central Tube Problems

The esophagus is a long, muscular tube that extends from the throat to the stomach. It is bound on both ends by circular muscles or sphincters that act as valves to control the passage of food. The upper sphincter muscle remains closed except during swallowing, thereby preventing airflow into the esophagus and the stomach. The sphincter automatically opens when swallowing and then closes immediately afterward. Various disorders along the tube may disrupt normal swallowing, including muscle spasms or uncoordinated contractions as well as the stricture or narrowing of the tube caused by a scar from a previous injury, the ingestion of caustic chemicals, a tumor, or esophagitis. These problems hinder eating and require medical attention through stretching procedures or surgery to widen the tube in addition to drug therapy to heal the inflammation. The diet during such problems is liquid to soft in texture, depending on the extent of the problem and individual tolerance.

Lower Esophageal Sphincter Problems

Defects in the function of the lower esophageal sphincter (LES) may come from changes in the smooth muscle itself or from the nerve, muscle, and hormone control of peristalsis (see Chapter 5). Spasms occur when the LES muscles maintain an excessively high muscle tone, even while resting, thereby failing to open normally when the person swallows. This condition is medically termed *achalasia* because of its tense muscle state, but it is commonly called *cardiospasm* because of its proximity of the heart (although the condition does not relate to the heart at all). Symptoms include swallowing problems, frequent vomiting, a feeling of fullness in the chest, weight loss from eating difficulties, malnutrition, and pulmonary complications and infections caused by the aspiration of food particles, especially during sleep. Surgical treatment involves dilating the LES or cutting the muscle, which is called *esophagomyotomy*. Both procedures can improve the relaxation of the LES, but neither affects the lack of peristalsis. The postoperative nutrition therapy starts with oral liquids and progresses to a regular diet within a few days, depending on tolerance. Patients should avoid very hot or cold foods, citrus juices, and highly spiced foods to prevent irritation. It is also helpful for patients to eat frequent small meals as tolerated, to eat slowly, to take small bites, and to thoroughly chew food.

Gastroesophageal Reflux Disease

Impaired esophageal peristalsis and ongoing LES problems are the two primary contributors to chronic gastroesophageal reflux disease (GERD).[8] GERD is a serious and difficult problem that has been described as acid "setting up shop" in the esophagus. The prevalence of GERD is increasing in the United States, and it is the most common upper GI disorder among elderly patients.[9] In addition, elderly patients tend to experience more severe cases and complications of GERD compared with other segments of the population.[10]

---

speech-language pathologist a specialist in the assessment, diagnosis, treatment, and prevention of speech, language, cognitive communication, voice, swallowing, fluency, and other related disorders.

esophagitis inflammation of the esophagus

achalasia a disorder of the esophagus in which the muscles of the tube fail to relax, thereby inhibiting normal swallowing.

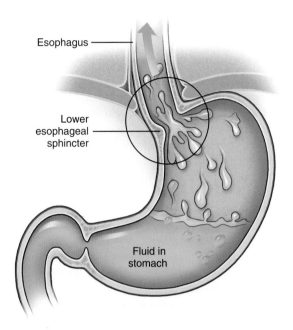

Esophagus

Lower esophageal sphincter

Fluid in stomach

Figure 18-3 Reflux of gastric acid up into the esophagus through the lower esophageal sphincter in a patient with gastroesophageal reflux disease. (Reprinted from Thibodeau GA, Patton KT. *Anatomy & physiology.* 6th ed. St. Louis: Mosby; 2007.)

TABLE 18-2 DIETARY CARE OF GASTROESOPHAGEAL REFLUX DISEASE

Goal	Action
Decrease esophageal irritation	Avoid common irritants such as coffee, strong tea, chocolate, carbonated beverages, tomato and citrus juices, spicy foods, smoking, and alcoholic beverages
Increase lower esophageal sphincter pressure	Increase lean protein foods
	Decrease fat to approximately 45 g/day or less; use nonfat milk
	Avoid peppermint and spearmint
Decrease reflux frequency and volume	Eat small, frequent meals
	Sip only a small amount of liquid with a meal; drink mostly between meals
	Avoid constipation by consuming adequate fiber; straining increases abdominal pressure reflux
	Avoid eating at least 3 to 4 hours before going to bed
Clear food materials from the esophagus	Sit upright at the table, and elevate the head of the bed
	Do not recline for 2 hours or more after eating
	Wear loose-fitting clothing, especially after a meal

The constant regurgitation of acidic gastric contents into the lower part of the esophagus results in erosive esophagitis in about half of the patients with this disease (Figure 18-3). Typical symptoms include frequent and severe heartburn that occurs 30 to 60 minutes after eating. The pain sometimes moves into the neck or jaw or down the arms. The most common complications are stenosis (i.e., a narrowing or stricture of the esophagus) and esophageal ulcer.

The risk for GERD symptoms and erosive esophagitis increase with overweight or obesity compared with a normal body mass index, thus indicating that overweight patients may respond well to weight-reduction strategies.[11] In addition, acid reflux may be attributed to pregnancy, pernicious vomiting, or the extended use of nasogastric tubes. In addition to weight loss, other conservative measures include acid control and a low-fat diet (high-fat diets make the closure of the esophageal sphincter less effective). Patients are advised to avoid lying down after eating and to sleep with the head of the bed elevated. The frequent use of antacids helps with the control of symptoms. The goals and actions of dietary care are outlined in Table 18-2. Laparoscopic fundoplication is a surgical procedure that restores LES function and esophageal peristalsis, thereby treating the condition and not just the symptoms. This procedure is highly successful, and it is recommended for patients whose symptoms are not relieved by weight loss or other conservative measures.[8]

Hiatal Hernia

The lower end of the esophagus normally enters the chest cavity through an opening in the diaphragm membrane called the *hiatus.* A hiatal hernia occurs when a portion of the upper stomach also protrudes through this opening, as shown in Figure 18-4. Hiatal hernias are not uncommon, especially in obese adults, for whom weight reduction is essential. Patients with hiatal hernias are advised to eat small amounts of food at a time, to avoid lying down after meals, and to sleep with the head of the bed elevated to prevent the reflux of acidic stomach contents. The frequent use of antacids helps to control the symptoms of heartburn, which is caused by the acid, enzyme, and food mixture irritating the lower esophagus and the

laparoscopic fundoplication a surgery that is used to treat gastroesophageal reflux disease; the upper portion of the stomach (i.e., the fundus) is wrapped around the esophagus and sewn into place so that the esophagus passes through the muscle of the stomach; this strengthens the esophageal sphincter to prevent acid reflux.

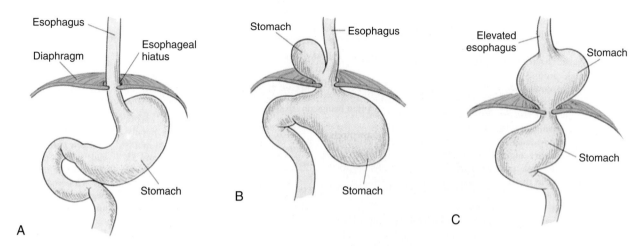

Figure 18-4 Hiatal hernia compared with normal stomach placement. **A,** Normal stomach. **B,** Paraesophageal hernia, with the esophagus in its normal position. **C,** Esophageal hiatal hernia, with an elevated esophagus. (Courtesy Bill Ober.)

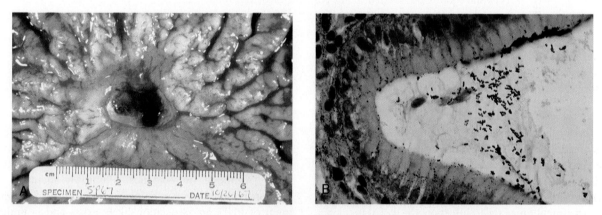

Figure 18-5   A, Gastric ulcer. **B,** *Helicobacter pylori (black particles)* infecting the stomach mucosa. (Reprinted from Thibodeau GA, Patton KT. *Anatomy & physiology.* 6th ed. St. Louis: Mosby; 2007.)

upper herniated area of the stomach. Large hiatal hernias or smaller sliding hernias require surgical repair.

Problems of the Stomach and Duodenum: Peptic Ulcer Disease

The mucosal lining of the stomach and duodenum protects the tissue from corrosive gastric acid. If the mucosa is weakened or disturbed and cannot protect against acidic gastric content, the tissue is damaged. The general term *peptic ulcer* refers to an eroded mucosal lesion in the central portion of the GI tract. This lesion can occur in the lower esophagus, the stomach, or the first portion of the duodenum (i.e., the duodenal bulb). Most ulcers occur in the duodenal bulb because the gastric contents emptying there are the most concentrated. A peptic ulcer is a crater-like lesion in the wall of the stomach or duodenum that results from the continuous erosion of the mucosal tissue through the mucosal layers down to the muscular layers (Figure 18-5).

Causes

The lesion results from an imbalance among the following three factors: (1) the amount of gastric acid and pepsin secretions; (2) the extent of *Helicobacter pylori* infection; and (3) the degree of tissue resistance to these secretions and the infection. The more acidic the environment, the more favorable the conditions are for *H. pylori* colonization. The two known causes of peptic ulcer disease (PUD) are *H. pylori* infection and the long-term use of nonsteroidal anti-inflammatory drugs (NSAIDs).[12]

Helicobacter pylori. *H. pylori* are common, spiraling, rod-shaped bacteria that inhabit the GI area around the pyloric valve (Figure 18-5, *B*). This muscular valve

CULTURAL CONSIDERATIONS

RISK FOR GASTRIC ULCER DISEASE: ENVIRONMENTAL OR GENETIC?

Before the bacteria *Helicobacter pylori* was shown in 1982 to be the causative organism of peptic ulcer disease, the disease was thought to be the result of excess stress, acid, and spicy food. Although these factors may still contribute to the disease, infection with *H. pylori* is now known to cause the majority of duodenal and gastric ulcers; the long-term use of nonsteroidal anti-inflammatory drugs is responsible for most of the other cases.

Infection with *Helicobacter Pylori*

H. pylori infection is more common among certain ethnic and age groups. In the United States, older adults, African Americans, and Hispanics have the highest prevalence of infection. In addition, individuals of a lower socioeconomic status have a higher risk of *H. pylori* infection compared with individuals of a higher socioeconomic status. The mechanism by which *H. pylori* infection is transmitted is not yet known; however, it is believed to be spread through the fecal-oral or oral-oral routes. However, not all carriers of the bacteria develop peptic ulcers.

Active *Helicobacter Pylori* Ulcers

H. pylori ulcers are more common among men than women in the United States. In countries such as Japan, where peptic ulcer disease is quite common, men are reported to have twice the prevalence of the condition compared with women. The risks for developing an ulcer are not easily defined by genetics, gender, ethnicity, or environment; a combination of all of these factors seems to lead to ulceration. Researchers believe that genetics are less important than environment with regard to determining the risk for ulceration, but both physiologic and psychologic factors are involved in the overall environmental risk.

Physiologic trauma and emotional stress can lead to excess acid secretions in the stomach. For individuals who are already infected with *H. pylori* bacteria, that may be the missing link for creating a perfect environment for rapid growth and inflammation that ultimately results in an ulcer. Therefore, the treatment of peptic ulcers must focus on eliminating the cause (i.e., bacteria or drugs) and focus on the environmental cues that are involved in the promotion of excessive acidic secretions.

---

connects the lower part of the stomach with the head of the small intestine (i.e., the duodenal bulb). Infection by *H. pylori* is a major determinant of chronic active gastritis, and it is a critical ingredient, along with gastric acid and pepsin, in the ulcerative process. As a result of aggressive treatment for *H. pylori* infection, the global incidence rate of PUD has decreased during recent years.[13] The Cultural Considerations box entitled "Risk for Gastric Ulcer Disease: Environmental or Genetic?" discusses additional risks factors for the development of PUD.

Nonsteroidal Anti-Inflammatory Drugs. NSAIDs are widely used medications. This drug class includes ibuprofen (Advil, Motrin) and aspirin (acetylsalicylic acid), which irritate the gastric mucosa and which may cause erosion, ulceration, and bleeding with prolonged or excessive use. The NSAIDs, including at least a dozen anti-inflammatory drugs, are so named to distinguish them from steroid drugs, which are synthetic variants of natural adrenal hormones.

Psychologic Factors. The influence of psychologic factors in the development of PUD varies. No distinct personality type is free from the disease. However, stress during the young and middle adult years, when personal and career striving are at their peaks, may contribute to the development of PUD in predisposed individuals. Several neurologic changes that result from severe or long-term stress have specific effects on the GI tract, such as increased colonic motor activity, slowed gastric emptying, and increased susceptibility to colonic inflammation.[14] Although no evidence definitively identifies a relationship between psychologic stress and the development of PUD, an association likely exists and is under investigation.[15,16]

Clinical Symptoms

General symptoms of PUD include increased gastric muscle tone and painful contractions when the stomach is empty. With duodenal ulcers, the amount and concentration of hydrochloric acid secretions are increased; with gastric ulcers, the secretions may be normal. Hemorrhage may be one of the first signs. Low plasma protein levels, anemia, and weight loss reveal nutrition deficiencies. Diagnosis is confirmed by radiographs and by visualization with gastroscopy.

---

gastroscopy an examination of the upper intestinal tract with a flexible tube with a small camera on the end; the tube is approximately 9 mm in diameter, and it takes color pictures as well as biopsy samples, if necessary.

Medical Management

There are four basic goals for the treatment of patients with PUD: (1) alleviate the symptoms; (2) promote healing; (3) prevent recurrences by eliminating the cause; and (4) prevent complications.

Rest. Adequate rest, relaxation, and sleep have long been the foundation of general care to enhance the body's natural healing process. Incorporating positive coping and relaxation skills into daily life may help patients to better deal with personal psychosocial stress factors. Habits that contribute to ulcer development (e.g., smoking, alcohol use) should be eliminated, and irritating drugs (e.g., aspirin, NSAIDs) should be avoided. Sometimes sedatives are prescribed to aid rest.

Drug Therapy. Advances in knowledge and therapy have provided physicians with the following four types of drugs for the management of PUD:

- Hydrochloric acid secretion controllers:
  - Histamine H_2-receptor antagonists (H_2-blockers) reduce hydrochloric acid production and secretion. These medications are available over the counter and include cimetidine (Tagamet), ranitidine (Zantac), famotidine (Pepcid), and nizatidine (Axid).
  - Proton pump inhibitors reduce hydrochloric acid production by inhibiting the hydrogen ion secretion that is needed to produce hydrochloric acid. These drugs include lansoprazole (Prevacid), omeprazole (Prilosec), esomeprazole (Nexium), pantoprazole (Protonix), and rabeprazole (Aciphex).
- Mucosal protectors, which inactivate pepsin and produce a gel-like substance to cover the ulcer and to protect it from acid and pepsin while it heals itself (e.g., sucralfate [Carafate]).
- Antibiotics, which address the *H. pylori* infection (e.g., amoxicillin, clarithromycin, tetracycline, metronidazole).
- Antacids, which counteract or neutralize the acid. Magnesium and aluminum compounds (e.g., Mylanta, Maalox) are the typical antacids of choice for the treatment of PUD.

Maintenance drug therapy is imperative to stabilize the growth rate of bacteria. A continuous low-dose drug therapy follows initial treatment, with intermittent full-dose treatment or symptomatic self-care with the same agents that are used to heal the initial ulcer infection. Success rates depend on the relative strengths of the risk factors that influence recurrence (Box 18-1).

See the Drug-Nutrient Interaction boxes entitled "Tetracycline and Mineral Absorption" and "Proton Pump

---

BOX 18-1 RISK FACTORS FOR RECURRING PEPTIC ULCER

High Risk
Medical/Physical
- *Helicobacter pylori* infection
- Previous recurrences of peptic ulcer with complications
- Hypersecretion of gastric acid
- Family history of peptic ulcer disease among close relatives

Emotional
- Continuous and unrelieved emotional stress
- Denial of emotional problems

Behavioral
- Poor dietary habits
- Failure to maintain prescribed diet and drug therapy
- Cigarette smoking of 10 or more per day
- Frequent use of aspirin and other nonsteroidal anti-inflammatory drugs

Moderate Risk
Medical/Physical
- Recurring discomfort after eating
- Age of 50 years old or older

Emotional
- Emotionally stressful environment
- Recognition of emotional problems

Behavioral
- Habitually skipping breakfast
- Distilled alcohol consumption
- Irregular meals

Inhibitors and Micronutrient Absorption" for more information about potential nutrient interactions with these commonly prescribed medications.

Dietary Management

In the past, a highly restrictive and bland diet was used for the care of patients with PUD. A bland diet has long since proved to be ineffective and lacking in adequate nutrition support for the healing process. Such a restrictive diet is unnecessary today, because more effective medication regimens are available to control acid secretions and to assist with healing. Thus, current diet therapy is based on a liberal individual approach that is guided by individual responses to food. As part of this positive nutrition support for medical management, two basic goals guide food habits.

Eating a Well-Balanced and Healthy Diet. Supply a well-balanced, regular, healthy diet to help with tissue

DRUG-NUTRIENT INTERACTION

TETRACYCLINE AND MINERAL ABSORPTION

Tetracycline is a broad-spectrum antibiotic that is used to treat conditions such as respiratory tract infections, acne, infections of the skin, and stomach ulcers. Minerals with a 2^+ charge—including magnesium, calcium, and iron—bond with tetracycline to form a new compound that the body can no longer absorb. Thus, tetracycline is less effective, and mineral absorption is poor.

To ensure optimal absorption, avoid the following foods or medications 1 hour before and 2 hours after taking tetracycline:

- Foods that contain high amounts of calcium (e.g., milk)
- Calcium supplements
- Antacids
- Laxatives that contain magnesium
- Iron supplements (these should be taken at least 2 hours before or 3 hours after tetracycline)

Sara Harcourt

DRUG-NUTRIENT INTERACTION

PROTON PUMP INHIBITORS AND MICRONUTRIENT ABSORPTION

Proton pump inhibitors are routinely prescribed for peptic ulcer disease. The long-term use of proton pump inhibitors is associated with the decreased absorption of some nutrients. This effect is largely as a result of the reduced acidity of the gastric environment. Gastric acid is required to separate bound nutrients in foods and to stabilize them for absorption. Vitamin B_{12} is naturally bound to protein in food. When acid production is reduced, vitamin B_{12} remains bound to protein carriers, and it is thus unavailable for absorption in the intestine.

Malabsorption is more likely to be a problem among elderly patients who already have a decrease in gastric acid production. Supplemental vitamin B_{12} is indicated for elderly patients who are receiving long-term proton pump inhibitor therapy. Reduced stomach acid may also affect the absorption of nonheme iron and vitamin C, which can lead to deficiencies of these nutrients. The effect on iron and vitamin C status is more marked when the patient is infected with *Helicobacter pylori;* thus, the supplementation of these nutrients may be indicated.[1]

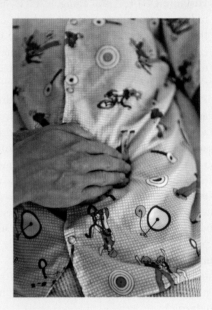

1. McColl KE. Effect of proton pump inhibitors on vitamins and iron. *Am J Gastroenterol.* 2009;104(Suppl 2):S5-S9.

healing and maintenance. Nutrient energy needs are outlined in the current Dietary Reference Intakes (see the inside front cover of this book) and expressed in the simple food choices of the MyPlate.gov guidelines (see Figure 1-3). Further focus is provided by the goals of the *Dietary Guidelines for Americans* (see Figure 1-4).

Avoiding Acid Stimulation. Avoid stimulating excess gastric acid secretion, which irritates the gastric mucosa.

Only the following few food-related habits are thought to affect acid secretion:

- *Food quantity:* To avoid stomach distension, do not eat large quantities at meals. Avoid eating right before going to bed, because food intake stimulates acid output.
- *Avoid irritants*: Individual tolerance is the rule, but some food seasonings such as hot chili peppers,

black pepper, and chili powder may irritate an already weakened mucosal layer. Caffeine, chocolate, and alcohol may increase acid secretions or prevent healing in some patients.

- *Smoking:* Complete smoking cessation is best, because smoking hinders ulcer healing. It also affects gastric acid secretion and hinders the effectiveness of drug therapy.

LOWER GASTROINTESTINAL TRACT

Small Intestine Diseases

Malabsorption

Malabsorption syndromes are characterized by a defect in the absorption of one or more of the essential nutrients. Malabsorption results from a disturbance in the normal digestive process or absorptive pathway, and the defect may include any of the following processes:

- *Digestion of macronutrients:* Carbohydrates, proteins, and fat are broken down into their basic building blocks (i.e., monosaccharides and disaccharides, amino acids, and fatty acids and glycerol, respectively) with the help of salivary and pancreatic enzymes and bile acid.
- *Terminal digestion at the brush border mucosa:* Disaccharides and peptides are hydrolyzed by disaccharidases and peptidases for the final step of digestion.
- *Absorption:* The end products of macronutrient digestion, micronutrients (i.e., vitamins, minerals, and electrolytes) and water are absorbed across the epithelium of the small intestine into the general or lymphatic circulation.

Several organ systems and functions are affected by malabsorption disorders. Chronic deficiencies of vitamins, minerals, and macronutrients can lead to several forms of anemia (e.g., iron, pyridoxine, folate, vitamin B_{12}); osteopenia and tetany from calcium, vitamin D, and magnesium deficiency; and other musculoskeletal, endocrine, and nervous system abnormalities. The most common symptoms of malabsorption disorders are chronic diarrhea, steatorrhea, or both.

Three specific malabsorption conditions—cystic fibrosis (CF), inflammatory bowel disease, and celiac sprue—are reviewed in this chapter. Other malabsorption syndromes are listed in Table 18-3. Diarrhea and steatorrhea are usually symptoms of a disease or disorder rather than a disease themselves. However, they are discussed in this section because they pertain to most malabsorption disorders.

Cystic Fibrosis

Disease Process. CF is the most common fatal genetic disease in North America; it occurs in approximately 1 in 3300 live Caucasian births and 1 in 15,300 African-American births.[17] Although the disease is characterized as a pulmonary disease, it is a multisystem disorder that has a profound GI tract impact. Because pulmonary diseases are outside of the scope of this text, only the nutrition implications of CF are discussed.

CF is a generalized genetic disease of childhood that is inherited as an autosomal recessive trait that can include multiple defects. Previously, children with CF lived to approximately the age of 10 years, dying from complications such as damaged airways and lung infections as well as a fibrous pancreas and malnutrition. However, the discovery of the CF gene and the underlying metabolic defect has improved the management of the disease and helped push the life expectancy of these individuals into adulthood. Nevertheless, mortality rates from CF have a strong correlation with poverty status. Minorities and individuals in the lowest socioeconomic category have a higher risk of complications, disease severity, and mortality, and they report a lower health-related quality of life compared with patients in the highest income category.[18-20] Identifying and addressing differences among socioeconomic classes with regard to disease self-management, environmental pollutants (e.g., cigarette smoke), and psychologic stress are important to improve the life of all patients with CF.

The metabolic defect of CF inhibits the normal movement of chloride and sodium ions in body tissue fluids (see Chapter 9). These ions become trapped in cells, and this causes thick mucus to form and clog ducts and passageways. Involved organ tissues are damaged so that they no longer function normally. The classic CF symptoms include the following:

- *Thick mucus in the lungs:* causes damaged airways, more difficult breathing, persistent coughing, and pulmonary infections (e.g., bronchitis, pneumonia)
- *Pancreatic insufficiency:* leads to a lack of normal pancreatic enzymes (see Chapter 5) to digest macronutrients and a progressive loss of insulin-

---

steatorrhea fatty diarrhea; excessive amount of fat in the feces, which is often caused by malabsorption diseases.

TABLE 18-3 MAJOR MALABSORPTION SYNDROMES

Symptoms	Causes
Defective Intraluminal Digestion	
Defective digestion of fats and proteins	Pancreatic insufficiency from pancreatitis or cystic fibrosis
	Zollinger-Ellison syndrome,* with the inactivation of pancreatic enzymes by excess gastric acid secretion
Solubilization of fat as a result of defective bile secretion	Ileal dysfunction or resection with decreased bile salt uptake
	Cessation of bile flow from obstruction or hepatic dysfunction
Nutrient preabsorption or modification	Bacterial overgrowth
Primary Mucosal Cell Abnormalities	
Defective terminal digestion	Disaccharidase deficiency (lactose intolerance)
	Bacterial overgrowth with brush border damage
Defective epithelial transport	Abetalipoproteinemia (an inherited disorder of fat metabolism from the inability to synthesize β lipoproteins)
	Primary bile acid malabsorption that results from mutations in the ileal bile acid transporter
Reduced small intestinal surface area	Gluten-sensitive enteropathy (celiac disease)
	Crohn's disease
Lymphatic obstruction	Lymphoma
	Tuberculosis and tuberculous lymphadenitis
Infection	Acute infectious enteritis
	Parasitic infestation
	Whipple's disease (bacterial infection)
General malabsorption that results from surgery	Subtotal or total gastrectomy
	Short gut syndrome after extensive surgical resection
	Distal ileal resection or bypass

*This is a rare disorder that causes tumors in the pancreas and duodenum and ulcers in the stomach and duodenum. The tumors secrete a hormone called *gastrin* that causes the stomach to produce too much hydrochloric acid, which in turn causes stomach and duodenal ulcers. The symptoms include signs of a peptic ulcer, such as the following: gnawing, burning pain in the abdomen; diarrhea; nausea; vomiting; fatigue; weakness; weight loss; and bleeding. From the National Digestive Disease Information Clearinghouse. *Zollinger-Ellison syndrome* (website): digestive.niddk.nih.gov/ddiseases/pubs/Zollinger. Accessed February 2011. Modified from Kumar V, Fausto N, Abbas A. *Robbins & Cotran pathologic basis of disease.* 7th ed. Philadelphia: Saunders; 2005.

producing β cells and eventual diabetes mellitus in approximately 15% of adult patients (see Chapter 20)

- *Malabsorption:* food is left undigested and unabsorbed, with consequential malnutrition, stunted growth, delayed puberty, and infertility
- *Liver and gallbladder disease:* from the progressive degeneration of functional liver tissue, which is initiated by clogged bile ducts
- *Inflammatory complications:* including arthritis, finger clubbing, and vasculitis
- *Increased salt concentration:* in body perspiration, thereby leading to salt depletion

Nutrition Management. Nutrition therapy is a critical component of the treatment regimen, and it can have a significant impact on normal growth. Patients who maintain an age-appropriate body mass index percentile have better overall health outcomes.[21] Treatment is augmented with the following: (1) increased knowledge of the disease process; (2) early newborn screening and diagnosis; and (3) improved pancreatic enzyme replacement products.

Enzyme-replacement products (e.g., pancrelipase [Pancrease]) contain the normal pancreatic enzymes for each energy nutrient (i.e., lipase for fat digestion; amylase for starch digestion; and the proteases trypsin, chymotrypsin, and carboxypeptidase [see Chapter 5]). These enzymes are processed into very small enteric-coated beads that are encased in capsules that have been designed not to open or dissolve until they reach the alkaline medium of the intestine. Generous doses of these enzyme-replacement capsules, which vary with a patient's age, weight, and symptoms, are divided among the day's meals; they are usually taken just before eating. Adequate enzyme replacement is the foundation that makes aggressive diet therapy a possibility for meeting growth needs.

Patients with CF who are older than 2 years of age require 110% to 200% of the recommended nutrients for their age, depending on the severity of the disease. A high-energy, nutritionally adequate diet is required and may include oral or enteral nutritional supplementation to maintain weight.[21] Routine care is based on regular nutrition assessment, diet counseling, food plans, enzyme and salt replacement, vitamin supplements (especially fat-soluble vitamins), nutrition education, and the exploration of individual problems. Box 18-2 outlines the current standards of nutritional care for the management of CF.

vasculitis the inflammation of the walls of blood vessels.

BOX 18-2 NUTRITION CARE FOR CYSTIC FIBROSIS

Evidence-Based Recommendations[1]:
1. Energy intake is increased to 110% to 200% of the standards for the healthy population
2. Optimal ranges of weight for age and stature for age for children and of body mass index for adults are indicated to support better lung function
   Optimal ranges:
   - *Children up to the age of 20 years:* ≥ 50th percentile recommended
   - *Women:* body mass index of ≥ 22
   - *Men:* body mass index of ≥ 23
3. Pancreatic enzyme preparations are required to ensure efficacy when treating cystic fibrosis–related pancreatic insufficiency

Nutrition Intervention During Cystic Fibrosis Should Focus on the Following[2]:
1. Increased calorie and fat intake
2. Maintenance of lean body mass

General Dietary Principles for Patients with Cystic Fibrosis[2]:
1. Provide three meals and two to three snacks per day
2. Provide pancreatic enzyme and vitamin supplementation
3. Provide an unrestricted diet that includes high-fat

foods and additives
4. Encourage a variety of whole grains, nuts, fruits, and vegetables to maintain adequate vitamin and mineral intake
5. Assess vitamin and mineral intake, including those that are received from supplements
6. Provide counseling to discuss ideas for calorie boosters, on the basis of the patient's usual intake, to meet energy needs
7. Understand that supplements and nutrient-dense nourishments may help to maintain adequate nutrient intake
8. Know that extra salt will be needed to replace the excess salt that is excreted in sweat, especially during hot weather, when exercising, or when febrile
9. Ensure adequate calcium, vitamin D, and vitamin K intake to promote optimal bone health

When Oral Intake is Inadequate and not Expected to Improve[2]:
1. Enteral nutrition support can provide a safe means of nutritional intake, maintain gut integrity, and possibly improve the patient's outcome
2. In severe cases and for patients with multisystem organ failure, parenteral nutrition support via a central line may be required

1. Stallings VA, Stark LJ, Robinson KA, et al; Clinical Practice Guidelines on Growth and Nutrition Subcommittee; Ad Hoc Working Group. Evidence-based practice recommendations for nutrition-related management of children and adults with cystic fibrosis and pancreatic insufficiency: results of a systematic review. *J Am Diet Assoc.* 2008;108(5):832-839.
2. American Dietetic Association. *ADA nutrition care manual.* Chicago: American Dietetic Association; 2010.

CLINICAL APPLICATIONS

CASE STUDY: PAUL'S ADAPTATION TO CYSTIC FIBROSIS

Paul is a 12-year-old boy with cystic fibrosis. He is hospitalized with pneumonia, and he has difficulty breathing. Paul is a thin child with little muscle development who tires easily, although he has a large appetite. His stools are large and frequent, and they contain undigested food material.

Questions for Analysis
1. What is cystic fibrosis? Account for the clinical effects of the disease as evidenced by Paul's appearance and symptoms.

2. What are the basic goals of the treatment of cystic fibrosis? Why is vigorous nutrition therapy a primary part of treatment?
3. Describe the role of enzyme replacement therapy in this aggressive nutrition support.
4. Why does Paul require therapeutic doses of multivitamins, including fat-soluble vitamins?

Try applying these principles of care while reading the Clinical Applications box entitled "Case Study: Paul's Adaptation to Cystic Fibrosis."

Inflammatory Bowel Disease

Inflammatory bowel disease is a general term that is used to describe chronic inflammation of the GI tract and the persistent activation of the mucosal immune system against the normal healthy gut flora. Chronic inflammation disrupts the protective epithelial barrier until ulceration of the mucosal surface destroys segments of the GI tract. As a result of lesions, portions of the GI tract are not functional, which causes malabsorption. The related condition of short-bowel syndrome may result if the

TABLE 18-4 CLINICAL MANIFESTATIONS OF CROHN'S DISEASE AND ULCERATIVE COLITIS

Manifestation	Common to Both Inflammatory Bowel Diseases	
Etiology	Unknown	
Genetics	15% of patients with inflammatory bowel disease have first-degree relatives with the condition	
Gut Flora	Intestinal gut flora plays a role, but there is no specific microbe that is the underlying causative factor	
Immune response	Linked to inappropriate T-cell activation or too little control by regulatory T lymphocytes	
Symptoms	Abdominal pain, diarrhea, and weight loss	
Risk factors	Females and Caucasians are affected more than other segments of the population	
Complications	Osteoporosis, dermatitis, ocular symptoms, liver and gallbladder complications, and kidney stones	
	SPECIFIC TO TYPE OF INFLAMMATORY BOWEL DISEASE	
	Crohn's Disease	**Ulcerative Colitis**
Incidence	3 per 100,000	4 to 12 per 100,000
Additional risk factors	Jewish ancestry and smoking	Former smokers are at higher risk than people who have never smoked
Bowel region affected	Ileum and colon	Colon only
Distribution	Skip lesions	Continuous from rectum
Inflammation	Mucosa and all underlying tissue layers	Mucosa and submucosal layers only
Ulceration	Deep, linear ulcerative lesions	Superficial ulcers
Fat-soluble vitamin malabsorption	If lesions are in ileum	No
Response to surgery	Poor to fair	Good
Long-term complications	Fibrosing strictures, fistulas to other organs, cancer, malabsorption (of vitamin B_{12} and bile salts, thereby causing pernicious anemia and steatorrhea), bowel obstruction, polyarthritis, sacroiliitis, ankylosing spondylitis, erythema nodosum, and clubbing of the fingertips	Perforation and toxic megacolon; these patients also have a high risk for cancer

repeated surgical removal of parts of the small intestine is necessary as the disease progresses.

One in 200 individuals of Northern European descent is affected by inflammatory bowel disease, and there is a genetic risk factor associated with it.[22] Crohn's disease and ulcerative colitis are the two most common forms of inflammatory bowel disease; both of these are idiopathic diseases. These diseases share many symptoms and management strategies, but they differ with regard to their clinical manifestations (Table 18-4).

Crohn's Disease. Crohn's disease may affect any portion of the GI tract from the esophagus to the anus, but it is most commonly localized to the ileum and the colon. Risk factors include a family history of the disease, Jewish ancestry, and smoking. Inflammation may skip sections of the GI tract and affect more than one section at a time (Figure 18-6). Symptoms will vary for patients, depending on the location of the inflammation, but they most commonly include the following: abdominal pain, fever, fatigue, anorexia, weight loss, painful defecation,

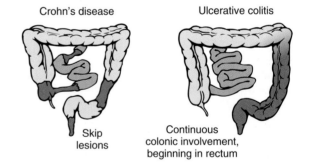

Figure 18-6 Comparison of the distribution pattern of Crohn's disease and ulcerative colitis. (Reprinted from Kumar V, Fausto N, Abbas A. *Robbins & Cotran pathologic basis of disease.* 7th ed. Philadelphia: Saunders; 2005.)

idiopathic of unknown cause.

and diarrhea.[23] Patients may experience long asymptomatic periods between flare-ups, or they may experience continuous and progressive attacks.

Iron-deficiency anemia is common among patients with Crohn's disease. Decreased intake, impaired absorption, and blood loss all contribute to iron deficiency in these patients.[24] Iron-deficiency anemia decreases quality of life, and it can have long-term negative cognitive consequences in children; thus, screening, early detection, and treatment are important parts of the management of this disease.

Ulcerative Colitis. Ulcerative colitis is an inflammatory disease that is limited to the colon. Symptoms include diarrhea with blood and mucus, abdominal pain, weight loss, fever, and rectal pain. The inflammation does not skip sections of the bowel; rather, it is progressive from the anus (see Figure 18-6).

All inflammatory bowel conditions can have severe and often devastating nutrition results as more and more of the absorbing surface area becomes involved. Malnutrition can exacerbate an attack and hinder the healing process. Restoring positive nutrition is a basic requirement for tissue healing and health. Enteral nutrition support of either polymeric formula or elemental formula is helpful for many patients (in addition to steroid treatment) to restore nutritional balance.[25] The diet is gradually advanced as tolerated to restore optimal nutrient intake. Principles of continuing dietary management include the following[26]:

During periods of inflammation:

- Use enteral or parenteral nutrition feedings, if necessary.
- Progress to low-fat, low-fiber, high-protein, high-kilocalorie, small, frequent meals when returning to a normal diet as tolerated.
- Vitamin and mineral supplementation should include vitamin D, zinc, calcium, magnesium, folate, vitamin B_{12}, and iron.

During periods of remission:

- Meet energy and protein needs that are specific for weight, and replenish nutrient stores.
- Avoid foods that are high in oxalates.
- Increase probiotic intake.
- Increase antioxidant intake, and consider supplementation with omega-3 fatty acids and glutamine.

Current studies and clinical practice indicate the benefit of a regular nourishing diet that reflects individual tolerances and disease status. A close working relationship among the physician, the dietitian, and the nurse is essential. The patient's appetite often is poor, but adequate nutrition intake is imperative. A range of feeding modes, including enteral and parenteral nutrition support as needed, are explored to achieve the vigorous nutrition care that is necessary for these individuals.

Diarrhea

Diarrhea typically is not a disease of the small intestine but rather a symptom or result of another underlying condition. In some cases, diarrhea may result from an intolerance to specific foods or nutrients, such as in lactose intolerance (see Chapter 2) or acute food poisoning from a specific food-borne organism or toxin (see Chapter 13). A variety of parasites (e.g., *Giardia lamblia, Cryptosporidium parvum, Cyclospora cayetanensis, Entamoeba histolytica*), bacteria (e.g., *Campylobacter, Clostridium difficile, Escherichia coli, Listeria monocytogenes, Salmonella enteritidis, Shigella*), and viral infections (HIV, rotavirus, Norwalk agent) are known causes of diarrhea. Traveler's diarrhea, which is often attributed to irregular meals, unfamiliar foods, and travel tensions, is also a well-known GI disturbance; bacterial infection is its most common cause.[27]

Chronic diarrhea (i.e., diarrhea that lasts for more than 2 weeks) can be a life-threatening illness, especially for young children or individuals with weak immune systems. Acute infectious diarrhea is the second most common cause of death among children in developing countries.[28] Intravenous fluid and electrolyte replacement may be necessary, or oral rehydration solutions such as Pedialyte, Resol, Ricelyte, CeraLyte, and Rehydralyte may be used. As soon as it is tolerated, a regular refeeding schedule is needed to avoid malnutrition. Nutrition therapy will depend on the underlying causative agent. Determining and treating the cause of diarrhea is paramount to restoring nutritional parameters.

polymeric formula a nutrition support formula that is composed of complete protein, polysaccharides, and fat as medium-chain fatty acids.

elemental formula a nutrition support formula that is composed of simple elemental nutrient components that require no further digestive breakdown and are thus readily absorbed; these formulas include protein as free amino acids and carbohydrate as the simple sugar glucose.

probiotic a food that contains live microbials, which are thought to benefit the consumer by improving intestinal microbial balance (e.g., lactobacilli in yogurt).

For severely malnourished patients, the resumption of nutrient intake should be carefully monitored. Refeeding syndrome is a potentially fatal metabolic disturbance that involves fluid and electrolyte imbalances and that can result in cardiac failure. When malnourished patients are started on a feeding schedule that is too aggressive, sudden shifts in electrolytes leave low serum levels of phosphate, potassium, magnesium, glucose, and thiamine. Malnourished patients require a slow reintroduction to nutrients and close monitoring.

Large Intestine Diseases

Diverticular Disease

Diverticulosis is a multifactorial disease that is characterized by the formation of many small pouches or diverticula along the mucosal lining in the colon (Figure 18-7). Segmental circular muscle contractions move waste down the colon to form feces for elimination. When pressures become sufficiently high in a segment with weakened bowel walls, small diverticula may develop. As the diverticula become infected, which is a condition called *diverticulitis*, the affected area becomes painful.

The commonly used collective term that covers diverticulosis and diverticulitis is *diverticular disease*. Epidemiologic studies have not found one specific cause for diverticular disease. It most often occurs among older people in Western societies, where it is estimated that half of the people who are older than 75 years of age will develop diverticulosis.[29] There is evidence that risks increase with age, a low-fiber diet, muscular abnormalities in the colon, and disordered intestinal motility (possibly as a result of neurotransmitter abnormalities).[30,31]

As the inflammatory process advances, increased pain and tenderness are localized in the lower left side of the abdomen, and they are accompanied by nausea, vomiting, distention, diarrhea, intestinal spasm, and fever. Perforation sometimes occurs, and surgery is indicated. Underlying malnutrition may also be present. The dietary management of chronic diverticular disease includes increasing dietary fiber (see Appendix B) to 6 to 10 g/day above the normal recommendations of 20 to 35 g/day along with adequate fluid intake.[26] Avoiding certain foods (e.g., nuts, seeds) that can accumulate in the small diverticula pouches was historically recommended, but little evidence suggests that this is truly protective against inflammation. Emerging therapies include the use of probiotics, nonabsorbable antibiotics, and anti-inflammatory medications (e.g., mesalamine).[32,33]

Irritable Bowel Syndrome

Irritable bowel syndrome (IBS) is the most commonly diagnosed GI disorder. The prevalence is hard to determine, because the definitions of IBS have varied throughout epidemiologic studies, because many people with symptoms do not seek medical attention, and because it often overlaps other GI-associated and non-GI disorders (e.g., psychiatric disorders, chronic fatigue syndrome, anxiety, mood disorders).[34] Medical guidelines define IBS as a benign functional and nonorganic disorder that displays three major types of symptoms: (1) chronic and recurrent pain in any area of the abdomen (Figure 18-8); (2) small-volume bowel dysfunction that varies from constipation or diarrhea to a combination of both; and (3) excess gas formation with increased distention and bloating that is accompanied by rumbling abdominal sounds, belching, and flatulence.

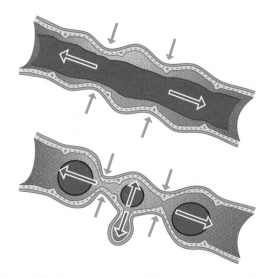

Figure 18-7 Mechanism by which low-fiber, low-bulk diets might generate diverticula. When the colon contents are bulky *(top)*, muscular contractions exert pressure longitudinally. If the lumen is small in diameter *(bottom)*, contractions can produce occlusions and exert pressure against the colon wall, which may produce a diverticular "blowout." (Reprinted from Mahan LK, Escott-Stump S. *Krause's food & nutrition therapy*. 12th ed. Philadelphia: Saunders; 2008.)

refeeding syndrome   a potentially lethal condition that occurs when severely malnourished individuals are fed high-carbohydrate diets too aggressively; a sudden shift in electrolytes and fluid retention and a drastic drop in serum phosphorus levels cause a series of complications that involves several organs.

diverticulitis   the inflammation of pockets of tissue (i.e., diverticula) in the lining of the mucous membrane of the colon.

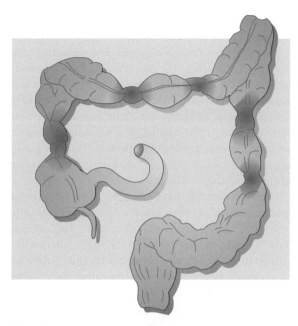

Figure 18-8 Irritable bowel syndrome. (Reprinted from Mahan LK, Escott-Stump S. *Krause's food, nutrition, & diet therapy.* 10th ed. Philadelphia: Saunders; 2000.)

Accumulating evidence indicates that IBS is a multi-component disorder that includes a genetic predisposition, environment, allergy, infection, inflammation, bacterial overgrowth, hormones, neurotransmitter disorders, and chronic stress.[26,35] Thus, treatment is designed to minimize symptoms, and it may include a combination of medications, cognitive behavioral therapy, probiotics, and diet therapy.[36-38] A highly individual and personal approach to nutrition care is essential, and it should be based on careful nutrition assessment. Guided by personal food preferences and symptom patterns, a reasonable food plan can be devised with the patient. In general, the food plan should give attention to the following basic principles[26]:

- *Normalize eating patterns:* A regular diet with an optimal energy and nutrient composition provides basic therapy. Assess the need for vitamin and mineral supplementation.
- *Eliminate food allergens and intolerances:* Along with any known intolerances, foods that contain the following should be specifically addressed: fructose, lactose, sorbitol, raffinose, caffeine, and alcohol.
- *Recognize and avoid gas formers:* Some foods are recognized gas formers as a result of known constituents (e.g., indigestible short chains of glucose [oligosaccharides] in the case of legumes). Others may cause gaseous discomfort on an individual basis.

- *Increase fiber and bulking agents:* Slowly increase dietary fiber (see Appendix B) intake to 25 to 35 g/day along with ample fluids. Use bulking agents as needed.
- *Consider the use of prebiotics or probiotics:* Emerging evidence supports the use of probiotics to manage IBS.
- *Consider the use of food diaries:* Tracking nutrient intake, environment, emotions, activity, and symptoms may help to narrow down instigating factors for future avoidance.

Patients are highly individualized with regard to the symptoms that they most often experience. For example, the predominant symptom may be diarrhea, constipation, abdominal pain, gas, or bloating (but not necessarily all of them). Therefore, the dietary recommendations are equally as individualized. Experienced practitioners have learned that, when helping patients to manage IBS, an honest and creative relationship is essential. Lifestyle and diet are highly personal, and wise nutrition management involves realistic counseling toward a healthier life.

Constipation

Americans spend a significant amount of health care resources each year on problems associated with constipation.[39] "Normal" intestinal elimination is ill defined and can vary greatly. This common short-term problem usually results from various sources of nervous tension and worry, neurologic or neuromuscular problems, changes in routines, side effects from medications, frequent laxative use, low-fiber diets, and lack of exercise.

The most important aspect of the treatment and prevention of constipation is risk assessment to identify the potential causes of constipation. Improved diet, exercise, and bowel habits usually help remedy the situation. Any regular laxative or enema routine should be avoided. The diet should include increased soluble fiber, naturally laxative fruits (e.g., dried prunes, figs), and adequate fluid intake.[40,41] Constipation occurs at all ages, but it is almost epidemic among elderly people. In all cases, a personalized approach to management is fundamental.

FOOD ALLERGIES AND INTOLERANCES

Food Allergies

The Problem

Several conditions may cause certain food allergies or intolerances. Intolerances—unlike true allergies—are not life threatening, and they are not immunologic in etiology.

The underlying problem of an allergic reaction is the body's immune system reacting to a protein as if it were a threatening foreign object and then launching a powerful attack against it. The word *allergy* comes from two Greek words meaning "altered reactivity," and it refers to the abnormal reactions of the immune system to a number of substances in the environment. A particular allergic condition results from a disorder of the immune system.

Common Food Allergens

The most common food allergens include the proteins in cow's milk, eggs, peanuts, tree nuts, fish, shellfish, wheat, soy, and sesame.[42] The prevalence of food allergies varies in accordance with many factors, including age, local diet, and early exposure. Table 18-5 presents estimated rates of food allergies in North America. Early foods of infancy and childhood are often offenders in sensitive individuals, especially if they are introduced to the child before the GI tract is fully capable of sophisticated digestion (i.e., approximately 6 months of age). In a child's diet, solid foods should be added one at a time, with common offenders excluded during early feedings.

If a patient shows signs of an allergic reaction, an oral food challenge, a skin prick test, an atopy patch test, or serum immunoassays (e.g., immunoglobulin E antibody response) may be used to identify offending foods.[42,43] If a given food causes an allergic reaction, the food is identified as an allergen for that individual and eliminated from the diet. The food may be tried again later to see if it still causes the same reaction, thereby validating the initial response. Individuals commonly outgrow allergies to milk, soy, and eggs. However, peanuts, tree nuts, and shellfish tend to elicit allergic responses—sometimes fatally—throughout life. Peanut allergy elicits the most severe form of food allergy and carries a high risk of anaphylaxis. Much effort has been devoted to understanding the immunologic response to peanuts and to developing effective methods for avoiding such severe reactions.[44,45]

Recognizing signs and symptoms of allergic reactions may save a life. The most common symptoms of food allergies are hives, nausea, diarrhea, and abdominal pain. Anaphylactic shock is the most severe form of allergic reaction, and it can result in death relatively quickly. Individuals who are in anaphylactic shock have swelling of the face and throat, difficulty breathing, anxiety, increased heart rate, and, if not treated, decreased blood pressure and loss of consciousness. The person's throat, lips, and tongue swell to the point of blocking the airway, ultimately suffocating the individual.

Nutrition care for food allergies is focused on two aspects: (1) avoiding offending foods; and (2) substituting nutritionally appropriate alternatives for the excluded foods.[26] Referring any person with food allergies to a dietitian to provide family support, education, and counseling may be helpful. Guidance regarding food substitutions or special food products and modified recipes to maintain nutrition needs for growth is necessary. Children tend to become less allergic as they grow older, but cooking guides and family education that addresses the deciphering of food product labels are essential from the beginning. Furthermore, if anaphylaxis is a known risk, patients should be under the care of a physician for the provision of self- or family-administered emergency medications if anaphylaxis occurs.

Celiac Disease

Disease Process. The pathology of celiac disease (CD) is attributed to a genetic predisposition and an autoimmune response to proteins that are found in wheat, barley, and rye.[46] The CD-activating proteins are known as *gluten*. However, gluten protein is only found in wheat products. The proteins in barley and rye that cause an adverse reaction are hordein and secalin, respectively. For simplicity, all dietary proteins involved in disease pathogenesis are referred to as *gluten* in this text in keeping with the general public's understanding. Oat products are not

TABLE 18-5 **ESTIMATED RATES OF FOOD ALLERGY IN NORTH AMERICA**

Prevalence	Infants and Children	Adults
Milk	2.5%	0.3%
Eggs	1.5%	0.2%
Peanuts	1%	0.6%
Tree nuts	0.5%	0.6%
Fish	0.1%	0.4%
Shellfish	0.1%	2%
Wheat and soy	0.4%	0.3%
Sesame	0.1%	0.1%
Overall	5%	3% to 4%

From Sicherer SH, Sampson HA. Food allergy. *J Allergy Clin Immunol.* 2010;125(2 Suppl 2):S116-S125.

allergy a state of hypersensitivity to particular substances in the environment that works on body tissues to produce problems in the functioning of the affected tissues; the agent involved (i.e., the allergen) may be a certain food that is eaten or a substance (e.g., pollen) that is inhaled.

atopy patch test a diagnostic test that is used to assess for allergic reactions on the skin.

anaphylaxis a severe and sometimes fatal allergic reaction that results from exposure to a protein that the body perceives as foreign and that elicits a systemic response that involves multiple organs.

problematic for all individuals with CD. However, oats often are processed in facilities that process wheat products, which can result in cross-contamination.

In reaction to the ingestion of a CD-activating protein, the mucosal surface is damaged; this leaves villi that are malformed and with few remaining functional microvilli (Figure 18-9). This injured mucosa effectively reduces the surface area for micronutrient and macronutrient absorption. In addition, the decreased release of peptide hormones, bile, and pancreatic secretions exacerbates malabsorption. CD is estimated to affect 1% of the U.S. population, most of whom have not been diagnosed.[47] About 25% of the population has the genetic polymorphism that leads to CD, but only 4% of people with this genetic predisposition will develop CD, thereby indicating the effects of other environmental factors.[48]

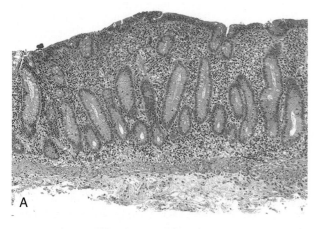

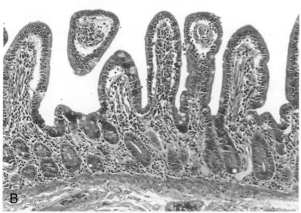

Figure 18-9 Celiac disease, gluten-sensitive enteropathy. **A,** Normal mucosal biopsy. **B,** A peroral jejunal biopsy specimen of diseased mucosa shows severe atrophy and the blunting of villi with a chronic inflammatory infiltrate of the lamina propria. (Reprinted from Kumar V, Fausto N, Abbas A. *Robbins & Cotran pathologic basis of disease.* 7th ed. Philadelphia: Saunders; 2005.)

Symptoms can vary greatly depending on the extent of the intestinal damage. The major symptoms of diarrhea, steatorrhea, and progressive malnutrition are secondary effects of the gluten reaction.

Nutrition Management. The goal of nutrition management is to avoid all dietary sources of gluten and to prevent malnutrition through healthy meal alternatives. Wheat, rye, and barley are eliminated from the diet, and corn, potato, and rice are used as substitutes. Some individuals with CD are sensitive to oats and also must eliminate oat-containing products. Careful label reading is important for parents and children, because many commercial products use gluten-containing grains as thickeners or fillers. Some commercial products have a gluten-free symbol on their labels to assist with the identification of acceptable foods (Figure 18-10). With the increasing number of processed foods and ethnic dishes available in the marketplace, detecting all food sources of gluten is difficult. Home test kits for gluten are available and may be beneficial for individuals who consume foods without standard ingredient lists. Adhering to a gluten-free diet is the only effective treatment for maintaining a healthy mucosa, and it must be followed for life (Table 18-6).

Because of the nature of the malabsorption disorder, patients with CD must be monitored for potential vitamin and mineral deficiencies and partake in supplementation as necessary. In addition, interference with medication absorption and action must be considered with any form of malabsorption disorder.

PROBLEMS OF THE GASTROINTESTINAL ACCESSORY ORGANS

Three major accessory organs—the liver, the gallbladder, and the pancreas—produce important digestive agents that enter the intestine and help with the handling of food substances (Figure 18-11). Diseases of these organs

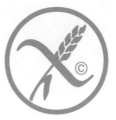

Figure 18-10 Two gluten-free symbols. (Copyright Coeliac UK, Bucks, UK, 2004.)

TABLE 18-6 GLUTEN-FREE DIET FOR INDIVIDUALS WITH CELIAC DISEASE

Food Groups	Foods Allowed	Foods Not Allowed*
Milk	Milk (plain or flavored with chocolate or cocoa), buttermilk, yogurt, ice cream, cottage cheese, and cream cheese	Malted milk; preparations such as Cocomalt, Hemo, Postum, and Nestlé chocolate
Meats and meat substitutes	Lean meat, trimmed well of fat Eggs, poultry, and fish Creamy peanut butter (if tolerated)	Luncheon meats, corned beef, frankfurters, and all common prepared meat products with any possible wheat filler (e.g., stuffed turkey) Fish canned in broth Meat prepared with bread, crackers, or flour
Fruits and juices	All cooked and canned fruits and juices Frozen or fresh fruits as tolerated, with no skins or seeds	Prunes and plums, unless tolerated
Vegetables	All cooked, frozen, and canned vegetables, as tolerated (prepared without wheat, rye, oat, or barley products); raw as tolerated	All prepared with wheat, rye, oat, or barley products (e.g., batter dipped)
Breads, flours, and cereal products	Hot and cold cereals made with amaranth, corn, quinoa, or rice products Breads, pancakes, and waffles made with tolerated flours (e.g., cornmeal, cornstarch, rice, soybean, lima bean, potato, buckwheat) Pasta made from beans, corn, peas, potatoes, quinoa, or rice; soy or rice flours	All bread and cereal products made with gluten; wheat, rye, oat, barley, macaroni, noodles, and spaghetti; any sauces, soups, or gravies prepared with gluten flour, wheat, rye, oat, or barley
Soups	Broth and bouillon (no thickening with wheat, rye, oat, or barley products); soups and sauces may be thickened with cornstarch	All soups that contain wheat, rye, oat, or barley products

*Oats and oat products are tolerated by some individuals and do not need to be avoided.
Dietary principles to be addressed include the following: (1) high kilocalories (approximately 20% above normal requirements) to compensate for fecal loss; (2) high protein as tolerated to promote growth in children and maintenance in adults; (3) low fat (but not fat free) because of impaired absorption; (4) simple carbohydrates, including easily digested sugars (e.g., fruits, vegetables), to provide approximately half of the day's kilocalories; (5) small, frequent feedings during ill periods; an afternoon snack for older children; (6) smooth and soft texture, initially avoiding irritating roughage; the use of strained foods for longer than usual for age, with whole foods added as tolerated and according to the age of the child; (7) supplements of B vitamins, vitamins A and E in water-miscible forms, and vitamin C; and (8) iron supplements if anemia is present.

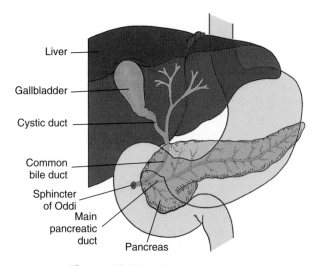

Figure 18-11 Biliary system organs.

negatively affect normal GI function and cause problems with the digestion and metabolism of nutrients.

Liver Disease

The liver plays several critical roles in basic metabolism and the regulation of body functions. Some essential functions include bile production; the synthesis of proteins and blood-clotting factors; the metabolism of hormones, medications, macronutrients, and micronutrients; the regulation of blood glucose levels; and urea production to remove the waste products of normal metabolism. Diseases of the liver have the potential to disrupt any of these functions.

Steatohepatitis

Fat accumulation ("steato") and inflammation in the liver ("hepatitis") is known as *steatohepatitis*. There are two primary types of steatohepatitis: alcoholic steatohepatitis (ASH) and nonalcoholic steatohepatitis (NASH). Steatohepatitis is most often associated with alcohol abuse and obesity.

Fat accumulates in the liver in response to high levels of fatty acids in the circulation, exaggerated lipogenesis, and impaired lipolysis. In other words, more fat is made and stored in the liver than is burned or oxidized by the liver. Alcohol-induced disturbances in the liver result in mass inflammation and malfunction. Disease progression in ASH is rapid, and it may advance to cirrhosis if it is left untreated. Genetic and environmental factors such as inflammation, oxidative stress, insulin resistance, metabolic syndrome, and obesity increase the risk for the development of NASH.[49,50]

Malnutrition is typical in patients with ASH, and aggressive enteral nutrition therapy is beneficial for reestablishing adequate nutrient intake.[51] Basic nutrition guidelines for steatohepatitis include a balanced diet, the avoidance of alcohol (if indicated), weight loss (if indicated), the consideration of antioxidant supplementation, and tight blood glucose control.

Hepatitis

Acute hepatitis is an inflammatory condition that is caused by viruses, alcohol, drugs, or toxins. Viral infections and alcohol abuse are the most common forms of hepatitis. Viral infections are often transmitted via the oral-fecal route (i.e., hepatitis A), which is common in many epidemic diseases that involve contaminated food or water. In other cases, the virus may be transmitted by transfusions of infected blood or by contaminated syringes or needles (i.e., hepatitis B). Symptoms of hepatitis include anorexia and jaundice with underlying malnutrition.

Treatment focuses on bed rest and nutrition therapy to support the healing of the liver tissue (see the Clinical Applications box, "Case Study: Bill's Bout With Infectious Hepatitis"). Dietary restrictions are not usually necessary during acute hepatitis, but they may be required for chronic inflammation. The following requirements govern the goals of the diet therapy[26]:

- Avoid substances that are hepatotoxic (e.g., alcohol, drugs, toxins).
- Achieve and maintain an optimal weight.
- Consume a diet that is adequate in macronutrients and micronutrients.
- *Protein:* Protein is essential for building new liver cells and tissues. It also combines with fats (lipoproteins) to remove them, thereby preventing damage from fatty infiltration in liver tissue. The diet should supply 1.0 to 1.2 g/kg of body weight of high-quality protein daily if no complications are present.

If the individual has complications and a positive nitrogen balance is desirable, 1.2 to 1.3 g/kg of protein may be warranted (Box 18-3).

- *Carbohydrates:* Available glucose restores protective glycogen reserves in the liver. It also helps to meet the energy demands of the disease process and prevents the breakdown of protein for energy, thus ensuring its use for the vital tissue building that is necessary for healing. The diet should supply 50% to 55% total kilocalories as carbohydrates. Glucose intolerance and hypoglycemia are sometimes problematic in patients with liver disease. Therefore, the amount of carbohydrates in the diet depends on individual needs and condition.
- *Fat:* Some fat helps to season food to encourage eating despite a poor appetite. A moderate amount of easily used fat from milk products and vegetable oil is beneficial. The diet should incorporate a maximum of 30% of total kilocalories from fat. Energy supply depends more on fat as the disease progresses.
- Cope with eating problems.
- *Meals and feedings:* Most patients will tolerate oral feedings, but enteral feedings or parenteral feedings (in severe cases) may be warranted. At first, liquid feedings (e.g., milkshakes that are high in protein and kilocalories [see Table 18-1] or special formula products) may be necessary.
- *A patient-centered plan:* As a patient's appetite and food tolerance improve, a full diet is needed while

---

BOX 18-3   EXAMPLE OF A HIGH-PROTEIN, HIGH-CARBOHYDRATE, MODERATE-FAT DAILY DIET

- 1 L (1 qt) low-fat milk
- ¼ cup egg substitute (e.g., Egg Beaters)
- 8 oz lean meat, fish, or poultry
- 4 servings vegetables:
  - 2 servings potato or substitute
  - 1 serving green leafy or yellow vegetable
  - 1 to 2 servings other vegetables, including 1 raw
- 3 to 4 servings fruit (including juices):
  - 1 to 2 citrus fruits (or other good source of ascorbic acid)
  - 2 servings other fruit
- 6 to 8 servings bread and cereal (whole grain or enriched):
  - 1 serving cereal
  - 5 to 6 slices bread or crackers
- 2 to 4 Tbsp butter or fortified margarine
- Additional jam, jelly, honey, and other carbohydrate foods as patient desires and as tolerated
- Sweetened fruit juices to increase both carbohydrates and fluid

CLINICAL APPLICATIONS

CASE STUDY: BILL'S BOUT WITH INFECTIOUS HEPATITIS

Bill is a college student who spent part of his summer vacation in Mexico. Shortly after he returned home, he began to feel ill. He had little energy, no appetite, and severe headaches, and nothing he ate seemed to agree with him. He felt nauseated, he began to have diarrhea, and he soon developed a fever. He began to show evidence of jaundice.

Bill was hospitalized for diagnosis and treatment, and his tests indicated impaired liver function. His liver and spleen were enlarged and tender. The physician's diagnosis was infectious hepatitis. Bill's hospital diet was high in proteins, carbohydrates, and kilocalories and moderately low in fats, but Bill had difficulty eating. He had no appetite, and food seemed to nauseate him even more.

Questions for Analysis

1. What are the normal functions of the liver in relation to the metabolism of carbohydrates, proteins, and fats? What other metabolic functions does the liver have?
2. What is the relationship of normal liver function to the effects or clinical symptoms that Bill had during his illness?
3. What vitamins and minerals would be significant aspects of Bill's nutrition therapy? Why?

---

observing his or her likes and dislikes and planning ways to encourage optimal food intake.

Cirrhosis

Cirrhosis is a chronic state of liver disease in which the liver is damaged beyond repair with scar tissue and fatty infiltration (Figure 18-12). Progressive cirrhosis or end-stage liver disease is a leading cause of death in the United States, and more than half of the cases are the result of alcoholism. Other causes include chronic hepatitis types B and C; autoimmune hepatitis; inherited diseases such as Wilson's disease and galactosemia; NASH; blocked bile ducts; and drugs, toxins, and infections.

One of the main functions of the liver is to remove ammonia—and hence nitrogen (see Chapter 5)—from the blood by converting it to urea (via the urea cycle) for urinary excretion. However, with steatohepatitis, the accompanying fatty infiltration kills liver cells and leaves only nonfunctioning fibrous scar tissue. When fibrous scar tissue replaces functional liver tissue, the blood can no longer circulate normally through the liver, which results in portal hypertension. The blood, which is carrying its ammonia load, cannot get to the liver for the normal removal of ammonia and nitrogen. Instead, it must follow the vessels that bypass the liver and proceed to the brain, thereby producing ammonia intoxication and hepatic encephalopathy. As a result of portal hypertension, the small blood vessels that surround the esophagus become distended with high pressure, which leads to the development of esophageal varices. The rupture of these enlarged veins with massive hemorrhage is often the cause of death.

Malnutrition is one of the most significant issues in patients with cirrhosis.[52,53] Low plasma protein levels

contribute to ascites. Nutrition therapy focuses on as much healing support as possible, as follows[26]:

- Avoid substances that are hepatotoxic (e.g., alcohol, drugs, toxins).
- Provide a balanced diet that is adequate in macronutrients and micronutrients.
    - *Energy:* Energy intake should equal basal energy needs plus approximately 20%. Practitioners must carefully distinguish body weight from fluid weight, because needs are based on dry weight. Adjustments are made if weight loss is desired.

Wilson's disease an autosomal recessive genetic disorder in which copper accumulates in tissue and causes damage to organs.

galactosemia an autosomal recessive genetic disorder in which the liver does not produce the enzyme that is needed to metabolize galactose.

portal hypertension high blood pressure in the portal vein

hepatic encephalopathy a condition in which toxins in the blood lead to alterations in brain homeostasis as a result of liver disease; this results in apathy, confusion, inappropriate behavior, altered consciousness, and eventually coma.

esophageal varices the pathologic dilation of the blood vessels within the wall of the esophagus as a result of liver cirrhosis; these vessels can continue to expand to the point of rupturing.

ascites fluid accumulation in the abdominal cavity

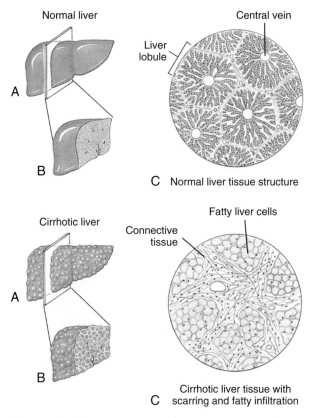

Figure 18-12 Comparison of a normal liver and a liver with cirrhotic tissue changes. **A,** Anterior view of the organ. **B,** Cross-sectional view. **C,** Tissue structure. (Copyright Medical and Scientific Illustration.)

- *Protein:* Protein in the amount of 0.8 to 1.2 g/kg of dry body weight should be given in the absence of impending hepatic encephalopathy. Sufficient protein is needed to correct severe malnutrition, to heal liver tissue, and to restore plasma proteins.
- Enteral or parenteral nutrition support, if indicated
- Vitamin and mineral supplementation
- Small, frequent meals
- Dietary restrictions should be implemented if cirrhosis-associated complications are present.
  - *Low sodium:* Sodium is restricted to less than 2000 mg/day to help reduce fluid retention in the presence of ascites
  - *Soft texture:* If esophageal varices develop, soft foods help to prevent the danger of rupture and hemorrhage.

- *Modest protein intake*: Avoid protein excess, which can exacerbate hepatic encephalopathy from nitrogen loading. Focus on plant proteins, and consider supplementing with branched chain amino acids.[54]
- *Fat restriction:* In the presence of steatorrhea, the dietary intake of fat should not exceed 30% of total kilocalories.
- *Fluid restriction:* In the presence of hyponatremia or ascites, this is required.
- Maintain regular physical activity, and achieve weight loss, if implicated.
- Address and correct any food or eating problems (e.g., anorexia, nausea, vomiting, bloating, gas, constipation).

Gallbladder Disease

The basic function of the gallbladder is to concentrate and store bile and then release the concentrated bile into the small intestine when fat is present there. Bile emulsifies fat in the intestine to prepare it for digestion and then helps carry it into the mucosal cells of the intestinal wall for preparation to enter the lymphatic circulation.

Cholecystitis and Cholelithiasis

Cholecystitis, which is the inflammation of the gallbladder, usually results from a low-grade chronic infection. Cholelithiasis, or gallstone formation, is attributed to both genetic and environmental factors.[55] Obesity is associated with a higher risk for both cholecystitis and cholelithiasis.[56] Of the two types of gallstones (those that contain bilirubin and those that contain cholesterol), cholesterol gallstones are more common. The non–water-soluble cholesterol in bile is normally kept in solution. If the amount of cholesterol is too concentrated, cholesterol may separate out and form gallstones. Most gallstones are asymptomatic, but a small percentage of gallstone carriers experience episodes of intense pain. The typical treatment in such painful and chronic cases is cholecystectomy, which is the surgical removal of the gallbladder.

As fat enters the intestine, the hormone cholecystokinin triggers gallbladder contractions to release bile. In patients with cholecystitis or cholelithiasis, the normal contraction of the gallbladder may cause pain. Diet therapy centers on controlling fat intake (i.e., less than 30% of calories from fat) and eating small, frequent meals.[26] Table 18-7 outlines a general low-fat diet guide, but the degree of its application depends on individual needs. Emerging recommendations for the prevention of gallstones include the following: reduced saturated fat and

TABLE 18-7 **LOW-FAT AND FAT-FREE DIETS**

Foods	Foods Allowed	Foods Not Allowed
Beverages	Skim milk, coffee, tea, carbonated beverages, and fruit juices	Whole milk, cream, and evaporated and condensed milk
Bread and cereals	Most all	Rich rolls or breads, waffles, and pancakes
Desserts	Gelatin, sherbet, water ices, fruit whips made without cream, angel food cake, and rice and tapioca puddings made with skim milk	Pastries, pies, rich cakes and cookies, and ice cream
Fruits	All fruits as tolerated	Avocado
Eggs	Three allowed per week, cooked any way except fried	Fried eggs
Fats	3 tsp butter or margarine daily	Salad and cooking oils and mayonnaise
Meats	Lean meat such as beef, veal, lamb, liver, lean fish, and fowl that has been baked, broiled, or roasted without added fat	Fried meats, bacon, ham, pork, goose, duck, fatty fish, fish canned in oil, and cold cuts
Cheese	Dry or fat-free cottage cheese	All other cheeses
Potato or substitute	Potatoes, rice, macaroni, noodles, and spaghetti prepared without added fat	Fried potatoes and potato chips
Soups	Bouillon or broth without fat and soups made with skim milk	Cream soups
Sweets	Jam, jelly, and sugar candies without nuts or chocolate	Chocolate, nuts, and peanut butter
Vegetables	All vegetables as tolerated	Omit the following if causing distress: broccoli, cauliflower, corn, cucumber, green pepper, radishes, turnips, onions, dried peas, and beans
Miscellaneous	Salt in moderation	Pepper, spices, highly spiced foods, olives, pickles, cream sauces, and gravies

Foods are prepared without the addition of fat. Fatty meats, gravies, oils, cream, lard, avocados, and desserts that contain eggs, butter, cream, and nuts are avoided.

Suggested food patterns for a low-fat diet are as follows: *Breakfast:* fruit, cereal, toast, jelly, 1 tsp butter or margarine, egg (three times per week), 1 cup skim milk, and coffee with sugar. *Lunch and dinner:* broiled or baked meat, potato, vegetable, salad with fat-free dressing, bread, jelly, 1 tsp butter or margarine, fruit or dessert (as allowed), 1 cup skim milk, and coffee with sugar. This pattern contains approximately 85 g protein, 50 g fat, 220 g carbohydrates, and 1670 kcal.

A relatively fat-free diet omits meat, eggs, and butter or margarine; a substitute for meat at the noon and evening meals is 3 oz of fat-free cottage cheese.

cholesterol intake; replacing saturated fat with monounsaturated or polyunsaturated fat; supplementing with fish oil; and reducing refined sugar intake. Other protective dietary factors may include dietary fiber, nuts, caffeine, and following a vegetarian diet.[57]

Pancreatic Disease

The pancreas is a key organ in normal digestion and metabolism, and it acts as both an exocrine gland and an endocrine gland. Digestive enzymes and bicarbonate, which are necessary for the breakdown of carbohydrates, proteins, and fats, are excreted by the pancreas under hormonal control during digestion. The endocrine functions of the pancreas are primarily related to blood glucose regulation by glucagon and insulin.

Pancreatitis

Inflammation of the pancreas, which is known as *pancreatitis,* inhibits normal pancreatic function, including the secretion of digestive enzymes and pancreatic hormones. Subsequently, digestion and blood glucose control are severely affected. Mild or moderate episodes may completely subside, but the condition tends to recur, which can lead to chronic pancreatitis. Excessive alcohol consumption is the major causative factor of pancreatitis in the United States. Other causes of chronic pancreatitis include a blocked or narrowed pancreatic duct, heredity, autoimmune disorders, and other unknown causes.

The inability to digest food leads to malnutrition. Supplementing with pancreatic enzymes immediately after diagnosis is important for the overall outcome of the patient.[58] Initial care includes the following measures[26]:

- *Nothing by mouth with hydration support during acute phases:* This allows for pancreatic rest while providing fluids and correcting for electrolyte and acid-base disturbances.
- *Provide adequate energy and nutrient needs when acute symptoms subside:*
  - Energy needs should be based on patient requirements to prevent weight loss.
  - Advance to liquid or solid foods as tolerated.

- The diet should be relatively high in calories (35 kcal/kg) and protein (1 to 1.5 g/kg) and low in fiber.[59]
- Assess the need for vitamin and mineral supplementation.
- Moderate to severe cases of pancreatitis may require enteral or parenteral nutrition support.
- Avoid alcohol.

SUMMARY

- The nutrition management of GI diseases is based on the degree of interference in the normal processes of ingestion, digestion, absorption, and metabolism that the disease causes.
- Problems in the upper GI tract relate to conditions that hinder chewing, swallowing, or transporting the food mass down the esophagus into the stomach. Esophageal problems such as muscle constriction, acid reflux that causes esophagitis, and hiatal hernias interfere with the passage of food into the stomach. These problems cause general tissue irritation and discomfort after eating. PUD, which is a common GI problem, involves the acidic erosion of the mucosal lining of the stomach or the duodenal bulb. The ulcerated tissue causes nutrition problems such as anemia and weight loss. Diet therapy is liberal and individual, with the goal of correcting malnutrition and supporting the healing process.
- Problems of the lower GI tract include common functional disorders such as malabsorption and diarrhea, for which symptomatic and personalized treatment is indicated. CD and CF require extensive individualized nutrition support. The inflammatory bowel diseases (e.g., Crohn's disease, ulcerative colitis) involve widespread tissue damage that often requires surgical resection and that results in decreased absorbing surface area. Large intestine problems (e.g., diverticular disease, IBS, constipation) often involve anxiety and stress and thus are more difficult to resolve. Nutrition therapy is specific to each condition and generally warrants the assistance of a registered dietitian.
- Diseases of the GI accessory organs also contribute to nutrition problems. Common liver disorders include hepatitis and cirrhosis. Uncontrolled cirrhosis leads to hepatic encephalopathy and eventual liver failure and death. Nutrient and energy levels of the necessary diet therapy vary with the progression of the disease process. Gallbladder disease, infection, and stones involve some limit to fat tolerance, which is modified in accordance with individual need. The treatment for gallstones is the surgical removal of the gallbladder followed by the moderate use of dietary fat. Pancreatitis is a serious condition that requires immediate measures to counter the symptoms of shock followed by restorative nutrition support.

CRITICAL THINKING QUESTIONS

1. What general nutrition guidance would you give to a person with esophageal reflux? What would be the basic goal of your suggestions?
2. What are the basic principles of diet planning for patients with PUD? What elements other than nutrition therapy may be involved in the treatment process?
3. Describe the causes, clinical signs, and treatments of diverticular disease, CD, and IBS.
4. Considering the nutrients that are digested and absorbed in the small intestine, what long-term deficiencies would you expect to encounter in a patient with chronically inflamed Crohn's disease that affects more than 40% of the gut? Explain why this may happen, and discuss what alternative method of feeding would be beneficial.
5. What is the rationale for treatment during the progressive course of liver disease (e.g., hepatitis, cirrhosis, hepatic encephalopathy)?

CHAPTER CHALLENGE QUESTIONS

True-False

Write the correct statement for each statement that is false.

1. *True or False:* A high-fiber diet that is rich in raw vegetables is appropriate for a person with dental problems.
2. *True or False:* Remaining upright after eating helps to prevent discomfort in a person with esophageal reflux.
3. *True or False:* The primary cause of PUD is a bacterial infection.
4. *True or False:* A low-fiber diet (i.e., no more than 12 g/day) is encouraged for the treatment of diverticulosis.
5. *True or False:* All food sources of wheat must be eliminated as part of the gluten-free diet for the treatment of CD.
6. *True or False:* The nutrition objectives for patients with CF are to meet growth needs and to help compensate for nutrient losses and enzyme replacement therapy.

Multiple Choice

1. In a gluten-free diet for CD, which of the following foods is eliminated?
   a. Eggs
   b. Milk
   c. Rice
   d. Whole-wheat crackers

2. The symptoms of anemia in patients with malabsorption diseases are caused by the poor absorption of which of the following nutrients?
   a. Vitamins B_2 and C
   b. Iron and folic acid
   c. Calcium and phosphorus
   d. Fats and protein

3. Treatment for hepatic encephalopathy includes
   a. increasing protein intake to help with the healing of liver cells.
   b. avoiding excess protein to reduce ammonia levels in the blood.
   c. increasing fat intake to reduce the metabolic load.
   d. increasing fluid intake to stimulate output.

4. Which of the following is a swallowing disorder?
   a. Dysphagia
   b. Xerostomia
   c. CD
   d. CF

5. Crohn's disease differs from ulcerative colitis in that
   a. Crohn's disease is progressive from the rectum up.
   b. Crohn's disease is temporary and easily treated with medication.
   c. Crohn's disease skips lesions throughout the small and large intestine.
   d. Crohn's disease only affects the small intestine.

⊖volve Please refer to the Students' Resource section of this text's Evolve Web site for additional study resources.

REFERENCES

1. Walsh T, Worthington HV, Glenny AM, et al. Fluoride toothpastes of different concentrations for preventing dental caries in children and adolescents. *Cochrane Database Syst Rev.* 2010;(1):CD007868.
2. Savoca MR, Arcury TA, Leng X, et al. Severe tooth loss in older adults as a key indicator of compromised dietary quality. *Public Health Nutr.* 2010;13(4):466-474.
3. Ervin RB, Dye BA. The effect of functional dentition on Healthy Eating Index scores and nutrient intakes in a nationally representative sample of older adults. *J Public Health Dent.* 2009;69(4):207-216.
4. Sue Eisenstadt E. Dysphagia and aspiration pneumonia in older adults. *J Am Acad Nurse Pract.* 2010;22(1):17-22.
5. Altman KW, Yu GP, Schaefer SD. Consequence of dysphagia in the hospitalized patient: impact on prognosis and hospital resources. *Arch Otolaryngol Head Neck Surg.* 2010;136(8):784-789.
6. Rofes L, Arreola V, Almirall J, et al. Diagnosis and management of oropharyngeal dysphagia and its nutritional and respiratory complications in the elderly. *Gastroenterol Res Pract.* 2011; 2011. pii: 818979.
7. Germain I, Dufresne T, Gray-Donald K. A novel dysphagia diet improves the nutrient intake of institutionalized elders. *J Am Diet Assoc.* 2006;106(10):1614-1623.
8. Herbella FA, Patti MG. Gastroesophageal reflux disease: from pathophysiology to treatment. *World J Gastroenterol.* 2010;16(30):3745-3749.
9. El-Serag HB. Time trends of gastroesophageal reflux disease: a systematic review. *Clin Gastroenterol Hepatol.* 2007;5(1):17-26.

10. Chait MM. Gastroesophageal reflux disease: important considerations for the older patients. *World J Gastrointest Endosc.* 2010;2(12):388-396.

11. Prachand VN, Alverdy JC. Gastroesophageal reflux disease and severe obesity: Fundoplication or bariatric surgery? *World J Gastroenterol.* 2010;16(30):3757-3761.

12. Yeomans ND. The ulcer sleuths: the search for the cause of peptic ulcers. *J Gastroenterol Hepatol.* 2011;26(Suppl 1):35-41.

13. Sung JJ, Kuipers EJ, El-Serag HB. Systematic review: the global incidence and prevalence of peptic ulcer disease. *Aliment Pharmacol Ther.* 2009;29(9):938-946.

14. Bhatia V, Tandon RK. Stress and the gastrointestinal tract. *J Gastroenterol Hepatol.* 2005;20(3):332-339.

15. Jones MP. The role of psychosocial factors in peptic ulcer disease: beyond *Helicobacter pylori* and NSAIDs. *J Psychosom Res.* 2006;60(4):407-412.

16. Choung RS, Talley NJ. Epidemiology and clinical presentation of stress-related peptic damage and chronic peptic ulcer. *Curr Mol Med.* 2008;8(4):253-257.

17. Merck & Co., Inc. *The Merck manual for healthcare professionals.* Whitehouse Station, NJ: Merck & Co., Inc; 2009-2010.

18. Schechter MS, McColley SA, Silva S, et al; Investigators and Coordinators of the Epidemiologic Study of Cystic Fibrosis; North American Scientific Advisory Group for ESCF. Association of socioeconomic status with the use of chronic therapies and healthcare utilization in children with cystic fibrosis. *J Pediatr.* 2009;155(5):634-639 e1-e4.

19. O'Connor GT, Quinton HB, Kneeland T, et al. Median household income and mortality rate in cystic fibrosis. *Pediatrics.* 2003;111(4 Pt 1):e333-e339.

20. Quittner AL, Schechter MS, Rasouliyan L, et al. Impact of socioeconomic status, race, and ethnicity on quality of life in patients with cystic fibrosis in the United States. *Chest.* 2010;137(3):642-650.

21. Stallings VA, Stark LJ, Robinson KA, et al; Clinical Practice Guidelines on Growth and Nutrition Subcommittee; Ad Hoc Working Group. Evidence-based practice recommendations for nutrition-related management of children and adults with cystic fibrosis and pancreatic insufficiency: results of a systematic review. *J Am Diet Assoc.* 2008;108(5):832-839.

22. Kumar V, Fausto N, Abbas A. *Robbins & Cotran pathologic basis of disease.* 7th ed. Philadelphia: Saunders; 2005.

23. National Center for Biotechnology Information. Crohn's disease (website): www.ncbi.nlm.nih.gov/pubmedhealth/PMH0001295#adam_000249.disease.causes. Accessed February 2011.

24. Kulnigg S, Gasche C. Systematic review: managing anaemia in Crohn's disease. *Aliment Pharmacol Ther.* 2006; 24(11-12):1507-1523.

25. Smith PA. Nutritional therapy for active Crohn's disease. *World J Gastroenterol.* 2008;14(27):4420-4423.

26. American Dietetic Association. *ADA nutrition care manual.* Chicago: American Dietetic Association; 2010.

27. Hill DR, Beeching NJ. Travelers' diarrhea. *Curr Opin Infect Dis.* 2010;23(5):481-487.

28. Black RE, Cousens S, Johnson HL, et al. Child Health Epidemiology Reference Group of WHO and UNICEF. Global, regional, and national causes of child mortality in 2008: a systematic analysis. *Lancet.* 2010;375(9730):1969-1987.

29. Commane DM, Arasaradnam RP, Mills S, et al. Diet, ageing and genetic factors in the pathogenesis of diverticular disease. *World J Gastroenterol.* 2009;15(20):2479-2488.

30. Matrana MR, Margolin DA. Epidemiology and pathophysiology of diverticular disease. *Clin Colon Rectal Surg.* 2009;22(3):141-146.

31. Jeyarajah S, Papagrigoriadis S. Review article: the pathogenesis of diverticular disease - current perspectives on motility and neurotransmitters. *Aliment Pharmacol Ther.* 2011;33(7): 789-800:

32. Lamiki P, Tsuchiya J, Pathak S, et al. Probiotics in diverticular disease of the colon: an open label study. *J Gastrointestin Liver Dis.* 2010;19(1):31-36.

33. Trivedi CD, Das KM. Emerging therapies for diverticular disease of the colon. *J Clin Gastroenterol.* 2008;42(10): 1145-1151.

34. Choung RS, Locke GR 3rd. Epidemiology of IBS. *Gastroenterol Clin North Am.* 2011;40(1):1-10.

35. Chang L. The role of stress on physiologic responses and clinical symptoms in irritable bowel syndrome. *Gastroenterology.* 2011;140(3):761-765.

36. Oerlemans S, van Cranenburgh O, Herremans PJ, et al. Intervening on cognitions and behavior in irritable bowel syndrome: A feasibility trial using PDAs. *J Psychosom Res.* 2011;70(3):267-277.

37. Jones M, Koloski N, Boyce P, Talley NJ. Pathways connecting cognitive behavioral therapy and change in bowel symptoms of IBS. *J Psychosom Res.* 2011;70(3):278-285.

38. Parkes GC, Sanderson JD, Whelan K. Treating irritable bowel syndrome with probiotics: the evidence. *Proc Nutr Soc.* 2010;69(2):187-194.

39. Singh G, Lingala V, Wang H, et al. Use of health care resources and cost of care for adults with constipation. *Clin Gastroenterol Hepatol.* 2007;5(9):1053-1058.

40. Attaluri A, Donahoe R, Valestin J, et al. Randomised clinical trial: dried plums (prunes) vs. psyllium for constipation. *Aliment Pharmacol Ther.* 2011;33(7):822-828.

41. Suares NC, Ford AC. Systematic review: the effects of fibre in the management of chronic idiopathic constipation. *Aliment Pharmacol Ther.* 2011;33(8):895-901.

42. Sicherer SH, Sampson HA. Food allergy. *J Allergy Clin Immunol.* 2010;125(2 Suppl 2):S116-S125.

43. Cudowska B, Kaczmarski M. Atopy patch test in the diagnosis of food allergy in children with gastrointestinal symptoms. *Adv Med Sci.* 2010;55(2):153-160.

44. Flinterman AE, Pasmans SG, den Hartog Jager CF, et al. T cell responses to major peanut allergens in children with and without peanut allergy. *Clin Exp Allergy.* 2010;40(4): 590-597.

45. Li XM. Beyond allergen avoidance: update on developing therapies for peanut allergy. *Curr Opin Allergy Clin Immunol.* 2005;5(3):287-292.

46. Schuppan D, Junker Y, Barisani D. Celiac disease: from pathogenesis to novel therapies. *Gastroenterology.* 2009; 137(6):1912-1933.

47. Kagnoff MF. Celiac disease: pathogenesis of a model immunogenetic disease. *J Clin Invest.* 2007;117(1):41-49.

48. Tjon JM, van Bergen J, Koning F. Celiac disease: how complicated can it get? *Immunogenetics.* 2010;62(10):641-651.

49. Feldstein AE. Novel insights into the pathophysiology of nonalcoholic fatty liver disease. *Semin Liver Dis.* 2010; 30(4):391-401.

50. Fabbrini E, Sullivan S, Klein S. Obesity and nonalcoholic fatty liver disease: biochemical, metabolic, and clinical implications. *Hepatology*. 2010;51(2):679-689.
51. Stickel F, Seitz HK. Alcoholic steatohepatitis. *Best Pract Res Clin Gastroenterol*. 2010;24(5):683-693.
52. Tsiaousi ET, Hatzitolios AI, Trygonis SK, Savopoulos CG. Malnutrition in end stage liver disease: recommendations and nutritional support. *J Gastroenterol Hepatol*. 2008;23(4): 527-533.
53. Ferreira LG, Anastacio LR, Correia MI. The impact of nutrition on cirrhotic patients awaiting liver transplantation. *Curr Opin Clin Nutr Metab Care*. 2010;13(5):554-561.
54. Chadalavada R, Sappati Biyyani RS, Maxwell J, Mullen K. Nutrition in hepatic encephalopathy. *Nutr Clin Pract*. 2010;25(3):257-264.
55. Wittenburg H. Hereditary liver disease: gallstones. *Best Pract Res Clin Gastroenterol*. 2010;24(5):747-756.
56. Tsai CJ. Steatocholecystitis and fatty gallbladder disease. *Dig Dis Sci*. 2009;54(9):1857-1863.
57. Gaby AR. Nutritional approaches to prevention and treatment of gallstones. *Altern Med Rev*. 2009;14(3):258-267.
58. Sikkens EC, Cahen DL, Kuipers EJ, Bruno MJ. Pancreatic enzyme replacement therapy in chronic pancreatitis. *Best Pract Res Clin Gastroenterol*. 2010;24(3):337-347.
59. Duggan S, O'Sullivan M, Feehan S, et al. Nutrition treatment of deficiency and malnutrition in chronic pancreatitis: a review. *Nutr Clin Pract*. 2010;25(4):362-370.

FURTHER READING AND RESOURCES

American Academy of Allergy, Asthma, & Immunology. www.aaaai.org

Asthma and Allergy Foundation of America. www.aafa.org

Celiac Sprue Association. www.csaceliacs.org

Crohn's and Colitis Foundation of America. www.ccfa.org

Cystic Fibrosis Foundation. www.cff.org

Cystic Fibrosis.com. www.cysticfibrosis.com

Dysphagia Resource Center. www.dysphagia.com

International Foundation for Functional Gastrointestinal Disorders. www.iffgd.org

National Digestive Diseases Information Clearinghouse, Irritable Bowel Syndrome. digestive.niddk.nih.gov/ddiseases/pubs/ibs/

These organizations provide support for individuals who are affected by disorders of the gastrointestinal tract. Health care providers should be familiar with these organizations and their Web sites to refer patients to organizations that can continue to give them support, understanding, and up-to-date information about their diseases.

Nowak-Wegrzyn A, Sampson HA. Future therapies for food allergies. *J Allergy Clin Immunol*. 2011;127(3):558-573, quiz 574-575.

Peyrin-Biroulet L, Loftus Jr EV, Colombel JF, Sandborn WJ. The natural history of adult Crohn's disease in population-based cohorts. *Am J Gastroenterol*. 2010;105(2):289-297.

CHAPTER 19

Coronary Heart Disease and Hypertension

KEY CONCEPTS

- Cardiovascular disease is the leading cause of death in the United States.
- Several risk factors contribute to the development of coronary heart disease and hypertension, many of which are preventable by improved food habits and lifestyle behaviors.
- Other risk factors are nonmodifiable, such as age, gender, family history, and race.
- Hypertension (i.e., chronically elevated blood pressure) may be classified as primary or secondary hypertension.
- Hypertension damages the endothelium of the blood vessels.
- Early education is critical for the prevention of cardiovascular disease.

Cardiovascular disease (CVD) is the leading cause of death in the United States, and it accounts for more than 615,000 deaths each year (Figure 19-1).[1] A similar situation exists in most other developed Western societies. Every day, thousands of people have heart attacks and strokes, and more than 1 million others continue to live with various forms of rheumatic and congestive heart disease.

This chapter discusses the primary underlying disease processes of atherosclerosis and hypertension as well as the various risk factors involved, and it explores ways to use nutrition therapy to reduce risk factors and to help prevent disease.

CORONARY HEART DISEASE

Atherosclerosis

Disease Process

The major cause of CVD and the underlying pathologic process in coronary heart disease is atherosclerosis. This process is characterized by fatty fibrous plaques that may begin as early as childhood and that develop into fatty streaks, which are largely composed of cholesterol, on the inside lining of major blood vessels. When tissue is examined, cholesterol can be seen with the unaided eye in the debris of advanced lesions. This fatty, fibrous plaque gradually thickens over time and narrows the interior part of the blood vessel. The thickening of the vessel or the development of a blood clot may eventually cut off blood flow (Figure 19-2).

Cells die when they are deprived of their normal blood supply. The local area of dying or dead tissue is called an *infarct*. If the affected blood vessel is a major artery that supplies vital nutrients and oxygen to the heart muscle (i.e., the myocardium), then the event is called a *myocardial infarction* (MI) or *heart attack*. If the affected vessel is a major artery that goes to the brain, then the event is called a *cerebrovascular accident* or *stroke*. The major arteries and their many branches that serve the heart are called *coronary arteries*, because they lie across the brow of the heart and resemble a crown. Thus, the overall disease process is identified as *coronary heart disease*. A common symptom of its presence is *angina pectoris* or

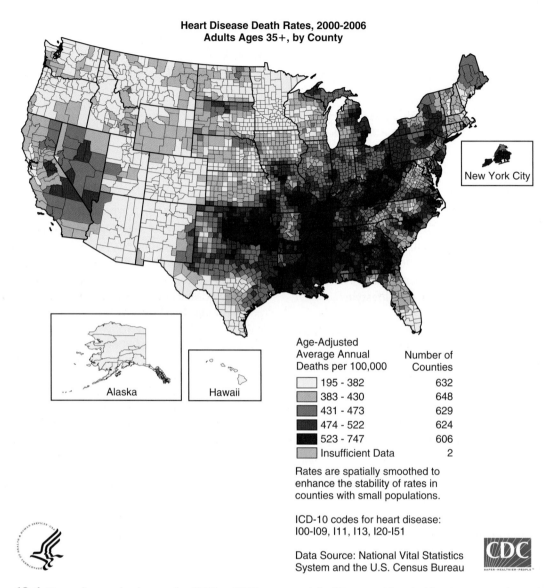

Figure 19-1 Heart disease death rates for 2000 to 2006 among adults 35 years old and older, by county. (From the Centers for Disease Control and Prevention. *Heart disease death rates, 2000-2006, adults ages 35+, by county* (website): www.cdc.gov/DHDSP/maps/pdfs/hd_all.pdf. Accessed March 2011.)

atherosclerosis the underlying pathology of coronary heart disease; a common form of arteriosclerosis that is characterized by the formation of fatty streaks that contain cholesterol and that develop into hardened plaques in the inner lining of major blood vessels such as the coronary arteries.

myocardial infarction (MI) a heart attack; a myocardial infarction is caused by the failure of the heart muscle to maintain normal blood circulation as a result of the blockage of the coronary arteries with fatty cholesterol plaques that cut off the delivery of oxygen to the affected part of the heart muscle.

cerebrovascular accident a stroke; a stroke is caused by arteriosclerosis within the blood vessels of the brain that cuts off oxygen supply to the affected portion of brain tissue, thereby paralyzing the actions that are controlled by the affected area.

coronary heart disease the overall medical problem that results from the underlying disease of atherosclerosis in the coronary arteries, which serve the heart muscle with blood, oxygen, and nutrients.

angina pectoris a spasmodic, choking chest pain caused by a lack of oxygen to the heart; this is a symptom of a heart attack, and it also may be caused by severe effort or excitement.

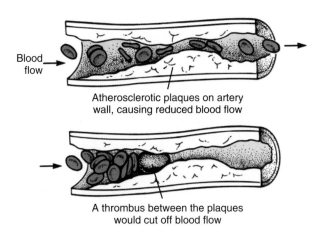

Atherosclerotic plaques on artery
wall, causing reduced blood flow

A thrombus between the plaques
would cut off blood flow

Figure 19-2 An atherosclerotic plaque in an artery.

chest pain that usually radiates down the left arm and that is sometimes brought on by excitement or physical effort.

Relation to Fat Metabolism

Elevated blood lipids are associated with CVD. Lipid substances involved in the disease process are described in detail in Chapter 3, and three of these substances are discussed again in this chapter.

Triglycerides. The chemical name for fat that describes its basic structure is *triglyceride.* All simple fats, whether in the body or in food, are triglycerides (see Chapter 3). The blood test for total triglycerides measures circulating levels in the blood. Studies that assesses the effect of dietary fat on blood lipid profiles show adverse results from diets that are high in saturated and trans fats.[2] Conversely, diets that are low in overall fat and diets that replace saturated fats with monounsaturated fats produce more desirable profiles and lower inflammatory markers.[3,4] In addition, supplementing with omega-3 fatty acids (i.e., eicosapentaenoic acid and docosahexaenoic acid) effectively reduces circulating levels of triglycerides in individuals with hypertriglyceridmia.[5]

Body fat assessment and the measurement of fat distribution with methods such as the body mass index, waist circumference, waist-hip circumference ratio, dual-energy x-ray absorptiometry, and ultrasonography help to identify people who are more likely to have CVD risk factors and elevated triglyceride levels.[6-8]

Cholesterol. Cholesterol is a fat-related compound that is both consumed in the diet and produced in the liver. It is an important part of normal cell functioning. Dietary cholesterol is found in foods of animal origin only (e.g., meat, dairy, butter). Although cholesterol is an essential compound in the body, excess total blood levels increase the risk of heart disease in predisposed individuals. High blood cholesterol levels increase the risk for the deposition of cholesterol, fats, fibrous tissue, and

macrophages in arteries throughout the body, which is the beginning of atherosclerosis. The Centers for Disease Control and Prevention reports that 14.9% of American adults 20 years old and older have high total blood cholesterol levels of more than 240 mg/dL.[1] Many patients with hypercholesterolemia have the related problems of obesity and hypertension; these require medical counseling and intervention, with diet as the primary treatment. A total blood cholesterol level of less than 200 mg/dL is desirable.[9]

Lipoproteins. Because fat is not soluble in water, it is carried in the bloodstream in small packages wrapped with protein called *lipoproteins.* These compounds are produced in the intestinal mucosal cells after a meal that contains fat and in the liver as part of the ongoing process of fat metabolism. Lipoproteins carry fat and cholesterol to tissues for cell metabolism and then back to the liver for breakdown and excretion as needed. Lipoproteins are grouped and named in accordance with their protein, fat, and cholesterol content (i.e., their density) (Figure 19-3). Those with the highest protein content have the highest density and vice versa. Five lipoproteins are significant in relation to heart disease risk as follows:

1. *Chylomicrons:* These are made predominantly (≈85%) from dietary triglycerides after absorption from the gastrointestinal tract. Chylomicrons are lipoprotein particles that transport absorbed dietary (i.e., exogenous) triglycerides to plasma and tissues (Figure 19-3, *A*).
2. *Very low-density lipoproteins (VLDLs):* These are formed in the liver from endogenous fat. VLDLs carry a relatively large load of triglycerides to cells, and they also contain approximately 12% cholesterol (Figure 19-3, *B*).

lipids the chemical group name for fats and fat-related compounds such as cholesterol and lipoproteins.

waist circumference the measurement of the waist at its narrowest point width-wise, just above the navel; waist circumference is a rough measurement of abdominal fat and a predictor of risk factors for cardiovascular disease; this risk factor increases with a waist measurement of more than 40 inches in men and of more than 35 inches in women.

dual-energy x-ray absorptiometry radiography that makes use of two beams (i.e., dual) that measure bone density and body composition.

ultrasonography an ultrasound-based diagnostic imaging technique that is used to visualize the muscles and internal organs; also referred to as *sonography.*

hypercholesterolemia elevated blood cholesterol levels.

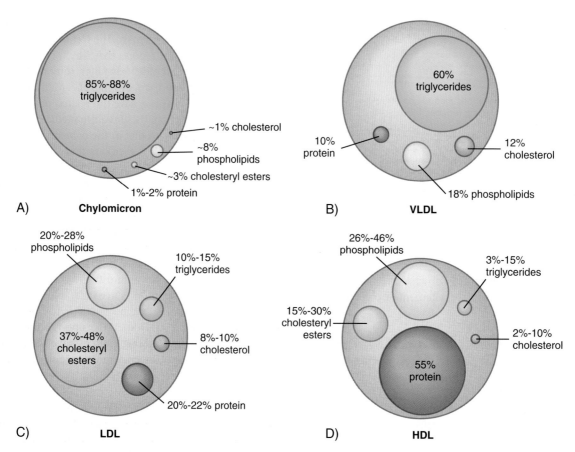

Figure 19-3 Serum lipoprotein factions showing lipid composition. **A,** Chylomicron. **B,** Very low-density lipoprotein. **C,** Low-density lipoprotein. **D,** High-density lipoprotein.

3. *Intermediate-density lipoproteins (IDLs):* Like VLDLs, IDLs deposit triglycerides throughout the body; degradation leaves IDLs in the circulation. IDLs continue delivering endogenous triglycerides to cells and tissue.

4. *Low-density lipoproteins (LDLs):* LDLs carry, in addition to other lipids, at least two thirds of the total plasma cholesterol to body tissues. LDLs are formed endogenously in the liver and in serum from the catabolism of VLDLs and IDLs. Because LDLs constantly send cholesterol to tissues, they can be considered "the source of bad cholesterol." With regard to cardiovascular health, LDL cholesterol is the major lipoprotein of concern[10] (Figure 19-3, *C*).

5. *High-density lipoproteins (HDLs):* HDLs carry less total fat and more protein (Figure 19-3, *D*). They transport cholesterol from the tissues to the liver for catabolism, and they are endogenously produced in the liver. Compared with LDL cholesterol, HDL often is considered "good cholesterol," and higher serum levels are protective against CVD. Values of

less than 40 mg/dL imply increased risk for CVD, and a value of 60 mg/dL or more contributes protection and decreased risk. Unlike other lipoproteins, HDL cholesterol is more closely associated with regular exercise and lean body mass than diet, which is one of the reasons that the Expert Panel on Detection, Evaluation, and Treatment of High Blood Cholesterol in Adults recommends regular physical activity.[2,9]

Table 19-1 outlines the recommended blood levels of each lipid component.

Risk Factors

The underlying disease process of atherosclerosis is caused by multiple risk factors (Box 19-1). Note the modifiable risk factors over which people have some control compared with those that individuals cannot control (i.e., nonmodifiable):

- *Gender:* CVD occurs more often among men than women until women reach menopause, at which time the relative risks are the same for both genders. Researchers have not concluded whether the

TABLE 19-1 CHOLESTEROL AND LIPOPROTEIN PROFILE CLASSIFICATION

Cholesterol Reading	Classification
Total Cholesterol (mg/dL)	
< 200	Desirable
200 to 239	Borderline high
≥ 240	High
Low-Density Lipoprotein Cholesterol (mg/dL)	
< 100	Optimal
100 to 129	Near optimal
130 to 159	Borderline high
160 to 189	High
≥ 190	Very high
High-Density Lipoprotein Cholesterol (mg/dL)	
≥ 60	Optimal
< 40	Low (elevated risk)
Triglycerides (mg/dL)	
< 150	Optimal
150 to 199	Borderline high
200 to 499	High
≥ 500	Very high

Data from National Cholesterol Education Program. *Third report of the NCEP Expert Panel on Detection, Evaluation, and Treatment of High Blood Cholesterol in Adults (Adult Treatment Panel III).* Washington, DC: National Institutes of Health; 2002.

increased risk for women is solely the result of menopause, because separating risks associated with age from those associated with menopause is difficult.[11,12]

- *Age:* General risk for CVD increases with the aging process. It is greater for men who are older than 45 years old and for women who are older than 55 years old.
- *Family history:* A positive family history is defined as a history of premature CVD (i.e., before the age of 55 years in a male first-degree relative or before the age of 65 years in a female first-degree relative). Early screening for children and adolescents with a high-risk family history is important so that appropriate diet and lifestyle modifications may begin before fatty streaks develop in the coronary arteries.
- *Heredity:* Certain ethnic groups (i.e., African Americans, Mexican Americans, Native Americans, Native Hawaiians, and some Asian Americans) have a higher incidence of risk factors and CVD. Genetic defects that result in abnormally high serum lipid levels include familial hypercholesterolemia and familial hypertriglyceridemia.

Both conditions require diet and drug therapy to begin during the second or third decade of life.

- *Compounding diseases:* Comorbidities associated with obesity such as type 2 diabetes, hypertension, and metabolic syndrome (Table 19-2) increase the risk for the development of CVD.[9,13]
- *Blood cholesterol profile:* High total and LDL cholesterol and low HDL cholesterol are major risk factors for the disease process, which is worsened by obesity, physical inactivity, diets that are high in trans fat and saturated fat, stress, and smoking. The National Cholesterol Education Program recommends cholesterol screening every 5 years for adults without existing risk factors and more often for those with higher risks.

Dietary Recommendations for Reduced Risk

Dietary Guidelines. Because the control of dietary fat and cholesterol is important to reduce risks for heart disease, the Dietary Guidelines for Americans (see Chapter 1) and the American Heart Association (Box 19-2) recommend the dietary restriction of both fat and cholesterol.

Adult Treatment Panel III Guidelines. The National Heart, Lung, and Blood Association's National Cholesterol Education Program (NCEP) began a campaign against high blood cholesterol in 1988 with the release of its "Report of the Expert Panel on Detection, Evaluation, and Treatment of High Blood Cholesterol in Adults, Adult Treatment Panel (ATP)." The NCEP designed the Step I and Step II diets, which were also endorsed by the American Heart Association, to lessen the risk of CVD by reducing high blood cholesterol levels. Since the inception of the Step I and Step II diets, the NCEP has released two follow-up reports. In the most recent report (ATP

familial hypercholesterolemia a genetic disorder that results in elevated blood cholesterol levels despite lifestyle modifications; this condition is caused by absent or nonfunctional low-density lipoprotein receptors, and it requires drug therapy.

familial hypertriglyceridemia a genetic disorder that results in elevated blood triglyceride levels despite lifestyle modifications; it requires drug therapy.

metabolic syndrome a combination of disorders that, when they occur together, increases the risk of cardiovascular disease and diabetes; it is also known as *syndrome X* and *insulin resistance syndrome*.

BOX 19-1 RISK FACTORS FOR CARDIOVASCULAR DISEASE

Lipid Risk Factors
- Low-density lipoprotein cholesterol > 130 mg/dL
- High-density lipoprotein cholesterol < 40 mg/dL*
- Total cholesterol > 200 mg/dL
- Triglycerides > 150 mg/dL
- Atherogenic dyslipidemia†

Nonlipid Risk Factors
Nonmodifiable
- Male gender
- Age (men ≥ 45 years, women ≥ 55 years)
- Heredity (including race)
- Family history of premature cardiovascular disease (i.e., myocardial infarction or sudden death at 55 years of age or less in a male first-degree relative or at 65 years of age or less in a female first-degree relative)
- Estimated glomerular filtration rate of < 60 mL/min or microalbuminuria
- Type 1 diabetes mellitus

Modifiable
- Cigarette smoking
- Hypertension (blood pressure > 140/90 mm Hg or taking antihypertensive medication)

- Physical inactivity
- Obesity (body mass index of > 30 kg/m^2) and overweight (body mass index of 25 to 29.9 kg/m^2)
- Type 2 diabetes mellitus
- Atherogenic diet (i.e., a high intake of saturated fat and cholesterol)

Emerging Risk Factors
Emerging Lipid Risk Factors
- Elevated lipoprotein remnants
- Elevated lipoprotein(a)
- Small low-density lipoprotein particles
- Elevated apolipoprotein B
- Low apolipoprotein A-I
- High total cholesterol/high-density lipoprotein cholesterol ratio

Emerging Nonlipid Risk Factors
- Hyperhomocysteinemia
- Thrombogenic or hemostatic factors
- Inflammatory markers (e.g., C-reactive protein)
- Impaired fasting glucose level

*High-density lipoprotein level of > 60 mg/dL counts as a "negative" risk factor; its presence removes one risk factor
†Atherogenic dyslipidemia is a disorder with four components: borderline high-risk low-density lipoprotein cholesterol level (i.e., 130 to 159 mg/dL), moderately raised (often high normal) triglyceride level, small low-density lipoprotein particles, and low high-density lipoprotein cholesterol level.
Modified from the National Cholesterol Education Program. *Third report of the NCEP Expert Panel on Detection, Evaluation, and Treatment of High Blood Cholesterol in Adults (Adult Treatment Panel III),* Washington, DC: National Institutes of Health; 2002.

BOX 19-2 AMERICAN HEART ASSOCIATION DIETARY GUIDELINES

Weight and Physical Activity
- Burn at least as many calories as consumed.
- Aim for at least 30 minutes of physical activity on most if not all days. To lose weight, do enough activity to burn more calories than eaten every day.

Foods to Focus On
- Eat a variety of nutritious foods from all food groups.
- Choose foods like vegetables, fruits, whole-grain products, and fat-free or low-fat dairy products most often.
- Choose lean meats and poultry without skin, and prepare them without added saturated and trans fats.
- Eat fish at least twice a week.
- Select fat-free, 1% fat, and low-fat dairy products.

Foods to Limit or Consume in Moderation
- Cut back on foods that contain partially hydrogenated vegetable oils to reduce trans fats in the diet.

- Cut back on foods that are high in dietary cholesterol. Aim to eat less than 300 mg of cholesterol each day.
- Eat less of the nutrient-poor foods.
- Cut back on beverages and foods with added sugars.
- Choose and prepare foods with little or no salt. Aim to eat less than 1500 mg of sodium per day.
- Drink alcohol in moderation, if at all. That means one drink per day for women and two drinks per day for men.

General Recommendations
- Follow the American Heart Association recommendations when eating out, and keep an eye on portion sizes.
- Don't smoke tobacco, and stay away from tobacco smoke.

Source: American Heart Association, Inc. Modified from the American Heart Association. *Diet and lifestyle recommendations* (website): www. heart.org/HEARTORG/GettingHealthy/Diet-and-Lifestyle-Recommendations_UCM_305855_Article.jsp. Accessed March 2011.

TABLE 19-2 DIAGNOSTIC CRITERIA FOR METABOLIC SYNDROME

Measure*	Categoric Cut points
Increased waist circumference†‡	≥ 102 cm (≥ 40 in) in men ≥ 88 cm (≥ 35 in) in women
Elevated triglycerides	≥ 150 mg/dL (1.7 mmol/L) or drug treatment for elevated triglycerides§
Reduced HDL cholesterol	< 40 mg/dL (1.03 mmol/L) in men < 50 mg/dL (1.3 mmol/L) in women or drug treatment for reduced high-density lipoprotein cholesterol§
Elevated blood pressure	≥ 130 mm Hg systolic or ≥ 85 mm Hg diastolic or drug treatment for hypertension
Elevated fasting glucose	≥ 100 mg/dL or drug treatment for elevated glucose

*Any three of these five criteria constitute a diagnosis of metabolic syndrome.

†To measure waist circumference, locate the top of the right iliac crest. Place a measuring tape in a horizontal plane around the abdomen at the level of the iliac crest. Before reading the tape measure, ensure that the tape is snug but that it does not compress the skin, and be sure that it is parallel to the floor. The measurement is made at the end of a normal expiration.

‡Some U.S. adults of non-Asian origin (e.g., Caucasian, African American, Hispanic) with marginally increased waist circumferences (e.g., 94 to 101 cm [37 to 39 in] in men and 80 to 87 cm [31 to 34 in] in women) may have a strong genetic contribution to insulin resistance and should benefit from changes in lifestyle habits; this is similar for men with categoric increases in waist circumference. A lower waist circumference cut point (e.g., 90 cm [35 in] in men and 80 cm [31 in] in women) appears to be appropriate for Asian Americans.

§Fibrates and nicotinic acid are the most commonly used drugs for elevated triglycerides and reduced high-density lipoprotein cholesterol. Patients who are taking one of these drugs are presumed to have a high triglyceride level and a low high-density lipoprotein cholesterol level.

From Grundy SM, Cleeman JI, Daniels SR, et al; American Heart Association; National Heart, Lung, and Blood Institute. Diagnosis and management of metabolic syndrome: an American Heart Association/National Heart, Lung, and Blood Institute Scientific Statement. *Circulation.* 2005;112:2735-2752.

TABLE 19-3 AMERICAN HEART ASSOCIATION AND NATIONAL CHOLESTEROL EDUCATION PROGRAM RECOMMENDATIONS FOR LOWERING CHOLESTEROL

Nutrient*	Recommended Intake as Percent of Total Calories
Total fat	25% to 35%
Saturated	< 7%
Polyunsaturated	Up to 10%
Monounsaturated	Up to 20%
Carbohydrate	50% to 60%
Protein	≈ 15%
Cholesterol	< 200 mg/day
Total fiber	25 to 30 g
Soluble fiber	10 to 25 g
Total calories	Balance energy intake and expenditure to maintain a desirable body weight and to prevent weight gain

*Calories from alcohol not included.
Modified from the National Cholesterol Education Program. *Third report of the NCEP Expert Panel on Detection, Evaluation, and Treatment of High Blood Cholesterol in Adults (Adult Treatment Panel III).* Washington, DC: National Institutes of Health; 2002.

- Total fat intake should not exceed 25% to 35% of total kilocalories, with saturated fats contributing no more than 7%, polyunsaturated fats contributing up to 10%, and monounsaturated fats contributing up to 20%. Individuals with metabolic syndrome or diabetes can increase their intake of monounsaturated and polyunsaturated fats in place of carbohydrates.
- Avoid trans fatty acids.
- Carbohydrates—mainly from complex carbohydrates such as whole grains, fruits, and vegetables—should make up 50% to 60% of the total energy intake per day. The diet should allow for a total of 25 to 30 g of fiber (of which 10 to 25 g should be from soluble fiber) and 2 g of plant-derived sterols or stanols per day.
- Total protein intake should account for approximately 15% of the total energy intake. Soy protein is encouraged as a low-fat alternative to other animal products (see the For Further Focus box, "Soy Protein and Heart Disease").

Therapeutic Lifestyle Changes (TLC) an intensive lifestyle intervention that is focused on appropriate weight, diet, physical activity, and other controllable risk factors to reduce cholesterol levels and to prevent other complications of heart disease.

III), the organization moved toward an intensive lifestyle habit intervention that was focused on appropriate weight, diet, physical activity, and other controllable risk factors.[9] This comprehensive approach is referred to as the Therapeutic Lifestyle Changes (TLC) diet. Table 19-3 outlines the recommendations for the TLC diet. Essential components of the approach are as follows[9]:

- Total energy intake should reflect energy expenditure to maintain a desirable body weight and to prevent weight gain.
- Include enough exercise to expend at least 200 kcal/day.

FOR FURTHER FOCUS

SOY PROTEIN AND HEART DISEASE

In recent years, soy protein has been linked to a reduced risk for coronary heart disease. The ingestion of soy protein has led to a reduction in low-density lipoprotein cholesterol levels, an increase in high-density lipoprotein cholesterol levels, and a reduction in triglyceride levels. The findings are so significant that the U.S. Food and Drug Administration (FDA) has approved an official health claim to link soy protein consumption with a reduced risk of coronary heart disease.[1]

One of the main focuses of research in this area is to narrow the recommendations for the amount and type of phytosterols and phytostanols needed on a daily basis to receive the most beneficial results. Phytosterols and phytostanols are the molecules that are found in plant foods that have the cholesterol-lowering effects. One way in which they work is by preventing the absorption of cholesterol in the digestive tract. Previous research had found a huge range (i.e., 18 to 124 g/day) in the amount of soy protein needed to achieve the desired results. One reason for this large difference is the low water solubility of the compounds. Because the compound requires fat as a carrier, consuming that amount of soy protein could drastically increase total fat consumption. (Even if it is the heart-healthy fat, it still carries the potential for causing weight gain.) The FDA recommends consuming four servings per day of soy protein, with each serving containing a minimum of 6.25 g for a total of 25 g/day.

Researchers are exploring alternative methods for introducing the protein without drastically changing diet or fat intake. One study found that a soy protein supplement of soybean β-conglycinin (a component of soy protein isolate) in the form of candy produced a significant reduction in triglyceride concentrations and may be an effective alternative or addition to soy-protein foods.[2] A similar study combined soy protein with small amounts of lecithin, dried it, and added it to otherwise fat-free foods as an alternative source of phytosterols and phytostanols.[3] β-Sitosterol and lecithin increased the water solubility of the compound and allowed for better absorption without the fat. In both cases, the beneficial effects of soy protein were seen in the form of lowered cholesterol levels and improved lipid profiles.

Incorporating soy protein into a low-fat, high-fiber diet with plenty of fruits and vegetables is a sound start to reducing the risk for coronary heart disease.[4] Soy protein can be found in the following foods:

- Soy-based meat alternatives
- Miso
- Nondairy frozen desserts
- Okara (not okra)
- Soy beverages
- Soy cheese
- Soy nut butter
- Soy yogurt
- Soybeans
- Soybean oil
- Soy milk
- Soy nuts
- Tempeh
- Textured vegetable protein
- Tofu

1. U.S. Food and Drug Administration. *Health claims: soy protein and risk of coronary heart disease (CHD), Electronic Code of Federal Regulations.* Washington, DC: U.S. Food and Drug Administration; 2011.
2. Kohno M, Hirotsuka M, Kito M, et al. Decreases in serum triacylglycerol and visceral fat mediated by dietary soybean beta-conglycinin. *J Atheroscler Thromb.* 2006;13(5):247-255.
3. Spilburg CA, Goldberg AC, McGill JB, et al. Fat-free foods supplemented with soy stanol-lecithin powder reduce cholesterol absorption and LDL cholesterol. *J Am Diet Assoc.* 2003;103(5):577-581.
4. Sacks FM, Lichtenstein A, Van Horn L, et al. Soy protein, isoflavones, and cardiovascular health: an American Heart Association Science Advisory for professionals from the Nutrition Committee. *Circulation.* 2006;113(7):1034-1044.

- Total cholesterol intake should be less than 200 mg/ day.

A diet that is rich in vegetables, fruits, and whole grains; low in saturated and trans fatty acids; and that includes the moderate use of polyunsaturated and monounsaturated food fats (i.e., mostly olive oil, corn oil, and other vegetable oils and products) is the basic guideline. Low-fat and fat-free dairy products as well as lean meat, fish, and poultry are used instead of their high-fat alternatives.

When the risk factor of obesity is present, weight loss via negative energy balance is encouraged. Interestingly, studies show that weight loss attempts are largely unsuccessful among patients with CVD; however, when a physician officially diagnoses a patient as overweight, weight loss attempts are more successful.[14] Negative energy balance should be achieved through reduced energy intake and increased energy expenditure as a result of regular physical activity (see Chapter 15). A treadmill exercise tolerance test is ideal to determine the exercise limit for individuals who are older, who are obese, or who have a history of CVD or hypertension before they start an exercise program (Figure 19-4).

Drug Therapy

In the event that the LDL cholesterol level is above the goal range, the NCEP ATP III guidelines recommend cut points for the TLC diet and drug therapy, depending on

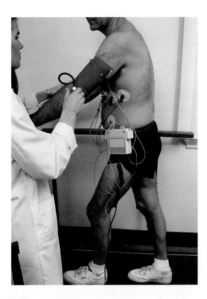

Figure 19-4 A patient with a history of cardiac disease is evaluated for exercise tolerance with a treadmill test. (Copyright PhotoDisc.)

the level of risk. As the number and severity of risk factors increase, the point at which TLC and drug therapy should begin declines. For example, a person with few or no risk factors associated with CVD may wait to initiate drug therapy until LDL levels exceed 190 mg/dL, whereas an individual with significant risk for CVD should consider drug therapy when LDL levels rise to more than 100 mg/dL. At any level of drug therapy, the TLC dietary guidelines should be continued as adjunct therapy.

Acute Cardiovascular Disease

When CVD progresses to the point of cutting off the blood supply to major coronary arteries, a critical vascular event (i.e., MI) may occur. During the initial acute phase of the attack, additional diet modifications are necessary for healing.

Objective: Cardiac Rest

The term *infarction* means tissue death from a lack of oxygen. Blood tests reveal enzymes and proteins that are released from the damaged heart muscle after infarction; these cardiac markers are one of the tests used for diagnosis. During the care immediately after an MI, patients are treated with the MONA protocol and given analgesics (e.g., *M*orphine), supplemental *O*xygen, intravenous *N*itroglycerine, and *A*spirin. All care, including the diet, is directed toward ensuring cardiac rest so that the damaged heart may be restored to normal functioning.

Principles of Medical Nutrition Therapy

Medical nutrition therapy goals for patients after MI are as follows: (1) promote recovery and strength; and (2) lower LDL cholesterol and other known risk factors to prevent the progression of CVD.[15] Patients who have experienced an MI are encouraged to follow the TLC diet (if they are not already doing so) to reduce further risk factors for CVD.

Initially, the diet is modified with regard to energy value and texture as well as for fat and sodium content (see the Clinical Applications box, "Case Study: The Patient With a Myocardial Infarction").

Energy. A brief period of reduced energy intake during the first day after the heart attack reduces the metabolic workload on the damaged heart. The metabolic demands for the digestion, absorption, and metabolism of food require a generous cardiac output. Thus, to decrease the level of metabolic activity that the weakened heart can handle, small feedings are spread over the day when an oral diet is started. The patient progresses to eating more as healing occurs. During the recovery period, caloric intake is adjusted to meet the energy needs of the person's ideal body weight.

Texture. Early feedings may include foods that are relatively soft in texture or easily digested to avoid excess effort during eating or the discomfort of gas formation. Some patients benefit from assistance during the feeding process for a short period, especially those with poor appetite or weakness or who become short of breath from the exertion of eating. Smaller and more frequent meals may provide needed nourishment without undue strain or pressure. Depending on the patient's condition, gasforming foods, caffeine-containing beverages, and hot or cold temperature extremes in foods in both solids and liquids should be avoided.

Fat. The TLC diet controls the amounts and types of fat and cholesterol consumed (see Table 19-3). Research supports the adoption of a Mediterranean-type diet (see Figure 14-8) for patients who have had an MI. Adherence to the Mediterranean diet reduces risk factors for CVD, reduces inflammatory markers after an MI, and increases the life span.[16-18] The basic components of a Mediterranean diet are plant-based foods; fish and poultry, with limited red meat; up to 4 eggs per week; moderate amounts of dairy products; olive oil as the primary source of fat; the use of herbs and spices in place of salt; moderate red wine intake with meals; fresh fruit as dessert; and minimal intake of processed foods.[19]

Sodium. General attention to reduced sodium content in food selection is important as well (Box 19-3). If the patient has hypertension, sodium restriction to

CLINICAL APPLICATIONS

CASE STUDY: THE PATIENT WITH A MYOCARDIAL INFARCTION

Charles Carter is a young businessman who works long hours and who carries the major responsibilities of his struggling small business. At his last physical checkup, the physician cautioned him about his pace, because he was already showing mild hypertension. His blood cholesterol was elevated, and he was overweight, with a body mass index of 28.5. At his desk job, he gets little exercise, and he finds himself smoking more and eating irregularly as a result of the stress of his increasing financial pressures.

One day while commuting in heavy freeway traffic, Charles felt a pain in his chest, and he became increasingly apprehensive. When he arrived home, the pain increased. He broke out into a cold sweat, and he felt nauseated. When he became more ill after trying to eat dinner, his wife called their physician, and Charles was admitted to the hospital.

After emergency care and tests, the physician placed Charles in the coronary care unit at the hospital. His test results showed elevated total cholesterol, low-density lipoprotein cholesterol, and triglyceride levels and a low high-density lipoprotein cholesterol level. The electrocardiogram revealed an infarction of the posterior myocardium wall.

When Charles was first able to take oral nourishment, he could only consume a liquid diet. As his condition stabilized, his diet was increased to 1200 kcal (soft diet) with low cholesterol and low fat. By the end of the first week, his diet was increased to 1600 kcal (full diet), with low cholesterol,

only 25% of the total kilocalories from fat, and a polyunsaturated fat to saturated fat ratio of 1:1.

Charles gradually improved over the next few days and was able to go home. The physician, the nurse, and the dietitian discussed with Charles and his wife the need for care at home during a period of convalescence. They explained that Charles had an underlying lipid disorder and that he needed to continue his weight loss and follow the TLC diet.

Questions for Analysis

1. Identify factors in this patient's personal and medical history that place him at high risk for coronary heart disease. Give reasons why each factor contributes to heart disease.
2. Why did Charles receive only a liquid diet at first? What is the reason for each modification in his first diet of solid food?
3. What occurs during the underlying disease process that causes a heart attack? What relationship do fat and cholesterol have to this underlying process?
4. What needs might Charles have when he goes home? How would you help him to prepare to go home? Name some community resources that you might use to help him understand his illness and plan self-care.

---

approximately 2400 mg/day may be indicated to control edema.[15] This restriction can be achieved by using little or no salt in cooking, adding no salt when eating, and avoiding salty processed foods. Appendix C provides a salt-free seasoning guide. Nutrition Facts labels provide specific information about the sodium content per serving of any food (see Chapter 13).

Heart Failure

Congestive heart failure is a form of chronic heart disease. The progressively weakened heart muscle is unable to maintain an adequate cardiac output to sustain normal blood circulation. The resulting fluid imbalances make basic functions of living (e.g., breathing, eating, walking, sleeping) difficult to perform. The most common causes of heart failure are coronary heart disease, MI, and chronic hypertension.

Control of Pulmonary Edema

The basic objective of diet therapy for a patient with congestive heart failure is to control the fluid imbalance that results in pulmonary edema. The primary causes of fluid

accumulation are altered fluid shift mechanisms and inappropriate hormonal responses.

Fluid Shift Mechanism. With decreased heart function, blood accumulates in the vascular system. This buildup offsets the delicate balance of filtration pressures and causes fluid to collect within intracellular spaces instead of flowing among fluid compartments.

Hormonal Alterations. Kidney nephrons sense decreased renal blood flow, which is normally an indication of dehydration, and they respond by triggering the vasopressin and renin-angiotensin-aldosterone systems to increase blood pressure (see Chapter 9). Unlike

---

congestive heart failure a chronic condition of gradually weakening heart muscle; the muscle is unable to pump normal blood through the heart–lung circulation, which results in the congestion of fluids in the lungs.

pulmonary edema an accumulation of fluid in the lung tissues.

> **BOX 19-3   SODIUM-RESTRICTED DIET RECOMMENDATIONS**
>
> - Choose low- or reduced-sodium or no-salt-added versions of foods and condiments, when available.
> - Choose fresh, frozen, or canned low-sodium or no-salt-added vegetables.
> - Cook without salt, and avoid adding salt to prepared meals.
> - Avoid salt-preserved foods such as salted or smoked meat (e.g., bacon, bacon fat, bologna, dried or chipped beef, corned beef, frankfurters, ham, kosher meats, luncheon meats, salt pork, sausage), salted or smoked fish (e.g., anchovies, caviar, salted and dried cod, herring, sardines), sauerkraut, and olives. Use fresh poultry, fish, and lean meats instead.
> - Avoid highly salted foods such as crackers, pretzels, potato chips, corn chips, salted nuts, and salted popcorn. Choose products that are lower in sodium.
> - Limit spices and condiments such as bouillon cubes, ketchup, chili sauce, celery salt, garlic salt, onion salt, monosodium glutamate, meat sauces, meat tenderizers, pickles, prepared mustard, relishes, Worcestershire sauce, and soy sauce.*
> - Limit processed foods and convenience foods (e.g., cheese, peanut butter, flavored rice and pasta, frozen dinners, canned soups) that are usually high in salt, or choose reduced-sodium versions.*

These restrictions are for a mild, low-sodium diet (i.e., 2 to 4 g/day).
*Low-sodium brands may be used.

dehydration, reduced blood flow is caused by the inadequate pumping of the heart rather than by low blood volume. Vasopressin from the pituitary gland, which is also known as *antidiuretic hormone,* stimulates the resorption of water in the kidneys. In addition, aldosterone, which is secreted by the adrenal glands, causes the resorption of sodium (and thus water) in the kidneys. Consequently, fluid retention is increased, and edema is exacerbated.

Principles of Medical Nutrition Therapy

Medical nutrition therapy focuses on achieving nutritional adequacy of the diet while limiting sodium and fluid intake to control edema.[15]

The main source of dietary sodium is common table salt or sodium chloride. The taste for salt is acquired. Some people heavily salt their food out of habit without tasting it first, thereby habituating their taste to high salt levels. Others acquire a taste for less salt by gradually using smaller and smaller amounts. The Adequate Intake for sodium is 1500 mg per day for adults up to the age of 50 years, and then it declines slightly.[20] Daily adult intakes

of sodium range widely in the typical American diet; men consume an average of 4043 mg/day, and women consume an average of 2884 mg/day.[21] Other than the salt that is used in cooking or added at the table, a large amount is used as a preservative in processed food. Remaining sources of sodium include that found as a naturally occurring mineral in certain foods.

Nutrition therapy focuses the following[15]:

- *Sodium restriction (2 g per day):* No salt is served with meals. Fresh foods are encouraged and should include sodium-free flavorings such as herbs. Salty processed foods are avoided (e.g., pickles, olives, bacon, ham, corn chips, potato chips). Some processed foods with low sodium are available in food markets.
- *Fluid restriction:* Fluid is limited to 2 L per day for patients with mild symptoms of heart failure. For advanced stages of heart failure, fluid is restricted to 1000 to 1500 mL per day as indicated.
- *Texture and timing:* Patients may tolerate soft foods better if eating is laborious or uncomfortable. Frequent small meals (e.g., five to six per day) are better suited than large meals to prevent fatigue from eating.
- *Nutritional adequacy:* Care should be taken to ensure that diet restrictions do not result in nutrient inadequacies in the diet.
- *Alcohol:* Alcohol intake is limited or avoided if it contributes to heart disease.

ESSENTIAL HYPERTENSION

The Problem of Hypertension

Incidence and Nature

Hypertension or high blood pressure is one of the most common vascular diseases worldwide. The Centers for Disease Control and Prevention reports that 31% of American adults who are older than 20 years old have hypertension, with an additional 18% of the population at risk with elevated blood pressure. The incidence is highest among African-American women, with a 44.4% prevalence rate.[1] When speaking of the chronic condition of elevated blood pressure, the term *hypertension* is more appropriate than *high blood pressure,* because blood pressure may occasionally be elevated during situations that involve overexertion or stress. With essential (or primary) hypertension, the specific cause is unknown, although injury to the inner lining of the blood vessel wall appears to be an underlying link. More than 90% of cases are considered to be essential hypertension. Secondary

TABLE 19-4 CLASSIFICATION OF BLOOD PRESSURE FOR ADULTS

Blood Pressure Classification	Systolic Blood Pressure (mm Hg)	Diastolic Blood Pressure (mm Hg)	Lifestyle Modification	INITIAL DRUG THERAPY	
				Without Compelling Indication	With Compelling Indication
Normal	< 120	and < 80	Encourage		
Prehypertension	120 to 139	or 80 to 89	Yes	No antihypertensive drug indicated	Drugs for compelling indications*
Stage 1 hypertension	140 to 159	or 90 to 99	Yes	Thiazide-type diuretics for most; may consider ACEI, ARB, BB, CCB, or combination	Drugs for compelling indications,* other antihypertensive drugs as needed (diuretics, ACEI, ARB, BB, or CCB)
Stage 2 hypertension	≥ 160	or ≥ 100	Yes	Two-drug combination for most† (usually thiazide-type diuretic and ACEI, ARB, BB, or CCB)	Drugs for compelling indications and other antihypertensive drugs as needed (diuretics, ACEI, ARB, BB, or CCB)

Information for adults 18 years old and older. Treatment is determined by the highest blood pressure category.
ACEI, Angiotensin-converting enzyme inhibitor; *ARB*, angiotensin receptor blocker; *BB*, β-blocker; *CCB*, calcium channel blocker.
*Patients with chronic kidney disease or diabetes should be treated with a blood pressure goal of < 130/80 mm Hg.
†Initial combined therapy should be used cautiously for individuals who are at risk for orthostatic hypotension.
Modified from the National Institutes of Health; National Heart, Lung, and Blood Institute. *Seventh report of the Joint National Committee on Prevention, Detection, Evaluation, and Treatment of High Blood Pressure (JNC 7) express, NIH publication No.03-5233.* Bethesda, Md: National Institutes of Health; 2003.

hypertension is the result of a known cause; it is a symptom or side effect of another primary condition. For example, individuals with kidney disease often have secondary hypertension.

Hypertension has been called "the silent killer," because no signs indicate its presence. It can have serious effects if it is not detected, treated, and controlled. Hypertension is a highly inherited disorder; children of hypertensive parents may develop the condition at an early age, often during their adolescent years. Obesity worsens the condition by forcing the heart to work harder to circulate blood through excess tissue, thereby maintaining higher pressure. Smoking also increases blood pressure, because nicotine constricts the small blood vessels. Other risk factors include increasing age, ethnicity, physical inactivity, chronic stress, alcohol abuse, a diet that is high in saturated fat and sodium, and a low potassium intake.

Hypertensive Blood Pressure Levels

Common blood pressure measurements indicate the pressure of the blood surge in the arteries of the upper arm with each heartbeat. The power of each surge is measured in millimeters of mercury (mm Hg). Two forces are counted and represented by separate numbers. The numerator of the fraction (i.e., the top value) measures the force of the blood surge when the heart contracts, which is known as the *systolic pressure.* The denominator of the fraction (i.e., the bottom value) measures the pressure that remains in the arteries when the heart relaxes between beats; this is known as the *diastolic pressure.* Adult blood pressure is considered normal if it is less than 120/80 mm Hg. Current hypertension screening and treatment programs identify people with hypertension according to the degree of severity of these pressures (Table 19-4).[22] Specific care is then outlined, depending on the severity.

Prehypertension. The initial focus of hypertension treatment is on lifestyle modifications. Lifestyle choices

---

essential (or primary) hypertension an inherent form of high blood pressure with no specific identifiable cause; it is considered to be familial.

secondary hypertension an elevated blood pressure for which the cause can be identified and which is a symptom or side effect of another primary condition.

TABLE 19-5 **LIFESTYLE MODIFICATIONS TO PREVENT AND MANAGE HYPERTENSION**

Modification	Recommendation	Approximate Systolic Blood Pressure Reduction (Range)*
Weight reduction	Maintain a healthy body weight (i.e., body mass index of 18.5 to 24.9 kg/m²)	5 to 20 mm Hg/10 kg
Adopt the DASH eating plan#	Consume a diet that is rich in fruits, vegetables, and low-fat dairy products with a reduced content of saturated and total fat	8 to 14 mm Hg
Dietary sodium reduction	Reduce dietary sodium intake to no more than 2.4 g of sodium or 6 g of salt per day	2 to 8 mm Hg
Physical activity	Engage in regular aerobic physical activity such as brisk walking at least 30 minutes per day most days of the week	4 to 9 mm Hg
Moderation of alcohol consumption	Limit alcohol consumption to no more than two drinks per day (e.g., 24 oz of beer, 10 oz of wine, 3 oz of 80-proof whiskey) for most men and to no more than one drink per day for women and lighter-weight men	2 to 4 mm Hg

For overall cardiovascular risk reduction, stop smoking.
*The effects of implementing these modifications are dependent on dose and time and could be greater for some individuals.
#DASH eating plan is discussed later in this chapter.
Modified from the National Institutes of Health; National Heart, Lung, and Blood Institute National High Blood Pressure Education Program. *The seventh report of the Joint National Committee on Prevention, Detection, Evaluation, and Treatment of High Blood Pressure, NIH Publication No. 04-5230.* Bethesda, Md: National Institutes of Health; 2004.

that are encouraged include the following: (1) weight loss, if indicated; (2) increased fruit, vegetable, and low-fat dairy consumption; (3) reduced salt and increased potassium and calcium intake; (4) reduced total fat, saturated fat, and cholesterol intake; (5) moderation of alcohol use; (6) regular aerobic physical fitness; and (7) quitting smoking, if indicated.[22] Such lifestyle changes are able to reduce the risk of chronic disease and improve the blood pressure (Table 19-5).[23-25]

Stage 1 Hypertension. In addition to the diet therapy for prehypertension, drugs are used according to need and usually include a diuretic. The continuous use of some—although not all—diuretic drugs causes a loss of potassium along with the increased loss of water from the body. Because potassium is necessary for maintaining normal heart muscle action, depletion could become dangerous. Potassium replacement is sometimes necessary. Dietary replacement with the increased use of potassium-rich foods (e.g., fruits, especially bananas and orange juice; vegetables; legumes; nuts; whole grains) is an important part of therapy. The sodium and potassium values of various foods can be found on Evolve.

Stage 2 Hypertension. In addition to the diet for stage 1 hypertension, vigorous drug therapy is necessary for stage 2 hypertension. See the Drug-Nutrient Interaction box entitled "Grapefruit Juice and Drug Metabolism" for more information about potential interactions with the medications that are often used for hypertension.

Nutrition therapy is important for all types of hypertension, along with other nondrug therapies such as physical activity and stress reduction.

Principles of Medical Nutrition Therapy

Weight Management. In accordance with individual need, weight management requires losing excess weight and maintaining a healthy weight for one's height. A sound approach to managing weight loss is discussed in Chapter 15, and guidance for increasing physical activity is given in Chapter 16. Because excess weight is closely associated with hypertension risk factors, a wisely planned personal program of weight reduction and physical activity is a cornerstone of therapy.

Sodium Control. About half of the American population with hypertension is salt sensitive, which means that their blood pressure is significantly affected by dietary sodium intake. Substantial evidence exists to support a direct correlation with decreasing sodium intake and decreasing blood pressure, even in patients with resistant hypertension.[26,27] However, achieving a palatable diet with sodium restrictions set at less than

resistant hypertension the presence of high blood pressure despite treatment with three antihypertensive medications

DRUG-NUTRIENT INTERACTION

GRAPEFRUIT JUICE AND DRUG METABOLISM

A common pathway for drug metabolism makes use of the enzyme CYP3A. This enzyme oxidizes lipid-soluble drugs, thereby making them more water soluble in preparation for urinary excretion. As more of the drug is oxidized, less is absorbed. This system is anticipated when standard dosages of drugs are determined. It is expected that only a percentage of the therapeutic agent will actually reach the circulation.

Compounds in grapefruit juice known as *furanocoumarins* inhibit CYP3A, thereby increasing the amount of the associated drug that enters the circulation. As little as 8 oz of grapefruit juice can increase the absorption of certain drugs

for up to 72 hours after consumption. The increased absorption of these medications may cause adverse events and can, in some cases, be fatal.[1] Patients essentially experience drug toxicity from their prescribed dose as a result of the drastic increase in absorption of the active ingredient.

Several cardiovascular drugs make use of the CYP3A pathway for metabolism. The table below shows some of the cardiovascular agents that are influenced by grapefruit's inhibition of CYP3A and their side effects. Hospitals and inpatient facilities do not serve grapefruit juice, and patients who are taking drugs that use the CYP3A pathway for metabolism should avoid drinking it at home.

DRUG NAME	DRUG CLASS	DRUG ACTION	SIDE EFFECTS	ADDITIONAL COMMENTS
Amiodarone (Cordarone)	Antiarrhythmic	Broad-spectrum antiarrhythmic, vasodilator	Anorexia, nausea, vomiting, constipation	High levels may cause fatal pulmonary toxicity
Amlodipine (Norvasc) Nifedipine (Procardia) Nisoldipine	Calcium channel blockers	Antihypertensive	Nausea, dyspepsia, constipation, peripheral edema, muscle cramps, flushing	Alternative calcium channel blockers (e.g., Verapamil) are available that do not interact with grapefruit juice
Atorvastatin (Lipitor) Lovastatin (Mevacor) Simvastatin (Zocor)	3-hydroxy-3methylglutaryl coenzyme A inhibitors/statins	Antihyperlipidemic	Nausea, dyspepsia, abdominal pain, constipation, diarrhea, possible myopathy	Alternative medications in this class are available that do not have significant interactions with grapefruit juice (e.g., fluvastatin, pravastatin, rosuvastatin)

Kelli Boi

1. Seden K, Dickinson L, Khoo S, Back D. Grapefruit-drug interactions. *Drugs*. 2010;70(18):2373-2407.

---

2 g/day may be difficult for some patients with the current food supply, which is rich in processed foods. A dietary restriction of sodium of between 1500 mg/day and 2400 mg/day is advised.[15] Keep in mind that 2.4 g of sodium is equivalent to approximately 6 g of sodium chloride (i.e., table salt). See Box 19-3 for ideas on ways to limit sodium intake.

Other Nutrients. In addition to sodium control, other nutrients have been discussed in relation to hypertension. Evidence suggests that the increased intake of the minerals calcium, potassium, and magnesium is beneficial for everyone, especially those with hypertension. The *Dietary Guidelines for Americans* and the American Heart Association encourage a diet that includes a wide variety of fruits, vegetables, and low-fat dairy products to ensure the adequate intake of these nutrients. Other nutrients that appear to have a link with blood pressure are vitamin D, polyunsaturated fatty acids, protein, and fiber intake.

However, studies are controversial with regard to the efficacy of these recommendations and their results on lowering blood pressure.[28-30]

The DASH Diet. The DASH diet is the result of the successful Dietary Approaches to Stop Hypertension landmark study, which was able to lower blood pressure significantly by diet alone within a 2-week period.[31] The diet recommends eating four to six servings of fruits, four to six servings of vegetables, and two to three servings of low-fat dairy foods per day in addition to lean meats and high-fiber grains. Studies have found that individuals who follow the diet have an average decrease in systolic blood pressure of 6 to 11 mm Hg.[31] When combining the DASH diet with a low-sodium diet, the blood–pressure-lowering effects are even greater.[32] Combining the DASH diet with exercise and weight loss also produces a significant reduction in total and LDL cholesterol, a reduced risk for coronary heart disease and heart failure, and improvements in insulin sensitivity.[33-36] Giving patients dietary supplements of potassium, magnesium, and fiber to match the amount provided by the DASH diet does not produce the same blood–pressure-lowering as actually following the diet and getting those nutrients through food.[37]

The DASH diet is recommended for individuals with high blood pressure, blood pressure in the prehypertension range, and a family history of high blood pressure; it is also recommended for those who are trying to eliminate the use of blood–pressure-lowering medications. The first step in following the DASH diet is to determine the appropriate energy level (in kilocalories) on the basis of the desired weight and activity level (see Chapter 6). The appropriate number of servings per day of each food group should then be based on the total energy need. Table 19-6 outlines the DASH diet and its associated serving sizes; Box 19-4 provides a 1-day sample menu that is based on a 2000-calorie diet.

Additional Lifestyle Factors

The National High Blood Pressure Education Program recommends limiting alcohol intake to 1 oz per day of ethanol for men and 0.5 oz per day of ethanol for most women and smaller men. One ounce of ethanol is equal to 24 oz of regular beer, 10 oz of wine, or 2 oz of 100-proof whiskey. Additional recommendations to prevent or treat hypertension include stopping smoking, replacing saturated fats with polyunsaturated fats (e.g., eicosapentaenoic acid, docosahexaenoic acid), and increasing aerobic physical activity to a minimum of 30 to 45 minutes per day on most days of the week.[22,38]

EDUCATION AND PREVENTION

Practical Food Guides

Food Planning and Purchasing

The *Dietary Guidelines for Americans, 2010* (see Chapter 1), provides a basic outline to guide sound food habits.[39] The food exchange list, which is described in Chapter 20, demonstrates the food groups and includes the fat and sodium modifications discussed in this chapter. These lists also provide a guide for controlling energy intake to help with weight-management planning.

An important part of purchasing food is carefully reading labels. The Nutrition Facts labels provide basic nutrition information in a standard format that is easily recognized and clearly expressed (see Chapter 13). All food products that make health claims must follow the strict guidelines provided by the U.S. Food and Drug Administration. A good general guide is to primarily use fresh, whole foods, with an informed selection of

---

BOX 19-4 SAMPLE 1-DAY MENU ON THE DASH DIET, 2000 CALORIES

Breakfast
- ¾ cup bran flakes cereal
- 1 medium banana
- 1 cup low-fat milk
- 1 slice whole-wheat bread
- 1 tsp unsalted soft (tub) margarine
- 1 cup orange juice

Lunch
- ¾ cup chicken salad
- 2 slices whole-wheat bread
- 1 Tbsp Dijon mustard
- Salad with the following:
  - ½ cup fresh cucumber slices
  - ½ cup tomato wedges
  - 1 Tbsp sunflower seeds
  - 1 tsp Italian dressing, low calorie
- ½ cup fruit cocktail, juice packed

Dinner
- 3 oz beef, eye of round
- 2 Tbsp beef gravy, fat free
- 1 cup green beans, sautéed with ½ tsp canola oil
- 1 small baked potato with the following:
  - 1 Tbsp sour cream, fat free
  - 1 Tbsp grated natural cheddar cheese, reduced fat
  - 1 Tbsp chopped scallions
- 1 small whole-wheat roll
- 1 tsp unsalted soft (tub) margarine
- 1 small apple
- 1 cup low-fat milk

Snacks
- ⅓ cup almonds, unsalted
- ¼ cup raisins
- ½ cup fruit yogurt, fat free, no sugar added

Modified from the National Institutes of Health; National Heart, Lung, and Blood Institute. *Your guide to lowering your blood pressure with DASH, NIH Publication No. 06-4082,* Washington, DC: U.S. Department of Health and Human Services; 2006.

---

processed foods used as necessary. Refer to Chapter 13 for background material regarding food supply and health.

Food Preparation

The public is more aware than ever before of the need to prepare foods with less fat and salt. Consequently, the cookbook industry has responded by providing an abundance of guides and recipes for various age groups and customs. Many seasonings (e.g., herbs, spices, lemon, wine, onion, garlic, nonfat milk and yogurt, fat-free/low-sodium broth) can help to train taste preferences for less

TABLE 19-6 THE DASH EATING PLAN

CALORIES PER DAY	SERVINGS PER DAY (UNLESS OTHERWISE SPECIFIED)							
	Grains*	Vegetables	Fruits	Fat-free or Low-Fat Milk and Milk Products	Lean Meats, Poultry, and Fish	Nuts, Seeds, and Legumes	Fats and Oils†	Sweets and added Sugars
1600	6	3 to 4	4	2 to 3	3 to 6	3 per week	2	0
2000	6 to 8	4 to 5	4 to 5	2 to 3	6	4 to 5 per week	2 to 3	≤ 5 per week
2600	10 to 11	5 to 6	5 to 6	3	6	1	3	≤ 2
3100	12 to 13	6	6	3 to 4	6 to 9	1	4	≤ 2
Serving sizes	1 slice bread; 1 oz dry cereal‡; ½ cup cooked rice, pasta, or cereal	1 cup raw leafy vegetables, ½ cup cut-up raw or cooked vegetables, ½ cup vegetable juice	1 medium fruit; ¼ cup dried fruit; ½ cup fresh, frozen, or canned fruit; ½ cup fruit juice	1 cup milk or yogurt, 1½ oz cheese	1 oz cooked meat, poultry, or fish; 1 egg§	⅓ cup or 1½ oz nuts, 2 Tbsp peanut butter, 2 Tbsp or ½ oz seeds, ½ cup cooked legumes (dry beans and peas)	1 tsp soft margarine, 1 tsp vegetable oil, 1 Tbsp mayonnaise, 2 Tbsp salad dressing	1 Tbsp sugar, 1 Tbsp jelly or jam, ½ cup sorbet, gelatin; 1 cup lemonade

*Whole grains are recommended for most grain servings as a good source of fiber and nutrients.
†Fat content changes the serving amount for fats and oils. For example, 1 Tbsp of regular salad dressing equals one serving, whereas 1 Tbsp of a low-fat dressing equals a half serving and 1 Tbsp of a fat-free dressing equals zero servings.
‡Serving sizes vary between ½ cup and 1¼ cups, depending on the cereal type. Check the product's Nutrition Facts label.
§Because eggs are high in cholesterol, limit egg yolk intake to no more than four per week; two egg whites have the same protein content as 1 oz of meat.
Modified from the National Institutes of Health; National Heart, Lung, and Blood Institute. *Your guide to lowering your blood pressure with DASH, NIH Publication No. 06-4082.* Washington, DC: U.S. Department of Health and Human Services; 2006.

CULTURAL CONSIDERATIONS

INFLUENCE OF ETHNICITY AND SOCIODEMOGRAPHICS ON A PERSON'S RISK FOR HEART DISEASE

Although the mortality rate from heart disease has declined since the 1960s, it is still the leading cause of death in the United States. The major conditions of heart disease, hypertension and high blood cholesterol, are more prevalent among certain ethnic and sociodemographic groups than others within the United States. Unlike weight and dietary habits, certain aspects constitute nonmodifiable risk factors for cardiovascular disease (e.g., ethnicity, gender), as shown in the graph.

Distinguishing between environmental factors and the genetics associated with a culture is important to help identify the specifics regarding the cause of disease. Only when those factors have been recognized can prevention and treatment programs be directed on an individual basis. A complex combination of such risk factors contributes to an individual's risk for death from cardiovascular disease. By acknowledging the risks associated with certain sociodemographic factors, warning signs may be detected earlier than they would be otherwise.

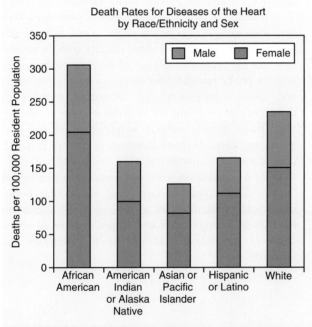

Death Rates for Diseases of the Heart by Race/Ethnicity and Sex

From the National Center for Health Statistics. *Health, United States, 2010: with special feature on death and dying.* Hyattsville, Md: U.S. Government Printing Office; 2011.

RISK FACTOR[1]	PREVALENCE OF MULTIPLE RISK FACTORS FOR HEART DISEASE AND STROKE BY SELECTED CHARACTERISTIC* (%)
Education	
Did not complete high school	52.5
High school graduate or equivalent	43.8
Some college	36.9
College graduate	25.9
Annual Household Income	
< $10,000	52.5
$10,000 to $19,999	49.3
$20,000 to $34,999	42.8
$35,000 to $49,999	37.0
≥ $50,000	28.8
Employment Status	
Unable to work	69.3
Retired	45.1
Unemployed	43.4
Homemaker	34.3
Employed	34.0
Student	31.0

*Two or more of the following: high blood pressure, high cholesterol, diabetes, obesity, current smoking, or physical inactivity.

For further reading: Moe GW, Tu J. Heart failure in the ethnic minorities. *Curr Opin Cardiol.* 2010;25(2):124-130.

1. Centers for Disease Control and Prevention. Racial/ethnic and socioeconomic disparities in multiple risk factors for heart disease and stroke–United States, 2003. *MMWR Morb Mortal Wkly Rep.* 2005;54(5):113-117.

salt and fat. Less meat in leaner and smaller portions can be combined with more complex carbohydrate foods (e.g., starches such as potatoes, pastas, rice, bulgur, and beans) to make more healthful main dishes. Whole-grain breads and cereals provide needed fiber, and an increased use of fish can add healthier forms of fat in smaller quantities. A variety of vegetables may be used (e.g., in salads or steamed and lightly seasoned), and fruits add interest, taste appeal, and nourishment to meals. The American Heart Association publishes several cookbooks that are excellent guides to newer, lighter, more tasteful, and healthier food preparation (www.americanheart.org).

Special Needs

The individual adaptation of diet principles is important in all nutrition teaching and counseling. Special attention must be given to personal desires, ethnic diets, individual situations, and food habits (see Chapter 14). Successful diet planning must meet both personal and health needs.

Education Principles

Starting Early

The prevention of hypertension and heart disease begins during childhood, especially with children from high-risk families. Preventive measures in family food habits relate to healthy weight maintenance and the limited use of foods that are high in salt, saturated fats, and trans fats. For adults with heart disease and hypertension, learning should be an integral part of all therapy. If a heart attack occurs, education should begin early during convalescence (rather than at hospital discharge) to give patients and their families clear and practical knowledge regarding positive diet and lifestyle needs.

Focusing on High-Risk Groups

Education about heart disease and hypertension should be particularly directed toward individuals and families with one or more high-risk factors (see Box 19-1). For example, hypertension has been closely associated with certain high-risk groups, including African Americans and Native Americans, people with a strong family history of the disease, and obese individuals (see the Cultural Considerations box, "Influence of Ethnicity and Sociodemographics on a Person's Risk for Heart Disease").

Using a Variety of Resources

As researchers learn more about heart disease and hypertension, the American Heart Association and other health agencies are able to provide many excellent resources. The Academy of Nutrition and Dietetics provides a Web site (www.eatright.org) for the public as well as for health professionals with helpful client education tools, several of which are applicable to heart disease. As professionals and the public have become more aware of health needs and disease prevention, an increasing number of resources and programs are available in most communities. These include various weight-management programs, registered dietitians in private practice or in health care centers who provide nutrition counseling, and practical food-preparation materials found in a number of "light cuisine" cooking classes and cookbooks. Bookstores and public libraries as well as health education libraries in health centers and clinics provide an abundance of materials that address health promotion and self-care.

SUMMARY

- Coronary heart disease is the leading cause of death in the United States. Atherosclerosis is the underlying blood vessel disease. If fatty buildup on the interior surfaces of the blood vessels becomes severe, it cuts off the supply of oxygen and nutrients to the cells, which in turn die. When this occurs in a major coronary artery, the result is an MI.
- The risk for atherosclerosis increases with the amount and type of blood lipids (fats) or lipoproteins in circulation. An elevated serum cholesterol level is a primary risk factor for the development of atherosclerosis.

- Current recommendations to help prevent coronary heart disease involve a low-fat and balanced diet, weight management, and increased physical activity.
- Dietary recommendations for acute CVD include measures to ensure cardiac rest. People with chronic heart disease that involves congestive heart failure benefit from a low-sodium diet to control pulmonary edema.
- People with hypertension may improve their condition with weight control, exercise, sodium restriction, and a diet that is rich in fruits, vegetables, whole grains, lean meats, and low-fat dairy products.

CRITICAL THINKING QUESTIONS

1. Why are fat and cholesterol the primary factors in heart disease? How are they carried in the bloodstream? Which of these lipoproteins carry so-called "good cholesterol," and which carry "bad cholesterol" (i.e., the cholesterol of concern)?
2. How can people influence the relative amounts of fat and cholesterol in the blood? Describe the food changes that are involved.
3. Identify the risk factors for heart disease. What control do people have over these risk factors?

4. Identify four dietary recommendations for a patient who has had a heart attack. Describe how each recommendation facilitates recovery.
5. Discuss the three levels of hypertension and the treatment options for each.
6. What does the term *essential hypertension* mean? Why would weight control and sodium restriction contribute to its control? What other nutrient factors may be involved in hypertension?

CHAPTER CHALLENGE QUESTIONS

True-False
Write the correct statement for each statement that is false.
1. *True or False:* In the disease process that underlies heart disease (i.e., atherosclerosis), the fatty deposits in blood vessel linings are made up mainly of cholesterol.
2. *True or False:* Hypertension occurs more frequently among Caucasians than among African Americans.
3. *True or False:* The problem of CVD could be solved if cholesterol could be removed entirely from the body.
4. *True or False:* Cholesterol is a dietary essential for adults, because people depend entirely on food sources for their supply.

5. *True or False:* Lipoproteins are the major transport form of lipids in the blood.
6. *True or False:* One of the initial clinical objectives when treating an acute heart attack is cardiac rest.
7. *True or False:* In a patient with chronic congestive heart disease, the heart eventually may fail, because its weakened muscle must work at a faster rate to pump the body's necessary blood supply.
8. *True or False:* The taste for salt is instinctive to ensure a sufficient supply.
9. *True or False:* Reduced sodium intake is an effective therapy for congestive heart failure and hypertension.

Multiple Choice
1. A low-cholesterol diet restricts which of the following foods? *(Circle all that apply.)*
   a. Fish
   b. Liver
   c. Butter
   d. Nonfat milk
2. Helpful seasonings to use as part of a sodium-restricted diet include which of the following? *(Circle all that apply.)*
   a. Lemon juice
   b. Soy sauce
   c. Herbs and spices
   d. Seasoned salt

3. Prehypertension is defined as a blood pressure of _____ (systolic)/_____ (diastolic) mm Hg.
   a. < 120; < 80
   b. 120 to 139; 80 to 89
   c. 140 to 159; 90 to 99
   d. > 160; > 100
4. Which of the following foods may be eaten freely as part of a low-sodium diet?
   a. Fruits
   b. Milk
   c. Cured meats
   d. Canned vegetables

⊖volve **Please refer to the Students' Resource section of this text's Evolve Web site for additional study resources.**

REFERENCES

1. National Center for Health Statistics. *Health, United States, 2010: with special feature on death and dying.* Hyattsville, Md: U.S. Government Printing Office; 2011.

2. Katcher HI, Hill AM, Lanford JL, et al. Lifestyle approaches and dietary strategies to lower LDL-cholesterol and triglycerides and raise HDL-cholesterol. *Endocrinol Metab Clin North Am.* 2009;38(1):45-78.
3. Marin C, Ramirez R, Delgado-Lista J, et al. Mediterranean diet reduces endothelial damage and improves the regenerative capacity of endothelium. *Am J Clin Nutr.* 2011; 93(2):267-274.
4. Jenkins DJ, Chiavaroli L, Wong JM, et al. Adding monounsaturated fatty acids to a dietary portfolio of cholesterol-

lowering foods in hypercholesterolemia. *CMAJ.* 2010; 182(18):1961-1967.

5. Skulas-Ray AC, Kris-Etherton PM, Harris WS, et al. Dose-response effects of omega-3 fatty acids on triglycerides, inflammation, and endothelial function in healthy persons with moderate hypertriglyceridemia. *Am J Clin Nutr.* 2011; 93(2):243-252.

6. Canoy D. Distribution of body fat and risk of coronary heart disease in men and women. *Curr Opin Cardiol.* 2008;23(6): 591-598.

7. Taylor AE, Ebrahim S, Ben-Shlomo Y, et al. Comparison of the associations of body mass index and measures of central adiposity and fat mass with coronary heart disease, diabetes, and all-cause mortality: a study using data from 4 UK cohorts. *Am J Clin Nutr.* 2010;91(3):547-556.

8. dos Santos RE, Aldrighi JM, Lanz JR, et al. Relationship of body fat distribution by waist circumference, dual-energy x-ray absorptiometry and ultrasonography to insulin resistance by homeostasis model assessment and lipid profile in obese and non-obese postmenopausal women. *Gynecol Endocrinol.* 2005;21(5):295-301.

9. National Cholesterol Education Program (NCEP) Expert Panel on Detection, Evaluation, and Treatment of High Blood Cholesterol in Adults (Adult Treatment Panel III). Third Report of the National Cholesterol Education Program (NCEP) Expert Panel on Detection, Evaluation, and Treatment of High Blood Cholesterol in Adults (Adult Treatment Panel III) final report. *Circulation.* 2002; 106(25):3143-3421.

10. Stone NJ, Bilek S, Rosenbaum S. Recent National Cholesterol Education Program Adult Treatment Panel III update: adjustments and options. *Am J Cardiol.* 2005;96(4A): 53E-59E.

11. ESHRE Capri Workshop Group. Hormones and cardiovascular health in women. *Hum Reprod Update.* 2006; 12(5):483-497.

12. Polotsky HN, Polotsky AJ. Metabolic implications of menopause. *Semin Reprod Med.* 2010;28(5):426-434.

13. Lavie CJ, Milani RV, Ventura HO. Obesity and cardiovascular disease: risk factor, paradox, and impact of weight loss. *J Am Coll Cardiol.* 2009;53(21):1925-1932.

14. Singh S, Somers VK, Clark MM, et al. Physician diagnosis of overweight status predicts attempted and successful weight loss in patients with cardiovascular disease and central obesity. *Am Heart J.* 2010;160(5):934-942.

15. American Dietetic Association. *ADA nutrition care manual.* Chicago: American Dietetic Association; 2010.

16. Panagiotakos DB, Dimakopoulou K, Katsouyanni K, et al; AIRGENE Study Group. Mediterranean diet and inflammatory response in myocardial infarction survivors. *Int J Epidemiol.* 2009;38(3):856-866.

17. Pérez-López FR, Chedraui P, Haya J, Cuadros JL. Effects of the Mediterranean diet on longevity and age-related morbid conditions. *Maturitas.* 2009;64(2):67-79.

18. Buckland G, González CA, Agudo A, et al. Adherence to the Mediterranean diet and risk of coronary heart disease in the Spanish EPIC Cohort Study. *Am J Epidemiol.* 2009; 170(12):1518-1529.

19. Walker C, Reamy BV. Diets for cardiovascular disease prevention: what is the evidence? *Am Fam Physician.* 2009; 79(7):571-578.

20. Food and Nutrition Board, Institute of Medicine. *Dietary reference intakes for water, potassium, sodium, chloride, and sulfate.* Washington, DC: National Academies Press; 2004.

21. U.S. Department of Agriculture, Agricultural Research Service. *Nutrient intakes from food: mean amounts consumed per individual, by gender and age. What we eat in America NHANES 2007-2008* (website): www.ars.usda.gov/ SP2UserFiles/Place/12355000/pdf/0708/Table_1_NIN_GEN_07.pdf. Accessed October 2010.

22. National Institutes of Health; National Heart, Lung, and Blood Institute; National High Blood Pressure Education Program. *The seventh report of the Joint National Committee on Prevention, Detection, Evaluation, and Treatment of High Blood Pressure.* Bethesda, Md: National Institutes of Health; 2004.

23. Dagogo-Jack S, Egbuonu N, Edeoga C. Principles and practice of nonpharmacological interventions to reduce cardiometabolic risk. *Med Princ Pract.* 2010;19(3):167-175.

24. Elmer PJ, Obarzanek E, Vollmer WM, et al; PREMIER Collaborative Research Group. Effects of comprehensive lifestyle modification on diet, weight, physical fitness, and blood pressure control: 18-month results of a randomized trial. *Ann Intern Med.* 2006;144(7):485-495.

25. Appel LJ, Champagne CM, Harsha DW, et al; Writing Group of the PREMIER Collaborative Research Group. Effects of comprehensive lifestyle modification on blood pressure control: main results of the PREMIER clinical trial. *JAMA.* 2003;289(16):2083-2093.

26. Pimenta E, Gaddam KK, Oparil S, et al. Effects of dietary sodium reduction on blood pressure in subjects with resistant hypertension: results from a randomized trial. *Hypertension.* 2009;54(3):475-481.

27. Kanbay M, Chen Y, Solak Y, Sanders PW. Mechanisms and consequences of salt sensitivity and dietary salt intake. *Curr Opin Nephrol Hypertens.* 2011;20(1):37-43.

28. Savica V, Bellinghieri G, Kopple JD. The effect of nutrition on blood pressure. *Annu Rev Nutr.* 2010;30:365-401.

29. Berry SE, Mulla UZ, Chowienczyk PJ, Sanders TA. Increased potassium intake from fruit and vegetables or supplements does not lower blood pressure or improve vascular function in UK men and women with early hypertension: a randomised controlled trial. *Br J Nutr.* 2010;104(12): 1839-1847.

30. He FJ, Marciniak M, Carney C, et al. Effects of potassium chloride and potassium bicarbonate on endothelial function, cardiovascular risk factors, and bone turnover in mild hypertensives. *Hypertension.* 2010;55(3):681-688.

31. Appel LJ, Moore TJ, Obarzanek E, et al. A clinical trial of the effects of dietary patterns on blood pressure. DASH Collaborative Research Group. *N Engl J Med.* 1997;336(16): 1117-1124.

32. Sacks FM, Svetky LP, Vollmer WM, et al. Effects on blood pressure of reduced dietary sodium and the Dietary Approaches to Stop Hypertension (DASH) diet. DASH-Sodium Collaborative Research Group. *N Engl J Med.* 2001;344(1):3-10.

33. Harsha DW, Sacks FM, Obarzanek E, et al. Effect of dietary sodium intake on blood lipids: results from the DASH-sodium trial. *Hypertension.* 2004;43(2):393-398.

34. Chen ST, Maruthur NM, Appel LJ. The effect of dietary patterns on estimated coronary heart disease risk: results

from the Dietary Approaches to Stop Hypertension (DASH) trial. *Circ Cardiovasc Qual Outcomes.* 2010;3(5):484-489.

35. Blumenthal JA, Babyak MA, Sherwood A, et al. Effects of the dietary approaches to stop hypertension diet alone and in combination with exercise and caloric restriction on insulin sensitivity and lipids. *Hypertension.* 2010;55(5): 1199-1205.

36. Levitan EB, Wolk A, Mittleman MA. Consistency with the DASH diet and incidence of heart failure. *Arch Intern Med.* 2009;169(9):851-857.

37. Al-Solaiman Y, Jesri A, Mountford WK, et al. DASH lowers blood pressure in obese hypertensives beyond potassium, magnesium and fibre. *J Hum Hypertens.* 2010;24(4): 237-246.

38. Hall WL. Dietary saturated and unsaturated fats as determinants of blood pressure and vascular function. *Nutr Res Rev.* 2009;22(1):18-38.

39. U.S. Department of Agriculture, U.S. Department of Health and Human Services. *Dietary guidelines for Americans, 2010.* Washington, DC: U.S. Government Printing Office; 2010.

FURTHER READING AND RESOURCES

American Heart Association. www.americanheart.org

National Center for Chronic Disease Prevention and Health Promotion. Heart disease prevention: what you can do. www.cdc.gov/HeartDisease/prevention.htm

National Cholesterol Education Program. www.nhlbi.nih.gov/about/ncep/

National Cholesterol Education Program. Risk assessment tool for estimating 10-year risk of developing coronary heart disease. hp2010.nhlbihin.net/atpiii/calculator. asp?usertype=prof

These organizations are valuable sources of information regarding the most current recommendations for healthy lifestyles to prevent and treat heart disease. The Web sites also provide educational materials for both health care professionals and the public.

Huang CL, Sumpio BE. Olive oil, the Mediterranean diet, and cardiovascular health. *J Am Coll Surg.* 2008;207(3):407-416.

Walker C, Reamy BV. Diets for cardiovascular disease prevention: what is the evidence? *Am Fam Physician.* 2009;79(7):571-578.

These two articles discuss the following: (1) How olive oil in the traditional Mediterranean diet helps to improve cardiovascular health; and (2) how the Mediterranean diet compares with other common diets (e.g., Atkins, Zone, South Beach) in the area of overall cardiovascular health.

CHAPTER 20

Diabetes Mellitus

KEY CONCEPTS

- Diabetes mellitus is a metabolic disorder of glucose metabolism that has many causes and forms.
- A consistent and sound diet is a major keystone of diabetes care and control.
- Daily self-care skills enable a person with diabetes to remain healthy and reduce risks for complications.

- Blood glucose monitoring is a critical practice for effective blood glucose control.
- A personalized care plan that balances food intake, exercise, and insulin regulation is essential to successful diabetes management.

The National Center for Health Statistics reported that 11% of the American adult population older than the age of 20 years has diabetes. Diabetes is currently the seventh leading cause of death in the United States.[1] Historically, diabetes mellitus claimed the lives of its victims at a young age. Greater knowledge of the disease and proper self-care practices have enabled people with diabetes to live long and fulfilling lives. However, diabetes has no cure, and individuals without health care and access to proper medication continue to die early in life. With professional guidance and support, individuals with diabetes can remain in a state of good health and reduce the risk of long-term complications by consistently practicing good self-care skills.

This chapter examines the nature of diabetes and explains why daily self-care is essential for the health of those with the condition.

THE NATURE OF DIABETES

Defining Factor

Glucose is the primary and preferred source of energy for the body. As discussed in Chapter 2, carbohydrate foods break down during digestion in the gastrointestinal tract, and they are absorbed into the bloodstream mainly as glucose. Glucose is then circulated throughout the body. For glucose to be used as energy by the cells in the body, it first has to be taken out of the blood and transported into the cells. For this process to happen in most cells, the hormone insulin must be present. Insulin is produced by the β cells of the pancreas (see the For Further Focus box, "The History and Discovery of Insulin"). Individuals with diabetes either do not produce insulin or cannot effectively use the insulin produced. Without insulin, glucose accumulates in the bloodstream. The American Diabetes Association defines diabetes as a group of metabolic diseases that are characterized by hyperglycemia that results from defects in insulin secretion, insulin action, or both.[2]

Classification of Diabetes Mellitus and Glucose Intolerance

Various types of diabetes mellitus are classified according to the pathogenic process of the disease.

FOR FURTHER FOCUS

THE HISTORY AND DISCOVERY OF INSULIN

Early History and Name
The symptoms of diabetes were first described on an Egyptian papyrus, the Ebers Papyrus, which dates to approximately 1500 BC. During the first century, the Greek physician Areatus wrote of a malady in which the body "ate its own flesh" and gave off large quantities of urine. He named it *diabetes,* from the Greek word meaning "to siphon" or "to pass through." During the seventeenth century, the word *mellitus* from the Latin word meaning "honey" was added because of the sweetness of the urine. The addition of *mellitus* distinguished the disorder from another disorder, *diabetes insipidus,* in which large urine output also was observed. However, diabetes insipidus is a much more rare and quite different disease that is caused by a lack of the pituitary antidiuretic hormone. Today, the term *diabetes* is almost always in reference to diabetes mellitus.

Diabetic Dark Ages
Throughout the Middle Ages and the dawning of the scientific era, many early scientists and physicians continued to puzzle over the mystery of diabetes, but the cause remained obscure. For physicians and their patients, these years could be called the "Diabetic Dark Ages." Patients had short life spans and were maintained on a variety of semistarvation and high-fat diets.

Discovery of Insulin
The first breakthrough came from a clue that pointed to the involvement of the pancreas in the disease process. This clue was provided by a young German medical student, Paul Langerhans (1847-1888), who found special clusters of cells scattered throughout the pancreas forming little islands of cells. Although he did not yet understand their function,

Langerhans could see that these cells were different from the rest of the tissue and assumed that they must be important. When his suspicions later proved true, these clusters of cells were named the *islets of Langerhans* for their young discoverer. In 1922, with the use of this important clue, two Canadian scientists—Frederick Banting and his assistant, Charles Best, together with two other research team members, physiologists J.B. Collip and J.J.R. Macleod—extracted the first insulin from animals. It proved to be a hormone that regulates the oxidation of blood glucose and that helps to convert it to heat and energy. They called the hormone *insulin* from the Latin word *insula,* meaning "island." Insulin did prove to be the effective agent for the treatment of diabetes. Leonard Thompson was the first child to be treated with insulin, in January 1922. He lived to adulthood, but he died at the age of 27 years—not from his diabetes but from coronary heart disease caused by the diabetic diet of the day, which obtained 70% of its total kilocalories from fat. Unsurprisingly, his autopsy showed marked atherosclerosis.

Successful Use of Diet and Insulin
The insulin discovery team was more successful on their third try with a young girl who was diagnosed with diabetes at the age of 11 years. She initially had been put on a starvation diet, and her weight fell from 75 to 45 pounds (34 to 21 kg) over a 3-year period. However, the medical research team fortunately had learned the importance of a well-balanced diet for normal growth and health. Thus, with a good diet and the new insulin therapy, this child, Elizabeth Hughes, gained weight and vigor and lived a normal life. She married, had three children, took insulin for 58 years, and died of heart failure at the age of 73 years.

Type 1 Diabetes Mellitus

Type 1 diabetes mellitus accounts for 5% to 10% of all cases of diabetes. It develops rapidly, and it tends to be more severe and unstable than other forms of diabetes. Type 1 diabetes is caused by the autoimmune destruction of the β cells in the pancreas. At least four autoantibodies have been identified as the causes of this destruction: islet cell autoantibodies, autoantibodies to insulin, autoantibodies to glutamic acid decarboxylase, and autoantibodies to the tyrosine phosphatases IA-2 and IA-2β.[2] The rate of destruction determines the onset of diabetes. The initial onset of type 1 diabetes occurs rapidly among children and adolescents (hence its former name *juvenile-onset diabetes*), but it can occur at any age. For some individuals, the rate of destruction is slower, and symptoms may not appear until adulthood. Individuals with this type of diabetes rely on exogenous insulin for

survival (hence its other former name *insulin-dependent diabetes*). At the time of diagnosis, individuals with type 1 diabetes are often underweight and at higher risk for acidosis.

Type 2 Diabetes Mellitus

Approximately 90% to 95% of individuals with diabetes have type 2 diabetes. This form has a strong genetic link, and it is more prevalent among obese individuals.[2-4] Box 20-1 lists additional risk factors for the development of type 2 diabetes. Unlike type 1 diabetes, type 2 diabetes is not caused by an autoimmune response. This form of diabetes results from an insulin resistance or insulin defect: either the body is not producing enough insulin or the insulin that it is producing cannot be used. These individuals usually do not need exogenous insulin for survival; rather, they rely on diet, exercise, and oral

CULTURAL CONSIDERATIONS

PREVALENCE OF TYPE 2 DIABETES

Type 2 diabetes was known for years as *adult-onset diabetes,* because it rarely affected anyone who was younger than 40 years old. However, this form of diabetes has rapidly become a health care concern among children and adolescents. As with the occurrence of type 2 diabetes in adults, it has been reported in all races and ethnic populations, with a disproportionate burden on minority groups. Diabetes, impaired glucose tolerance, obesity, and even cardiovascular disease are beginning to plague the children of America in a similar fashion as they do adults.

Children

In an effort to define the contributing factors responsible for the increased prevalence of type 2 diabetes in children, researchers have investigated fetal exposure to maternal diabetes and obesity and found such exposures to be strong contributing factors among diverse ethnic groups.[1] Ethnic

groups with pronounced risks are African Americans, Hispanic and Latino Americans, Native Americans, and some Asian Americans, Native Hawaiians, and other Pacific Islanders. The estimated prevalence of type 2 diabetes in children younger than 20 years old is 24.3 cases per 100,000 youth,[2] of which 10.4% were overweight and 79% were obese at the time of study.[3]

Adults

The Centers for Disease Control and Prevention reported the number of people diagnosed with diabetes from 2007 to 2009 who were 20 years old or older to have the following prevalence by race and ethnicity[4]:

- 7.1% of non-Hispanic whites
- 8.4% of Asian Americans
- 11.8% of Hispanics
- 12.6% of non-Hispanic blacks

1. Dabelea D, Mayer-Davis EJ, Lamichhane AP, et al. Association of intrauterine exposure to maternal diabetes and obesity with type 2 diabetes in youth: the SEARCH Case-Control Study. *Diabetes Care.* 2008;31(7):1422-1426.
2. Writing Group for the SEARCH for Diabetes in Youth Study Group; Dabelea D, Bell RA, D'Agostino Jr RB, et al. Incidence of diabetes in youth in the United States. *JAMA.* 2007;297(24):2716-2724.
3. Liu LL, Lawrence JM, Davis C, et al. Prevalence of overweight and obesity in youth with diabetes in USA: the SEARCH for Diabetes in Youth study. *Pediatr Diabetes.* 2010;11(1):4-11.
4. Centers for Disease Control and Prevention. *National diabetes fact sheet: national estimates and general information on diabetes and prediabetes in the United States, 2011.* Atlanta: U.S. Department of Health and Human Services, Centers for Disease Control and Prevention; 2011.

BOX 20-1	RISK FACTORS FOR TYPE 2 DIABETES MELLITUS

- A family history of diabetes
- Age of 45 years or more
- Overweight (i.e., a body mass index of 25 kg/m² or more)
- Not physically active on a regular basis
- Race/ethnicity (non-Hispanic African American, Hispanic American, Native American, Alaska Native, Asian American, and Pacific Islander)
- Women with a history of gestational diabetes or who have delivered an infant who weighed more than 9 pounds
- Previously identified as having impaired glucose tolerance
- Low high-density lipoprotein cholesterol level or high triglyceride level; high blood pressure

youth between the ages of 10 and 14 years and 11.8 cases per 100,000 youth between the ages of 15 and 19 years).[5] The Cultural Considerations box entitled "Prevalence of Type 2 Diabetes" discusses this issue in more depth. Many adults and children with type 2 diabetes can improve or reduce their symptoms with weight loss and thus require only diet therapy and balanced exercise programs.

Table 20-1 summarizes the differences between type 1 and type 2 diabetes mellitus.

Gestational Diabetes

Gestational diabetes mellitus (GDM) is a temporary form of diabetes that occurs during pregnancy, with normal blood glucose control usually recovered after delivery. Women who have type 1 or type 2 diabetes before conception do not fall into this category during pregnancy. GDM

---

insulin a hormone that is produced by the pancreas, attaches to insulin receptors on cell membranes, and allows the absorption of glucose into the cell.

hyperglycemia an elevated blood glucose level.

exogenous originating from outside the body.

medications for disease management. This form of diabetes, which was previously called *adult-onset diabetes* or *non–insulin-dependent diabetes,* has an onset primarily in adults who are older than 40 years old. However, as children get heavier, the prevalence of type 2 diabetes among young people is on the rise (i.e., 8.1 cases per 100,000

TABLE 20-1   **DIFFERENTIATING TYPE 1 AND TYPE 2 DIABETES MELLITUS**

Factor	Type 1	Type 2
Ethnicity	Increased rates among persons with Northern European heritage	Increased rates among persons with heritages from equatorial countries; the highest rates are found in those with Native American, Hispanic, African-American, Asian, Pacific Islander, and Mediterranean heritages
Age of onset	Generally younger than 30 years of age, with the peak onset before puberty	Generally older than 40 years of age, although genetic predisposition and obesity may cause onset to occur at younger ages
Weight	Usually normal or underweight; unintentional weight loss often precedes diagnosis	Usually overweight, but may be of normal weight
Treatment	Insulin injections are necessary for life; food and exercise must be balanced with insulin	Weight loss is usually the first goal; a reduction in sugar and fat and an increase in soluble fiber are helpful; oral hypoglycemic agents, insulin, or both may be necessary for good blood glucose management, but they are not necessary to prevent imminent death; exercise is important
β-cell functioning	Totally absent (i.e., no insulin is produced) after the "honeymoon period"; residual insulin is produced for approximately 1 year after diagnosis	Excess insulin production is usually evident (i.e., hyperinsulinemia), but insulin resistance occurs at the cellular level; insulin production may also be normal or below normal

Modified from Peckenpaugh NJ. *Nutrition essentials and diet therapy.* 10th ed. Philadelphia: Saunders; 2007.

BOX 20-2   **SCREENING FOR AND DIAGNOSIS OF GESTATIONAL DIABETES MELLITUS**

- Perform a 75-g oral glucose tolerance test with a plasma glucose measurement at baseline (fasting) and at 1 and 2 hours at 24 to 28 weeks' gestation in women who were not previously diagnosed with overt diabetes.
- The oral glucose tolerance test should be performed in the morning after an overnight fast of at least 8 hours.
- The diagnosis of gestational diabetes mellitus is made if any of the following plasma glucose values are exceeded:
  - Fasting: 92 mg/dL (5.1 mmol/L)
  - 1 hour: 180 mg/dL (10.0 mmol/L)
  - 2 hour: 153 mg/dL (8.5 mmol/L)

From American Diabetes Association. Diagnosis and classification of diabetes mellitus. *Diabetes Care.* 2011;34(Suppl 1):S62-S69.

can present complications for both the mother and the infant if it is not carefully monitored and controlled. Persistent hyperglycemia is associated with an increased risk of intrauterine fetal death and macrosomia.

GDM develops in approximately 7% of all pregnant women.[2] Risk factors for GDM are the same as for type 2 diabetes (see Box 20-1). Pregnant women who are at high risk for developing GDM should be screened with a fasting plasma glucose and glycosylated hemoglobin A1c test during the first prenatal visit. All women who are not

otherwise known to have diabetes should be screened with a glucose tolerance test between 24 and 28 weeks' gestation.[2,6] The screening protocol for GDM is provided in Box 20-2.[2]

Women with GDM have their blood glucose levels carefully monitored and are taught to follow a tightly managed program of diet and to self-test blood glucose, blood pressure, and urinary protein. For women who are unable to maintain blood glucose levels within an acceptable range (i.e., 92 mg/dL or less fasting, 180 mg/dL or less 1 hour postprandial, or 153 mg/dL or less 2 hours postprandial), insulin therapy is recommended. Oral hypoglycemic agents were not used for GDM in the past for fear of teratogenic effects. However, recent research indicates that selective oral hypoglycemic agents are as appropriate for use in this population as exogenous insulin.[7,8]

Complications of GDM for mother and baby are greatly reduced (if not eliminated) by the tight control of blood glucose levels. Women with GDM are also advised to maintain a balanced diet, a regular exercise schedule, and a healthy body mass index and to attend all follow-up visits with their physicians. Women with GDM have a 41.5% chance of having subsequent pregnancies that are

macrosomia excessive fetal growth that results in an abnormally large infant; this condition carries a high risk for perinatal death.

complicated by diabetes, and the risk for developing type 2 diabetes later in life is significantly higher among women with a history of GDM.[9]

Other Types of Diabetes

Secondary diabetes may be caused by a number of conditions or agents that affect the pancreas, including the following:

- *Genetic defects:* Defects in the β cells or insulin action may result in several forms of diabetes. These forms are not characteristic of the autoimmune destruction found in patients with type 1 diabetes. Mutations on at least six genetic loci have been identified, and these result in impaired insulin secretion (although not the action of the insulin). Other less common defects in the action of the insulin (but not in the amount secreted) also result in hyperglycemia and diabetes. Two such syndromes that have been identified in the pediatric population are leprechaunism and Rabson-Mendenhall syndrome.[2]
- *Pancreatic conditions or diseases:* Any condition that causes damage to the pancreatic cells can result in diabetes. Such conditions include tumors that affect the islet cells; acute viral infection by a number of agents, such as the mumps virus; acute pancreatitis from biliary disease and gallstones; chronic pancreatic insufficiency, such as that which occurs with cystic fibrosis; pancreatic surgery; and severe traumatic abdominal injury. One of the most common causes of chronic pancreatitis is alcohol abuse. Approximately one third to one half of patients with acute pancreatitis develop disorders such as diabetes and steatorrhea.[10]
- *Endocrinopathies:* Insulin works in conjunction with several other hormones in the body. Hormones such as growth hormone, cortisol, glucagon, and epinephrine are all antagonistic to the functions of insulin. Therefore, for patients with disorders in which excessive amounts of antagonistic hormones are produced, the action of insulin is hindered, and hyperglycemia ensues. Cushing's syndrome, glucagonoma, pheochromocytoma, hyperthyroidism, and aldosteronoma are examples of endocrinopathies that ultimately cause symptoms of diabetes. When the primary disorder (i.e., excessive antagonistic hormone secretion) is removed, the resulting hyperglycemia is usually resolved.
- *Drug- or chemical-induced diabetes:* Certain drugs and toxins can impair insulin secretion or insulin action. The following drugs and toxins have been linked to impaired glucose tolerance (IGT) and diabetes: Vacor (rat poison), pentamidine, nicotinic acid, glucocorticoids, thyroid hormone, thiazides, diazoxide, phenytoin (Dilantin), β-adrenergic agonist, and α-interferon.[2]

Impaired Glucose Tolerance

Individuals whose fasting blood glucose is higher than normal (i.e., 110 mg/dL or more) but less than the level for the clinical diagnosis of diabetes (i.e., 126 mg/dL or more) are given the IGT classification, which is also referred to as *prediabetes.* IGT is a risk factor for the development of type 2 diabetes. Treatment guidelines follow those that are designed for patients with type 2 diabetes, and they can help to prevent or prolong the progression into full-blown diabetes. Individuals with IGT often have a complicated assortment of underlying conditions (e.g., dyslipidemia, obesity, hypertension) that build on one another to create the condition known as *metabolic syndrome.* The prevalence of cardiovascular disease (CVD) with the diagnosis of type 2 diabetes in patients with metabolic syndrome is approximately 20.1%, and metabolic syndrome is thought to be an independent risk factor for CVD and mortality.[11-13] See Table 19-2 for the diagnostic criteria for metabolic syndrome.

Symptoms of Diabetes

Initial Signs

Early signs of diabetes include three primary symptoms: (1) increased thirst (polydipsia); (2) increased urination (polyuria); and (3) increased hunger (polyphagia). Unintentional weight loss occurs with type 1 diabetes. Additional signs include blurred vision, dehydration, skin irritation or infection, and general weakness and loss of

---

Cushing's syndrome the excess secretion of glucocorticoids from the adrenal cortex; symptoms and complications include protein loss, obesity, fatigue, osteoporosis, edema, excess hair growth, diabetes, and skin discoloration.

pheochromocytoma a tumor of the adrenal medulla or the sympathetic nervous system in which the affected cells secrete excess epinephrine or norepinephrine and cause headache, hypertension, and nausea.

aldosteronoma the excess secretion of aldosterone from the adrenal cortex; symptoms and complications include sodium retention, potassium wasting, alkalosis, weakness, paralysis, polyuria, polydipsia, hypertension, and cardiac arrhythmias.

strength. Older adults also may demonstrate poor wound healing.

Laboratory Test Results

Various laboratory tests show glucosuria (i.e., glucose in the urine), hyperglycemia (i.e., elevated blood glucose), and abnormal glucose tolerance tests. Although the urinary excretion of glucose is correlated with increasing levels of blood glucose, it is not as sensitive in patients with type 2 diabetes.[14] Glycosylated hemoglobin A1c, which is usually abbreviated as *HbA1c* or *A1C,* represents blood glucose levels over a 3-month period. HbA1c levels of 6.5% or more are indicative of diabetes mellitus.[2]

Progressive Results

If the disease is left uncontrolled, chronic hyperglycemia causes progressive deterioration. These results may include water and electrolyte imbalance, ketoacidosis, and coma.

THE METABOLIC PATTERN OF DIABETES

Energy Supply and Control of Blood Glucose

Energy Supply

Diabetes has been called a disease of carbohydrate metabolism, but it is a general metabolic disorder that involves all three of the energy-yielding nutrients: carbohydrate, fat, and protein. Diabetes is especially related to the metabolism of the two main fuels, carbohydrate and fat, in the body's overall energy system. The three basic stages of normal glucose metabolism are as follows:

1. Initial interchange with glycogen (glycogenolysis) and reduction to a smaller central compound (glycolysis pathway)
2. Joining with the other two energy-yielding nutrients, fat and protein (pyruvate link)
3. Final common energy production (citric acid cycle and electron transport chain)

Blood Glucose Control

The control of blood glucose within its normal range of 70 to 110 mg/dL is important for general health. Normal control mechanisms ensure sufficient circulating blood glucose to meet the constant energy needs (even the basal metabolic energy needs during sleep), because glucose is the body's preferred fuel. Figure 20-1 shows the balanced sources and uses of blood glucose.

Sources of Blood Glucose. To ensure a constant supply of the body's main fuel, the following two sources provide the body with glucose:
- *Dietary intake:* the energy-yielding nutrients in food (i.e., dietary carbohydrates and the carbon backbones of fat and protein, as needed)
- *Glycogen:* the backup source from the constant turnover of stored glycogen in the liver and muscles (i.e., glycogenolysis)

Uses of Blood Glucose. The body uses glucose as needed in the following actions:
- Burning it during cell oxidation for immediate energy needs (i.e., glycolysis)
- Changing it to glycogen (i.e., glycogenesis), which is briefly stored in the muscles and liver and then withdrawn and changed back to glucose for short-term energy needs
- Converting it to fat, which is stored for longer periods in adipose tissue (i.e., lipogenesis)

Figure 20-2 summarizes the pathways that are involved in glucose metabolism.

Pancreatic Hormonal Control

The specialized cells of the islets of Langerhans in the pancreas provide three hormones that work together to regulate blood glucose levels: insulin, glucagon, and somatostatin. Insulin is produced in the β cells of the islets, which fill its central zone and make up about 60% of each islet gland. The specific arrangement of human islet cells is illustrated in Figure 20-3.

Insulin. Insulin is the major hormone that controls the level of blood glucose. It accomplishes this through the following metabolic actions:
- Helping to transport circulating glucose into cells by binding to insulin receptors and activating glucose transporters
- Stimulating glycogenesis
- Stimulating lipogenesis
- Inhibiting the breakdown of tissue fat (lipolysis) and protein degradation
- Promoting the uptake of amino acids by skeletal muscles, thereby increasing tissue protein synthesis

---

ketoacidosis the excess production of ketones; a form of metabolic acidosis that occurs with uncontrolled diabetes or starvation from burning body fat for energy fuel; a continuing uncontrolled state can result in coma and death.

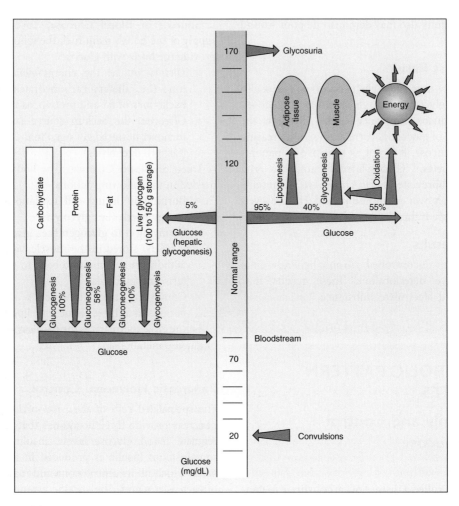

Figure 20-1 Sources of blood glucose (e.g., food, stored glycogen) and normal routes of control.

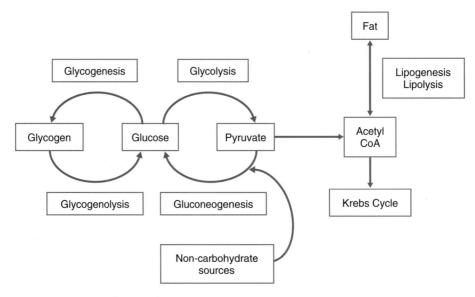

Figure 20-2 Glucose metabolism.

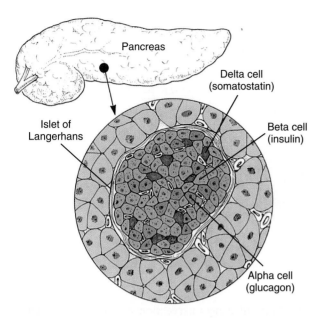

Figure 20-3 The islets of Langerhans, which are located in the pancreas.

- Influencing the burning of glucose for constant energy as needed

Glucagon. Glucagon is a hormone that acts in an opposite manner of insulin to balance the overall blood glucose control. It can rapidly break down stored glycogen (i.e., glycogenolysis). This action raises blood glucose concentrations as needed to protect the brain and other tissues during sleep or fasting. Glucagon is produced in the α cells of the pancreatic islets, which are arranged around the outer rim of each of these glands and make up about 30% of the gland's total cell mass.

Somatostatin. Somatostatin is the pancreatic hormone that acts as a referee for several other hormones that affect blood glucose levels. Somatostatin is produced in the δ cells of the pancreatic islets, which are scattered between the α and β cells and make up approximately 10% of each islet's cells. Somatostatin inhibits the secretion of insulin, glucagon, and other gastrointestinal hormones (e.g., gastrin, cholecystokinin). Because it has more generalized functions in the regulation of circulating blood glucose, somatostatin also is produced in other parts of the body (e.g., the hypothalamus).

Abnormal Metabolism in Uncontrolled Diabetes

When insulin activity is insufficient, such as it is in a patient with uncontrolled diabetes, the normal controls for blood glucose levels do not function properly. As a result, abnormal metabolic changes and imbalances occur among the three macronutrients.

Glucose

In the presence of hyperglycemia, glucose is absorbed into the pancreatic cells (no insulin is needed for transport in the pancreas) and triggers the secretion of insulin into the bloodstream. Insulin is then circulated throughout the blood, and it attaches to insulin receptor sites on cell membranes throughout the body. Once bound, a signaling cascade begins that phosphorylates GLUT4 vesicles (within the cell) and results in the migration of GLUT4 vesicles to the cell membrane. Ultimately, GLUT4 transporters allow for the uptake of glucose into the cell (Figure 20-4). If this process cannot happen, cells are essentially starved for glucose.

Fat

In the absence of functioning insulin, fat tissue formation (lipogenesis) decreases, and fat tissue breakdown (lipolysis) increases. However, normal lipolysis requires an adequate supply of glucose, which in turn relies on the help of insulin to accept glucose into the cell. Therefore, intermediate products of fat breakdown, called *ketones*, accumulate in the body. Ketones are acids, and their excess accumulation leads to diabetic ketoacidosis. The appearance of the ketone *acetone* in the urine is one indicator of poor glucose control as well as of the adverse development of ketoacidosis.

---

glucagon a hormone secreted by the α cells of the pancreatic islets of Langerhans in response to hypoglycemia; it has an effect opposite to that of insulin in that it raises the blood glucose concentration and thus is used as a quick-acting antidote for a low blood glucose reaction; it also counteracts the overnight fast during sleep by breaking down liver glycogen to keep blood glucose levels normal and to maintain an adequate energy supply for normal nerve and brain function.

GLUT4 an insulin-regulated protein that is responsible for glucose transport into cells.

ketones the chemical name for a class of organic compounds that includes three keto acid bases that occur as intermediate products of fat metabolism.

acetone a major ketone compound that results from fat breakdown for energy in individuals with uncontrolled diabetes; persons with diabetes periodically take urinary acetone tests to monitor the status of their diabetes control.

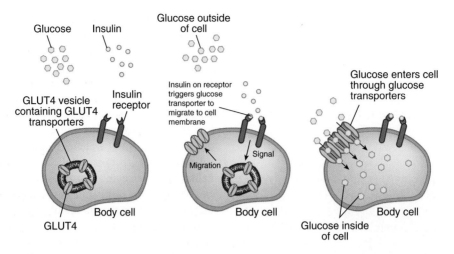

Figure 20-4 Insulin allows glucose to enter the cell through the glucose channel.

Protein

Protein tissues are also broken down in the body's effort to secure energy sources, thereby causing weight loss, muscle weakness, and urinary nitrogen loss.

Long-Term Complications

The long-term complications associated with diabetes result from continuous hyperglycemia. These health problems mainly relate to microvascular and macrovascular dysfunction in the vital organs. Individuals with good blood glucose control can avoid many such complications.

Retinopathy

Retinopathy involves small hemorrhages from broken arteries in the retina that involve yellow, waxy discharge or retinal detachment. Diabetic retinopathy is the leading cause of new cases of blindness in adults between the ages of 20 and 74 years. The risk for retinopathy significantly increases with incessant hyperglycemia (i.e., a fasting blood glucose of 120 mg/dL or more). Retinopathy has few warning signs; however, 28.5% of people with diabetes who are older than 40 years old have diabetic retinopathy.[15] Some treatment modalities (e.g., laser photocoagulation therapy) can prevent or at least delay the onset of this condition; thus, ongoing eye evaluations are an important part of the care plan. The American Diabetes Association recommends that individuals with type 1 diabetes go for a first-time eye examination within 5 years after diagnosis and that those with type 2 diabetes have their first eye examination shortly after diagnosis. Examinations with dilation should continue annually from that point forward.[16] The strict control of the blood glucose

level and intensive intervention can reduce retinopathy progression and decrease the development of severe diabetic retinopathy.[17]

Retinopathy should not be confused with the blurry vision that sometimes occurs as one of the first signs of diabetes. Blurry vision is caused by the increased glucose concentration in the fluids of the eye, which bring about brief changes in the curved, light-refracting surface of the eye.

Nephropathy

Diabetes is the leading cause of end-stage renal disease in the United States, and it accounts for 44% of all new kidney failure cases.[15] As with retinopathy, nephropathy is exacerbated by poor blood glucose control. The primary symptom is microalbuminuria. Nephropathy and end-stage renal disease cannot be cured, but, with better blood glucose control and antihypertensive therapy, disease progression can be slowed.[17] Recommendations for screening are the same as for retinopathy: within 5 years of diagnosis for type 1 and at diagnosis for type 2, with annual follow-up.[16]

Neuropathy

Current estimates are that 60% to 70% of people with diabetes have mild to severe forms of nervous system damage.[15] Changes in the nerves involve injury and disease in the peripheral nervous system, especially in the legs and feet, that cause prickly sensations, increasing

microalbuminuria low but abnormal levels of albumin in the urine.

pain, and the eventual loss of sensation from damaged nerves. The loss of nerve reaction can lead to further tissue damage and infection from unfelt foot injuries such as bruises, burns, and deeper cellulitis. Amputations and foot ulcerations are the most common results of severe neuropathy. The risk for such complications is increased for individuals who have had diabetes for more than 10 years; those who are male; those who have poor glucose control; and those who have concurrent complications such as cardiovascular, retinal, or renal disease.[18] Diabetic neuropathy is also linked to chronic problems such as motor deficits, cardiac ischemia, hypotension, gastroparesis, bladder dysfunction, and sexual dysfunction. As with other microvascular complications, annual screening is recommended.

Heart Disease

CVD is the major cause of death for people with diabetes, and it occurs two to four times more frequently in this population compared with the general population.[15] The standards of medical care for individuals with diabetes include recommendations for the prevention and management of CVD that are specifically aimed at blood lipid levels, blood pressure, aspirin use, and smoking cessation.[16] Glycemic control is not as strongly related to dyslipidemia and hypertension as it is to other long-term microvascular complications of diabetes (i.e., retinopathy, nephropathy, and neuropathy). However, the comorbid conditions of hyperglycemia and dyslipidemia greatly increase the risk of CVD; thus, evaluation and treatment must be part of the overall health care plan for individuals with diabetes.

Dyslipidemia. Elevated triglyceride levels and decreased high-density lipoprotein (HDL) cholesterol levels are characteristic of dyslipidemia in patients with type 2 diabetes. The management of dyslipidemia is prioritized as follows: (1) lifestyle modifications that focus on the reduction of saturated fats, trans fats, and cholesterol intake; weight loss, if indicated; and increased physical activity; (2) lowering low-density lipoprotein cholesterol levels; (3) raising HDL cholesterol levels; and (4) lowering triglyceride levels. Intensive glycemic control reduces the development of coronary artery calcification, which is an index of atherosclerosis, especially among patients with high triglyceride levels and poor glucose control.[19] Recommendations for lipid profiles for adults with diabetes are as follows[16]:

- *Low-density lipoprotein cholesterol:* less than 100 mg/dL; if the patient has advanced CVD, reduce the low-density cholesterol level to less than 70 mg/dL

- *HDL cholesterol:* more than 40 mg/dL for men and more than 50 mg/dL for women
- *Triglycerides:* less than 150 mg/dL

Hypertension. Hypertension affects the majority of adults with diabetes, and it is a major risk factor for microvascular complications. CVD mortality is doubled for people with both diabetes and hypertension, thereby making blood pressure evaluation and treatment an important part of the health care plan. The recommendation for blood pressure in adults with diabetes is less than 130/80 mm Hg. To achieve such a level of blood pressure, patients are encouraged to adopt lifestyle modifications such as reducing sodium intake; losing weight (if indicated); increasing the consumption of fruits, vegetables, and low-fat dairy products (i.e., following the DASH diet; see Chapter 19); moderating alcohol intake; and increasing physical activity levels.[16]

GENERAL MANAGEMENT OF DIABETES

Early Detection and Monitoring

The guiding principles for the treatment of diabetes are early detection and the prevention of complications. Community screening programs and annual physical examinations help to identify people with elevated blood glucose levels who may benefit from a glucose tolerance test (e.g., fasting and 2-hour tests with a measured glucose dose) and medical evaluation. An additional monitoring aid is the HbA1c assay (normal range, 4% to 6%), which provides an effective tool for evaluating the long-term management of diabetes and the degree of control. Because glucose attaches itself to the hemoglobin molecule over the life of the red blood cell, this test reflects the average level of blood glucose over the preceding 3 months. Other tests such as fructosamine and C-peptide are sometimes used for diagnostic purposes. However, HbA1c is currently the most accurate assessment tool for monitoring ongoing blood glucose control and the risk for complications. Box 20-3 outlines the criteria for the diagnosis of diabetes mellitus, and Table 20-2 gives the correlation between HbA1c values and plasma glucose.

---

cellulitis the diffuse inflammation of soft or connective tissues (e.g., in the foot) from injury, bruises, or pressure sores that leads to infection; poor care may result in ulceration and abscess or gangrene.

BOX 20-3 CRITERIA FOR THE DIAGNOSIS OF DIABETES MELLITUS

- HbA1c ≥ 6.5%. The test should be performed in a laboratory using a method that is National Glycohemoglobin Standardization Program (NGSP) certified and standardized to the Diabetes Control and Complications Trial (DCCT) assay.*

  or

- Fasting plasma glucose level of at least 126 mg/dL (7.0 mmol/L)

  The term *fasting* is defined as no caloric intake for at least 8 hours.*

  or

- A 2-hour plasma glucose level of at least 200 mg/dL (11.1 mmol/L) during an oral glucose tolerance test

  The oral glucose tolerance test should be performed as described by the World Health Organization with the use of a glucose load that contains the equivalent of 75 g of anhydrous glucose dissolved in water.*

  or

- In a patient with classic symptoms of hyperglycemia or hyperglycemic crisis, a random plasma glucose level of at least 200 mg/dL (11.1 mmol/L)

*In the absence of unequivocal hyperglycemia, results should be confirmed by repeat testing.
Modified from American Diabetes Association. Standards of medical care in diabetes–2011. *Diabetes Care*. 2011;34(1 suppl):S11-S62.

TABLE 20-2 CORRELATION BETWEEN GLYCOSYLATED HEMOGLOBIN A1C AND PLASMA GLUCOSE LEVELS

HbA1c	MEAN PLASMA GLUCOSE LEVEL	
	mg/dL	mmol/L
6	126	7.0
7	154	8.6
8	183	10.2
9	212	11.8
10	240	13.4
11	269	14.9
12	298	16.5

From American Diabetes Association. Standards of medical care in diabetes–2011. *Diabetes Care*. 2011;34(1 Suppl):S11-S62.

Basic Goals of Care

General Objectives

The health care team is guided by three basic objectives when working with patients with diabetes: maintaining optimal nutrition, avoiding symptoms, and preventing complications.

TABLE 20-3 SUMMARY OF RECOMMENDATIONS FOR ADULTS WITH DIABETES

Parameter	Recommendation
Glycosylated hemoglobin A1c level	< 7.0%
Preprandial capillary plasma glucose level	70 to 130 mg/dL (3.9 to 7.2 mmol/L)
Peak postprandial capillary plasma glucose level*	< 180 mg/dL (< 10.0 mmol/L)
Blood pressure	< 130/80 mm Hg
Low-density lipoprotein level	< 100 mg/dL (< 2.6 mmol/L) for individuals without overt cardiovascular disease
	< 70 mg/dL (< 1.8 mmol/L) for individuals with overt cardiovascular disease
Triglyceride level	< 150 mg/dL (< 1.7 mmol/L)
High-density lipoprotein level	> 40 mg/dL (> 1.0 mmol/L) for men
	> 50 mg/dL (> 1.3 mmol/L) for women

- Goals should be individualized on the basis of the following:
  - Duration of diabetes
  - Patient's age and life expectancy
  - Comorbid conditions
  - Known cardiovascular disease or advanced microvascular complications
  - Hypoglycemia unawareness
  - Individual patient considerations
- More or less stringent glycemic goals may be appropriate for individual patients.
- Postprandial glucose may be targeted if HbA1c level goals are not met despite reaching preprandial glucose goals.

*Postprandial glucose measurements should be made 1 to 2 hours after the beginning of the meal; this is generally when peak levels are seen in patients with diabetes.
From the American Diabetes Association. Standards of medical care in diabetes—2011. *Diabetes Care*. 2011;34(1 Suppl):S11-S62.

Maintaining Optimal Nutrition. The first objective is to sustain a high level of nutrition for general health promotion, adequate growth and development, and the maintenance of an appropriate weight.

Avoiding Symptoms. This objective seeks to keep a person relatively free from symptoms of hyperglycemia, hypoglycemia, and glycosuria, which indicate poor blood glucose control.

Preventing Complications. The consistent control of blood glucose levels helps to reduce the risks of chronic complications. Table 20-3 summarizes recommendations for adults with diabetes as defined by the American Diabetes Association.

Importance of Good Self-Care Skills

To accomplish these objectives, a person with diabetes must learn and regularly practice good self-care. Daily self-discipline and informed self-care are necessary for sound diabetes management, because all people with diabetes must ultimately treat themselves, with the support of a good health care team. More emphasis is now being given to comprehensive diabetes education programs that encourage more self-care responsibility.

Basic Elements of Diabetes Management

Balancing three basic elements is essential for the good control of blood glucose levels. First, the healthy diet described here is essential for good glucose management. Second, physical activity provides an important balance to maintain good blood glucose control. Third, to ensure adequate insulin activity, some people require medications (e.g., insulin injections or oral hypoglycemic agents). However, a fourth element—stress management—may well be added in today's stressful world.

Special Objectives During Pregnancy

When a woman with diabetes becomes pregnant or when the pregnancy induces GDM, her body metabolism changes to meet the increased physiologic needs of the pregnancy while battling the manifestations of diabetes (see Chapter 10). A team of specialists usually works closely with the mother. Careful team monitoring of the mother's diabetes management is essential to ensure her health and the health of her baby. Potential problems of fetal damage, perinatal death, stillbirth, prematurity, and macrosomia are serious concerns during this time.

MEDICAL NUTRITION THERAPY FOR INDIVIDUALS WITH DIABETES

Glycemic control is the primary focus of diabetes management for all patients with diabetes. Medical nutrition therapy (MNT) will be discussed below in terms of recommendations, energy balance, nutrient balance, food distribution, and diet management.

Medical Nutrition Therapy

The MNT recommendations and interventions for all people with diabetes or who are at high risk for developing diabetes are as follows[16,20]:

Prediabetes

For individuals at risk for type 2 diabetes or with prediabetes: decrease the risk of diabetes and CVD by promoting healthy food choices and at least 150 minutes per week of physical activity to promote and maintain weight loss of 5% to 10% of body weight.

Diabetes

For individuals with diagnosed type 1 or type 2 diabetes, the MNT goals are as follows:
1. Achieve and maintain the following:
   - Blood glucose levels in the normal range or as close to normal as is safely possible
   - A lipid and lipoprotein profile that reduces the risk for vascular disease
   - Blood pressure levels in the normal range or as close to normal as is safely possible
2. Prevent or at least slow the rate of the development of the chronic complications of diabetes by modifying nutrient intake and lifestyle.
3. Address individual nutrition needs by taking into account personal and cultural preferences and willingness to change.
4. Maintain the pleasure of eating by only limiting food choices when indicated by scientific evidence.

Additional Considerations

The goals of MNT that apply to specific situations include the following:
1. For youth with type 1 diabetes, youth with type 2 diabetes, pregnant and lactating women, and older adults with diabetes, meet the nutrition needs of these unique times of the life cycle.
2. Provide self-management training for the safe conducting of exercise, including the prevention and treatment of hypoglycemia and diabetes treatment during acute illness.

Total Energy Balance

Normal Growth and Weight Management

Type 1 diabetes most commonly begins during childhood; therefore, the normal height/weight charts for children provide a standard for adequate growth and development. During adulthood, maintaining a lean weight continues to be a basic goal. Because type 2 diabetes usually occurs in overweight adults, a major goal is weight reduction and control.

Energy Intake

The total energy value of the diet for a person with diabetes should be sufficient to meet individual needs for normal growth and development, physical activity and exercise, and the maintenance of a desirable lean weight. Exercise is always an important factor in diabetes control, because it improves the cellular uptake of glucose. Energy intake is adjusted to equal energy output, or a negative energy balance should be achieved if weight loss is the goal. The Dietary Reference Intakes for children and adults (see the inside cover of this text) can serve as guides for total energy needs, with appropriate reductions in kilocalories made for overweight adults (see Chapter 15).

Nutrient Balance

The ratios of carbohydrate, fat, and protein in the diet are based on current recommendations for ideal glucose regulation and lower fat intake to reduce the risks of cardiovascular complications. There is not a specific set ratio of calories from each of the macronutrients that is recommended for all individuals with diabetes. The Dietary Reference Intake recommendations for the Acceptable Macronutrient Distribution Range are the basic guide for planning daily food intake: 45% to 65% from carbohydrate, 20% to 35% from fat, and 10% to 35% from protein. The diet for any person with diabetes is always based on the normal nutrition needs of that person for positive health, with a consideration of personal preferences, appetite, and schedule of meals and physical activity.

Carbohydrate

The primary focus in diabetes care is glycemic control, which involves the regulation of the body's primary fuel: blood glucose. The American Diabetes Association recommends a diet that includes carbohydrates from fruits, vegetables, whole grains, legumes, and low-fat milk for good health (Box 20-4). Carbohydrate intake should be consistently distributed throughout the day on a day-to-day basis and adjusted in response to blood glucose self-monitoring. Low-carbohydrate diets that involve the intake of less than 130 g/day of total carbohydrates are not recommended for the management of diabetes.[16,21]

Starch and Sugar. Carbohydrate-containing foods make up a large portion of the food supply. The most obvious of these are breads, cereals, grains, and sugary sweets. Almost all of the calories provided by fruits and vegetables are carbohydrate as well. Individuals with diabetes should not avoid carbohydrate-containing foods, because these represent an important source of energy, vitamins, minerals, and fiber. Monitoring carbohydrate

intake—whether by carbohydrate counting, exchanges, or experience-based estimation—remains a key strategy for achieving and maintaining glycemic control. Sucrose-containing foods do not have to be eliminated from the diet completely. For individuals with diabetes who choose to eat such foods, the sucrose-containing foods can be substituted for other carbohydrate-containing foods for a specific meal or snack.[21]

Glycemic Index. A food's glycemic index is determined by measuring the increase in blood glucose after the ingestion of a 50-g carbohydrate sample of the food compared with a 50-g sample of a known source, usually white bread or pure glucose. The rate of digestion and absorption determines the glycemic index value. The glycemic index theory of carbohydrate foods indicates that starchy foods greatly differ from one another with regard to their ability to raise plasma glucose levels, thereby contradicting the notion that all complex carbohydrates are created equal. Although carbohydrates differ with regard to their ability to raise blood glucose, no clear trend separates simple sugars from complex carbohydrates (see Chapter 2). For example, potatoes and white bread—both of which are complex carbohydrates—have glycemic indices that are similar to pure glucose. Therefore, the use of the glycemic index for individuals with diabetes may provide a modest benefit for glycemic control; however, there is conflicting evidence of its effectiveness.[16,21] For now, personal preference dictates the use of glycemic index values.

Fiber. As it is for all individuals, the consumption of dietary fiber is encouraged for patients with diabetes. There are no reasons for these individuals to consume greater amounts of fiber than what is recommended for the general public. Current recommendations are to consume approximately 25 to 30 g/day, with special emphasis on soluble fiber (i.e., 7 to 13 g/day).[21]

Sugar Substitutes and Sweeteners. Nutritive and nonnutritive sweeteners may be used in the diet in moderation. Various sugar substitutes are available. Approved noncaloric sweeteners include products such as saccharin, neotame, aspartame, acesulfame-K, and sucralose. Aspartame is made from two amino acids, phenylalanine and aspartic acid, and it is metabolized as such. The use of caloric sweeteners (e.g., sucrose, fructose, sorbitol) should be accounted for in a meal. However, many people

---

glycemic index the increase above fasting in the blood glucose level more than 2 hours after the ingestion of a constant amount of that food divided by the response to a reference food.

BOX 20-4   NUTRITION RECOMMENDATIONS FOR THE MANAGEMENT OF DIABETES

Carbohydrate

- A dietary pattern that includes carbohydrate from fruits, vegetables, whole grains, legumes, and low-fat milk is encouraged for good health.
- Monitoring carbohydrate—whether by carbohydrate counting, exchanges, or experienced-based estimation—remains a key strategy for the achievement of glycemic control.
- The use of the glycemic index and load in conjunction with carbohydrate counting may provide a modest additional benefit over that observed when total carbohydrate is considered alone.
- Sucrose-containing foods can be substituted for other carbohydrates in the meal plan or, if they are added to the meal plan, they can be considered with regard to the dosage of insulin or other glucose-lowering medications. Care should be taken to avoid excess energy intake.
- As for the general population, people with diabetes are encouraged to consume a variety of fiber-containing foods. However, evidence is lacking to recommend a higher fiber intake than that suggested for the population as a whole.
- Sugar alcohols and nonnutritive sweeteners are safe when they are consumed within the daily intake levels established by the U.S. Food and Drug Administration.

Fat

- Limit saturated fat to less than 7% of total calories.
- The intake of trans fats should be minimized.
- In individuals with diabetes, limit dietary cholesterol to less than 200 mg/day.
- Two or more servings of fish per week (with the exception of commercially fried fish filets) provide omega-3 polyunsaturated fatty acids and are recommended.

Protein

- For individuals with diabetes and normal renal function, evidence is insufficient to suggest that usual protein intake (i.e., 15% to 20% of energy) should be modified.
- For individuals with type 2 diabetes, ingested protein can increase the insulin response without increasing plasma glucose concentrations. Therefore, protein should not be used to treat acute hypoglycemia or to prevent nighttime hypoglycemia.
- High-protein diets are not recommended as a method for weight loss at this time. The long-term effects of protein intake of more than 20% of calories on diabetes management and its complications are unknown. Although such diets may produce short-term weight loss and improved glycemia, it has not been established that these benefits are maintained for the long term, and the long-term effects on the kidney functioning of persons with diabetes are unknown.

Alcohol

- If adults with diabetes choose to use alcohol, daily intake should be limited to a moderate amount (i.e., one drink per day or less for women and two drinks per day or less for men).
- To reduce the risk of nocturnal hypoglycemia among individuals who are using insulin or insulin secretagogues, alcohol should be consumed with food.
- For individuals with diabetes, moderate alcohol consumption (when ingested alone) has no acute effect on glucose and insulin concentrations, but carbohydrate ingested with alcohol (e.g., in a mixed drink) may raise blood glucose levels.

Micronutrients

- No clear evidence demonstrates a benefit from vitamin or mineral supplementation in people with diabetes (as compared with the general population) who do not have underlying deficiencies.
- Routine supplementation with antioxidants (e.g., vitamins E and C, carotene) is not advised because of a lack of evidence of efficacy and concern related to long-term safety.
- The benefits of chromium supplementation for individuals with diabetes or obesity have not been clearly demonstrated and therefore cannot be recommended.

Adapted from the American Diabetes Association. Nutrition recommendations and interventions for diabetes. *Diabetes Care.* 2008; 31(1 Suppl):S61-S78.

---

cannot tolerate a high intake of sorbitol, and they may have significant diarrhea when sorbitol is used in excess. Nutritive and nonnutritive sweeteners are safe to consume in moderation and as part of a nutritious and well-balanced diet.

Protein

Standard requirements as outlined in the Dietary Reference Intakes can be a guide for protein intake. In general, approximately 10% to 35% of the total energy as protein is sufficient to meet growth needs in children and to maintain tissue integrity in adults. Excessively high protein intake is not recommended because of its unnecessary stress on the kidneys for patients with diabetic nephropathy.

Fat

No more than 7% of the diet's total kilocalories should come from saturated fat. Lower cholesterol intake (i.e., no more than 200 mg/day) is also recommended. The control of fat-related foods, which contribute to the development of atherosclerosis and coronary heart disease, helps to lessen the increased risk for CVD. An emphasis is placed on polyunsaturated fats (e.g., fish oil) and the avoidance of trans fats.

Guidelines for macronutrient, micronutrient, and alcohol intake are based on the recommendations from the American Diabetes Association position statement and outlined in Box 20-4.

Food Distribution

As a general rule, fairly even amounts of food should be eaten at regular intervals throughout the day and adjusted in response to blood glucose levels. This basic pattern helps to provide a more even blood glucose supply and to prevent extremes in high and low levels. Snacks between meals may be needed. Physical activity and medication use are significant factors for determining ideal food distribution on an individual basis.

Daily Activity Schedule

Food distribution must be planned ahead, especially when using insulin, and adjusted according to each day's scheduled activities and blood glucose monitoring to prevent episodes of hypoglycemia. The careful distribution of food and snacks is especially important for children and adolescents with diabetes to balance with insulin during the growth spurts and changing hormone patterns of puberty. Practical consideration should be given to school and work schedules, athletics, social events, and stressful periods. A stressful event caused by any source (e.g., injury, anxiety, fear, pain) brings an adrenaline (epinephrine) rush. This fight-or-flight effect counteracts insulin activity and can contribute to a glycemic response.

Exercise

Current recommendations for people with type 1 or type 2 diabetes are to perform at least 150 minutes per week of moderate-intensity aerobic physical activity (i.e., 50% to 70% of maximum heart rate). In addition, people with type 2 diabetes should be encouraged to perform resistance training three times per week in the absence of contraindications.[16] Regular moderate-intensity exercise programs help individuals with type 2 diabetes to control their blood glucose levels and to reduce their risk for cardiovascular disease, hyperlipidemia, hypertension, and obesity.

For people who are using insulin, any exercise or additional physical activity must be covered in the food distribution plan (Table 20-4). The energy demands of exercise are discussed separately in Chapter 16. The following guidelines are recommended for regulating

TABLE 20-4 MEAL PLANNING GUIDE FOR ACTIVE PEOPLE WITH TYPE 1 DIABETES

Activity Level	Exchange Needs	Sample Menus
Moderate		
30 minutes	1 bread *or* 1 fruit	1 bran muffin *or* 1 small orange
1 hour	2 bread + 1 meat *or* 2 fruit + 1 milk	Tuna sandwich *or* ½ cup fruit salad + 1 cup milk
Strenuous		
30 minutes	2 fruit *or* 1 bread + 1 fat	1 small banana *or* ½ bagel + 1 tsp cream cheese
1 hour	2 bread + 1 meat + 1 milk *or* 2 bread + 2 meat + 2 fruit	Meat and cheese sandwich + 1 cup milk *or* Turkey sandwich + 1 cup orange juice

the glycemic response to exercise in individuals with diabetes[22]:

1. Achieve metabolic control before physical activity.
   - Avoid physical activity if fasting glucose levels are higher than 250 mg/dL and if ketosis is present, and use caution if glucose levels are higher than 300 mg/dL and if no ketosis is present.
   - Ingest added carbohydrate if glucose levels are less than 100 mg/dL.
2. Monitor blood glucose levels before and after physical activity.
   - Identify when changes in insulin or food intake are necessary.
   - Learn the glycemic response to different physical activity conditions.
3. Monitor food intake.
   - Consume added carbohydrate as needed to avoid hypoglycemia.
   - Carbohydrate-based foods should be readily available during and after physical activity.

hypoglycemia a low blood glucose level; a serious condition in diabetes management that requires immediate sugar intake to counteract, followed by a snack of complex carbohydrate (e.g., bread, crackers) and protein (e.g., lean meat, peanut butter, cheese) to maintain a normal blood glucose level.

Drug Therapy

The food distribution pattern is also influenced by any form of drug therapy (i.e., type, amount, and dose schedule of insulin or oral hypoglycemic agent) that is necessary for glucose control. Successful self-care means that the patient can adjust his or her diet, medications, and exercise on the basis of the result of blood glucose monitoring.

Diet Management

General Planning

The nature of an individual's diabetes, his or her treatment regime, and his or her health status largely determine the necessary personal diet management. Table 20-5 provides guidelines for dietary strategies for type 1 and type 2 diabetes.

Individual Needs

Every person with diabetes is unique, with a particular form and degree of diabetes as well as a different living situation, a different background, and different food habits. All of these personal needs must be considered (as discussed in Chapters 14 and 17) if appropriate and realistic care is to be planned. The nutrition counselor, who usually is the clinical dietitian or certified diabetes educator, should determine these various needs as part of a careful initial nutrition assessment that includes medical, socioeconomic, and psychosocial needs as well as personal lifestyle characteristics. This information provides the basis for determining the diet prescription.

A major principle of diabetes management is the variety of methods and dietary guidelines that the nutrition team can use when planning for and supporting patients. Of these dietary guides, carbohydrate counting and the food exchange method—when tailored to meet individual needs—remain the two most commonly used approaches. Materials that can be used for planning the diet are available from the American Diabetes Association and the Academy of Nutrition and Dietetics in both English and Spanish.

Carbohydrate Counting

Carbohydrate counting is a way to balance the carbohydrate intake with insulin injections (i.e., the insulin-to-carbohydrate ratio). Patients count the total number of carbohydrates for a meal and then inject an appropriate amount of insulin to process the glucose. One carbohydrate serving equals 15 g of carbohydrate. Insulin may be injected manually or with an insulin pump (Figures 20-5 and 20-6). There are multiple resources (e.g., books, online programs, handheld devices, phone applications)

TABLE 20-5 DIETARY STRATEGIES FOR TYPE 1 AND TYPE 2 DIABETES MELLITUS

Dietary Strategy	Type 1	Type 2
Decrease energy intake (kilocalories)	No	Yes, if weight loss is recommended
Increase frequency and number of feedings	Yes	Usually no
Have regular daily intake of kilocalories from carbohydrate, protein, and fat	Very important	Yes
Plan consistent daily ratio of protein, carbohydrate, and fat for each feeding	Desirable	Yes, but not as tightly controlled
Use extra or planned food to treat or prevent hypoglycemia	Very important	Usually not necessary
Plan regular times for meals and snacks	Very important	Yes
Use extra food for unusual exercise	Yes	Usually not necessary
During illness, use small, frequent feedings of carbohydrates to prevent starvation ketoacidosis	Important	Usually not necessary because of resistance to ketoacidosis

available that list grams of carbohydrates for thousands of foods. One benefit of carbohydrate counting is that meal plans are much less stringent and flexibility is more easily accommodated. For this type of meal and insulin planning to work, the patient must be well versed in calculating the total number of carbohydrate grams consumed per meal or snack.

Additional information and tool kits for dietary planning based on carbohydrate counting can be found on the American Diabetes Association Web site (www.diabetes.org) and the Academy of Nutrition and Dietetics Web site (www.eatright.org).

Food Exchange System

The dietitian uses the food exchange system to calculate a patient's energy and nutrient needs as well as to distribute foods in a balanced meal and snack pattern. The food exchange system is called this because people with diabetes use the system to select a variety of foods from the various food groups in accordance with their personal diet plans.

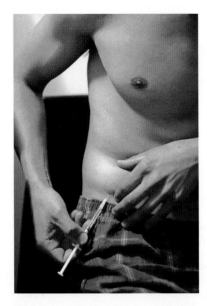

Figure 20-5 A man with diabetes injecting himself with insulin. (Copyright PhotoDisc.)

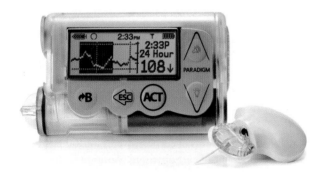

Figure 20-6 Insulin pump and monitor.

With this system, commonly used foods are grouped into basic exchange lists according to roughly equal macronutrient values in the portions indicated. Thus, a variety of foods may be chosen from these lists to fulfill the food plan while the basic diet prescription of total energy and a balanced ratio of nutrients are maintained. The designated food values for each of the food exchange groups are shown in Table 20-6. The booklet entitled "Choose Your Foods: Exchange Lists for Diabetes" is available for purchase from the Academy of Nutrition and Dietetics. Its colorful illustrations, clear content, and style provide a helpful tool for patient and client education. Table 20-7 illustrates a calculated 2200-kcal diet and food pattern example that uses the exchange system, and Box 20-5 outlines a sample menu that is based on this pattern.

Special Concerns

Special concerns come up in daily living and become an important part of ongoing dietary counseling. Some suggestions for these concerns are given in the following sections.

Special Diet Food Items. Little need exists for special "diabetic" foods. People with diabetes should eat the regular, well-balanced diet that is recommended for the general population to promote health and prevent disease. This kind of a healthful diet primarily makes use of regular fresh foods from all of the basic food groups, with the limited use of processed foods (noting the grams of carbohydrate per serving on the label) and an increased use of nonfat seasonings. The simple principles of moderation and variety should guide food choices and amounts.

Alcohol. The occasional use of alcohol in an adult diabetic diet can be planned, but caution must be exercised. Individuals with type 1 diabetes who consume alcohol must be reminded of the following: (1) to eat when they drink; and (2) to not increase their insulin doses, because the overall effect of alcohol is to lower the blood glucose level. Occasional use is defined as moderate intake: one drink or less per day for women and two drinks or less per day for men. Equivalent portions are 1 oz of liquor, 4 oz of wine, and 12 oz of beer. The same precautions for the use of alcohol that apply to the general public apply to people with diabetes.

A person with type 1 diabetes should not substitute alcohol for food exchanges in the diet. When a person's blood glucose levels begin to drop, the liver typically responds to the hormone glucagon and releases glucose into the blood to reestablish normal blood glucose levels. However, when alcohol is in the system, the liver's primary role is to detoxify the blood of alcohol, and it will not respond to impending hypoglycemia until the alcohol is cleared. Therefore, alcohol should only be consumed in moderation and in conjunction with food. Alcohol may be used in cooking as desired because it vaporizes in the cooking process and contributes only its flavor to the finished product.

Hypoglycemia. The brain depends on a constant supply of glucose for metabolism and proper function; a prolonged lack of glucose can lead to permanent brain damage. Hypoglycemia (i.e., a blood glucose level of less than 70 mg/dL) may occur from too much insulin or oral hypoglycemic agents that act by stimulating the islet cells in the pancreas to secrete more insulin. Hypoglycemia can also occur if a person with diabetes delays a meal or snack, does not eat enough carbohydrate, or exercises too much without sufficient food. Table 20-8 lists symptoms

TABLE 20-6   AMOUNT OF NUTRIENTS IN ONE SERVING FROM EACH EXCHANGE LIST

Food List	Carbohydrate (g)	Protein (g)	Fat (g)	Calories (g)
Carbohydrates				
Starch: breads, cereals, and grains; starchy vegetables; crackers and snacks; and beans, peas, and lentils	15	0 to 3	0 to 1	80
Fruits	15	—	—	60
Milk				
Fat free, low fat, 1%	12	8	0 to 3	100
Reduced fat, 2%	12	8	5	120
Whole	12	8	8	160
Sweets, desserts, and other carbohydrates	15	Varies	Varies	Varies
Nonstarchy vegetables	5	2	—	25
Meat and Meat Substitutes				
Lean	—	7	0 to 3	45
Medium fat	—	7	4 to 7	75
High fat	—	7	8+	100
Plant-based proteins	Varies	7	Varies	Varies
Fats	—	—	5	45
Alcohol	Varies	—	—	100

From the American Diabetes Association; American Dietetic Association: *Choose your foods: exchange lists for meal planning,* Chicago, and Alexandria, Va: American Diabetes Association and American Dietetic Association; 2008.

TABLE 20-7   CALCULATION OF A DIABETIC DIET USING THE EXCHANGE SYSTEM (2200 KCAL)

FOOD GROUP	TOTAL DAY'S EXCHANGES	CARBOHYDRATES: 275 g (50% kcal)	PROTEIN: 110 g (20% kcal)	FAT: 75 g (30% kcal)	BREAKFAST	LUNCH	DINNER	SNACKS Afternoon	Bedtime
Carbohydrates									
Starch	11.5	172	34.5	—	3	3	3	1	1.5
Fruits	3	45	—	—	1	1		1	
Milk									
Fat free	2	24	16		1	—	—	—	1
Sweets, Desserts and Other Carbohydrates	1	15	Varies	Varies	—	—	1		
Nonstarchy Vegetables	4	20	8	—	—	2	2		
Meat and Meat Substitutes									
Very lean	2	—	14	0 to 1	—	—	—	1	1
Lean	3	—	21	9	—	—	3		
Medium fat	2	—	14	10	1	1			
Fat	11	—	—	55	3	3	3	1	1
Total grams		276	107.5	75					

of both hyperglycemia and hypoglycemia. Because behavior is often irrational and movements are uncoordinated, patients in this state may be mistaken for being intoxicated. Thus, an identification bracelet or pendant is an ideal means of informing others about the true condition so that proper treatment—glucose replacement in the form of a food or beverage or an injection of glucagon—can be given. (Note the 15-g carbohydrate replacement portions listed in the bread/cereal [starch] and fruit exchange groups [see Table 20-6].) People with type 1 diabetes should always carry a convenient form of sugar (e.g., sugar lumps or glucose tablets) with them to take at the first sign of a hypoglycemic attack and then follow this sugar as soon as possible with a snack of

BOX 20-5 SAMPLE MENU PRESCRIPTION: 2200 KCAL

- 275 g carbohydrate (50% kcal)
- 110 g protein (20% kcal)
- 75 g fat (30% kcal)

Breakfast
- 1 medium fresh peach
- 1 serving shredded wheat cereal
- 1 poached egg on whole-grain toast
- 1 bran muffin
- 1 tsp margarine
- 1 cup low-fat milk
- Coffee or tea with nonnutritive sweetener only

Lunch
- Vegetable soup with wheat crackers
- Tuna sandwich on whole-wheat bread
  - Tuna (½ cup, drained)
  - Mayonnaise (2 tsp)
  - Chopped dill pickle
  - Chopped celery
- 1 fresh pear

Dinner
- Pan-broiled pork chop (well trimmed)
- 1 cup brown rice
- ½ cup green beans
- Tossed green salad
  - Italian dressing (1 to 2 Tbsp)
- ½ cup applesauce
- 1 bran muffin

Afternoon Snack
- 10 crackers with 2 Tbsp peanut butter
- 1 medium orange

Evening Snack
- 3 cups plain popped popcorn
- 1 oz cheese
- 1 cup low-fat milk

TABLE 20-8 SYMPTOMS OF HYPERGLYCEMIA AND HYPOGLYCEMIA

Factor	Hyperglycemia	Hypoglycemia
Cause	Too much food, not enough insulin, illness, or stress	Not enough food, too much insulin, too much exercise, or alcohol intake without food
Symptoms	Polydipsia	Sudden shaking
	Polyuria	Nervousness
	Polyphagia	Sweating
	Dry or itchy skin	Anxiety and irritability
	Blurred vision	
	Drowsiness	Dizziness
	Nausea	Impaired vision
	Fatigue	Weakness
	Shortness of breath	Headache
	Weakness	Hunger
	Confusion	Confusion
	Coma	Tingling sensations around the mouth
		Seizure

complex carbohydrate and protein (e.g., peanut butter crackers, granola bar and yogurt, ham and cheese sandwich).

Illness. When general illness occurs, food and insulin should be adjusted accordingly. The texture of the food can be modified to make use of easily digested and absorbed liquid foods. This type of liquid substitution can be used for meals that are not eaten. In general, people with diabetes who are ill should do the following:

- Maintain food intake every day; do not skip meals.
- Do not omit insulin; follow an adjusted dosage if needed.
- Monitor the blood glucose level frequently.
- Replace carbohydrate solid foods with equal liquid or soft foods, if necessary, and drink plenty of fluids.

- Contact a physician if the illness lasts for more than 24 hours.

Travel. When a trip is planned, the dietitian and client should confer to make decisions about food choices that depend on what will be available to the traveler. In general, preparation activities may include the following:

- Review meal-planning skills, the number and type of exchanges at each meal, basic portion sizes, and tips on eating out.
- Learn about foods that will be available (e.g., ordering a diabetic meal ahead from an airline).
- Select appropriate snacks to carry, and plan time intervals for their use.
- Plan for time-zone changes with regard to medication, exercise, and diet routines.
- Carry some quick-acting form of carbohydrate (e.g., sugar lumps, glucose tablets) at all times, and tell companions about the signs, symptoms, and treatment of hypoglycemia.
- Wear an identification bracelet or pendant.
- Secure a physician's letter that addresses syringes and insulin prescriptions.

Eating Out. In general, people with diabetes should plan ahead so that food that is eaten at home before and after a meal out can be accommodated to maintain the continuing day's balance. Choosing restaurants wisely also makes menu selection easier. Timing insulin doses to food arrival is important, because taking insulin too long before eating will result in hypoglycemia.

Stress. Any form of physiologic or psychosocial stress affects diabetes control because of the hormonal responses that are antagonistic to insulin. People with diabetes, especially those who use insulin, should learn useful stress-reduction exercises and activities as part of their self-care skills and practices. Stress-reducing activities can vary greatly from one person to the next (e.g., meditation, running, yoga, journaling, playing music). Finding the best coping mechanism may require trial and error.

DIABETES EDUCATION PROGRAM

Goal: Person-Centered Self-Care

During the past decade, the traditional roles of health care professionals and their patients have been changing. Patients are taking much more active and informed roles in their own health care. These actions are especially true of people with diabetes. As a result of the nature of the disease process and the necessity of daily survival skills, people with diabetes must practice regular daily self-care (see the Clinical Applications box, "Case Study: Richard Manages His Diabetes"). Thus, any effective and successful diabetes education program must focus on personal needs and informed self-care skills.

Diabetes Self-Management Education

The overall objectives of diabetes self-management education, as defined by the American Diabetes Association Standards of Medical Care, are to improve health status and quality of life by supporting informed decision making, self-care behaviors, problem solving, and active collaboration with the health care team.[23] Certified diabetes educators and the American Diabetes Association have developed guidelines for diabetes self-management education that are based on the learning needs, skills, and content areas that are necessary for the self-care of patients with diabetes.

Necessary Skills

The elements that are involved in a patient's diabetes self-management education program may involve any or all of the following content areas, depending on the specific needs of that individual.[23,24]

Healthy Eating. People with diabetes should develop a lifestyle that involves healthy eating choices that are based on individual nutrition needs, living and working situations, and food habits. Such planning includes understanding how the food plan relates to the maintenance of good blood glucose control and the promotion of positive health.

Being Active. A healthy lifestyle that includes regular physical activity is an important aspect of overall fitness, weight management, and blood glucose control. Patients can work with their health care providers to determine an appropriate activity plan and to discuss how to balance food intake with medications during exercise.

CLINICAL APPLICATIONS

CASE STUDY: RICHARD MANAGES HIS DIABETES

Richard Smith, who is 21 years old, has type 1 diabetes mellitus. He gives himself two injections per day, and each one is a combination of medium-acting insulin and regular short-acting insulin. He takes one injection before breakfast and one before dinner, and he usually tests his blood glucose level before each meal and at bedtime. Richard is a college student who is usually active in athletics.

However, this is final examination week, and Richard's schedule is irregular. He is putting in long hours of study, and he is under considerable stress. On the day before a particularly difficult examination, he is reviewing his study materials at home, and he forgets to check his blood glucose or eat lunch. During the middle of the afternoon, he begins to feel faint. He realizes that his blood glucose level is low and that an insulin reaction is imminent if he does not get a quick source of energy. He looks in the kitchen, but all he can find is orange juice, milk, a loaf of bread, and a jar of peanut butter.

Questions for Analysis
1. Which of the foods should Richard eat immediately? Why?
2. Later, when he is feeling better, Richard makes a peanut butter sandwich, pours a glass of milk, and eats his snack while he continues studying. What carbohydrate food sources of energy are in his snack?
3. Are these carbohydrate sources in a form that the cells can burn for energy? What changes must Richard's body make to these sources to get them into the basic carbohydrate fuel form?
4. What is the complex form of carbohydrate in his snack? Why is this a valuable form of carbohydrate in his diet?
5. If Richard did not take his insulin to provide the necessary control agent for metabolizing the carbohydrate, what would happen to him as the result of improper handling of fat and the accumulation of ketones?

Monitoring. The monitoring of blood glucose levels, urinary acetone levels (which indicate ketoacidosis), weight, and blood pressure is fundamental to diabetes management. This monitoring includes learning accurate self-testing procedures as well as understanding the meaning of the results and knowing what action to take in relation to food, insulin, or exercise. A variety of self-tests are now available for quick blood glucose monitoring. Small glucose testing kits can fit into purses, backpacks, and glove compartments for easy access and convenience. Some insulin pumps provide continuous interstitial blood glucose monitoring.

Medications. In accordance with their treatment plans, people with diabetes should have a thorough understanding of how their medications work and when to take them. Patients should understand the side effects, efficacy, toxicity, dosage, and effects of missed or delayed doses as well as how to store and travel with their medications. Although it is not within the scope of this book to extensively cover medications, a summary of basic information follows.

- *Insulin:* There are several types of insulin with different durations of action (Table 20-9), and there are multiple combinations of insulin use (see the For Further Focus box, "Comparative Types of Insulin"). Patients should know how insulin works in the body and how its action relates to the food plan. Learning good insulin injection technique is also an important part of the treatment plan. In addition to the standard injections, insulin can also be administered with a pump (see Figure 20-6). Newer forms of insulin-pump therapy continuously deliver insulin to the body in response to a programmed basal rate (Figure 20-7). Fast-acting insulin can then be delivered in a bolus immedi-

ately after a meal based on the number of carbohydrates that the meal contained.
- *Oral hypoglycemic agents:* Medications that stimulate insulin activity, their comparative types and effects (Table 20-10), and how to regulate them are key points that should be well understood by the patient and his or her caretakers. The Drug-Nutrient Interaction box, "Exenatide and Glucose Control," describes the action of one such hypoglycemic medication.

Problem Solving. The prevention, detection, and the treatment of acute complications require informed problem-solving skills. People should recognize the early signs of hypoglycemia and its causes and treatment. This recognition includes the following: (1) knowledge of hypoglycemia's relationship to the interactive balances among insulin, food, and exercise as the basis of the

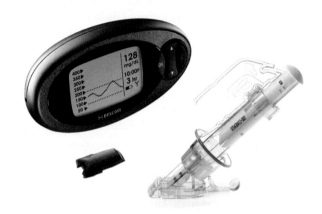

Figure 20-7 Insulin pump with optional continuous glucose monitoring functionality. (Courtesy DexCom, Inc., San Diego, Calif.)

TABLE 20-9 **TYPES OF INSULIN**

Type	Examples	Onset of Action	Peak Action	Duration of Action
Rapid acting	Humalog (Lispro) NovoLog (Aspart) Apidra (Glulisine)	<15 minutes	30 to 90 minutes	3 to 5 hours
Short acting (regular)	Humulin R Novolin R	30 to 60 minutes	2 to 4 hours	5 to 8 hours
Intermediate acting*	Humulin N (NPH) Novolin N (NPH)	1 to 3 hours	8 hours	12 to 16 hours
Long acting	Lantus (Glargine) Levemir (Detemir)	1 hour	None	20 to 26 hours

*Intermediate and short-acting mixtures are also available.
From the National Diabetes Information Clearinghouse. *Types of insulin* (website): diabetes.niddk.nih.gov/dm/pubs/medicines_ez/insert_C. htm. Accessed March 2011; and the American Dietetic Association. *ADA nutrition care manual.* Chicago: American Dietetic Association; 2010.

FOR FURTHER FOCUS

COMPARATIVE TYPES OF INSULIN

A common method of insulin use is a mixture of short-acting and longer-acting types injected twice a day (see figure). Persons with unstable diabetes or irregular mealtimes may inject short-acting insulin before each meal or snack and use a longer-acting type of insulin once or twice a day. Experienced patients self-test their blood glucose levels with finger pricks and glucose monitors. These patients have learned to adjust their insulin dosage to their test results; food patterns; work, school, and social activities; and exercise schedules. In some cases, an insulin pump that continuously delivers insulin into the bloodstream may be used to maintain better control over the body's varying insulin needs.

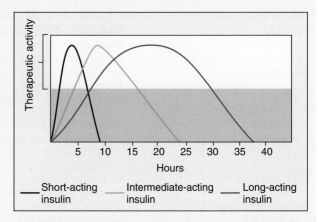

DRUG-NUTRIENT INTERACTION

EXENATIDE AND GLUCOSE CONTROL

Incretins are hormones that are secreted by intestinal cells in response to the presence of food. One of these incretins is known as *glucagon-like peptide 1* (GLP-1). This peptide acts by stimulating glucose-dependent insulin release by the pancreas and inhibiting glucagon secretion when glucose is present. The net effect is an overall reduction in plasma glucose.[1]

Exenatide (Byetta) is a member of the incretin mimetic class of drugs that is used for the treatment of type 2 diabetes. This drug resembles GLP-1, and it has similar effects when it is injected at mealtimes. In addition to reducing blood glucose levels, exenatide also slows gastric emptying and nutrient absorption, which enhances satiety and promotes mild weight loss. The most common side effects are nausea, vomiting, indigestion, abdominal pain, and diarrhea.[2]

The powerful interaction between exenatide and glucose is the reason for its effectiveness in the treatment of type 2 diabetes. Exenatide is shown to improve glycemic control and to reduce HbA1c by 1.0%, and it may prolong the time before insulin therapy is needed to control hyperglycemia. Patients who receive higher doses (i.e., 10 μg twice daily) are at risk for hypoglycemia, primarily when they are using exenatide with sulfonylureas.[1]

Kelli Boi

1. Norris SL, Lee N, Thakurta S, Chan BK. Exenatide efficacy and safety: a systematic review. *Diabet Med.* 2009;26(9):837-846.
2. Amylin Pharmaceuticals. *Byetta (exenatide) injection* (website): www.amylin.com/products/byetta.htm. Accessed March 2011.

diabetes care plan; (2) daily diabetic care and how to prevent such episodes; (3) the immediate emergency treatment with some form of quick-acting simple carbohydrate to counteract it; and (4) the need to follow the emergency sugar with a snack of complex carbohydrate and protein as soon as possible to sustain a normal blood glucose level. People with diabetes should learn how to deal with illness and other special needs, several of which have been discussed. This knowledge includes how to adjust one's diet and insulin intake and how to plan ahead for events of daily living such as travel, eating out, exercise, and stress.

Health Coping. Health care providers can help patients to address the psychologic and social issues that impede the patient's ability to manage his or her diabetes. Developing personal strategies to promote health and behavior changes may have significant and long-term effects on a patient's health status and quality of life. Patients should be able to identify appropriate coping mechanisms and support systems.

Reducing Risk. Prevention, detection, and a thorough knowledge of treatment options for chronic complications should be well understood by all patients with diabetes. Skills taught in diabetes self-management education programs include the following: blood glucose and blood pressure self-monitoring, smoking cessation, foot care, aspirin use, and the maintenance of personal care records.

TABLE 20-10 ORAL HYPOGLYCEMIC MEDICATIONS

Category of Medication	Examples	Action
α-Glucosidase inhibitor	Acarbose (Precose) Miglitol (Glyset)	Slows breakdown of starches, thereby delaying the rise in blood glucose that occurs after a meal
Biguanide	Metformin (Glucophage) Metformin extended release (Glucophage XR)	Suppresses hepatic glucose production
Meglitinide	Nateglinide (Starlix) Repaglinide (Prandin)	Stimulates the release of insulin from β cells
Sulfonylurea (first-generation)	Chlorpropamide (Diabinese)	Stimulates the release of insulin from β cells
Sulfonylurea (second-generation)	Glipizide (Glucotrol, Glucotrol XL) Glyburide (Micronase, Glynase PresTab, Diabeta) Glimepiride (Amaryl)	Stimulates the release of insulin from β cells
Thiazolidinedione	Pioglitazone (Actos) Rosiglitazone (Avandia)	Increases insulin sensitivity in muscle and fat
Dipeptidyl peptidase-4 inhibitor	Sitagliptin (Januvia) Saxagliptin (Onglyza)	Prevents the breakdown of hormones that increase insulin secretion and suppress glucagon production
Incretin mimetics	Exenatide (Byetta)	Improves the glucose-dependent secretion of insulin; decreases glucagon secretion after eating
Amylinomimetic	Pramlintide (Symlin)	Suppresses glucagon production

From the American Dietetic Association. *ADA nutrition care manual.* Chicago: American Dietetic Association; 2010.

Resources

A number of organizations with a wealth of health care tools are available, such as the American Diabetes Association, the Academy of Nutrition and Dietetics, and the American Association of Diabetes Educators. In addition, resources include certified diabetes educators, hospital and clinic dietitians, dietitians in private practice, public health nutritionists, and local chapters of the American Diabetes Association. Any resource materials used must be evaluated in terms of individual needs.

Staff Education

In the final analysis, the success of the diabetes education program in any health care facility depends on the sensitivity and training of the staff members who are conducting the program. Continuing education is essential for all professionals and their assistants. Certified diabetes educators are the recognized experts in diabetes education for both patient and staff training. The American Association of Diabetes Educators has a Web site at www.diabeteseducator.org where patients and health care providers can locate specialists.

SUMMARY

- Diabetes mellitus is a syndrome of varying forms and degrees that has the common characteristic of hyperglycemia. Its underlying metabolic disorder involves all three of the energy-yielding nutrients and influences energy balance. The major controlling hormone involved is insulin from the pancreas, and people with diabetes have either a lack of insulin or a resistance to its action.
- Type 1 diabetes affects approximately 5% to 10% of all people with diabetes; it usually presents itself first during childhood, and it is more severe and unstable. The treatment of type 1 diabetes involves regular meals and snacks that are balanced with insulin and exercise. The self-monitoring of blood glucose levels is a critical part of disease management.
- Type 2 diabetes occurs mostly among adults, especially those who are overweight. Acidosis is rare. Treatment involves weight reduction and maintenance along with regular exercise. Oral hypoglycemic medications or insulin may be needed.

- A significant keystone of care for all forms of diabetes is sound diet therapy. The basic food plan should be rich in complex carbohydrates and dietary fiber; low in simple sugars, fats (especially saturated fats), and cholesterol; and moderate in protein. Food should be distributed throughout the day in fairly regular amounts and at regular times, and it should be tailored to meet individual needs.
- Diabetes self-management education is a cornerstone of the overall success of patients who are managing their diabetes.

CRITICAL THINKING QUESTIONS

1. Define *diabetes mellitus*. Describe the nature of the underlying metabolic disorder. What is the common characteristic of all forms of diabetes mellitus?
2. Describe the major characteristics of the two main types of diabetes mellitus. Explain how these characteristics influence nutrition therapy.
3. Identify and explain the symptoms of uncontrolled diabetes mellitus. How would you explain to a patient the differences between hyperglycemia and hypoglycemia and how to recognize and treat these symptoms?
4. Describe the possible long-term complications of poorly controlled diabetes mellitus. Can these complications be avoided? If so, how?

CHAPTER CHALLENGE QUESTIONS

True-False

Write the correct statement for each statement that is false.

1. *True or False:* Most people with type 2 diabetes are underweight when the disease is diagnosed.
2. *True or False:* The two energy-yielding nutrients whose metabolism is most severely affected in patients with diabetes are fat and protein.
3. *True or False:* Insulin is a hormone that is produced by the pituitary gland.
4. *True or False:* Insulin action is influenced by both glucagon and somatostatin.
5. *True or False:* Acetone in the urine of a person with diabetes usually indicates that the diabetes is poorly controlled.
6. *True or False:* People with type 1 diabetes are taught to test their own blood glucose daily and to regulate their insulin, food, and exercise accordingly.
7. *True or False:* Coronary artery disease occurs in people with diabetes at a higher rate than that seen in the general population.
8. *True or False:* Chronic complications occur in a relatively small number of people with diabetes.
9. *True or False:* A diabetic diet involves a combination of specific foods that should remain constant.
10. *True or False:* People with unstable type 1 diabetes should follow a low-carbohydrate diet for better control.

Multiple Choice

1. The caloric value of the diet for a person with diabetes should be
   a. increased above normal requirements to meet the increased metabolic demand.
   b. decreased below normal requirements to prevent glucose formation.
   c. sufficient to maintain the person's appropriate lean weight.
   d. contributed mainly by fat to spare the carbohydrate for energy needs.

2. Carbohydrate counting is based on which of the following principles?
   a. Equivalent food exchange values
   b. The insulin-to-carbohydrate ratio
   c. Sucrose and fructose balance
   d. High fat content

3. Oral hypoglycemic agents are used for individuals with which kind of diabetes?
   a. Type 1 diabetes
   b. Type 2 diabetes
   c. Prediabetes
   d. All of the above

4. Which of the following conditions are potential long-term complications of uncontrolled diabetes? *(Circle all that apply.)*
   a. Retinopathy
   b. Nephropathy
   c. Neuropathy
   d. Heart disease

⊖volve Please refer to the Students' Resource section of this text's Evolve Web site for additional study resources.

REFERENCES

1. National Center for Health Statistics. *Health, United States, 2010: with special feature on death and dying.* Hyattsville, Md: U.S. Government Printing Office; 2011.
2. American Diabetes Association. Diagnosis and classification of diabetes mellitus. *Diabetes Care.* 2011;34(Suppl 1):S62-S69.
3. McCarthy MI. Genomics, type 2 diabetes, and obesity. *N Engl J Med.* 2010;363(24):2339-2350.
4. Petrie JR, Pearson ER, Sutherland C. Implications of genome wide association studies for the understanding of type 2 diabetes pathophysiology. *Biochem Pharmacol.* 2011;81(4):471-477.
5. Writing Group for the SEARCH for Diabetes in Youth Study Group; Dabelea D, Bell RA, D'Agostino Jr RB, et al. Incidence of diabetes in youth in the United States. *JAMA.* 2007;297(24):2716-2724.
6. Hadar E, Hod M. Establishing consensus criteria for the diagnosis of diabetes in pregnancy following the HAPO study. *Ann N Y Acad Sci.* 2010;1205:88-93.
7. Waugh N, Royle P, Clar C, et al. Screening for hyperglycaemia in pregnancy: a rapid update for the National Screening Committee. *Health Technol Assess.* 2010;14(45):1-183.
8. Nicholson W, Bolen S, Witkop CT, et al. Benefits and risks of oral diabetes agents compared with insulin in women with gestational diabetes: a systematic review. *Obstet Gynecol.* 2009;113(1):193-205.
9. Retnakaran R, Austin PC, Shah BR. Effect of subsequent pregnancies on the risk of developing diabetes following a first pregnancy complicated by gestational diabetes: a population-based study. *Diabet Med.* 2011;28(3):287-292.
10. Sekimoto M, Takada T, Kawarada Y, et al. JPN Guidelines for the management of acute pancreatitis: epidemiology, etiology, natural history, and outcome predictors in acute pancreatitis. *J Hepatobiliary Pancreat Surg.* 2006;13(1):10-24.
11. Doshi KB, Kashyap SR, Brennan DM, et al. All-cause mortality risk predictors in a preventive cardiology clinic cohort-examining diabetes and individual metabolic syndrome criteria: a PRECIS database study. *Diabetes Obes Metab.* 2009;11(2):102-108.
12. Findeisen HM, Weckbach S, Stark RG, et al. Metabolic syndrome predicts vascular changes in whole body magnetic resonance imaging in patients with long standing diabetes mellitus. *Cardiovasc Diabetol.* 2010;9:44.
13. Guzder RN, Gatling W, Mullee MA, Byrne CD. Impact of metabolic syndrome criteria on cardiovascular disease risk in people with newly diagnosed type 2 diabetes. *Diabetologia.* 2006;49(1):49-55.
14. Gerich JE. Role of the kidney in normal glucose homeostasis and in the hyperglycaemia of diabetes mellitus: therapeutic implications. *Diabet Med.* 2010;27(2):136-142.
15. Centers for Disease Control and Prevention. *National diabetes fact sheet: national estimates and general information on diabetes and prediabetes in the United States, 2011.* Atlanta: U.S. Department of Health and Human Services, Centers for Disease Control and Prevention; 2011.
16. American Diabetes Association. Standards of medical care in diabetes–2011. *Diabetes Care.* 2011;34(Suppl 1):S11-S61.
17. Mattila TK, de Boer A. Influence of intensive versus conventional glucose control on microvascular and macrovascular complications in type 1 and 2 diabetes mellitus. *Drugs.* 2010;70(17):2229-2245.
18. Mayfield JA, Reiber GE, Sanders LJ, et al; American Diabetes Association. Preventive foot care in diabetes. *Diabetes Care.* 2004;27(Suppl 1):S63-S64.
19. Cleary PA, Orchard TJ, Genuth S, et al; DCCT/EDIC Research Group. The effect of intensive glycemic treatment on coronary artery calcification in type 1 diabetic participants of the Diabetes Control and Complications Trial/Epidemiology of Diabetes Interventions and Complications (DCCT/EDIC) Study. *Diabetes.* 2006;55(12):3556-3565.
20. American Dietetic Association. *ADA nutrition care manual.* Chicago: American Dietetic Association; 2010.
21. Franz MJ, Powers MA, Leontos C, et al. The evidence for medical nutrition therapy for type 1 and type 2 diabetes in adults. *J Am Diet Assoc.* 2010;110(12):1852-1889.
22. Zinman B, Ruderman N, Campaigne BN, et al; American Diabetes Association. Physical activity/exercise and diabetes mellitus. *Diabetes Care.* 2003;26(Suppl 1):S73-S77.
23. Funnell MM, Brown TL, Childs BP, et al. National standards for diabetes self-management education. *Diabetes Care.* 2008;31(Suppl 1):S97-S104.
24. American Association of Diabetes Educators. AADE guidelines for the practice of diabetes self-management education and training (DSME/T). Chicago: American Association of Diabetes Educators; 2010.

FURTHER READING AND RESOURCES

American Association of Diabetes Educators. www.diabeteseducator.org

American Diabetes Association. www.diabetes.org

Diabetes.com. www.diabetes.com

National Institute of Diabetes and Digestive and Kidney Diseases. www.niddk.nih.gov

The preceding organizations are dedicated to providing the most current information about the evaluation, treatment, and prevention of diabetes. These Web sites are excellent resources for both health care professionals and patients.

Waryasz GR, McDermott AY. Exercise prescription and the patient with type 2 diabetes: a clinical approach to optimizing patient outcomes. *J Am Acad Nurse Pract.* 2010;22(4):217-227.

CHAPTER 21

Kidney Disease

KEY CONCEPTS

- Kidney disease interferes with the normal capacity of nephrons to filter the waste products of metabolism.
- Short-term kidney disease requires basic nutrition support for healing rather than dietary restriction.
- The progressive degeneration of chronic kidney disease requires dialysis treatment and nutrient modification in accordance with each individual's disease status.
- Current therapy for kidney stones depends more on basic nutrition and health support for medical treatment than on major food and nutrient restrictions.

More than 100,000 Americans are diagnosed with end-stage renal disease (ESRD) annually, and this results in 84,000 deaths per year.[1] Decreased kidney function often goes undiagnosed. A review of the National Health and Nutrition Examination Survey found that less than 6% of individuals with compromised kidney function were aware of their condition.[2] These kidney problems are costly as a result of lost work, time, pay, and quality of life.

This chapter looks at the nutrition care of people with kidney disease and primarily focuses on the extensive medical nutrition therapy (MNT) of chronic kidney disease (CKD). Dialysis extends the lives of patients with this irreversible disease; however, it does so at an emotional, physical, and financial cost.

BASIC STRUCTURE AND FUNCTION OF THE KIDNEY

Tremendous quantities of fluid (approximately 1.2 L) are filtered through the kidneys every minute. Most of this fluid is reabsorbed back into the vascular system to maintain circulating blood volume. As the blood circulates through the kidneys, these twin organs repeatedly "launder" it to monitor and maintain its quantity and quality. Indeed, the composition of various body fluids is determined not as much by what the mouth takes in as by what the kidneys keep; they are the master chemists of the internal environment.

Structures

The basic functional unit of the kidney is the nephron. Each human kidney is made up of approximately 1 million nephrons, all of which are independently capable of forming urine. Key parts of the nephron include the glomerulus and the tubules (Figure 21-1).

Glomerulus

At the head of each nephron, a cup-shaped membrane referred to as Bowman's capsule holds the entering blood capillary and its clump of smaller vessels. Within Bowman's capsule, the afferent arteriole branches into a

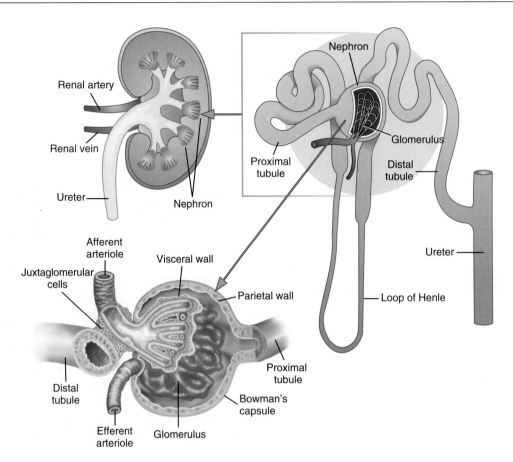

Figure 21-1 Anatomy of the kidney. (*Top,* Reprinted from Peckenpaugh NJ: *Nutrition essentials and diet therapy,* ed 10, Philadelphia, 2002; *Bottom,* reprinted from Thibodeau GA, Patton KT. *Anatomy & physiology.* 6th ed. St. Louis: Mosby; 2007.)

cluster of capillaries to form the glomerulus (see Figure 21-1). Only the larger blood proteins and cells remain behind in the circulating blood as it leaves the glomerulus via the efferent arteriole. The rate at which blood is filtered through the glomerulus, which is called the *glomerular filtration rate* (GFR), is the preferred method for monitoring kidney function and for defining stages of kidney disease. CKD is defined as a GFR of less than 60 mL/min (adjusted to a standard body surface area of 1.73 m²) for 3 or more months or a urinary albumin-to-creatinine ratio of more than 30 mg/g.[3]

Tubules

From the cupped head of each nephron, a small tubule carries the filtered fluid through its winding pathway and empties into the central area of the kidney medulla. Specific substances are reabsorbed and secreted along the way in each of the four parts of these tubules (Table 21-1).

Proximal Tubule. Most of the needed nutrients are reabsorbed in this first part of the tubule and returned to the blood. The surface area of the tubule is greatly

dialysis the process of separating crystalloids (i.e., crystal-forming substances) and colloids (i.e., glue-like substances) in solution by the difference in their rates of diffusion through a semipermeable membrane; crystalloids (e.g., blood glucose, other simple metabolites) pass through readily, and colloids (e.g., plasma proteins) pass through slowly or not at all.

nephron the functional unit of the kidney that filters and reabsorbs essential blood constituents, secretes hydrogen ions as needed to maintain the acid-base balance, reabsorbs water, and forms and excretes a concentrated urine for the elimination of wastes.

Bowman's capsule the membrane at the head of each nephron; this capsule was named for the English physician Sir William Bowman, who in 1843 first established the basis of plasma filtration and consequent urine secretion in the relationship of the blood-filled glomeruli and the filtration across the enveloping membrane.

TABLE 21-1 **REABSORPTION AND SECRETION IN PARTS OF THE NEPHRON**

Part	Function	Substance Moved
Proximal tubule	Reabsorption (active)	Sodium, glucose, amino acids
	Reabsorption (passive)	Chloride, phosphate, urea, water, other solutes
Loop of Henle		
Descending limb	Reabsorption (passive)	Water
	Secretion (passive)	Urea
Ascending limb	Reabsorption (active)	Sodium
	Reabsorption (passive)	Chloride
Distal tubule	Reabsorption (active)	Sodium
	Reabsorption (passive)	Chloride, other anions, water (in the presence of antidiuretic hormone)
	Secretion (passive)	Ammonia
	Secretion (active)	Potassium, hydrogen, some drugs
Collecting duct	Reabsorption (active)	Sodium
	Reabsorption (passive)	Urea, water (in the presence of antidiuretic hormone)
	Secretion (passive)	Ammonia
	Secretion (active)	Potassium, hydrogen, some drugs

From Thibodeau GA, Patton KT. *Anatomy & physiology*. 6th ed. St Louis: Mosby; 2007.

increased by a brush border membrane that contains thousands of microvilli. Glucose and amino acids as well as approximately 80% of the water and other substances are usually reabsorbed here. Approximately 20% of the filtered fluid remains to enter the next section of the tube.

Loop of Henle. The tubule's midsection narrows and dips down into the central part of the kidney. Here, the important exchange of sodium, chloride, and water occurs. This fluid environment maintains the necessary osmotic pressure to concentrate the urine as it passes through the distal tubule and ureter on its way to the bladder for elimination.

Distal Tubule. The latter part of the tubule winds back up into the outer area of the kidney cortex. Here, the

secretion of hydrogen ions occurs as needed to control the acid-base balance. Sodium is also reabsorbed as needed under the influence of the adrenal hormone aldosterone.

Collecting Tubule. In this final section of the tubule, concentrated urine is produced by the following water-reabsorbing actions: (1) the influence of the antidiuretic hormone; and (2) the osmotic pressure from the more dense surrounding fluid in the central area of the kidney. The urine, which is now concentrated and ready for excretion, only amounts to 0.5% to 1% of the original fluid and materials that have been filtered through the glomerulus.

Function

Nephron structure is adapted in fine detail to balance the internal fluids that are necessary for life. At birth, each person has far more nephrons than are actually needed, but they are gradually lost with advancing age. Diabetes and long-term use of high-protein diets tend to exacerbate damage to the glomerulus and to increase the rate of lost functioning nephrons.[4]

Excretory and Regulatory Functions

The following tasks are performed while blood flows through the nephron:

- *Filtration:* Most particles in blood are filtered out, except for the larger components of red blood cells and proteins.
- *Reabsorption:* As the filtrate continues through the winding tubules, substances that the body needs are

glomerulus the first section of the nephron; a cluster of capillary loops that are cupped in the nephron head that serves as an initial filter.

glomerular filtration rate (GFR) the volume of fluid that is filtered from the renal glomerular capillaries into Bowman's capsule per unit of time; this term is used clinically as a measure of kidney function.

aldosterone a hormone of the adrenal glands that acts on the distal nephron tubule to stimulate the reabsorption of sodium in an ion exchange with potassium; the aldosterone mechanism is essentially a sodium-conserving mechanism, but it also indirectly conserves water, because water absorption follows sodium resorption.

antidiuretic hormone a hormone of the pituitary gland that acts on the distal nephron tubule to conserve water by reabsorption; also called *vasopressin*.

selectively reabsorbed and returned to the blood to maintain the electrolyte, acid-base, and fluid balances.

- *Secretion:* Along the tubules, additional hydrogen ions are secreted as needed to maintain the acid-base balance.
- *Excretion:* Waste materials are excreted in the now-concentrated urine.

Endocrine Functions

In addition to major functions in the regulation of the blood constituents and the making and excreting of concentrated urine, the kidneys perform the following other functions:

- *Renin secretion:* When the arteriole pressure falls, the kidneys activate and secrete renin, which is an enzyme that initiates the renin-angiotensin-aldosterone mechanism to reabsorb sodium and to maintain hormonal control of the body water balance (see Chapter 9).
- *Erythropoietin secretion:* The kidneys are responsible for producing the body's major supply (80% to 90%) of erythropoietin, which is a circulating hormone that is the principal factor in stimulating red blood cell production within the bone marrow in response to decreased tissue oxygen.
- *Vitamin D activation:* The kidneys convert an intermediate inactive form of vitamin D into the final active vitamin D hormone in the proximal tubules of the nephrons (see Chapter 7). This action is stimulated by the parathyroid hormone.

DISEASE PROCESS AND DIETARY CONSIDERATIONS

General Causes of Kidney Disease

Several disease conditions may interfere with the normal functioning of nephrons and result in kidney disease.

Infection and Obstruction

Symptoms of bacterial urinary tract infection may range from the mild discomfort of bladder infections to more involved chronic disease and obstruction from kidney stones. Obstruction anywhere in the urinary tract blocks drainage and may cause further infection and general tissue damage.

Damage From Other Diseases

Diabetes mellitus is the leading cause of ESRD in the United States[1] (Figure 21-2). Hyperglycemia and hypertension associated with diabetes can damage small renal

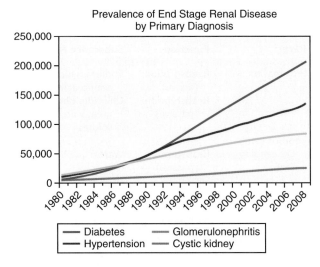

Figure 21-2 Prevalence of chronic kidney disease by primary diagnosis. (Data from the US Renal Data System. *USRDS 2010 annual data report: atlas of chronic kidney disease and end-stage renal disease in the United States.* Bethesda, Md: National Institutes of Health, National Institute of Diabetes and Digestive and Kidney Diseases; 2010.)

arteries, thereby leading to glomerulosclerosis (i.e., the loss of functioning nephrons) and eventual CKD.[5] Circulatory disorders such as prolonged and poorly controlled hypertension can cause the degeneration of the small arteries within the kidney and interfere with normal nephron function. More than 80% of patients with advanced CKD have hypertension.[1] Increased demands on other nephrons may in turn cause further hypertension and additional damage to nephrons. Other major causes are glomerulonephritis and cystic kidney disease. Autoimmune diseases such as systemic lupus erythematosus may also lead to compromised function or kidney disease.

Toxins

Various environmental agents (e.g., chemical pesticides, solvents), animal venom, certain plants, heavy metals, and some drugs (e.g., nonsteroidal anti-inflammatory drugs, aminoglycoside antibiotics, radiographic contrast dye) are nephrotoxic and can cause kidney damage.

---

arteriole the smallest branch of an artery that connects with the capillaries.

erythropoietin hormone that stimulates the production of red blood cells in the bone marrow.

nephrotoxic poisonous to the kidney.

Genetic or Congenital Defects

Cystic diseases (e.g., polycystic kidney disease, medullary cystic disease) are genetically linked kidney diseases that often lead to ESRD later in life. Congenital abnormalities of both kidneys can contribute to kidney disease with extensive distortion of kidney structure. Individuals who are born with only one kidney do not necessarily have kidney disease or even impaired function. People with a single kidney are often unaware of the fact and usually lead full lives without compromised kidney function.

Risk Factors

Risks for CKD are higher among individuals who have diabetes, hypertension, or cardiovascular disease (CVD); who are older than 60 years old; who smoke or are obese; and who have a family history of kidney disease. Malnutrition can exacerbate the rate of renal tissue destruction and increase susceptibility to infection. The prevalence of CKD is also higher among individuals with low income or education and among racial and ethnic minority populations.[6] Box 21-1 lists risk factors and common causes of kidney disease.

Medical Nutrition Therapy in Kidney Disease

During the treatment of kidney disease, appropriate MNT is based on the severity of the disease, the GFR, the presence of metabolic abnormalities, and the medical treatment (e.g., renal replacement therapy, medications).

Length of Disease

During short-term acute disease that results from infection, drug therapy with antibiotics usually controls the disease. Nutrition therapy is aimed at optimal nutrition support for healing and normal growth. More specific nutrient modifications may be necessary if the patient is a child or if the disease progresses to become chronic.

Degree of Impaired Kidney Function and Clinical Symptoms

For milder acute disease with few nephrons involved, less interference occurs with general kidney function, because the large number of backup nephrons can meet basic needs. However, with progressive chronic disease, more and more nephrons become involved, which results in CKD. In such cases, extensive MNT is required to help maintain kidney function as long as possible. With continuing disease, nutrient modifications are designed to meet individual needs to address clinical symptoms.

BOX 21-1   RISK FACTORS AND COMMON CAUSES OF KIDNEY DISEASE

Sociodemographic Factors
- Older age
- Family history of chronic kidney disease
- Member of racial or ethnic minority group
- Exposure to certain chemical and environmental conditions
- Low income or education level

Clinical Factors
- Poor glycemic control in diabetes
- Hypertension
- Autoimmune disease
- Systemic infection
- Urinary tract infection
- Urinary stones
- Lower urinary tract obstruction
- History of acute kidney injury
- Reduction in kidney mass
- Exposure to certain nephrotoxic drugs
- Low birth weight or hereditary diseases

From Levey AS, Eckart KU, Tsukamoto Y, et al. Definition and classification of chronic kidney disease: a position statement from Kidney Disease: Improving Global Outcomes (KDIGO). *Kidney Int.* 2005;67(6):2089-2100.

Working closely with a registered dietitian for personalized nutrition therapy is especially important when advanced kidney disease is treated with dialysis.

This chapter's discussion focuses primarily on the serious degenerative process of CKD and dialysis that requires MNT. Clinical practice guidelines are discussed for each type of kidney disease in the following sections.

NEPHRON DISEASES

Acute Glomerulonephritis or Nephritic Syndrome

Disease Process

This inflammatory process affects the glomeruli, which are the small blood vessels in the cupped membrane at the head of the nephron. Glomerulonephritis is one of the three most common causes of stage 5 CKD, which is also known as *ESRD.*[1]

Clinical Symptoms

Classic symptoms include hematuria and proteinuria, although edema and mild hypertension also may occur. These patients may experience anorexia in advanced stages, which contributes to feeding problems and

TABLE 21-2 **GLOMERULAR SYNDROMES**

Syndrome	Clinical Manifestations
Acute nephritic syndrome	Hematuria, azotemia, variable proteinuria, oliguria, edema, and hypertension
Rapidly progressive glomerulonephritis	Acute nephritis, proteinuria, and acute kidney failure
Nephrotic syndrome	> 3.5 g proteinuria, hypoalbuminemia, hyperlipidemia, and lipiduria
Chronic kidney failure	Azotemia and uremia that progress for years
Asymptomatic hematuria or proteinuria	Glomerular hematuria and subnephrotic proteinuria

From Kumar V, Fausto N, Abbas A. *Robbins and Cotran pathologic basis of disease*. 7th ed. Philadelphia: Saunders; 2005.

malnutrition. If the disease progresses to more kidney involvement, signs of oliguria or anuria may develop. Table 21-2 outlines the five glomerular syndromes and their respective clinical manifestations.

Medical Nutrition Therapy

Nephrologists and dietitians favor overall optimal nutrition support for growth with adequate protein. Diet modifications are not crucial in most patients with acute short-term disease. Fluid intake is adjusted to output and insensible losses.

Nephrotic Syndrome

Disease Process

Nephrotic syndrome or nephrosis results from nephron tissue damage to the major filtering membrane of the glomerulus, thereby allowing protein to pass into the tubule. This high protein concentration may cause further damage to the tubule. Both filtration and reabsorption functions of the nephron are disrupted. Nephrosis may be caused by infection, medications, neoplasms, preeclampsia, progressive glomerulonephritis, or diseases such as diabetes and systemic lupus erythematosus.

Clinical Symptoms

Nephrotic syndrome is characterized by a group of symptoms that result from nephron tissue damage and impaired function. The large protein losses (i.e., 3.5 g/day or more in adults) lead to hypoalbuminemia, edema, and ascites. The abdomen becomes distended as fluid accumulates, and the plasma protein level is greatly reduced because of losses in the urine. As protein loss continues, tissue proteins are broken down, and general malnutrition follows. Severe edema and ascites often mask the extent of body

tissue wasting. Other clinical manifestations include hyperlipidemia and lipiduria.

Medical Nutrition Therapy

Diets with moderate amounts of protein reduce albuminuria and albumin catabolism, with no change in the GFR. Nutrition therapy is directed toward controlling major symptoms and replacing the nutrients that are lost in the urine. Current standards of care are as follows[7]:

- *Protein:* The diet is usually moderate in protein (0.8 to 1.0 g/kg of body weight/day), with at least 50% of the protein from high biologic value sources, including soy protein. Total protein intake may be modified on the basis of blood urea nitrogen and GFR results. If blood urea nitrogen is elevated and urine output is decreased, dietary protein may be restricted.
- *Energy:* Total energy intake should be adequate to support nutrition status. Needs may be as high as 35 kcal/kg/day. To provide sufficient energy in kilocalories, complex carbohydrates should be given liberally, which also helps to combat the catabolism of tissue protein and to prevent starvation ketosis.

---

hematuria the abnormal presence of blood in the urine.

proteinuria an abnormal excess of serum proteins (e.g., albumin) in the urine.

edema the excess accumulation of fluid in the body tissues.

oliguria the secretion of small amounts of urine in relation to fluid intake (i.e., 0.5 mL/kg per hour or less).

anuria the absence of urine production; anuria indicates kidney shutdown or failure.

nephrosis degenerative lesions of the renal tubules of the nephrons and especially of the thin basement membrane of the glomerulus that helps to support the capillary loops; marked by edema, albuminuria, and a decreased serum albumin level.

ascites the accumulation of serous fluid (i.e., blood and lymph serum) in the abdominal cavity.

lipiduria lipid droplets found in the urine that are composed mostly of cholesterol esters.

blood urea nitrogen a test of nephron function that measures the ability to filter urea nitrogen, which is a product of protein metabolism, from the blood.

ketosis the accumulation of ketones, which are intermediate products of fat metabolism, in the blood.

Decreasing the dietary intake of fat and cholesterol may help to alleviate dyslipidemia and the resulting risk for CVD. Total fat intake should not exceed 30% total kcals/day, 7% of kcals or less should come from saturated fat, cholesterol intake should not exceed 200 mg/day, trans fats should be limited, and up to 10% of kcals should come from polyunsaturated fats, including fish.

- *Sodium and potassium:* Edema is common among patients with glomerular diseases. To reduce symptoms, a sodium restriction of 1 to 2 g/day is advised to maintain the sodium and fluid balance. Sodium overload is difficult to treat because of the characteristic hypoalbuminuria and hypotension; therefore, careful monitoring is necessary. The renal clearance of potassium is impaired with oliguria. Thus, potassium intake must be monitored and carefully adjusted in accordance with individual needs.

- *Calcium and phosphorus:* Some calcium is bound to albumin in the blood. As albumin is lost through the tubule, bound calcium is also lost. In addition, low serum vitamin D decreases calcium absorption. Thus, the recommendations are to consume 1 to 1.5 g of calcium per day and to limit phosphorus to 12 mg/kg/day.

- *Fluid:* Fluid intake may be restricted in response to urine output and insensible losses. If restriction is not indicated, fluids can be consumed as desired.

KIDNEY FAILURE

The two types of kidney failure—acute and chronic—have a number of symptoms that reflect interference with normal nephron functions in nutrient metabolism. Both forms are addressed with similar nutrition therapy, depending on the extent of renal tissue damage and the treatment method used.

Acute Kidney Injury

Disease Process

Healthy kidneys may suddenly shut down after metabolic insult or traumatic injury, thereby causing a life-threatening situation. Baseline risk factors for the development of in-hospital acute kidney injury (also known as *acute renal failure*) include older age, diabetes, underlying renal insufficiency, and heart or liver failure.[8] This is a medical emergency in which the dietitian and the nurse play important supportive roles. Depending on the underlying cause, acute kidney injury (AKI) is divided into three categories[7]:

1. *Prerenal:* Prerenal AKI involves inadequate blood flow to the kidneys and subsequent reduced GFR. Common causes include severe dehydration, hypotension, shock, congestive heart failure, and renal vasoconstriction or occlusion.

2. *Intrinsic:* Intrinsic AKI results from damage to a part of the kidney. Common causes include hypertension, infection, acute tubular necrosis or interstitial nephritis, obstruction, or nephrotoxicity from antibiotics, antimicrobial agents, or other drugs.

3. *Postrenal obstruction:* Postrenal obstruction involves the obstruction of urine flow. Common causes include benign prostatic hypertrophy with urinary retention, cancer, ureteral stones, and other obstructions.

AKI can last from days to weeks, with normal function returning when the condition that is causing the failure is resolved. Depending on the extent of renal tissue damage, regaining full function may take months. However, some individuals do not regain normal kidney function, and the disease then progresses to CKD. Patients with a particularly high risk for advancing to CKD are those with diabetes, those of advanced age, those with low serum albumin levels, and those with severe AKI (i.e., chiefly those who require dialysis).[9]

Clinical Symptoms

AKI is classified according to the RIFLE classification system, which assesses the severity of **R**isk, **I**njury, **F**ailure, and the outcomes of either **L**oss or **E**SRD.[10] The major sign of AKI is an increase in serum creatinine levels and oliguria, which is caused when cellular debris from the tissue damage blocks the tubules. Diminished urine output may be accompanied by proteinuria or hematuria. Researchers are working to define more sensitive markers for diagnosing AKI, because there are weaknesses involved in the use of the traditional markers of creatinine and urine output.[11] Other symptoms include nausea, vomiting, fatigue, muscle weakness, swelling in the lower extremities, itchy skin, and confusion. Water balance also becomes a crucial factor. Continuous renal replacement therapy, which is a type of dialysis, may be needed to support kidney function.

Medical Nutrition Therapy

Basic Objectives. The major challenge during AKI is to improve or maintain nutrition status while the patient

---

hypotension   low blood pressure.

creatinine   a nitrogen-carrying product of normal tissue protein breakdown; it is excreted in the urine; serum creatinine levels are an indicator of renal function.

is faced with marked catabolism. Current standards indicate the need for highly individualized therapy that is focused on the following: (1) treating the underlying cause; (2) preventing further kidney damage and complications from nutrient deficiencies; and (3) correcting any fluid, electrolyte, or uremic abnormalities.[7] Loss of appetite is common, and enteral nutrition may be required. If enteral nutrition is contraindicated, parenteral nutrition may then be necessary (see Chapter 22).

Principles. Preventing protein catabolism, electrolyte and hydration disturbances, acidosis, and uremic toxicity through individualized MNT is thought to play a role in maintaining kidney function while reducing the complications of CVD and progressive kidney deterioration.[12] General recommendations for AKI are presented below. Keep in mind that kidney function and treatment modality may vary greatly among patients; thus, MNT should be adjusted accordingly.[7]

- *Protein:* Adequate protein is important for supporting kidney function and for preserving lean tissue. For patients who are not receiving dialysis and who are not experiencing catabolism, a protein intake of 0.8 to 1.2 g/kg is recommended. For patients who are experiencing catabolism or who are on dialysis, 1.2 to 1.5 g/kg of daily protein is recommended to allow for nutrient replenishment and to account for losses.
- *Energy:* Energy intake in the range of 25 to 35 kcal/kg is suggested. This amount needs to be adjusted on an individual basis, depending on metabolic stress and the nutritional status of the patient. If the patient is on dialysis, energy intake from the dialysate should be included in the total energy intake.
- *Sodium and potassium:* During a diuretic phase, patients may lose excessive electrolytes. Losses of both sodium and potassium (2 to 3 g/day each) should be replaced during this phase. These levels are further adjusted depending on blood pressure and the presence of edema.
- *Phosphate and calcium:* Dietary phosphorus intake is determined on the basis of body weight, with a range of 8 to 15 mg/kg of phosphorus. The MNT goal for calcium is to maintain serum value levels within normal limits and to adjust dietary intake accordingly.
- *Vitamins and minerals:* A patient's diet should be balanced to prevent nutrient deficiencies by meeting the Dietary Reference Intakes for all other vitamins and minerals. If the patient is experiencing catabolism or other complications, nutrient intakes may be modified to meet specific needs.

- *Fluid:* Individual fluid needs are highly variable with AKI, and treatment modality, hydration, and fluid loss should be considered. Insensible fluid loss may increase as a result of fever, and sensible fluid loss (e.g., urine output, vomit, diarrhea) will vary considerably among patients. A starting point recommendation is 500 mL of fluid plus urine output daily.

Chronic Kidney Disease

Disease Process

CKD is caused by the progressive breakdown of kidney tissue, which impairs all kidney functions. Few functioning nephrons remain and they gradually deteriorate. CKD develops slowly, and no cure exists.

CKD is most commonly a result of the following:
- Primary glomerular disease
- Metabolic diseases with kidney involvement (e.g., diabetes, hypertension, CVD)
- Inherited diseases (e.g., polycystic kidney disease, congenital abnormality)
- Other causes: immune disease such as lupus, obstructions such as kidney stones, chronic urinary tract infections, and hypertension

Modifiable risk factors include controlling blood pressure, proteinuria, or albuminuria; addressing the HbA1C level and dyslipidemia; and quitting smoking.[6,13] In its clinical practice guidelines, the National Kidney Foundation categorizes CKD into five stages on the basis of the GFR (Table 21-3).

TABLE 21-3 STAGES OF CHRONIC KIDNEY DISEASE

Stage	Description	Glomerular Filtration Rate (mL/min/1.73 m²)
1	Kidney damage with normal or elevated GFR	≥ 90
2	Kidney damage with mild decrease in GFR	60 to 89
3	Moderate decrease in GFR	30 to 59
4	Severely decreased GFR	15 to 29
5	Kidney failure or end-stage renal disease	< 15 (or dialysis)

GFR, Glomerular filtration rate.
Chronic kidney disease is defined as either kidney damage or a glomerular filtration rate of less than 60 mL/min per 1.73 m² for 3 or more months. Kidney damage is defined as pathologic abnormalities or markers of damage, including abnormalities in blood or urine tests or imaging studies.
From Levey AS, Eckart KU, Tsukamoto Y, et al. Definition and classification of chronic kidney disease: a position statement from Kidney Disease: Improving Global Outcomes (KDIGO). *Kidney Int.* 2005;67(6):2089-2100.

Clinical Symptoms

Depending on the nature of the underlying kidney disease, chronic kidney changes may involve the extensive scarring of renal tissue, which distorts the kidney structure and brings vascular changes as a result of prolonged hypertension. As nephrons are lost one by one, the remaining nephrons gradually lose their ability to sustain metabolic balance.

Water Balance. During the early stages of chronic kidney failure, the kidneys are unable to reabsorb water or to properly concentrate urine. Therefore, large amounts of dilute urine are produced (i.e., polyuria). Dehydration is a risk factor at this point, and it may become critical. As the disease progresses, urine production declines to a point of oliguria and finally anuria. Without the urinary excretion of waste products, dangerous levels of urea accumulate in the blood.

Electrolyte Balance. Several imbalances among electrolytes result from decreasing nephron function. The failing kidney cannot appropriately maintain the vital sodium and potassium balance that guards body water (see Chapter 9). A concentration of materials (e.g., phosphate, sulfate, organic acids) is produced by the metabolism of nutrients. Without appropriate filtering, these materials accumulate in the blood, thereby causing metabolic acidosis. The disturbed metabolism of calcium and phosphorus, the abnormal levels of parathyroid hormone, and the lack of activated vitamin D (a process that occurs in the kidneys) leads to bone pain, abnormal bone metabolism, and chronic kidney disease-mineral and bone disorder or osteodystrophy.

Nitrogen Retention. An increasing loss of nephron function results in elevated nitrogenous metabolites such as urea and creatinine. Protein-energy malnutrition is a common complication of protein catabolism.

Anemia. The damaged kidney cannot accomplish its normal initiation of red blood cell production through erythropoietin. Therefore, fewer red blood cells are produced, and those that are produced have a decreased survival time.

Hypertension. When blood flow to the kidney tissues is increasingly impaired, renal hypertension develops. In turn, hypertension causes cardiovascular damage and the further deterioration of the nephrons.

Azotemia. Elevated blood urea nitrogen, serum creatinine, and serum uric acid levels are reflected in the characteristic laboratory finding of azotemia.

General Signs and Symptoms

Increasing loss of kidney function causes progressive weakness, shortness of breath, general lethargy, and fatigue. Thirst, anorexia, weight loss, diarrhea, and vomiting may occur. Increasing capillary fragility may cause skin, nose, oral, and gastrointestinal bleeding. Nervous system involvement brings muscular twitching, burning sensations in the extremities, and convulsions. Irregular cyclic breathing (i.e., Cheyne-Stokes respiration) indicates acidosis. Acidosis may cause mouth ulcers, a foul taste, and bad breath in the patient. Malnutrition lowers resistance to infection, and some patients may experience bone and joint pain.

Medical Nutrition Therapy

Basic Objectives. Treatment must always be individual and adjusted according to the progression of the illness, the type of treatment, and the patient's response. The Kidney Disease Outcomes Quality Initiative dietary guidelines recommend monitoring the nutrition status of patients with CKD at regular intervals: every 1 to 3 months for patients with a GFR of less than 30 mL/min per 1.73 m^2 and every 6 to 12 months for patients with a GFR of 30 to 59 mL/min per 1.73 m^2 to identify anorexia and to help prevent malnutrition.[14]

Principles. Nutrition for CKD involves several nutrient adjustments that should be made in accordance with individual need. The MNT recommendations for patients with CKD are as follows[7]:

- *Protein:* The goal is to provide adequate protein to maintain tissue integrity while avoiding excess. Protein is generally limited to 0.6 to 0.8 g/kg/day for individuals who are not on dialysis with a GFR of less than 50 mL/min per 1.73 m^2. Patients with GFRs of

---

dialysate the cleansing solution used in dialysis; contains dextrose and other chemicals similar to those in the body.

chronic kidney disease-mineral and bone disorder a clinical syndrome that develops as a systemic disorder of mineral and bone metabolism in patients with chronic kidney disease; results from abnormalities of calcium, phosphorus, parathyroid hormone, or vitamin D metabolism; causes abnormalities in bone turnover, mineralization, volume, linear growth, strength, and soft-tissue calcification.

osteodystrophy an alteration of bone morphology found in patients with chronic kidney disease.

urea the chief nitrogen-carrying product of dietary protein metabolism; urea appears in the blood, lymph, and urine.

azotemia an excess of urea and other nitrogenous substances in the blood.

less than 20 mL/min per 1.73 m^2 may be limited to dietary protein of 0.3 to 0.5 g/kg/day with additional keto acid analogs (i.e., nitrogen-free copies of essential amino acids) to meet protein requirements.[15] At least 50% of this amount should come from high biologic value protein (see Chapter 4) to ensure an adequate intake of essential amino acids.

- *Energy:* Carbohydrate and fat must provide sufficient nonprotein kilocalories to supply energy and spare protein for tissue synthesis. For individuals who are younger than 60 years old with CKD and GFRs of less than 25 mL/min per 1.73 m^2, the recommended energy intake is 35 kcal/kg/day. Energy needs are less for individuals who are 60 years old or older (30 to 35 kcal/kg/day). Because cardiovascular disease is accelerated in patients with CKD, the remaining calories should support cardiovascular health principles (e.g., substitute monounsaturated and polyunsaturated fats for saturated and trans fats, reduce total cholesterol intake; see Chapter 19).

- *Sodium and potassium:* If hypertension and edema are present, sodium intake must be restricted. Sodium intake is usually limited to 1 to 3 g/day. As CKD advances, potassium is not cleared adequately from the blood. Dietary intake is determined by assessing laboratory values. If blood levels of potassium are elevated and other nondietary causes are eliminated, then a potassium-restricted diet may be indicated.

- *Phosphorus and calcium:* Inappropriate blood phosphorus and calcium levels negatively affect bone composition. As the kidney loses function, the activation of vitamin D and the control of blood calcium levels decline. This problem is worsened by excess blood phosphorus, which results in calcium resorption from the bone. Thus, moderate dietary phosphorus restriction depends on laboratory values in the patient who is not undergoing dialysis, and it is generally limited to 800 to 1000 mg/day when serum phosphorus is 4.6 mg/dL or more or when the parathyroid hormone level is elevated. Calcium recommendations are 1.0 to 1.5 g/day and not to exceed 2 g/day, including both dietary and supplemental calcium sources.

- *Vitamins and minerals:* A protein-restricted diet does not contribute the full daily requirement of all essential nutrients (review the Clinical Applications box, "Case Study: A Patient with CKD"). Supplemental fat-soluble vitamins A and E are not recommended, because they may accumulate to toxic levels in patients with kidney failure. Excesses of vitamins D and K are contraindicated, because the kidney cannot convert vitamin D to its active form, and vitamin K can adversely affect clotting time. The specific MNT recommendations are to help patients meet their Dietary Reference Intakes for the B-complex vitamins and vitamin C and to determine the patient-specific needs for vitamin D, iron, and zinc.

- *Fluid:* Fluid intake should be sufficient to maintain adequate urine volume in patients who are not undergoing dialysis. Intake usually is balanced with output, and it is not otherwise restricted.

End-Stage Renal Disease

Disease Process

When CKD advances to its end stages, life-support decisions face the patient, the family, and the physician. ESRD occurs when the patient's GFR decreases to less than 15 mL/min per 1.73 m^2. This decrease is caused by irreversible damage to a majority of the kidneys' nephrons. At this point, the patient has two options: long-term kidney dialysis or kidney transplant. The lives of an estimated 500,000 people in the United States are prolonged by dialysis and kidney transplants annually.[1] Dialysis is the chief treatment for ESRD.

Two forms of dialysis are used: hemodialysis and peritoneal dialysis. For a thorough understanding of the treatment options that are available for ESRD, please refer to the article listed in the "Further Reading and Resources" section at the end of this chapter.

Treatment Options and Respective Medical Nutrition Therapy

Hemodialysis. Hemodialysis is the use of an "artificial kidney machine" to remove toxic substances from the blood and to restore nutrients and metabolites to normal blood levels (Figure 21-3). To prepare a patient for hemodialysis therapy, vascular access must be established. This procedure ideally takes place 4 to 16 weeks before treatments begin to allow for adequate healing. The three basic kinds of vascular access for hemodialysis are arteriovenous fistula, arteriovenous graft, and a venous catheter (Figure 21-4). An arteriovenous fistula is the preferred access for long-term dialysis, and it is made by joining an artery and a vein on the forearm just beneath the skin.[16] After the fistula has healed, a cannula (i.e., a large-bore needle) is inserted through the tissue and connected by tubes to the dialysis machine.

A patient with ESRD who is on hemodialysis usually receives three treatments per week, each of which lasts 3

CLINICAL APPLICATIONS

CASE STUDY: A PATIENT WITH CHRONIC KIDNEY DISEASE

Gary, who is 49 years old, is an active man who works at a large company and has begun to tire more easily. He has little appetite, and he generally feels ill most of the time. He recently noticed some ankle swelling and blood in his urine. At his family's insistence, he finally decided to see his physician.

After a complete workup, the physician's findings included the following:

- No prior illness except a case of the flu with a throat infection during his overseas service in the Army
- Laboratory tests: presence of albumin, red blood cells, and white blood cells in the urine; high blood potassium, phosphorus, creatinine, and urea levels; and low glomerular filtration rate of 20 mL/min per 1.73 m^2
- Other symptoms: hypertension, edema in the lower legs, headache, occasional vision blurring, and low-grade fever

The physician discussed the findings and the serious prognosis of stage 4 chronic kidney disease with Gary and his wife. Together with the dietitian, they explored the immediate medical and nutrition needs for treatment. They also discussed the ultimate need for medical management with dialysis or transplantation. The physician prescribed medications to control Gary's growing symptoms and discomfort.

Over the next 10 months, Gary's symptoms worsened. He lost more weight, became anemic, and had increased bone and joint pain and gastrointestinal bleeding. Nausea increased, and he had occasional muscle twitching and spasms. Small mouth ulcers made eating a painful effort. Gary and his wife made an appointment with their dietitian to learn how to manage his present predialysis diet at home.

Questions for Analysis

1. What metabolic imbalances in chronic kidney disease do you think account for Gary's symptoms?
2. What are the objectives of the treatment of chronic kidney disease?
3. What are the basic principles of Gary's predialysis diet? Describe this type of diet. What foods would be included? Plan a 1-day menu for Gary with the use of the dietary analysis program that is included with this text.

---

to 4 hours. However, a recent study found that patients who were receiving hemodialysis up to six times per week with shorter sessions (i.e., about 2.5 hrs/each) experienced significant health benefits with no reported loss in quality of life as a result of the frequency of treatments. However, the patients who received frequent hemodialysis in this study did require more interventions related to vascular access.[17]

During each treatment, the patient's blood makes several complete cycles through the dialyzer, which removes excess waste to maintain normal blood levels of life-sustaining substances, a function the patient's own kidneys can no longer accomplish. Two compartments in the machine are separated by a filter. One compartment contains blood from the patient with all of the excess fluids and waste; the other contains the dialysate, which is a type of "cleaning fluid." As during normal capillary filtration, the blood cells are too large to pass through the pores in the filter. However, the remaining smaller molecules in the blood pass through the filter and are carried away by the dialysate. If the patient's blood is deficient in certain nutrients, these may be added to the dialysate.

Medical Nutrition Therapy for Hemodialysis. The diet of a patient who is undergoing hemodialysis is an important aspect of maintaining biochemical control. Registered dietitians who specialize in renal care are heavily involved with meal planning and diet education.

The goal of the nutrition therapy during hemodialysis is to maintain optimal nutrition while preventing the buildup of waste products in between treatments. In most cases, MNT can be planned with more liberal nutrient allowances, as follows[7]:

- *Protein:* Protein energy malnutrition, as indicated by dietary intake and the biomarkers of protein status, is a major concern for patients on dialysis, and it is considered one of the most significant predictors of overall malnutrition and adverse outcomes.[18-20] For most adult patients on dialysis, a protein allowance of at least 1.2 g/kg is ideal to prevent protein malnutrition. This amount provides nutrition needs, maintains positive nitrogen balance, does not produce excessive nitrogenous waste, and replaces the amino acids that are lost during each dialysis treatment. At least 50% of this daily allowance should consist of protein foods of high biologic value (e.g., eggs, meat, fish, poultry).
- *Energy:* MNT recommendations for energy intake are 35 kcal/kg/day for individuals who are younger than 60 years old and 30 to 35 kcal/kg/day for individuals who are older than 60 years old. Interestingly, the mortality rate decreases as the body mass index increases above normal ranges (i.e., 23 kg/m^2 or more), purportedly as the result of a complex association between malnutrition and clinical

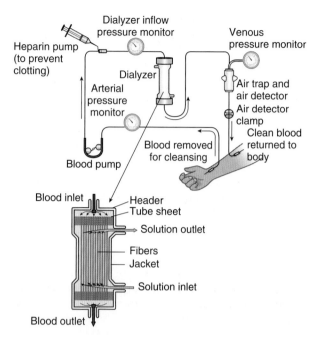

Figure 21-3 Hemodialysis cleans and filters blood with a special filter called a *dialyzer* that functions as an artificial kidney. Blood travels through tubes into the dialyzer, which filters out wastes and extra water, and then the cleaned blood flows through another set of tubes and back into the body. (From the National Institute of Diabetes and Digestive and Kidney Diseases. *Treatment methods for hemodialysis.* National Institutes of Health Publication No. 07-4666. Bethesda, Md: National Institutes of Health; 2006.)

outcomes.[21,22] The unfortunate combination is that ESRD is closely related to a decrease in appetite when the GFR falls below 60 mL/min per 1.73 m². A generous amount of carbohydrates with some fat continues to supply needed kilocalories for energy and protein sparing.

- *Sodium and potassium:* To control body fluid retention and hypertension, sodium is limited to 1 to 3 g/day. Sodium intake is not as stringently regulated for patients on dialysis as it is for those with CKD and not yet on dialysis, because the dialysis process rids the body of excess sodium. To prevent potassium accumulation, which can cause cardiac problems, intake is restricted to 2 to 3 g/day, with adjustments that are based on serum levels.
- *Phosphorus and calcium:* With careful monitoring to control for comorbid bone conditions such as chronic kidney disease-mineral and bone disorder, the dietary intake of phosphorus is limited to 800 to 1000 mg/day or 8 to 15 mg/kg when serum phosphorus levels exceed 5.5 mg/dL or when parathyroid hormone is elevated. Calcium intake should not exceed 2 g/day, including the amount received through medications such as binders.
- *Vitamins and minerals:* The general recommendation for all water-soluble vitamins is to achieve the Dietary Reference Intakes. Iron and vitamin D intake are individualized per patient on the basis of

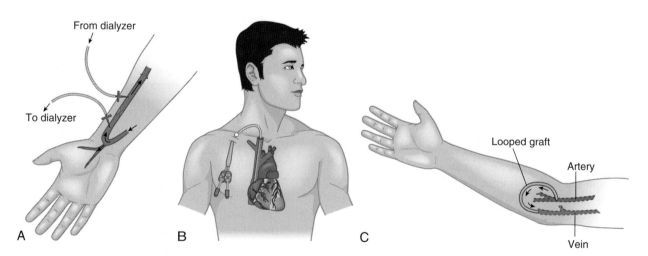

Figure 21-4 Types of access for hemodialysis. **A,** Forearm arteriovenous fistula. **B,** Venous catheter for temporary hemodialysis access. **C,** Artificial loop graft. (From the National Institute of Diabetes and Digestive and Kidney Diseases. *Kidney failure: choosing a treatment that's right for you.* National Institutes of Health Publication No. 00-2412. Bethesda, Md: National Institutes of Health; 2007.)

biochemical markers. Other micronutrients of special interest are as follows:

- Vitamin C: 60 to 100 mg/day
- Vitamin B_6: 2 mg/day
- Folate: 1 mg/day
- Vitamin B_{12}: 3 µg/day
- Vitamin E: 15 IU/day
- Zinc: 15 mg/day
- *Fluid:* Fluid intake is limited to 1000 mL/day plus an amount equal to urine output.

Peritoneal Dialysis. An alternative form of treatment is peritoneal dialysis, which has the convenience of mobility. Approximately 6% of patients with ESRD who are on dialysis use this form of dialysis.[1] During this process, the patient introduces the dialysate solution directly into the peritoneal cavity, where it can be exchanged for fluids that contain the metabolic waste products. Because this form of dialysis is continuous within the body, the process is called *continuous ambulatory peritoneal dialysis.*

First, the patient is prepared by surgically inserting a permanent catheter into the peritoneal cavity. Treatments are then carried out by doing the following: (1) attaching a disposable bag that contains the dialysate solution to the abdominal catheter, which leads into the peritoneal cavity; (2) allowing 4 to 6 hours for the solution exchange; (3) lowering the bag to allow gravity to pull the waste-containing fluid into it; and (4) repeating the procedure (Figure 21-5). When the bag is empty, it can be folded around the waist or tucked into a pocket to provide the patient with mobility. The intermittent use of peritoneal dialysis that is self-administered at home gives the patient a sense of control. An automated device is often used to

---

peritoneal cavity a serous membrane that lines the abdominal and pelvic walls and the undersurface of the diaphragm to form a sac that encloses the body's vital visceral organs.

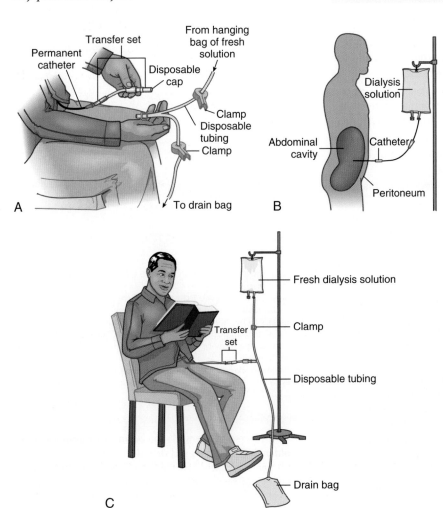

Figure 21-5 Continuous ambulatory peritoneal dialysis. **A,** A soft tube catheter is used to fill the abdomen with a cleansing dialysis solution. **B,** The walls of the abdominal cavity are lined with a peritoneal membrane that allows waste products and extra fluid to pass from the blood into the dialysis solution. **C,** Wastes and fluid then leave the body when the dialysis solution is drained. The time during which the dialysis solution remains in the abdominal cavity (i.e., dwell time) ranges from 4 to 6 hours, and the patient can be mobile during this time. An exchange takes approximately 30 to 40 minutes, and a typical schedule calls for four to five exchanges every day. (From the National Institute of Diabetes and Digestive and Kidney Diseases. *Treatment methods for kidney failure: peritoneal dialysis.* National Institutes of Health Publication No. 06-4688. Bethesda, Md: National Institutes of Health; 2006.)

provide several solution exchanges during sleep hours and one continuous exchange during the day for a technique that is called *continuous cyclic peritoneal dialysis*.

Medical Nutrition Therapy for Peritoneal Dialysis. A slightly more liberal diet may be used with peritoneal dialysis, as follows[7]:

- *Protein:* Increase protein intake slightly to at least 1.2 to 1.3 g/kg with at least 50% of that intake coming from foods with high biologic value protein.
- *Energy:* Maintain a lean body weight by accounting for the energy provided by the dialysate solution in the meal plan.
- *Sodium and potassium:* Sodium intake is slightly more liberal and contingent on fluid balance, with a recommended intake ranging from 2 to 4 g/day. Potassium may be increased to 3 to 4 g/day, depending on serum levels, by eating a wide variety of fruits and vegetables each day.
- *Phosphorus and calcium:* Recommendations for phosphorus and calcium intake remain the same as for hemodialysis: phosphorus, 800 to 1000 mg/day or 8 to 15 mg/kg when serum phosphorus levels exceed 5.5 mg/dL or when parathyroid hormone is elevated; calcium, less than 2 g/day, including the amount received through medications such as binders.
- *Vitamins and minerals:* All recommendations are the same as for hemodialysis, as described previously, with the following exception: patients may need 1.5 to 2 mg/day of thiamin (vitamin B_1) as a result of losses that occur during dialysis.
- *Fluid:* Fluid intake should be adequate to maintain balance.

Table 21-4 presents nutrition laboratory parameter outcome goals for patients with CKD who are either on hemodialysis or peritoneal dialysis.

Transplantation. Kidney transplantation, which is another treatment modality, improves affected individuals' quality of life and survival rates, and it is more cost effective than maintenance dialysis.[1,23] Kidney transplantation has several advantages. Current advances in surgical techniques, immunosuppressive drugs to prevent rejection, and antibiotics to control infection have helped to ensure successful outcomes (see the Drug-Nutrient Interaction box, "Immunosuppressive Therapies After Kidney Transplantation"). Patients who are undergoing kidney transplantation have significantly lower rates of CVD progression, despite the disadvantages of immunosuppressive therapy.

The difficulty with transplantation is that waiting lists can be long and donor matches difficult to find, even when using expanded-criteria donors (matches with more liberal criteria).[24] See the Cultural Considerations

TABLE 21-4   NUTRITION LABORATORY PARAMETER OUTCOME GOALS FOR STAGE 5 CHRONIC KIDNEY DISEASE (HEMODIALYSIS AND PERITONEAL DIALYSIS)

Nutrition Laboratory Parameter	Goal	Outcome Prevention Focus
Serum albumin (g/dL)	≥ 4.0	Protein energy malnutrition
Serum prealbumin (mg/dL)	> 30	Protein energy malnutrition
Predialysis serum creatinine (mg/dL)	> 10	Protein energy malnutrition
Serum cholesterol (mg/dL)	> 150 to 180	Protein energy malnutrition
	< 200	Hyperlipidemia
Hemodialysis Prognostic Nutrition Index	≥ 0.8	Increased mortality and morbidity rates
Subjective Global Assessment: 4-item, 7-point scale	≥ 6 to 7	Malnutrition
Serum phosphorus (mg/dL)	3.5 to 5.5	Bone disease
Serum calcium (mg/dL)	8.4 to 10.5	Bone disease
Serum calcium-phosphorus product	≤ 55	Bone disease
Serum bicarbonate (mmol/L)	≥ 22	Metabolic acidosis
Lipid Profile		
Low-density lipoprotein cholesterol (mg/dL)	< 100	Cardiovascular disease
High-density lipoprotein cholesterol (mg/dL)	> 40	Cardiovascular disease
Triglycerides (mg/dL)	< 150	Cardiovascular disease

Based on the Kidney Disease Outcome Quality Initiative recommendations.
Also applicable to stages 1 through 4 of chronic kidney disease, with individualization to the appropriate level of kidney function. Parameters to be monitored monthly, with the exception of the Hemodialysis Prognostic Nutrition Index, the Subjective Global Assessment (quarterly or when changes are indicated), and the lipid profile (annually).
From Beto JA, Bansal VK. Medical nutrition therapy in chronic kidney failure: integrating clinical practice guidelines. *J Am Diet Assoc.* 2004;104:404-409.

expanded-criteria donors any brain-dead donor who is older than 60 years old or a donor who is older than 50 years old with two of the following conditions: history of hypertension, a terminal serum creatinine level of at least 1.5 mg/dL, or death from a cerebrovascular accident.

DRUG-NUTRIENT INTERACTION

IMMUNOSUPPRESSIVE THERAPIES AFTER KIDNEY TRANSPLANTATION

The kidney is the most common solid organ that is transplanted worldwide, and the need for kidney transplantation has grown over the past decade. Survival after kidney transplant is largely dependent on a successful immunosuppressive regimen.[1] Several antirejection medications are used after an organ transplant. Most kidney transplant recipients undergo multidrug immunosuppressive therapy that includes corticosteroids to reduce the risk of acute rejection. Over time, the patient may be weaned from steroid use but continue on long-term maintenance regimens that include other antirejection medications. The use of corticosteroids is associated with a number of adverse side effects that specifically affect overall nutritional status, such as the following:

- Peptic ulcer disease
- Hypertension
- Hyperglycemia
- Bone disease
- Increased appetite and weight gain
- Growth retardation (in children)

Corticosteroids also increase the excretion of several nutrients. Additional consumption of vitamins A, B_6, and C; potassium; magnesium; zinc; and protein may be needed in the diet or as supplements. Supplemental calcium and vitamin D are recommended with long-term corticosteroid use. Other antirejection medications are often used concomitantly with corticosteroids, and these may also interact with some of these nutrients. For example, cyclosporine and tacrolimus (Prograf) are calcineurin inhibitors. These immunosuppressants may cause hyperkalemia; thus, high potassium intake from food or supplements should be avoided when these drugs are included in the drug regimen. When the patient is taking these medications, serum drug levels and electrolytes are monitored and the dosage is adjusted for optimal therapeutic benefit. Azathioprine (Imuran) and mycophenolate (CellCept) are other antirejection medications that do not have significant nutrient interactions, but they can cause nausea, vomiting, abdominal pain, and diarrhea in some patients. This can become a concern if the patient is unable to consume adequate nutrition, so the side effects are generally managed by reducing the dose.[2]

Research continues to explore more potent immunosuppressive regimens that avoid or reduce corticosteroid and cyclosporine use. In 2008, only 59% of patients were discharged on corticosteroids and 8% on cyclosporine compared with 96% and 63%, respectively, in 1999.[3] Newer therapies have been associated with fewer episodes of acute rejection, and steroid avoidance is associated with improved growth outcomes in children.[4,5] Further research is needed before new protocols can be accepted.

Kelli Boi

1. Wolfe RA, Roys EC, Merion RM. Trends in organ donation and transplantation in the United States, 1999-2008. *Am J Transplant*. 2010;10(4 Pt 2):961-972.
2. Peters TG. *Transplant drugs: medicines that prevent rejection* (website): www.aakp.org/aakp-library/Transplant-Drugs/. Accessed March 2011.
3. Axelrod DA, McCullough KP, Brewer ED, et al. Kidney and pancreas transplantation in the United States, 1999-2008: the changing face of living donation. *Am J Transplant*. 2010;10(4 Pt 2):987-1002.
4. Grenda R. Effects of steroid avoidance and novel protocols on growth in paediatric renal transplant patients. *Pediatr Nephrol*. 2010;25(4):747-752.
5. Heldal K, Hartmann A, Leivestad T, et al. Risk variables associated with the outcome of kidney recipients >70 years of age in the new millennium. *Nephrol Dial Transplant*. 2011;26(8):2706-2711.

box entitled "Cultural Disparities in Kidney Transplant Availability and Success in Certain Ethnic and Racial Groups" for more details.

MNT for patients who choose kidney transplantation will be highly individualized. Table 21-5 summarizes nutrition parameters for various levels of kidney disease and treatments.

Complications

Long-term complications of dialysis include bone disorders, malnutrition, anemia, hormonal and blood pressure imbalances, psychologic depression, and diminished quality of life as a result of constant dependence on treatments.

Nutrition Support. There are special considerations for patients on dialysis who are in medical need of nutrition support via enteral or parenteral feedings. A medical necessity of nutrition support usually means that the patient is experiencing severe malnutrition, inflammation, and anorexia. The type of and tolerance of dialysis must be considered when choosing an appropriate nutrition support modality, and the current GFR, metabolic state, stress, and nitrogen balance must also be considered. The American Society for Parenteral and Enteral Nutrition has published clinical guidelines for administering and evaluating nutrition support specifically for patients with CKD.[25]

Osteodystrophy. Bone disease and disorders are prevalent in CKD, and they are an important cause of morbidity. A combination of factors contribute to renal osteodystrophy and chronic kidney disease-mineral and bone disorder. The decreased activation of vitamin D has

CULTURAL CONSIDERATIONS

CULTURAL DISPARITIES IN KIDNEY TRANSPLANT AVAILABILITY AND SUCCESS IN CERTAIN ETHNIC AND RACIAL GROUPS

Kidney transplantation is generally considered the optimal treatment for patients with end-stage renal disease. In 2010, nearly 17,000 kidney transplantations were performed in the United States. Almost half of those transplants went to Caucasian recipients; however, Caucasians only make up 38% of those on the waiting list to receive a transplant.[1] Advances in both medical technology and immunosuppressive therapies have led to longer lives for transplant recipients among all ethnic groups over the past 30 years. Despite this increase in survival rates, African-American kidney transplant recipients continue to have a higher incidence of the transplant failing within 10 years as well as a higher rate of death among transplant recipients compared with their white counterparts. Hispanic and Asian transplant recipients are reported to have the best outcomes.[2,3] Several theories exist to explain these disparities in transplantation rates and survival among various ethnic groups.

Racial variation with regard to transplant success can be attributed in part to differences in immunologic function among different racial and ethnic groups. There are also social factors that affect the disparity of transplantation (see figure). Minorities are less likely to pursue live donor kidney transplants as a result of lack of knowledge, discomfort with talking to family members or individuals from other social networks about the procedure, difficulty with finding suitable donors, insufficient education from health care providers, lower availability of health insurance, and health care provider discrimination.[4] Provider inequity is related to variations in the consensus regarding the appropriate and just allocation of organs. Many providers believe that an organ should go to the recipient who is likely to receive the greatest benefit or live the longest as a result of the transplant. Factors such as African-American ethnicity, lower socioeconomic status, comorbid diseases, and limited access to health care all decrease survival rate and length of life despite transplantation. To compound this issue, the longer that a recipient is on dialysis while waiting for a transplant, the lower the success rate of the transplant.[5]

To decrease these disparities, many interventions have been suggested. Immunosuppression regimens should be modified for different racial groups. Education methods and materials should also be culturally sensitive and consider the patients' cultural beliefs, values, language, socioeconomic status, and social context.[2] In addition, dialysis providers should be educated regarding kidney transplantation so that they can supply quality education to both potential transplant patients and potential live donors. Education about live donor kidney transplant should be offered to families of patients with end-stage renal disease to increase the donor pool and thus ease the matching process for donors for these groups. Research indicates that education that is provided early during the course of treatment and frequently throughout treatment leads to an increase across all ethnic groups with regard to patients' pursuit of transplantation.[4,5]

Jennifer E. Schmidt

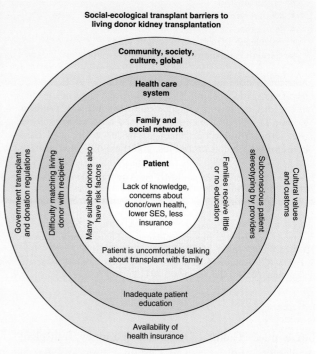

From Waterman AD, Rodrigue JR, Purnell TS, et al. Addressing racial/ethnic disparities in live donor kidney transplantation: priorities for research and intervention. *Semin Nephrol.* 2010;30(1):90-98.

1. Organ Procurement and Transplantation Network: *Transplants in the U.S. by recipient ethnicity: U.S. transplants performed January 1, 1988-January 31, 2011.* Washington, DC: U.S. Department of Health and Human Services; 2011.
2. Gordon EJ, Ladner DP, Caicedo JC, Franklin J. Disparities in kidney transplant outcomes: a review. *Semin Nephrol.* 2010;30(1):81-89.
3. US Renal Data System: *USRDS 2010 annual data report: atlas of chronic kidney disease and end-stage renal disease in the United States.* Bethesda, Md: National Institutes of Health, National Institute of Diabetes and Digestive and Kidney Diseases; 2010.
4. Waterman AD, Rodrigue JR, Purnell TS, et al. Addressing racial and ethnic disparities in live donor kidney transplantation: priorities for research and intervention. *Semin Nephrol.* 2010;30(1):90-98.
5. Courtney AE, Maxwell AP. The challenge of doing what is right in renal transplantation: balancing equity and utility. *Nephron Clin Pract.* 2009;111(1):c62-c67; discussion c68.

TABLE 21-5   **SELECTED NUTRITION PARAMETERS FOR VARIOUS LEVELS OF KIDNEY FAILURE***

Parameter	Normal Kidney Function	Stages 1 Through 4 of Chronic Kidney Disease	Stage 5 Hemodialysis	Stage 5 Peritoneal Dialysis	Transplant
Energy	30 to 37 kcal/kg of body weight	35 kcal/kg if < 60 years old	35 kcal/kg if < 60 years old	35 kcal/kg if < 60 years old	30 to 35 kcal/kg initial
		30 to 35 kcal/kg if ≥ 60 years old	30 to 35 kcal/kg if ≥ 60 years old	30 to 35 kcal/kg if ≥ 60 years old; include calories from dialysate	25 to 30 kcal/kg for maintenance
Protein	0.8 g/kg	0.6 to 0.75 g/kg ≥ 50% HBV	≥ 1.2 g/kg ≥ 50% HBV	≥ 1.2 to 1.3 g/kg ≥ 50% HBV	1.3 to 1.5 g/kg initial 1.0 g/kg for maintenance
Fat (% total kcal)	30% to 35%	Patients considered at highest risk for cardiovascular disease; emphasis on MUFA, PUFA, and 250 to 300 mg of cholesterol per day			< 10% saturated fat
Sodium	Unrestricted	1 to 3 g/day	1 to 3 g/day	2 to 4 g/day; monitor fluid balance	Unrestricted; monitor medication effects
Potassium	Unrestricted	Unrestricted unless serum level is high	2 to 3 g/day; adjust to serum levels	3 to 4 g/day; adjust to serum levels	Unrestricted; monitor medication effects
Calcium	Unrestricted	1 to 1.5 g/day and not to exceed 2 g/day with binder load	≤2 g/day from diet and medications, including binder load	≤ 2 g/day from diet and medications, including binder load	1.2 g/day
Phosphorus	Unrestricted	800 to 1000 mg/day when serum phosphorus level is > 4.6 mg/dL or when parathyroid hormone is elevated	800 to 1000 mg/day when serum phosphorus level is > 5.5 mg/dL or when parathyroid hormone is elevated	800 to 1000 mg/day when serum phosphorus level is > 5.5 mg/dL or when parathyroid hormone is elevated	Unrestricted unless indicated
Fluid	Unrestricted	Unrestricted with normal urine output	1000 mL plus urine output	Maintain balance	Unrestricted unless indicated

*These are guidelines for initial assessment only; individualization to the patient's metabolic status and coexisting metabolic conditions is essential for optimal care.
HBV, High biologic value; *MUFA,* monounsaturated fatty acids; *PUFA,* polyunsaturated fatty acids.
Modified from Beto JA, Bansal VK. Medical nutrition therapy in chronic kidney failure: integrating clinical practice guidelines. *J Am Diet Assoc.* 2004;104:404-409; and the American Dietetic Association. *ADA nutrition care manual.* Chicago: American Dietetic Association; 2010.

a cascading effect that results in elevated parathyroid hormone and reduced serum calcium levels. Patients also have elevated serum phosphorus levels as a result of the inability of the kidney to excrete phosphorus. This combination causes abnormal changes in bone structure and function. Hyperphosphatemia is associated with increased mortality risk; thus, phosphate binders are an important management aspect of CKD. Patients with any level of kidney dysfunction should be evaluated for bone disease and disorders of calcium and phosphorus metabolism.

Treatment strategies for bone disorders require a highly individualized management plan and continue to evolve in the light of new research.[26]

Neuropathy. Central and peripheral neurologic disturbances are common among patients at the initiation of dialysis, and they are even more prevalent in patients with diabetes. Symptoms of neuropathy may not be present until the GFR falls to less than 12 to 20 mL/min per 1.73 m^2; however, patients should be periodically assessed for implications of uremia or disease progression.[14]

KIDNEY STONE DISEASE

In the United States, approximately 5% of women and 12% of men form kidney stones at some point during their lives.[27] The basic cause of nephrolithiasis is unknown, but many factors that relate to the nature of the urine itself or to conditions of the urinary tract environment contribute to stone formation. Genetics, urine calcium excretion, and urine pH are three factors that are closely linked with the risk for stone formation.[28] The most common types of kidney stones are calcium, struvite, and uric acid. Figure 21-6 illustrates various types of stones. In addition, Box 21-2 lists risk factors that are associated with kidney stone development.

Disease Process

Calcium Stones

Calcium oxalate and calcium phosphate stones are the most common types, and they account for approximately 80% of all kidney stones. High levels of urinary oxalate increase the risk of an individual forming a calcium oxalate stone. Oxalates are derived from endogenous synthesis (relative to lean body mass) and dietary sources (see Box 21-3). Oxalic acid is a metabolite of ascorbic acid. Therefore, the long-term megadosing of vitamin C supplements (more than 3 g/day) may pose a potential health risk for kidney stone formation. A small percentage of the population are "hyperabsorbers" of dietary oxalate and thus are at higher risk of forming stones. The supersaturation of kidney stone materials in the urine may result from the following[29]:

- Excess calcium in the blood (hypercalcemia) or urine (hypercalciuria)
- Excess oxalate (hyperoxaluria) or uric acid in the urine (hyperuricosuria)
- Low levels of citrate in the urine (hypocitraturia)
- Excess animal protein and sodium intake

Significant dietary calcium intake from food or supplements equaling up to 2 g/day is inversely associated with calcium oxalate stones. Essentially, individuals with a low dietary intake of calcium are at a *higher* risk for calcium oxalate stone formation than those who adequately consume calcium. It is a common misunderstanding to restrict the calcium intake of those patients who form calcium oxalate stones.[29,30]

Struvite Stones

Struvite stones, which account for approximately 10% of all stones, are composed of magnesium ammonium phosphate and carbonate apatite. They often are called

---

nephrolithiasis the formation of a kidney stone.

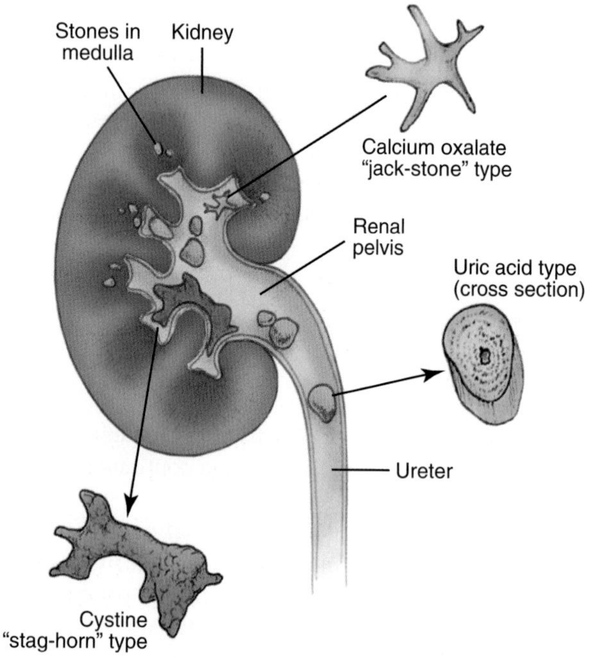

Figure 21-6 Renal calculi: stones in the kidney, renal pelvis, and ureter.

BOX 21-2 **RISK FACTORS FOR THE DEVELOPMENT OF KIDNEY STONES**

- High dietary intake of the following:
  - Animal protein
  - Purines
  - Oxalate
  - Vitamin C
  - Sodium
- Inadequate intake of the following:
  - Fiber
  - Potassium
  - Fluid
- Family history
- Urinary tract infections
- Kidney disorders such as cystic kidney diseases
- Metabolic disorders such as the following:
  - Hyperparathyroidism
  - Chronic inflammation of the bowel
  - Intestinal bypass or ostomy surgery
  - Higher body mass index

From the American Dietetic Association. *ADA nutrition care manual.* Chicago: American Dietetic Association; 2010.

BOX 21-3   HIGH-OXALATE FOODS AND DRINKS

Drinks
Chocolate drink mixes, soymilk, Ovaltine, instant iced tea, fruit juices of the fruits listed in this table

Fruits
Apricots (dried), red currants, figs, kiwi, rhubarb

Vegetables
Beans (wax, dried), beets and beet greens, chives, collard greens, eggplant, escarole, dark greens of all kinds, kale, leeks, okra, parsley, green peppers, potatoes, rutabagas, spinach, Swiss chard, tomato paste, watercress, zucchini

Breads, Cereals, and Grains
Amaranth, barley, white corn flour, fried potatoes, fruitcake, grits, soybean products, sweet potatoes, wheat germ and bran, buckwheat flour, All-Bran cereal, graham crackers, pretzels, whole wheat bread

Meat, Meat Replacements, Fish, and Poultry
Dried beans, peanut butter, soy burgers, miso

Desserts and Sweets
Carob, chocolate, marmalades

Fats and Oils
Nuts (peanuts, almonds, pecans, cashews, hazelnuts), nut butters, sesame seeds, tahini (a paste made from sesame seeds)

Other Foods
Poppy seeds

From the American Dietetic Association. *ADA nutrition care manual.* Chicago: American Dietetic Association; 2010.

infection stones because they are primarily caused by urinary tract infections and because they are not associated with any specific nutrient. Thus, no particular diet therapy is involved. Struvite stones are usually large "staghorn" stones that are surgically removed.

Uric Acid Stones

The excess excretion of uric acid may be caused by some impairment that involves the metabolism of purine, which is a nitrogen end product of the dietary protein from which uric acid is formed. This impairment occurs with diseases such as gout, and it can also occur with rapid tissue breakdown during wasting disease. Other conditions that are associated with persistently acid urine and uric acid stone formation are diarrheal illness, diabetes, obesity, and metabolic syndrome.[29] Roughly 9% of kidney stones are uric acid stones.

Other Stones

Other rare forms of kidney stones are often reflective of inherited disorders or complications of medications. For example, cystine stones are caused by a genetic defect in the renal reabsorption of the amino acid cystine (as well as other dibasic amino acids), thereby causing an accumulation in the urine (cystinuria). Cystine is not soluble and thus high levels may result in stone formation.

Clinical Symptoms

The main symptom of kidney stones is severe pain. Many other urinary symptoms may result from the presence of the stones, and general weakness and sometimes fever are present. Laboratory examination of the urine and of any passed stones helps to determine treatment.

Medical Nutrition Therapy

General Objectives

MNT may include several aspects, and it will vary depending on the type of stone. General MNT recommendations are as follows[7]:

- *Protein:* Excessive protein intake, especially from animal sources, is a risk factor for stone formation. Thus, patients should normalize their intake to healthy population standard recommendations of 0.8 to 1.0 g/kg/day and should not exceed the Dietary Reference Intake.
- *Calcium:* Low dietary calcium intake is a risk for calcium oxalate stone formation. Thus, patients should be encouraged to normalize calcium intake to 800 mg/day for men and 1200 mg/day for women and balance intake throughout the day.
- *Sodium:* High sodium intake increases the amount of calcium excretion in the urine, thereby precipitating hypercalciuria, and it is associated with an increased risk of stone formation. Sodium intake should not exceed 2300 to 3450 mg/day.
- *Oxalates:* Limiting urinary oxalate significantly reduces the risk of calcium oxalate stone formation.[31] Thus, avoiding foods that are high in oxalates is advised. Intake should be less than 40 to 50 mg/day; see Box 21-3.
- *Vitamins and minerals:* Vitamin C should be limited to the Dietary Reference Intake, and all other vitamin and mineral intake should meet the Dietary Reference Intake standards.
- *Fluid:* A large fluid intake of 2 L/day or more helps to produce more dilute urine and thus to prevent the accumulation of materials that form stones.

TABLE 21-6   SUMMARY OF DIETARY PRINCIPLES IN KIDNEY STONE DISEASE

Stone Chemistry	Nutrient Modification
All types of stones	Increase fluid intake enough to produce ≥ 2.5 L/day of clear urine
Calcium oxalate	Reduce sodium, animal protein, and oxalate-containing food intake; continue normal calcium intake; increase fiber intake; avoid high doses of vitamin C
Calcium phosphate	Reduce phosphorus intake
Uric acid	Reduce animal protein intake and purine intake
Cystine	Reduce sodium intake; avoid excess protein; maintain fluid intake at 4 L/day

Exact fluid intake needs vary by patient, but enough fluids—preferably water—should be ingested to produce at least 2.5 L of clear urine daily. For patients who consume soft drinks, reducing soft-drink intake may lower the risk of recurrent stone formation.[32]

General dietary principles that involve kidney stone disease are summarized in Table 21-6.

Objectives Specific to Type of Stone

The nutrition care plan may be further individualized relative to the nature of the specific stone formed. A variety of medications are useful for the treatment of kidney stones in combination with diet therapy. For medications to be most effective, the specific type of stone must be identified. This is not always possible and therefore limits drug therapy in some individuals.

Calcium Stones.   In some cases, dietary control of the stone constituents may help to reduce the recurrence of such stone formation. If a stone is made of calcium oxalate, then foods that are high in oxalate (see Box 21-3) should be limited. If a stone is made of calcium phosphate, additional sources of phosphorus (e.g., meats, legumes, nuts) should be controlled.

In addition to the recommendations listed previously, fiber intake should be considered in the case of calcium stones. Materials that bind potential stone elements in the intestine can prevent their absorption and eliminate them from the body. For example, phytate can bind calcium and thus help to prevent the crystallization of oxalate calcium salts. Phytates are found in high-fiber plant foods such as whole wheat, bran, and soybeans.

Uric Acid Stones.   The alkalinization of the urine helps to prevent the formation of uric acid stones. Dietary attempts to alter urinary pH with acidic or alkaline diets are unsuccessful.[33] However, potassium salts may be used to raise the urinary pH, which decreases the supersaturation of uric acid.[29] Establishing and maintaining a healthy weight and limiting animal protein (including red meat, fish, and poultry) intake to 40 to 50 g/day are also advisable.[31]

Cystine Stones.   Dietary modifications are geared toward reducing urinary cystine concentrations by decreasing intake and diluting the urine. Diluting the urine may require the intake of 4 to 5 L/day of water in adults.[31]

acidic or alkaline diets **diets based on the theory that diets high in acidic foods (e.g., animal protein, caffeine, simple sugars) will disrupt the body's normal pH balance, which is slightly alkaline.**

SUMMARY

- The nephrons are the functional units of the kidneys. Through these unique structures, the kidney maintains homeostasis in the blood of the materials that are required for life and health. The nephrons accomplish their tremendous task by constantly cleaning the blood, returning necessary elements to the blood, and eliminating the remainder in concentrated urine.

- Various diseases that interfere with the vital function of nephrons can cause kidney disease. Kidney diseases have predisposing factors, such as diabetes, recurrent urinary tract infections that may lead to

renal calculi, and progressive glomerulonephritis that may lead to chronic nephrotic syndrome and kidney failure.

- At its end stage, CKD is treated by dialysis or kidney transplantation. Patients who are undergoing dialysis require close monitoring for protein, water, and electrolyte balance.

- Kidney stones may be formed from a variety of substances. For some patients, a change in the dietary intake of the identified substance (e.g., sodium, oxalate, purine) may decrease stone formation.

CRITICAL THINKING QUESTIONS

1. For each of the following conditions, outline the nutrition components of therapy, and explain the effect of each on kidney function: glomerulonephritis, nephrotic syndrome, and CKD.
2. Consider the nutrition factors that must be monitored in patients who are undergoing kidney dialysis. How would you suggest a client self-monitor fluid intake to meet hydration needs while not exceeding restrictions?
3. Outline the medical and nutrition therapy for patients who are on hemodialysis and peritoneal dialysis. What are the critical differences, and why?

CHAPTER CHALLENGE QUESTIONS

True-False

Write the correct statement for each statement that is false.

1. *True or False:* The basic functional unit of the kidney is the nephron.
2. *True or False:* Only a few nephrons are present in each kidney, so metabolic stress can easily cause problems.
3. *True or False:* The functioning of the nephrons relates little to the rest of the body.
4. *True or False:* The main function of the glomerulus is filtration.
5. *True or False:* The tasks of the various parts of the nephron tubules are reabsorption, secretion, and excretion.
6. *True or False:* Dietary modifications in acute glomerulonephritis usually involve crucial restrictions of protein and sodium.
7. *True or False:* The primary symptom in nephrotic syndrome is massive albuminuria.
8. *True or False:* Nephrotic syndrome is best treated by a very-low-protein diet.
9. *True or False:* The multiple symptoms of advanced CKD result from metabolic imbalances in the body's inability to handle protein, electrolytes, and water.
10. *True or False:* Prolonged immobilization (e.g., with full body casts or disability) may lead to the withdrawal of bone calcium and the formation of calcium kidney stones.

Multiple Choice

1. Acute glomerulonephritis is best treated with which of the following methods? *(Circle all that apply.)*
   a. Reducing protein because filtration is impaired
   b. Using a normal amount of protein for optimal tissue nutrition and growth
   c. Restricting sodium to 1500 mg/day
   d. Restricting potassium intake
2. Diet therapy for patients with nephrotic syndrome is designed to perform which of the following functions? *(Circle all that apply.)*
   a. Increase protein to replace the massive losses
   b. Normalize protein intake to reduce albumin losses
   c. Provide adequate kilocalories for energy and spare protein for tissue needs
   d. Moderately restrict sodium to help prevent edema
3. The general diet needs for a patient in stage 5 CKD who is on hemodialysis includes which of the following? *(Circle all that apply.)*
   a. Increased protein intake
   b. Reduced protein intake
   c. Careful control of sodium and potassium according to need
   d. Increased fluids to stimulate kidney function

---

evolve Please refer to the Students' Resource section of this text's Evolve Web site for additional study resources.

REFERENCES

1. US Renal Data System. *USRDS 2010 annual data report: atlas of chronic kidney disease and end-stage renal disease in the United States.* Bethesda, Md: National Institutes of Health, National Institute of Diabetes and Digestive and Kidney Diseases; 2010.
2. Plantinga LC, Boulware LE, Coresh J, et al. Patient awareness of chronic kidney disease: trends and predictors. *Arch Intern Med.* 2008;168(20):2268-2275.
3. Levey AS, de Jong PE, Coresh J, et al. The definition, classification and prognosis of chronic kidney disease: a KDIGO Controversies Conference report. *Kidney Int.* 2011; 80(1):17-28.
4. Tuttle KR, Anderberg RJ, Cooney SK, et al. Oxidative stress mediates protein kinase C activation and advanced glycation end product formation in a mesangial cell model of diabetes and high protein diet. *Am J Nephrol.* 2009;29(3): 171-180.

5. Choudhury D, Tuncel M, Levi M. Diabetic nephropathy—a multifaceted target of new therapies. *Discov Med.* 2010; 10(54):406-415.

6. Levey AS, Eckhardt KU, Tsukamoto Y, et al. Definition and classification of chronic kidney disease: a position statement from Kidney Disease: Improving Global Outcomes (KDIGO). *Kidney Int.* 2005;67(6):2089-2100.

7. American Dietetic Association. *ADA nutrition care manual.* Chicago: American Dietetic Association; 2010.

8. Leblanc M, Kellus JA, Gibney RT, et al. Risk factors for acute renal failure: inherent and modifiable risks. *Curr Opin Crit Care.* 2005;11(6):533-536.

9. Chawla LS, Amdur RL, Amodeo S, et al. The severity of acute kidney injury predicts progression to chronic kidney disease. *Kidney Int.* 2011;79(12):1361-1369.

10. Dirkes S. Acute kidney injury: not just acute renal failure anymore? *Crit Care Nurse.* 2011;31(1):37-49; quiz 50.

11. Ricci Z, Cruz DN, Ronco C. Classification and staging of acute kidney injury: beyond the RIFLE and AKIN criteria. *Nat Rev Nephrol.* 2011;7(4):201-208.

12. Moore H, Reams SM, Wiesen K, et al; National Kidney Foundation Council on Renal Nutrition. National Kidney Foundation Council on Renal Nutrition survey: past-present clinical practices and future strategic planning. *J Ren Nutr.* 2003;13(3):233-240.

13. Beto JA, Bansal VK. Medical nutrition therapy in chronic kidney failure: integrating clinical practice guidelines. *J Am Diet Assoc.* 2004;104(3):404-409.

14. National Kidney Foundation. K/DOQI clinical practice guidelines for chronic kidney disease: evaluation, classification, and stratification. *Am J Kidney Dis.* 2002;39(2 Suppl 1):S1-S266.

15. American Dietetic Association. *Chronic kidney disease evidence-based nutrition practice guideline.* American Dietetic Association; 2011.

16. Crawford PW, Lerma EV. Treatment options for end stage renal disease. *Prim Care.* 2008;35(3):407-432, v.

17. FHN Trial Group; Chertow GM, Levin NW, Beck GJ, et al. In-center hemodialysis six times per week versus three times per week. *N Engl J Med.* 2010;363(24):2287-2300.

18. Jahromi SR, Hosseini S, Razeghi E, et al. Malnutrition predicting factors in hemodialysis patients. *Saudi J Kidney Dis Transpl.* 2010;21(5):846-851.

19. Kovesdy CP, Shinaberger CS, Kalantar-Zadeh K. Epidemiology of dietary nutrient intake in ESRD. *Semin Dial.* 2010;23(4):353-358.

20. Herselman M, Esau N, Kruger JM, et al. Relationship between serum protein and mortality in adults on long-term hemodialysis: exhaustive review and meta-analysis. *Nutrition.* 2010;26(1):10-32.

21. Yen TH, Lin JL, Lin-Tan DT, et al. Association between body mass and mortality in maintenance hemodialysis patients. *Ther Apher Dial.* 2010;14(4):400-408.

22. Kalantar-Zadeh K, Abbott KC, Salahudeen AK, et al. Survival advantages of obesity in dialysis patients. *Am J Clin Nutr.* 2005;81(3):543-554.

23. Nolan CR. Strategies for improving long-term survival in patients with ESRD. *J Am Soc Nephrol.* 2005;16(Suppl 2):S120-S127.

24. Pascual J, Zamora J, Pirsch JD. A systematic review of kidney transplantation from expanded criteria donors. *Am J Kidney Dis.* 2008;52(3):553-586.

25. Brown RO, Compher C; American Society for Parenteral and Enteral Nutrition Board of Directors. A.S.P.E.N. clinical guidelines: nutrition support in adult acute and chronic renal failure. *JPEN J Parenter Enteral Nutr.* 2010;34(4): 366-377.

26. Moe SM, Drüeke T. Improving global outcomes in mineral and bone disorders. *Clin J Am Soc Nephrol.* 2008;3(Suppl 3):S127-S130.

27. Pearle MS, Calhoun EA, Curhan GC. Urologic diseases in America project: urolithiasis. *J Urol.* 2005;173(3):848-857.

28. Evan AP. Physiopathology and etiology of stone formation in the kidney and the urinary tract. *Pediatr Nephrol.* 2010;25(5):831-841.

29. Worcester EM, Coe FL. Nephrolithiasis. *Prim Care.* 35(2):369-391, vii, 2008.

30. Heaney RP. Calcium supplementation and incident kidney stone risk: a systematic review. *J Am Coll Nutr.* 2008; 27(5):519-527.

31. Johri N, Cooper B, Robertson W, et al. An update and practical guide to renal stone management. *Nephron Clin Pract.* 2010;116(3):c159-c171.

32. Fink HA, Akornor JW, Garimella PS, et al. Diet, fluid, or supplements for secondary prevention of nephrolithiasis: a systematic review and meta-analysis of randomized trials. *Eur Urol.* 2009;56(1):72-80.

33. Koff SG, Paquette EL, Cullen J, et al. Comparison between lemonade and potassium citrate and impact on urine pH and 24-hour urine parameters in patients with kidney stone formation. *Urology.* 2007;69(6):1013-1016.

FURTHER READING AND RESOURCES

American Urological Association. www.urologyhealth.org

National Institute of Diabetes and Digestive and Kidney Diseases. www.niddk.nih.gov

National Kidney Foundation. www.kidney.org
These Web sites provide additional information about various forms of kidney disease. Several national organizations provide free education and support for health care providers, patients, and family members. Dietary restrictions for patients with kidney disease can sometimes be overwhelming. To fully understand such diets, continuous follow-up and feedback are needed.

Crawford PW, Lerma EV. Treatment options for end stage renal disease. *Prim Care.* 2008;35(3):407-432, v.

Kalista-Richards M. The kidney: medical nutrition therapy—yesterday and today. *Nutr Clin Pract.* 2011;26(2): 143-150.

CHAPTER 22

Surgery and Nutrition Support

KEY CONCEPTS

- Surgical treatment requires added nutrition support for tissue healing and rapid recovery.
- Nutrition problems related to gastrointestinal (GI) surgery require diet modifications because of the surgery's effect on the normal passage of food.
- To ensure optimal nutrition for surgery patients, diet management may involve enteral and parenteral nutrition support.

Malnutrition continues to burden hospitalized patients. A review of the literature from 12 countries indicates that 38.7% of hospitalized elderly patients and 50.5% of elderly patients in rehabilitation facilities have clinical signs of malnutrition, which hinders healing.[1] Effective nutrition support should reverse malnutrition, improve prognosis, and speed recovery in a cost-effective manner. The surgical process also places physiologic and psychologic stress on patients, which causes added nutrition demands and increases the risk for clinical problems.

This chapter looks at the nutrition needs of surgical patients and the enteral and parenteral feeding methods of providing nutrition support. Careful attention to both preoperative and postoperative nutrition support can reduce complications and provide essential resources for healing and health.

NUTRITION NEEDS OF GENERAL SURGERY PATIENTS

A patient who is undergoing surgery often faces significant physical and psychologic stress. As a result, nutrition demands are increased during this period, and deficiencies can develop that lead to malnutrition and clinical complications. Therefore, careful attention must be given to a patient's nutrition status in preparation for surgery as well as to the individual nutrition needs that follow to address wound healing and recovery. A significant amount of research has been dedicated to understanding the association between malnutrition and clinical outcomes. Poor nutrition status and the following clinical problems are well documented[2,3]:

- Impaired wound healing and increased risk of postoperative infection
- Impaired functioning of the GI tract, cardiovascular system, respiratory system, and immune system
- Reduced quality of life and increased mortality rate
- Longer hospital stay and increased medical cost

FOR FURTHER FOCUS

PROTEIN ENERGY MALNUTRITION AFTER SURGERY

Protein energy malnutrition (PEM) compromises quality of life and the ability to recover from surgery and injury. As general health declines with age and the risk for unplanned surgery increases, so does the prevalence of PEM. Actively evaluating the nutritional status of older people in the home, the hospital, or the nursing home may provide valuable information about the preoperative needs of these individuals. Oral supplements or enteral feedings for malnourished elderly patients before surgery is a cost-effective way to improve outcome, reduce hospital stay, and reduce the risk of complications associated with surgery.

Even without a formal nutrition assessment, PEM can be identified by monitoring unplanned weight loss. Unplanned weight loss is indicative of PEM as well as of the inability to deal with physiologic stress. An unplanned weight loss of up to 5% over a 1-month period or of 10% over a 6-month period is considered a significant loss. Unintentional weight loss of more than 5% in 1 month or 10% in 6 months is classified as severe. Identifying and treating those individuals who are at risk for PEM may also prevent poor outcomes in the event of surgery or injury.

The following table provides a quick guide to evaluate weight loss:

Initial Weight (lb)	WEIGHT LOSS AND RESULTING WEIGHT (LB)	
	5%	10%
80	76	72
85	81	77
90	86	81
95	90	86
100	95	90
110	105	99
120	114	108
130	124	117
140	133	126
150	143	135
160	152	144
170	162	153
180	171	162

Preoperative Nutrition Care: Nutrient Reserves

When the surgery is elective (i.e., not necessary or emergent), body nutrient stores can be built up to fortify a patient for the demands of the surgery and the period that immediately follows, when food intake may be limited. Particular needs center on protein, energy, vitamins, and minerals.

Protein

Protein deficiencies among pediatric and adult hospital patients are common.[4] Every patient facing surgery must be equipped with adequate body protein to counteract blood losses that occur during surgery and to prevent tissue catabolism during the immediate postoperative period (see the For Further Focus box, "Protein Energy Malnutrition After Surgery"). For example, extensive bone healing may be involved in orthopedic surgery. Protein is essential for establishing healthy bone mineral density, and it is especially relevant with the occurrence of bone fractures among the growing U.S. population of elderly people.[5,6] The adequate dietary consumption of high-quality complete proteins (i.e., those that contain all of the essential amino acids) is associated with the maintenance of lean tissue, bone mineral density, and bone mineral content.[6]

Energy

Sufficient energy must be provided when increased protein is necessary for tissue building. The increased source of kilocalories supports the added energy demands and spares protein for its tissue-building work. For example, carbohydrate intake should be adequate to maintain optimal glycogen stores in the liver as a necessary resource for immediate energy, thereby directing protein to its tissue synthesis task. If a person is underweight, extra energy may be required to increase weight to an ideal maintenance level before surgery. If a person is overweight and the surgery is elective, some weight reduction may help to reduce surgical complications.

Vitamins and Minerals

When increased protein and energy are necessary, the appropriate intake of vitamins and minerals involved

---

enteral a mode of feeding that makes use of the gastrointestinal tract through oral or tube feedings.

parenteral a mode of feeding that does not involve the gastrointestinal tract but that instead provides nutrition support via the intravenous delivery of nutrient solutions.

catabolism the metabolic process of breaking down large substances to yield the smaller building blocks.

TABLE 22-1   **NONRESIDUE DIET***

Food Type	Foods Allowed	Foods Not Allowed
Beverages	Carbonated beverages, coffee, tea	Milk, milk drinks
Bread	Crackers, Melba or Rusk	Whole-grain bread
Cereals	Refined as Cream of Wheat, farina, fine cornmeal, Malt-O-Meal, Pablum, rice, strained oatmeal, cornflakes, or puffed rice	Whole-grain and other cereals
Cheese		None allowed
Desserts	Plain cakes and cookies, gelatin desserts, water ices, angel food cake, arrowroot cookies, tapioca puddings made with fruit juice only	Pastries, all others
Eggs	As desired, preferably hard cooked	Fried eggs
Fats	Butter or substitute, small amount of cream	All others
Fruits	Strained fruit juices	All others
Meat, fish, and poultry	Tender beef, chicken, fish, lamb, liver, veal; crisp bacon	Fried or tough meat, pork
Potatoes or substitutes	Only macaroni, noodles, spaghetti, refined rice	Potatoes, corn, hominy, unrefined rice
Soups	Bouillon and broth only	All others
Sweets†	Hard candy, fondant, gumdrops, jelly, marshmallows, sugar, syrup, honey	Other candy, jam, marmalade
Vegetables	Tomato juice	All others
Miscellaneous	Salt	Pepper

*Presurgery nonresidue diet: This diet includes only foods that are free from fiber, seeds, and skins and with a minimal amount of residue. Fruits and vegetables are omitted except for strained fruit juices. Milk is omitted. The diet should be adequate in protein and energy, but it is likely to be inadequate in vitamin A, calcium, and riboflavin. If patients are to remain on this diet for a long period, supplementary vitamins and minerals should be administered. Postsurgery nonresidue diet: This diet is slightly higher in residue, but it has greater variety and includes potatoes (without skin), white bread products (without bran), processed cheeses, sauces, desserts made with milk (but no fruits or nuts), and cream (2 oz) for coffee, cereal, and gravy. The average daily menu contains slightly more protein, energy, vitamins, and minerals compared with the presurgery nonresidue diet.
†Fruit juice and hard candies may be consumed between meals to increase caloric intake.

in protein and energy metabolism (e.g., B-complex vitamins) must also be supplied. Any specifically identified deficiency states (e.g., iron-deficiency anemia) should be corrected. Electrolyte and water balance are necessary to prevent dehydration.

Immediate Preoperative Period

The usual preparation for surgery calls for nothing to be taken orally for at least 8 hours before the procedure. This protocol is necessary to ensure that the stomach retains no food during surgery, because the presence of food may cause complications such as the aspiration of food particles during anesthesia or during recovery from anesthesia in the event that the patient vomits. In addition, any food present in the stomach may interfere with the surgical procedure or increase the risk for postoperative gastric retention and expansion. Before GI surgery, a nonresidue diet may be followed for several days to clear the surgical site of any food residue (Table 22-1). Commercial nonresidue elemental formulas can provide a complete diet in liquid form. These formulas can be administered by tube or made more palatable for oral use with various flavorings.

Emergency Surgery

If the surgery is urgent, no time is available for building up ideal nutrition reserves, which is another reason to maintain good nutrition status through a healthy diet at all times. If optimal nutrition is maintained, then reserves are available to supply needs during times of stress.

Postoperative Nutrition Care: Nutrient Needs for Healing

Adequate nutrition support is necessary to help with recovery from surgery when nutrient losses are great. At the same time, food intake may be diminished or even absent for a period. If a patient is not able to resume

elemental formula a nutrition support formula composed of simple elemental nutrient components that require no further digestive breakdown and are thus readily absorbed (e.g., glucose, amino acids, medium-chain triglycerides).

adequate oral intake within 3 to 5 days, an alternative form of nutrition support such as enteral or parenteral routes must be considered. Several nutrients require particular attention during this time.

Protein

Optimal protein intake during the postoperative recovery period is of primary concern for all patients. Protein is needed to replace losses that occur during surgery and to supply increased demands of the healing process. During the period immediately after surgery, body tissues usually undergo considerable catabolism, which means that the process of tissue breakdown and loss exceeds the process of tissue buildup. Weight loss and malnutrition are common among patients who are experiencing catabolic stress. Although the maintenance of lean body mass improves the survival of catabolic patients, malnutrition or marginal nutritional states are common among hospitalized surgical patients. Some research supports the use of branched-chain amino acids in particular to help alleviate the burden of muscle wasting and to improve recovery time during this phase.[7]

In addition to protein losses from tissue breakdown, other losses of protein from the body may occur. These losses include plasma protein loss from hemorrhage, bleeding, and various body fluid losses or exudates. The increased loss of plasma protein from extensive tissue destruction, inflammation, infection, and trauma should be monitored. If any degree of prior malnutrition or chronic infection existed, a patient's protein deficiency could easily become severe and cause complications. Several reasons exist for this increased protein demand, and these will be detailed in the following paragraphs.

Building Tissue. The process of wound healing requires building a great deal of new body tissue, which depends on an adequate amount of essential amino acids. Necessary amino acids must come from dietary protein (either oral or tube feedings) or from parenteral nutrition if a patient cannot eat or tolerate enteral feedings for an extended period. Dietary protein recommendations may increase above normal needs to restore lost protein and to build new tissues at the wound site.

Controlling Edema. When serum protein levels are low, osmotic pressure is lost, and edema develops. Edema is characterized by puffiness or swelling of the tissue from the excess fluid being held there instead of returning to circulation. Generalized edema may adversely affect heart and lung function. Local edema at the wound site also interferes with the closure of the wound, and it hinders the normal healing process.

Controlling Shock. A sufficient supply of plasma protein—mainly albumin—is necessary to maintain

blood volume. If the plasma albumin level drops, pressure to keep tissue fluid circulating between the capillaries and cells is insufficient. Without adequate pressure, water leaves the capillaries, and it cannot be drawn back into circulation; this results in edema. Shock symptoms result from a loss of blood volume and the body's efforts to restore it.

Healing Bone. Protein and mineral matter are essential to the foundation of bone tissue for proper formation and healing. Protein provides a matrix for calcium and phosphorus, and these are required for strong bones.

Resisting Infection. Protein tissues are the major components of the body's immune system, and they provide the body's defense against infection. These defense agents include specialized white cells called *lymphocytes* as well as antibodies and various other blood cells, hormones, and enzymes. Tissue strength is a major defense barrier against infection at all times.

Transporting Lipids. Fat is also an important component of tissue structure. It forms the lipid bilayer of cell membranes, and it participates in many other necessary metabolic activities. Protein (e.g., lipoproteins) is necessary for fat transportation via the bloodstream to all tissues and to the liver for metabolism.

Because protein has many important functions during recovery from surgery, protein deficiency at this time can lead to many clinical complications. Such problems include poor wound healing, the rupture of the suture lines (i.e., dehiscence), the delayed healing of fractures,

---

branched-chain amino acids amino acids with branched side chains; three of the essential amino acids are branched-chain amino acids: leucine, isoleucine, and valine.

exudate various materials such as cells, cellular debris, and fluids that have escaped from the blood vessels and that are deposited in or on the surface tissues, usually as a result of inflammation; the protein content of exudate is high.

osmotic pressure hydrostatic pressure across a semipermeable membrane that is necessary to maintain the normal movement of fluid between the capillaries and the surrounding tissue.

edema an unusual accumulation of fluid in the interstitial compartments (i.e., the small structural spaces between tissue parts) of the body.

dehiscence a splitting open; the separation of the layers of a surgical wound that may be partial, superficial, or complete and that involves total disruption and resuturing.

depressed heart and lung function, anemia, the failure of GI stomas, a reduced resistance to infection, liver damage, extensive weight loss, muscle wasting, and an increased risk of death.

Water

Surgery induces altered fluid distribution in the patient, which can reduce circulation and hinder recovery.[8] Sufficient fluid intake is necessary to prevent dehydration. Elderly patients, whose thirst mechanisms may be depressed, warrant special attention to total fluid intake and hydration status. During the postoperative period, large water losses may also occur from vomiting, hemorrhage, fever, infection, or diuresis. A variety of solutions are available for intravenous administration, depending on the patient's needs. Intravenous fluids after surgery supply some initial hydration needs, but oral intake should begin as soon as possible and be sufficiently maintained.

Energy

As always, when increased protein is demanded for tissue building, enough nonprotein kilocalories must be provided for energy to spare protein for its vital tissue-building function. Therefore, the fuel sources (i.e., carbohydrate and fat) must be sufficient in the total diet. For adults, a minimum of 130 g carbohydrates must be supplied on a daily basis to spare protein from catabolism.[9] In situations of acute metabolic stress (e.g., with extensive surgery or burns), energy needs may increase to as much as 1.2 to 2 kcal/kg body weight/day over basal energy requirements. Energy requirements can be estimated by first calculating the individual's basal energy needs with the Mifflin-St. Jeor equation (see Chapter 6) and then multiplying by an injury factor (1.2 to 2, depending on the patient's status) to meet the added energy needs of stress and sepsis:

Male: Basal metabolic rate = $(10 \times$ Weight in kg$) +$
$\qquad (6.25 \times$ Height in cm$) - (5 \times$ Age in years$) + 5$
Female: Basal metabolic rate = $(10 \times$ Weight in kg$) +$
$\qquad (6.25 \times$ Height in cm$) - (5 \times$ Age in years$) - 161$

Carbohydrates spare protein for tissue building and help to avoid liver damage by maintaining glycogen reserves in the liver tissue. Excessive fuel storage as body fat should be avoided, because fatty tissue heals poorly and is more susceptible to infection.

Vitamins

Several vitamins require particular attention during wound healing. Vitamin C is vital for building connective tissue and capillary walls during the healing process, but levels are often low in critically ill patients. Studies demonstrate that the parenteral administration of vitamin C protects microvascular functions and improves the risk for morbidity.[10] If extensive tissue building is necessary, as much as 1150 to 3000 mg/day of vitamin C may be beneficial during the postoperative period for patients who are critically ill.[11,12] (Long-term supplementation at this level is not recommended.) As energy and protein intake are increased, the B-complex vitamins that have important coenzyme roles in protein and energy metabolism (e.g., thiamin, riboflavin, niacin) must be increased. Other B-complex vitamins (e.g., folate, B_{12}, pyridoxine, and pantothenic acid) play important roles in building hemoglobin and thus must meet the demands of an increased blood supply and general metabolic stress. Vitamin K, which is essential for blood clotting, is usually present in a sufficient amount because it is synthesized by intestinal bacteria. However, patients who are treated with antibiotics may have decreased gut flora and vitamin K synthesis.

Minerals

Attention to any mineral deficiencies is essential. Tissue catabolism results in cell potassium and phosphorus loss. Electrolyte imbalances of sodium and chloride also result from fluid imbalances. Iron-deficiency anemia may develop from blood loss or inadequate iron absorption (see the Drug-Nutrient Interaction box, "Aspirin and Iron Absorption"). Another mineral that is important in wound healing is zinc. Adequate protein-rich food consumption usually meets this need, because most dietary zinc is found in protein foods of animal origin such as beef, crab, lobster, and oysters. However, even if patients have adequate dietary intake of zinc, surgical trauma and infection may lead to reduced serum zinc status. Studies that have evaluated zinc supplementation in wound healing indicate that oral zinc supplementation (17 mg/day) and topical zinc therapy may help to facilitate the healing process, particularly among patients with low zinc levels.[13,14]

stoma the opening that is established in the abdominal wall that connects with the ileum or the colon for the elimination of intestinal wastes after the surgical removal of diseased portions of the intestines.

diuresis the increased excretion of urine.

DRUG-NUTRIENT INTERACTION

ASPIRIN AND IRON ABSORPTION

Aspirin is one of the most common analgesics used in the United States today. Its use is implicated in the presence of other conditions as well, such as transient ischemic attacks (i.e., mini strokes), myocardial infarctions, arthritis and other inflammatory diseases, blood-clotting disorders, and insomnia.

Long-term aspirin use may lead to poor iron absorption. The acetylsalicylic acid found in aspirin can irritate the stomach lining and prevent or slow the normal excretion of gastric acid. Gastric acid is needed to keep iron in its Fe^{3+}

state until absorption can occur in the duodenum. When gastric acid levels are low, iron-deficiency anemia may result.

For the greatest absorption, aspirin should be taken on an empty stomach with a large glass of water. This dilutes the acetylsalicylic acid, thereby reducing the erosion of the stomach lining. Aspirin may be taken with other liquids but never with alcohol; it increases the bioavailability of alcohol and thus increases the risk for adverse side effects.

Sara Harcourt

GENERAL DIETARY MANAGEMENT

Initial Intravenous Fluid and Electrolytes

Routine intravenous fluids are used to supply hydration needs and electrolytes and not to sustain energy and nutrients. For example, a 5% dextrose solution with normal saline (i.e., 0.9% sodium chloride solution) contains only 5 g dextrose/dL or approximately 170 kcal/L (dextrose provides 3.4 kcal/g), although the patient's total energy need is more than 10 times that amount. A return to regular eating should be encouraged and maintained as soon as tolerated.

Methods of Feeding

The method of feeding used in the nutrition care plan depends on the patient's condition. Many patients are both energy and protein undernourished during hospital stays.[15] The appropriate and timely administration of nutrition support is an important predictor of overall health outcomes and quality of life.[16] The physician, the dietitian, and the nurse work together to manage the diet by using oral, enteral, or parenteral feeding as necessary:

- *Oral:* nourishment through the regular GI route by oral feedings; may include a variety of diet plans, textures, and meal replacement liquid supplements
- *Enteral:* technically refers to nourishment through the regular GI route either by regular oral feedings or tube feedings; however, in medical nutrition therapy, enteral feedings imply tube feedings
- *Parenteral:* nourishment through the veins (either small peripheral veins or a large central vein)

When a patient is capable of meeting his or her nutrient needs by oral feedings and when feedings are well tolerated, then that is the feeding method of choice. Table 22-2 lists conditions that often require nutrition support by tube feeding or parenteral nutrition. General criteria for selecting the most appropriate nutrition support method are listed in Box 22-1.

Oral Feedings

When the GI tract can be used, it is the preferred route of feeding: orally if possible and by feeding tube if not. Most general surgical patients can and should receive oral feedings as soon as feasible to provide adequate nutrition. Oral feedings provide needed nutrients and help to stimulate the normal action of the GI tract. Feedings within 24 hours after surgery are associated with reduced complications and earlier hospital discharge.[17] When oral feedings begin, the patient may begin with clear or full liquids and then progress to a soft or regular diet as indicated. Individual tolerance and needs are always the guide, but encouragement and help should be supplied as part of the general care of postsurgery patients to facilitate eating as soon as possible. If inadequate caloric intake is a concern, the energy value of foods in the regular diet may also be increased with added sauces, dried protein powder, and dressings. Alternatively, a general food supplement formula such as Boost or Ensure may be added orally with or between meals. More frequent, less bulky, and concentrated small meals may be helpful to make every bite count.

Routine House Diets. A schedule of routine "house" diets that is based on a cyclic menu is typically followed in most hospitals. The basic modification is in texture, and this ranges from clear liquid (no milk) to full liquid (including milk) and soft food to a full regular diet. Mechanically altered soft diets are designed for patients

TABLE 22-2   **CONDITIONS THAT OFTEN REQUIRE NUTRITION SUPPORT**

Recommended Route of Feeding	Condition	Typical Disorders
Enteral nutrition	Impaired nutrient ingestion	Neurologic disorders HIV/AIDS Facial trauma Oral or esophageal trauma Congenital anomalies Respiratory failure Cystic fibrosis Traumatic brain injury Anorexia and wasting with severe eating disorders
	Inability to consume adequate nutrition orally	Hyperemesis gravidarum Hypermetabolic states (e.g., burns) Comatose states Anorexia with congestive heart failure, cancer, chronic obstructive pulmonary disease, and eating disorders Congenital heart disease Impaired intake after orofacial surgery or injury Spinal cord injury
	Impaired digestion, absorption, and metabolism	Severe gastroparesis Inborn errors of metabolism Crohn's disease Short-bowel syndrome with minimal resection
	Severe wasting or depressed growth	Cystic fibrosis Failure to thrive Cancer Sepsis Cerebral palsy Myasthenia gravis
Parenteral nutrition	Gastrointestinal incompetence	Short-bowel syndrome or major resection Severe acute pancreatitis Severe inflammatory bowel disease Small-bowel ischemia Intestinal atresia Severe liver failure Major gastrointestinal surgery
	Critical illness with poor enteral tolerance or accessibility	Multiorgan system failure Major trauma or burns Bone marrow transplantation Acute respiratory failure with ventilator dependency and gastrointestinal malfunction Severe wasting with renal failure and dialysis Small-bowel transplantation, immediately after surgery

Adapted from Mahan LK, Escott-Stump S. *Krause's food & nutrition therapy*. 12th ed. St. Louis: Saunders; 2008.

with chewing or swallowing problems. Small amounts of liquid may be added to regular foods to achieve an appropriate consistency when pureed. These diets may be further modified, depending on the patient's needs. For example, low-sodium, low-fat, or high-protein requirements can still be met with mechanically altered diets. Therapeutic soft diets are used to transition between liquid and regular diets. Whole foods that are low in fiber and limited seasonings are included as tolerated. Table 22-3 summarizes the details of routine hospital diets.

Assisted Oral Feeding. In accordance with the patient's condition, assistance with eating may be needed. Patients usually like to maintain independence as much as possible and should be encouraged to do so with whatever degree of assistance that is necessary. Plate guards or special utensils to facilitate independence are usually welcomed by both the patient and the staff. The staff should try to learn each patient's needs and limitations so that little things (e.g., having the meat precut or the bread buttered before bringing the tray to the bedside) can be

BOX 22-1   CRITERIA FOR SELECTING A NUTRITION SUPPORT METHOD

The physician will make a decision about the most appropriate method of medical nutrition therapy for the patient with the use of the following criteria. Either the pharmacist or the registered dietitian will make the calculations for the formula or total parenteral nutrition solution that will be used.

Enteral nutrition support is indicated for patients with the following characteristics:

- They have functional gastrointestinal tracts.
- They have adequate digestive and absorptive capacity in their gastrointestinal tracts, but they cannot or will not eat enough to meet their needs. Examples: mechanical (e.g., neurologic disorder of swallowing, obstruction in the upper gastrointestinal tract, malabsorption or maldigestion that requires elemental formulas) or psychologic problems (e.g., eating disorders); unconsciousness; prematurity without suck reflex
- They are at risk for malnutrition without nutrition support. Examples: patients whose nutrient needs are elevated to the point that they are not capable of orally consuming enough energy (e.g., with severe trauma or burns)

Parenteral nutrition support is indicated for patients with the following characteristics:

- They do not have sufficient gastrointestinal tract function and they need nutrition support for more than 5 to 7 days. Examples: short-bowel syndrome, intestinal infarction, obstruction in the lower gastrointestinal tract, severe prolonged diarrhea, nothing by mouth before surgery for more than 7 days
- There is a need for bowel rest (e.g., enteral fistulas, acute inflammatory bowel disease).
- They do not have access for feeding tube placement and need nutrition support.
- They repeatedly pull out their feeding tubes.

Peripheral Parenteral Nutrition

- Length of therapy of less than 5 to 7 days
- Not hypermetabolic
- No fluid restriction

Central Parenteral Nutrition

- Length of therapy of more than 5 to 7 days
- Hypermetabolic
- Fluid restriction
- Poor peripheral access or central access already in place

BOX 22-2   ASSISTED ORAL FEEDING GUIDELINES

- Have the tray securely placed within the patient's sight.
- Sit down beside the bed if this is more comfortable, and make simple conversation or remain silent as the patient's condition indicates. Do not carry on a conversation with another patient or coworker or on the phone; this will exclude the patient whom you are helping.
- Offer small amounts, and do not rush the feeding.
- Allow ample time for a patient to chew and swallow or to rest between mouthfuls.
- Offer liquids between the solids, with a drinking straw if necessary.
- Wipe the patient's mouth with a napkin during and after each meal.
- Let the patient hold his or her bread if desired and if he or she is able to do so.
- When feeding a patient who is blind or who has eye dressings, describe the food on the tray so that a mental image helps create a desire to eat. Sometimes the analogy of the face of a clock helps a patient to visualize the position of certain foods on the plate (e.g., indicate that the meat is at 12 o'clock, the potatoes are at 3 o'clock, and so on).
- Warn the patient that soup feels particularly hot when it is taken through a straw.
- Identify each food that is being served beforehand.

done without making the patient feel inadequate. Box 22-2 provides guidelines for the times that complete assistance is needed.

Assisted feeding times provide a special opportunity for nutrition counseling and support. Important observations can be made during this time. The assistant can closely observe the patient's physical appearance and responses to the foods served, the patient's appetite and tolerance for certain foods, and the meaning of food to the person. These observations help the nurse and the dietitian to adapt the patient's diet to meet any particular individual needs. Helping patients learn more about their nutrition needs is an important part of personal care. People who understand the role of good food in health (e.g., that it helps them to regain strength and recover from illness) are more likely to accept the diet prescription. Patients also feel more encouraged to maintain sound eating habits after discharge from the hospital as well as to improve their eating habits in general.

Enteral Feedings

When a patient cannot eat orally but the remaining portions of the GI tract can be used, an alternate form of enteral feeding by tube provides nutrition support. Enteral tube feedings preserve gut function, they are noninvasive, and they are less expensive than parenteral nutrition. The most common route is the nasogastric tube, which is inserted through the patient's nasal cavity and down to the stomach. For patients who are at risk for aspiration,

TABLE 22-3   **ROUTINE HOSPITAL DIETS**

Food	Clear Liquid*	Full Liquid	Mechanical Soft†	Regular House Diet
Soup	Clear, fat-free broth; bouillon	Same as clear, plus strained or blended cream soups	Same as clear and full, plus all cream soups	All
Cereal	Not included	Cooked refined cereal	Cooked cereal, corn flakes, rice, noodles, macaroni, and spaghetti	All
Bread	Not included	Not included	White bread, crackers, Melba toast, and Zwieback	All
Protein foods	Not included	Milk, cream, milk drinks, and yogurt	Same as full, plus eggs (not fried), mild cheeses, cottage and cream cheeses, fowl, fish, tender beef, veal, lamb, liver, and bacon	All
Vegetables	Not included	Vegetable juices or pureed vegetables	Potatoes: baked, mashed, creamed, steamed, or scalloped; tender, cooked, whole, bland vegetables; fresh lettuce, and tomatoes	All
Fruit and fruit juices	Strained fruit juices as tolerated and flavored fruit drinks	Fruit juices	Same as clear and full, plus cooked fruit: peaches, pears, apple sauce, peeled apricots, and white cherries; ripe peaches, pears, and bananas; orange and grapefruit sections without membrane	All
Desserts and gelatin	Fruit-flavored gelatin, fruit ices, and popsicles	Same as clear, plus sherbet, ice cream, puddings, custard, and frozen yogurt	Same as clear and full, plus plain sponge cakes, plain cookies, plain cake, puddings, and pies made with allowed foods	All
Miscellaneous	Soft drinks as tolerated, coffee, tea, decaffeinated coffee and tea, cereal beverages such as Postum, sugar, honey, salt, hard candy, Polycose (Abbott Nutrition, Columbus, Ohio), and residue-free supplements	Same as clear, plus margarine and all supplements	Same as clear and full, plus mild salad dressings	All

*Seldom used.
†Mechanically altered diets can vary depending on the condition of the patient. This may include pureed foods, mechanically soft foods, or mechanically advanced diets that focus on foods with high moisture.

reflux, or continuous vomiting, a nasoduodenal or naso-jejunal tube may be more appropriate (Figure 22-1, *A*). In both cases, a tube is first inserted through the nose and into the stomach. It is then passed through the stomach and into the appropriate portion of the small intestine by peristaltic activity or endoscopic or fluoroscopic guidance. Correct placement of the tube is verified by radiography, auscultation, or gastric content aspiration. Modern small-bore nasoenteric feeding tubes are made of soft and flexible polyurethane and silicone materials. These feeding tubes are relatively comfortable for the patient, and they easily carry the variety of nutrient materials that are available in enteral nutrition support formulas.

Alternative Routes. The patient's disease state, GI anatomy, function, motility, and estimated length of enteral therapy are all important aspects to consider when determining the most appropriate access point for enteral feedings. The nasoenteric route is indicated for short-term therapy of 4 weeks or less in many clinical situations. For long-term feedings, however, an enterostomy (i.e., the

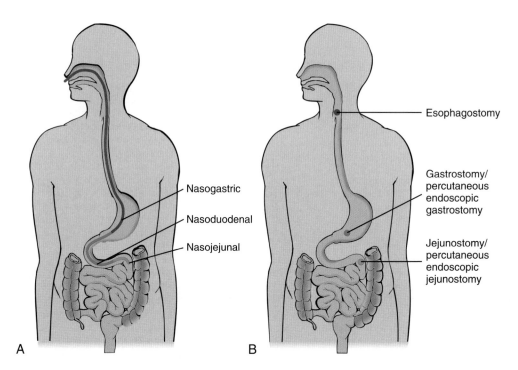

Figure 22-1 Types of enteral feeding. **A,** Nonsurgical routes accessed through the nasal cavity. **B,** Surgically placed feeding routes. (Copyright Rolin Graphics.)

surgical placement of the tube at progressive points along the GI tract) provides a more comfortable route, as follows (see Figure 22-1, *B*):

- *Esophagostomy:* A cervical esophagostomy is placed at the level of the cervical spine to the side of the neck after head and neck surgeries for cancer or traumatic injury. This placement removes the discomfort of the nasal route and enables the entry point to be easily concealed under clothing.
- *Percutaneous endoscopic gastrostomy:* A gastrostomy tube may be surgically placed through the abdominal wall into the stomach if the patient is not at risk for aspiration.
- *Percutaneous endoscopic jejunostomy:* A jejunostomy tube is surgically placed through the abdominal wall and passed through the duodenum into the jejunum. This procedure is indicated for patients with gastroparesis, gastric obstructions, or a history of reflux or aspiration or for those who otherwise cannot tolerate gastric feedings.

Formula. The tube-feeding formula is generally prescribed by the physician and the clinical dietitian in accordance with the patient's nutrition needs and tolerance. In addition to the immediate needs of the patient, other considerations include preexisting conditions,

comorbidities, food allergies, food intolerances, and other aspects of nutrient needs that are specific to the patient. Several varieties of commercial formulas are available and designed to meet particular needs. These products may be made from intact nutrients for use with a fully functioning GI system that is capable of digestion and absorption. Others may be made from predigested elemental or semi-elemental nutrients that are readily absorbed with only minimal residue. Still others may be formulated for special problems or single-nutrient modules of protein, carbohydrate, and fat mixed together as calculated by the dietitian or the pharmacist to meet a patient's specific needs.

With the development of improved formulas and feeding equipment, the question of using blender-mixed formulas of regular foods seldom arises. The use of pureed table food for tube feedings may present the following problems:

- *Physical form:* Foods that are broken down and mixed in a blender yield a sticky, larger-particle mixture that does not go through the small feeding tubes easily and thus requires the use of the more uncomfortable large-bore tubing.
- *Safety:* Blender-mixed formulas carry problems of bacterial growth and infection as well as

TABLE 22-4   **EXAMPLES OF ENTERAL FORMULAS AND MACRONUTRIENT COMPONENTS***

Brand Name	Manufacturer	MACRONUTRIENT SOURCES		
		Carbohydrate	Protein	Fat
Standard Complete Diets: Intact Macronutrients				
Ensure	Ross Products (Columbus, Ohio)	Sucrose	Casein	Soy oil and canola oil
Osmolite	Ross Products	Corn syrup	Casein and soy protein isolate	Canola oil, corn oil, and MCT
Jevity (1 Cal)	Ross Products	Maltodextrin and corn syrup	Casein	Canola oil, corn oil, and MCT
Standard Complete Diets: Semi-Elemental and Elemental				
Vital HN	Ross Products	Maltodextrin and sucrose	Whey protein concentrate	Safflower oil and MCT
Optimental	Ross Products	Maltodextrin and sucrose	Whey protein hydrolysate	Structured lipids (i.e., marine oil and MCT)

In addition to the standard formula examples provided, there are also specialty formulas that are intended to meet the needs of patients with unique requirements. Specialty diet formulas are available for trauma, cancer, HIV, renal conditions, and pediatric conditions.
*All formulas are enriched with essential vitamins and minerals as needed. There are many more formulas available; only a few examples are provided here.
MCT, Medium-chain triglycerides.

inconsistent nutrient composition because the solid components settle out.

- *Digestion and absorption:* Pureed food requires a fully functioning GI system to digest the food and absorb its released nutrients. Many patients have GI deficits that require nutrients with varying degrees of predigestion (i.e., hydrolysis) or smaller molecular structure.

For comparison, note that commercial formulas provide a sterile, homogenized solution that is suitable for small-bore feeding tubes and that ensures a fixed profile of nutrients in intact or elemental form. Formulas are available in varying caloric densities (e.g., 1 kcal/mL, 1.5 kcal/mL, 2 kcal/mL) to meet a patient's need for calories in a given volume of fluid. Some examples are given in Table 22-4. No matter what type of feeding tube or formula is used to meet a patient's physiologic needs, this feeding method may contribute to a patient's psychologic stress. Support for a patient's quality of life is an important part of the planning of patient care.

Rate. For any form of tube feeding, the amount of formula and the rate at which it is given must be regulated. See the Clinical Applications box entitled "Calculating a Tube Feeding," for details about setting the rate of administration for a tube feeding. Adults who are receiving bolus or gravity-controlled feedings that are introduced into the stomach generally tolerate full-strength formulas from the beginning if they are provided as three to eight feedings per day. The amount given is increased by 60 to 120 mL every 8 to 12 hours until the goal volume

for nutrient needs is met. Pump-assisted feedings are used for small-bowel feedings and for critically ill patients to allow for the slower administration of continuous feedings. Critically ill patients or those who have not been fed enterally for some time will not be able to tolerate large feedings at initiation and should start with slow rates (10 to 40 mL/hr), with gradual increases to the goal rate (e.g., increase by 10 to 20 mL/hr every 8 to 12 hours).[17]

Monitoring for Complications. Tube-fed patients require continuous monitoring for appropriate feeding schedules, tolerance, and potential complications. For patients who are fed by tube, diarrhea is the most frequently reported GI complication. Although a number of factors may contribute to diarrhea in tube-fed patients, the addition of fiber-rich formulas may improve bowel function and help to reduce the incidence of diarrhea.[18] However, fiber-supplemented formulas are contraindicated for patients with impaired gastric emptying.

---

auscultation listening to the sounds of the gastrointestinal tract with a stethoscope.

bolus feeding a volume of feeding from 250 mL to 500 mL over a short period of time (usually 10 to 15 minutes) that is given via several feedings per day.

continuous feeding an enteral feeding schedule with which the formula is infused via a pump over a 24-hour period.

CLINICAL APPLICATIONS

CALCULATING A TUBE FEEDING

To calculate the nutrient needs of a patient, the following information is required:

1. Ideal body weight in kilograms (lb/2.2)
   - Female: 100 lb ± 5 lb for every inch above or below 5 feet
   - Male: 106 lb ± 6 lb for every inch above or below 5 feet
2. Energy needs
   - Basal metabolic rate* × Injury factor (which depends on the condition of the patient)
3. Total formula needed (Energy need [kcal/day] ÷ Formula [kcal/mL])
4. Feeding schedule (Total formula ÷ Number of feedings)

Sample Calculation†
How many milliliters of formula does the following patient need at each feeding?

- She is a 37-year-old woman who is 5 feet and 7 inches tall.
- She is under considerable catabolic stress, with an injury factor of 1.8.
- Energy value of formula: 1.5 kcal/mL
- Schedule: 6 feedings per day

1. Ideal body weight: 100 lb + (7 in × 5 lb) = 135 lb/2.2 = 61.4 kg
2. Basal metabolic rate: (10 × 61.4 kg) + (6.25 × 170.2 cm) − (5 × 37) − 161 = 1332 kcal/day

   1332 kcal/day × 1.8 (injury factor) = 2398 kcal/day

3. Formula: 2398 kcal/day ÷ 1.5 kcal/mL = 1599 mL/day
4. Feeding schedule: 1599 mL/day ÷ 6 feedings/day = 266.5 mL/feeding

*As calculated by the Mifflin-St. Jeor equation: Female basal metabolic rate = (10 × Weight) + (6.25 × Height) − (5 × Age) − 161; male basal metabolic rate = (10 × Weight) + (6.25 × Height) − (5 × Age) + 5.
†These equations require the weight in kilograms, the height in centimeters, and the age in years.

Medications and *Clostridium difficile* enterocolitis are common culprits that cause diarrhea and should be ruled out before further changes are made to the enteral formula.[19]

Box 22-3 provides guidelines for an ideal monitoring schedule, and Table 22-5 gives problem-solving suggestions for common issues that may be encountered with tube feeding.

Parenteral Feedings

If a patient cannot tolerate food or formula moving through the GI tract, alternative methods of nutrition support are necessary. The term *parenteral nutrition* refers to any feeding method other than one that involves the normal GI route. In current medical terminology, parenteral nutrition specifically refers to the feeding of nutrients directly into the blood circulation through certain veins (i.e., a peripheral vein in the arm or the subclavian vein) when the GI tract cannot be used. Compared with enteral feeding, parenteral feedings are more invasive and expensive, and they introduce more risk. However, for patients in whom part or all of the GI tract or the accessory organs (e.g., liver, pancreas) are not functioning, it is necessary. Table 22-2 outlines indications for parenteral feedings. Depending on the nutrition support necessary, the following two routes are available:

- Peripheral parenteral nutrition is used when a solution of no more than 800 to 900 mOsm/L is sufficient to provide nutrient needs and when feeding is necessary for only a brief period of 5 to 7 days or less or as a supplement to enteral feedings. The osmolality (i.e., mOsm/L) of a solution depends on the concentration of its total particles, including dextrose, protein, and electrolytes. Small peripheral veins, usually in the arm, are used to deliver the less-concentrated solutions (Figure 22-2). Some catheters allow for an extended feeding period in a peripheral vein for individuals with large veins who can tolerate the extended dwell catheter.
- Total parenteral nutrition (TPN) is used when the energy and nutrient requirement is large or when full nutrition support is needed for longer periods. A large central vein (usually the subclavian vein that leads directly into the rapid flow of the superior vena cava to the heart) is used for the surgical placement of the catheter. The catheter may access the superior vena cava by direct access (Figure 22-3, *A*); a peripherally inserted central catheter (Figure 22-3, *B*); or a tunneled catheter (Figure 22-3, *C*). Nutrition support solutions of much higher osmolality are tolerated by the central veins.

TPN is used in cases of major surgery or complications, especially those that involve the GI tract or when the patient is unable to obtain sufficient nourishment enterally. TPN provides crucial nutrition support from solutions that contain glucose, amino acids, electrolytes,

BOX 22-3   MONITORING THE PATIENT WHO IS RECEIVING ENTERAL NUTRITION

Anthropometrics
- Weight (daily for 3 to 4 days until stable and then at least three times per week)
- Length or height in pediatric patients (monthly)

Physical Assessment
- Signs and symptoms of edema (daily)
- Fluid balance (daily)
- Adequacy of enteral intake (at least two times per week)
- GI motility (every 2-4 hours during initiation of feedings, every 8 hours when stable)
  - Abdominal distention and discomfort
  - Nausea and vomiting; risk for aspiration
  - Gastric residuals
  - Stool output and consistency
- Tube placement: make sure that the tube is in the desired location (daily for the short term or as needed if there are indications of migration)

Biochemical Measures
- Glucose (three times daily until stable, then two to three times per week)
- Serum electrolytes (daily until stable, then two to three times per week)
- Blood urea nitrogen (one to two times per week)
- Serum calcium, magnesium, and phosphorus (one to two times per week)
- Complete blood count and transferrin or prealbumin (once a week)

Adapted from Moore MC. *Nutrition assessment and care.* 6th ed. St Louis: Mosby; 2009; and Bankhead R, Boullata J, Brantley S, et al; A.S.P.E.N. Board of Directors. Enteral nutrition practice recommendations. *JPEN J Parenter Enteral Nutr.* 2009;33(2):122-167.

minerals, and vitamins. Fat in the form of lipid emulsions is also used to supply needed energy and the essential fatty acids. A basic TPN solution may contain between 3.5% and 15% crystalline amino acids and 5% to 70% dextrose, with additional micronutrients that are specific to patient needs. Each constituent of the parenteral solution contributes to the overall osmolality. Because the peripheral access point has a limited capacity for high osmolality, this must be considered when choosing an appropriate site for access.

A team of specialists including physicians, dietitians, pharmacists, and nurses works closely together during the administration of TPN. The physician and the clinical dietitian on the nutrition support team determine the individual formula that is needed on the basis of a detailed individual nutrition assessment and concurrent medication use (see the Drug-Nutrient Interaction box, "Propofol and Lipids in Nutrition Support"). The pharmacist

TABLE 22-5   PROBLEM-SOLVING TIPS FOR PATIENTS WHO ARE RECEIVING ENTERAL NUTRITION

Problem	Suggested Solutions
Thirst and oral dryness	Lubricate the lips Chew sugarless gum Brush the teeth Rinse the mouth frequently
Tube discomfort	Gargle with a mixture of warm water and mouthwash Gently blow the nose Clean the tube regularly with water or a water-soluble lubricant If persistent, gently pull out the tube, clean it, and reinsert it Request a smaller tube
Tension and fullness	Relax and breathe deeply after each feeding
Reflux or aspiration	Lift the head of the bed to 30 to 45 degrees
Constipation	Use a fiber-containing formula Assess for adequate fluid intake
Diarrhea	Take antidiarrheal medications if bacterial infections have been ruled out Avoid excess sorbitol and hypertonic solutions Use continuous feedings instead of bolus feedings Evaluate for lactose intolerance and intestinal mucosal atrophy
Gustatory Distress*	
General dissatisfaction with feeding	Warm or chill feedings *Caution:* Feedings that are too cold may cause diarrhea Serve favorite foods that have been liquefied
Persistent hunger	Chew gum Suck hard candy
Inability to drink	Rinse the mouth frequently with water and other liquids

*This refers to the frustration that is experienced when the sense of taste is not satisfied.

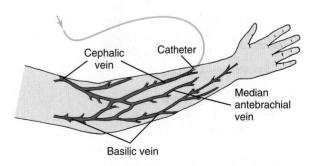

Figure 22-2 Peripheral parenteral nutrition feeding into the small veins of the arm.

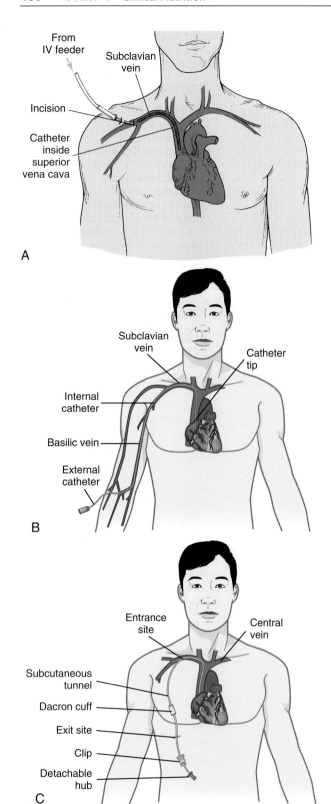

A

B

C

Figure 22-3 Catheter placement for total parenteral nutrition. **A,** A direct line via the subclavian vein to the superior vena cava. **B,** A peripherally inserted central catheter line. **C,** A tunneled catheter.

---

on the nutrition support team mixes the solutions in accordance with the prescription. The administration of the solution is an important nursing responsibility (Box 22-4).

The use of either TPN or enteral feedings via tube must first be discussed with the patient or the patient's family. The use of assisted medical technology in feeding is not always welcome and may be against the will of the patient for ethnic, cultural, religious, or personal reasons. See the Cultural Considerations box entitled "Cultural Differences in Advanced Care Planning" for more information.

SPECIAL NUTRITION NEEDS AFTER GASTROINTESTINAL SURGERY

Because the GI system is uniquely designed to handle food, a surgical procedure on any part of this system requires special dietary attention and modification.

DRUG-NUTRIENT INTERACTION

PROPOFOL AND LIPIDS IN NUTRITION SUPPORT

Propofol is a drug that is often used for sedation and anesthesia during surgery or to maintain sedation in mechanically ventilated patients in the intensive care unit. The drug is fat soluble, and it is emulsified in an oil and water solution for intravenous administration. During long-term sedation, patients often receive nutrition support in the form of enteral or total parenteral nutrition. One important consideration for the nutrition support team is the concurrent administration of propofol. The lipid emulsion contributes 1.1 kcal per mL; therefore, enteral or total parenteral nutrition solutions must provide reduced calories from fat to compensate for those that are provided with the propofol.

Propofol and other intravenous lipid emulsions are designed like chylomicrons. They are cleared from the bloodstream by the same enzyme: lipoprotein lipase. Elevated serum triglycerides may result if the infusion rate of propofol exceeds the clearance rate. This is more likely to occur with long-term use of propofol, when other risk factors are present (e.g. advanced age, previous diagnosis of cardiovascular disease, renal failure) or when the overall amount of lipid provided exceeds the patient's needs.[1] Serum triglycerides should be monitored during propofol infusion to prevent hypertriglyceridemia.

Kelli Boi

1. Mirtallo JM, Dasta JF, Kleinschmidt KC, Varon J. State of the art review: intravenous fat emulsions: current applications, safety profile, and clinical implications. *Ann Pharmacother*. 2010;44(4):688-700.

CULTURAL CONSIDERATIONS

CULTURAL DIFFERENCES IN ADVANCED CARE PLANNING

Advanced care planning is the process by which future treatment of a patient is determined before it is needed. Advanced directives and living wills are examples of documents that are recognized in the United States by all health care institutions. The Patient Self-Determination Act of 1991 was intended to promote the use of advanced care procedures and to strengthen the rights of patients during end-of-life medical procedures. Such documents are the only way that the treatment preferences of the patient can be ensured during times of unconsciousness or when there is otherwise an inability to communicate.

Some consider medical nutrition therapy in the form of enteral and parenteral nutrition to be a life-sustaining intervention. Several recent studies have compared the cultural discrepancies with regard to attitudes toward advanced care planning.[1-3] Researchers suggest that significant differences exist among various racial and ethnic patients and their caregivers with regard to advanced care planning and end-of-life decisions. When demographic values are examined, several factors are related to the completion of a living will, a do-not-resuscitate order, or orders that address the removal of life support. These values include the following:

- *Gender:* Females are more likely than males to complete advance directives.

- *Education:* Most individuals who complete advance directives have at least a high school education.
- *Religion:* Some religions (e.g., Catholicism, Judaism) encourage the completion of advance directives, whereas others promote the use of life-saving technology, even when the individual will not recover.
- *Age:* Individuals who have completed advance directives are more likely to be 85 years old or older.[3]
- *Ethnicity:* Researchers have also found African-American patients to be more likely than Caucasians to request life-supportive treatments.[1-3]

By recognizing such cultural differences in desired treatment and knowing the likelihood of patients having advanced care planning, health care professionals can assist the patient with greater awareness and sensitivity and provide more culturally appropriate education to patients and their families about advanced directives, living wills, and all methods of life support that may be available. Even if the patient has verbally expressed his or her wishes to the family, sometimes family members find it difficult to follow through with the patients wishes. Advanced care planning can alleviate the burden on the family and ensure that the patient's wishes are granted.

Jennifer E. Schmidt

1. Johnson RW, Newby LK, Granger CB, et al. Differences in level of care at the end of life according to race. *Am J Crit Care*. 2010;19(4):335-343; Quiz 344.
2. Sharma RK, Dy SM. Documentation of information and care planning for patients with advanced cancer: associations with patient characteristics and utilization of hospital care. *Am J Hosp Palliat Care*. 2011;28(8):543-549.
3. Alano GJ, Pekmezaris R, Tai JY, et al. Factors influencing older adults to complete advance directives. *Palliat Support Care*. 2010;8(3):267-275.

Mouth, Throat, and Neck Surgery

Surgery that involves the mouth, jaw, throat, or neck requires modification with regard to the mode of eating. These patients usually cannot chew or swallow normally, so accommodations must be made to address individual limitations.

Oral Liquid Feedings

Concentrated liquid feedings should be planned to ensure that adequate nutrition is supplied in a smaller amount of food. An enriched commercial formula can be used several times a day to supply needed nourishment.

Mechanical Soft Diets

Mechanical soft diets are used to transition between liquid and regular diets. Whole foods that are easy to chew and swallow are included as tolerated (see Table 22-3). Because high-fiber foods (e.g., vegetables) are often omitted as part of the mechanical soft diet, the overall fiber intake may be substantially lower than recommendations.

Enteral Feedings

For cases that involve radical neck or facial surgery or when a patient is severely debilitated, tube feedings may be indicated. For long-term needs, improved equipment and standardized commercial formulas have made continued home tube feeding possible for many patients. A nasogastric tube is often used, but the obstruction of the esophagus and other complications require the surgeon to make a gastrostomy at the time of surgery.

Gastric Surgery

Nutrition Problems

Because the stomach is the first major food reservoir in the GI tract, gastric surgery poses special problems for the maintenance of adequate nutrition. Some of these problems may develop immediately after the surgery, depending on the type of surgical procedure and the individual patient's response. Other physical or malabsorption complications may occur later, when the person begins to eat a regular diet.

Gastrectomy

Serious nutritional deficits may occur immediately after gastric surgery, especially after a total gastrectomy. Increased gastric fullness and distention may result if the gastric resection also involved a vagotomy. Because it lacks the normal nerve stimulus, the stomach becomes atonic and empties poorly. Food fermentation occurs,

and this produces discomfort, gas, and diarrhea. Weight loss is common after extensive gastric surgery.

To cover the immediate postoperative nutrition needs after a gastrectomy procedure, surgeons usually prepare a jejunostomy through which the patient can be fed an elemental formula. Frequent small oral feedings are resumed in accordance with the patient's tolerance. A typical pattern of simple dietary progression may cover approximately 2 weeks. The basic principles of such general diet therapy for the immediate postgastrectomy period involve both the size of the meals (which should be small and frequent) and the nature of the meals (which are generally simple, easily digested, bland, and low in bulk).

Dumping Syndrome

Dumping syndrome is a frequently encountered complication subsequent to extensive gastric resection. After the initial recovery from surgery, when the patient begins to feel better and eats a regular diet in greater volume and variety, discomfort may occur beginning 10 to 30 minutes after meals. A cramping and full feeling develops, the pulse becomes rapid, and a wave of weakness, cold sweating, and dizziness may follow. Nausea, vomiting, or diarrhea typically terminates the event.

This complex of symptoms constitutes a shock syndrome that results when a meal that contains a large proportion of readily soluble carbohydrates rapidly enters or "dumps" into the small intestine. When the stomach is bypassed, food quickly passes from the esophagus into the small intestine. This rapidly entering food mass is a concentrated solution with a higher osmolality compared with the surrounding circulation of blood. To achieve osmotic balance (i.e., a state of equal concentrations of fluids within the small intestine and the surrounding blood circulation), water is drawn from the circulatory system into the intestine. This water shift rapidly shrinks the vascular fluid volume, thereby causing shock. Blood pressure drops, and signs of rapid heart rate to rebuild the blood volume appear; these include a rapid pulse, sweating, weakness, and tremors.

If the meal consisted of simple carbohydrates, late dumping may occur approximately 2 hours after eating. The initial concentrated solution of simple carbohydrate has been rapidly absorbed, which results in a rapid rise in blood glucose and stimulates an overproduction of insulin. Blood sugar eventually drops below normal, with

---

vagotomy the cutting of the vagus nerve, which supplies a major stimulus for gastric secretions.

atonic without normal muscle tone.

CLINICAL APPLICATIONS

CASE STUDY: JOHN HAS A GASTRECTOMY

After a long experience with persistent peptic ulcer disease that involved more and more gastric tissue, John and his physician decided that surgery was needed. John then entered the hospital for a total gastrectomy. John weathered the surgery well and received some initial nutrition support from an elemental formula fed through a tube that the surgeon had placed into his jejunum. After a few days, the tube was removed. Over the next 2-week period, John was gradually able to take a soft diet in small oral feedings. He soon recovered enough to go home, and he gradually felt his strength returning. He was relieved to be free of his former ulcer pain, and he began to resume more and more of his usual activities, including eating a regular diet of increasing volume and variety.

However, as time went by, John began having more discomfort after meals. He felt a cramping sensation, an increased heartbeat, and then a wave of weakness with sweating and dizziness. John would often become nauseated and have diarrhea. As his anxiety increased, he began to eat less and less, and his weight began to drop. He was soon in a state of general malnutrition.

John finally returned to seek medical help. The physician and the clinical dietitian outlined a change in his eating habits, and a special food plan was developed for him. Although the diet seemed strange to him, John followed it

faithfully because he had felt so ill. To his surprise, he soon found that his previous symptoms after eating had almost completely disappeared. Because he felt so much better on the new diet plan, he formed new eating habits around it. His weight gradually returned to normal, and his state of nutrition markedly improved. John found that he always fared better if he would nibble on food items throughout the day rather than consume large meals as he used to do.

Questions for Analysis

1. What were John's nutrition needs immediately after surgery and for the next 2 weeks? Why did his feedings need to be resumed cautiously?
2. Why is emphasis given to postsurgical protein sources? How should this nutrient be provided?
3. Why is fluid therapy important after surgery?
4. After John began to feel better and resumed eating, why did he become ill? Describe why his symptoms developed.
5. Using the principles of the special diet that the dietitian provided to relieve John's symptoms, plan a day's meal and snack pattern for John that includes basic instructions and suggestions that you would discuss with him.

---

symptoms of hypoglycemia (e.g., weakness, shaky, sweating, confusion). These distressing reactions to food increase anxiety. As a result, less and less food is eaten. Weight loss and general malnutrition follow (see the Clinical Applications box, "Case Study: John Has a Gastrectomy").

Bariatric Surgery

Special considerations must be made after bariatric surgery, because patients typically have deficiencies in several micronutrients for an extended period (see the For Further Focus box, "Nutrient Deficiencies after Bariatric Surgery"). After gastric bypass, patients progress slowly from a clear liquid diet to a regular diet at approximately 6 weeks postsurgery, but they are limited to approximately 1 cup of food per meal from that point forward, and they are subject to dumping syndrome. Patients should avoid using a straw to reduce air swallowing, which can cause discomfort. Table 22-6 provides a general guideline for dietary advancement after bariatric surgery. The combination of severely reduced intake coupled with dumping syndrome dramatically reduces nutrient availability.[20]

Careful adherence to the postoperative diet allows dramatic relief from these distressing symptoms as well as the gradual stabilization of weight. The careful reintroduction of milk in small amounts may later be used to test tolerance. Patients may also find that eating slowly, eliminating fluids during meals, and lying down for 15 to 30 minutes after eating help to decrease the rate of gastric emptying.

Gallbladder Surgery

For patients with acute gallbladder inflammation (i.e., cholecystitis) or gallstones (i.e., cholelithiasis) (Figure 22-4), the treatment is usually the removal of the gallbladder (i.e., cholecystectomy). The modern procedure for this removal, called *laparoscopic cholecystectomy,* requires only minimal surgery that involves small skin punctures;

---

cholecystitis   acute gallbladder inflammation.

cholelithiasis   gallstones.

cholecystectomy   the removal of the gallbladder.

TABLE 22-6 **DIET STAGES AFTER BARIATRIC SURGERY***

Diet State	Postoperative Period	Fluids And Foods	Comments
1	1 to 2 days	Clear liquids[†]	Sugar-free, caffeine-free, noncarbonated
2	2 to 3 days	Clear and full liquids	Full liquids should have 15 g of sugar or less and 3 g of fat or less per serving. Examples: 1% or skim milk mixed with whey or soy protein powder (with a limit of 20 g of protein per serving) Lactaid milk or soymilk mixed with soy protein powder Light or plain yogurt Begin supplementation: chewable multivitamin with mineral supplementation, chewable or liquid calcium citrate, vitamin D, and vitamin B$_{12}$[‡]
3	10 to 14 days	Clear liquids; replace full liquids with pureed, diced, soft, and moist protein sources	Examples of protein sources: eggs; ground meat; poultry; fish; cooked beans; cottage cheese; low-fat yogurt Nonfat gravy or light mayonnaise can be added to moisten food. Continue to drink 48 to 64 oz of fluid per day at least 30 minutes before or after food intake.
	4 weeks[§]	Add well-cooked soft vegetables and soft, peeled fruit	Protein should be consumed first to ensure adequate protein intake before satiety. Continue to drink 48 to 64 oz of fluid per day at least 30 minutes before or after food intake.
	5 weeks[§]	Add crackers with protein	Continue to consume protein with some fruit or vegetable at every meal. Avoid pasta, rice, and bread. Continue to drink 48 to 64 oz of fluid per day at least 30 minutes before or after food intake.
4	6 weeks[§]	Healthy solid foods	Consume mixed meals of protein, fruits, vegetables, and whole-grain carbohydrates. Eat from small plates with small utensils for portion control. Continue to drink 48 to 64 oz of fluid per day at least 30 minutes before or after food intake.

*These diet stages are not standardized. The timing of diet advancement should be modified on the basis of the individual's tolerance for the previous diet stage.
†For procedures other than laparoscopic adjustable gastric banding, the diet can be started after a Gastrografin swallow test is performed to assess for leaks.
‡For biliopancreatic diversion with duodenal switch, at least 350 to 500 µg of oral vitamin B$_{12}$ daily is recommended; this may need to be administered intramuscularly.
§This is usually longer for biliopancreatic diversion with duodenal switch.

the previous surgery required a transverse right upper quadrant incision. Through these small openings, the surgeon can insert needed instruments and a laparoscope fitted with a miniature camera and bright fiber-optic lighting.

Because the function of the gallbladder is to concentrate and store bile, which helps with the digestion and absorption of fat, some moderation in dietary fat intake is usually indicated. After surgery, the control of fat in the diet (e.g., less than 30% of total energy intake as fat) facilitates wound healing and comfort, because the hormonal stimulus for bile secretion still functions in the surgical area, thereby causing pain with the high intake of fatty foods. The body also needs a period to adjust to

the more dilute supply of bile that is available to assist with fat digestion and absorption directly from the liver. Depending on individual tolerance and response, a low-fat diet may be needed; see the guide given for gallbladder disease in Table 18-7.

Intestinal Surgery

Intestinal disease that involves tumors, lesions, or obstructions may require the surgical resection of the affected intestinal area. For complicated cases that require the removal of large sections of the small intestine, the use of enteral nutrition support may be difficult at first. In such cases, TPN is used for nutrition support, with a

FOR FURTHER FOCUS

NUTRIENT DEFICIENCIES AFTER BARIATRIC SURGERY

Bariatric surgery for obese patients (i.e., those with a body mass index of 30 kg/m^2 or more) is becoming more common around the world. Although surgery is currently the most effective means of long-term weight loss and maintenance, it is not without drawbacks. Restrictive eating patterns, dumping syndrome, and nutrient deficiencies from malabsorption are common complications after surgery. The quality-of-life cost-benefit ratio of surgery is difficult to assess: obesity increases the mortality rate, but the complications of surgery can introduce a new set of risks.

The Roux-en-Y gastric bypass (see Chapter 15), in which the amount of bowel that is capable of absorbing nutrients is reduced, is the surgery of choice for obesity in the United States. Obese patients are at risk for complications during surgery from comorbid conditions such as diseases of the cardiovascular, endocrine, renal, pulmonary, gastrointesti-

nal, and musculoskeletal systems.[1] Therefore, special care must be taken to prepare the patient for surgery.

Bariatric surgery that induces malabsorption (e.g., gastric bypass, biliopancreatic diversion) presents particular nutritional problems. Protein energy malnutrition is a significant risk for many patients, and it results in hospitalization and the necessity of parenteral nutrition support in severe cases. Patients who have undergone bariatric procedures should be screened every 6 to 12 months for protein energy malnutrition.[2] In addition, significant micronutrient deficiencies warrant mineral and multivitamin supplementation postoperatively. There are also specific nutrients to be aware of and that should be supplemented for life[3]:

- Vitamins: A, B$_1$, B$_{12}$, C, D, K, and folate
- Minerals: copper, iron, selenium, and zinc

1. Eisenberg D, Duffy AJ, Bell RL. Update on obesity surgery. *World J Gastroenterol*. 2006;12(20):3196-3203.
2. Strohmayer E, Via MA, Yanagisawa R. Metabolic management following bariatric surgery. *Mt Sinai J Med*. 2010;77(5):431-445.
3. Shankar P, Boylan M, Sriram K. Micronutrient deficiencies after bariatric surgery. *Nutrition*. 2010;26(11-12):1031-1037.

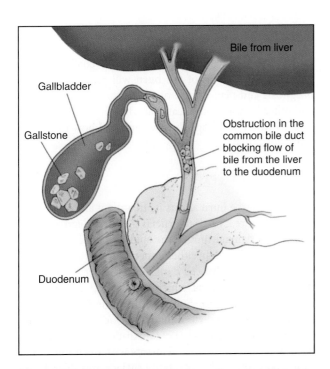

Figure 22-4 Gallbladder with stones (i.e., cholelithiasis).

small allowance of oral feeding for personal food desires when tolerated. After general resection for less severe cases, a diet that is relatively low in dietary fiber may be beneficial in the beginning to allow for healing and comfort.

Intestinal surgery sometimes requires making an opening in the abdominal wall to the intestine, called a *stoma,* for the elimination of fecal waste. If the opening is in the area of the ileum, which is the last section of the small intestine, it is called an *ileostomy* (Figure 22-5, *A*). The food mass is still fairly liquid at this point in the GI tract, and more problems are encountered with management. If the opening is farther along in the large intestine, it is called a *colostomy* (Figure 22-5, *B*). In the large intestine, the water is predominantly reabsorbed and the remaining feces are more solid, thereby making management easier. Patients with an ostomy begin a clear liquid diet during the immediate postoperative period. Patients progress toward small, frequent feedings of meals that are relatively low in dietary fiber, as tolerated. Encouraging patients to drink plenty of fluids between meals may help to reduce diarrhea. Lactose intolerance and fat malabsorption are common complications in patients with ileostomies and should be monitored, with dietary adjustments made as indicated.[21]

Patients need support and practical help to learning about self-care with an ostomy. Eliminating gas-producing foods, odor-causing foods, and foods that may cause an obstruction will help to facilitate maintenance. A relatively low-fiber diet is helpful at first, but the goal is to advance to an individualized diet that is acceptable to the patient as soon as tolerated. Progression to a regular diet is important for nutritional value and emotional support. Regular food provides psychologic comfort, and

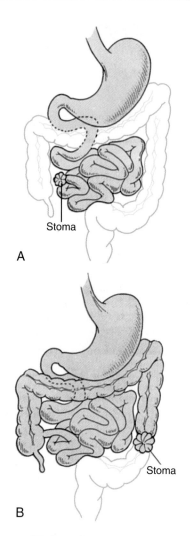

Figure 22-5 A, Ileostomy. **B,** Colostomy.

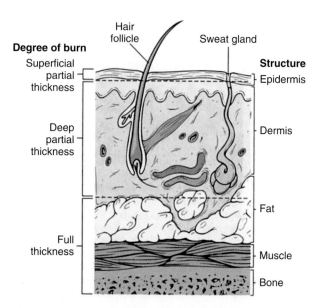

Figure 22-6 Depth of skin area involved in burns. (Reprinted from Lewis SM, Heitkemper MM, Dirksen SR. *Medical-surgical nursing: assessment and management of clinical problems.* 7th ed. St Louis: Mosby; 2007.)

dietary adjustments to individual preferences for specific foods can be made.

Rectal Surgery

For a brief period after rectal surgery or hemorrhoidectomy, a clear fluid or nonresidue diet (see Table 22-1) may be indicated to reduce painful elimination and to allow for healing. In some cases, a nonresidue commercial elemental formula may be used to delay bowel movements until the surgical area has healed. Return to a regular diet is usually rapid.

SPECIAL NUTRITION NEEDS FOR PATIENTS WITH BURNS

In the United States, there are approximately 450,000 visits to emergency departments and 3500 deaths per year

as a result of burn injuries.[22] The treatment of severe burns presents a tremendous nutrition challenge. The location and severity of the burn will greatly affect the prognosis and plan of care of the patient. Comorbidities and other injuries complicate care, but they must be considered when deciding when, where, and how to initiate nutrition support.

Type and Extent of Burns

The depth of the burn affects its treatment and its healing process (Figure 22-6). Superficial (i.e., first-degree) burns involve cell damage only to the epidermis. Second-degree burns are classified as either superficial partial-thickness burns, which involve cell damage to the dermis, or deep partial-thickness burns, which involve both the first and second layers of skin. Full-thickness (i.e., third-degree) burns result in complete skin loss, including the underlying fat layer. Subdermal (i.e. fourth-degree) burns leave bone and tendon exposed. Patients with burn injuries of more than 10% of the total body surface area (TBSA) are referred to a regional burn unit facility for specialized burn team care that includes nutrition support.

Stages of Nutrition Care

The nutrition care of patients with massive burns presents a great challenge and must be constantly adjusted to individual needs and responses. At each stage, critical attention is given to amino acid requirements for tissue rebuilding, fluid and electrolyte balance, and energy support. Energy expenditure in burned patients can be very high, and it will fluctuate depending on the stage of healing.

Burn Shock or Ebb Phase

From the first hours until approximately the second day after a burn, massive flooding edema occurs at the burn site. The destruction of protective skin leads to immediate losses of heat, water, electrolytes (mainly sodium), and protein. As water is drawn from surrounding blood to replace the losses, general loss continues, blood volume and pressure drop, and urine output decreases. Cell dehydration follows as intracellular water is drawn out to balance the loss of tissue fluid. Cell potassium is also withdrawn, and circulating serum potassium levels rise.

Immediate intravenous fluid therapy with a salt solution (e.g., 6% hetastarch in saline, balanced salt solution) or lactated Ringer's solution replaces water and electrolytes and helps to prevent shock. After approximately 12 hours, when vascular permeability returns to normal and losses begin to decrease at the burn site, albumin solutions or plasma can be used to help restore blood volume. Medical nutrition therapy is not the priority during the ebb phase. The stability of the patient and his or her resuscitation needs are greater during this phase and must be established before nutrition efforts are considered.

Acute or Flow Phase

After approximately 48 to 72 hours, tissue fluids and electrolytes are gradually reabsorbed, and the pattern of massive tissue loss is stabilized. A sudden diuresis occurs, and this indicates successful initial therapy. Constant attention to fluid intake and output with evaluation for any signs of dehydration or overhydration are essential. This state of hypermetabolism may last weeks to months. Toward the end of the first week after the burn, adequate bowel function returns, and a rigorous medical nutrition therapy program must begin. The following three major reasons exist for these increased nutrient and energy demands:

1. Tissue destruction brings large losses of protein and electrolytes that must be replaced.

2. Tissue catabolism follows the injury and involves a further loss of lean body mass and nitrogen.

3. Increased metabolism brings added nutrition needs to cover the energy costs of infection, fever, and the increased protein metabolism of tissue replacement and skin grafting.

Medical Nutrition Therapy

Most patients with burns of less than 20% of the TBSA are able to consume an oral meal plan that is adequate in nutrient needs, unless the burn site hinders eating. Successful nutrition therapy during this critical feeding period is based on vigorous protein and energy intake as follows[21]:

- *High protein:* The aggressive supplementation of protein is crucial to promote early wound healing and to support immune function. Depending on the extent of the burn and the associated catabolic losses, individual protein needs vary from 1.5 to 2 g/kg/day. This level of protein will equal 20% to 25% of energy intake. For obese individuals or patients with burns that cover less than 10% of the TBSA, protein intake is calculated at 1.2 g/kg.

- *High energy:* Energy needs are commonly between 25 to 30 kcal/kg. However, individual energy needs will vary greatly among patients and should be calculated with the most precise method available. Energy needs are calculated by using either the Harris-Benedict equation with a stress factor of 1.5; the Curreri equations on the basis of the amount of TBSA burned; or indirect calorimetry with an injury factor of 20% to 30%. The Harris-Benedict and indirect calorimetry methods were covered in Chapter 6. The Curreri equation is as follows: 25 kcal/kg body weight + (40 × Percentage of TBSA burned), with a maximum of 50% TBSA used. Beyond 50% of the TBSA being burned, little increase in total energy needs occurs.

- Overfeeding increases metabolic stress and should be avoided. Such high energy needs are necessary to spare the protein that is essential for tissue rebuilding and to supply the greatly increased metabolic demands that are essential for healing. A liberal portion of the total kilocalories should come from carbohydrate, with a moderate amount of fat supplying the remaining needs. The frequent recalculation of energy needs may be necessary if the patient is gaining or losing weight. One goal of medical nutrition therapy is for patients to not lose more than of 10% of their body weight from the point of admission.

---

lactated Ringer's solution a sterile solution of calcium chloride, potassium chloride, sodium chloride, and sodium lactate in water that is given to replenish fluid and electrolytes; this solution was developed by the English physiologist Sidney Ringer (1835-1910).

▪ *High vitamin, high mineral:* Increased vitamin C (500 mg/day) may be needed as a partner with amino acids for tissue rebuilding. Vitamin A (10,000 IU/day) and zinc are specifically important for optimal immune function, and they are often supplemented. Increased thiamin, riboflavin, and niacin are necessary for increased energy and protein metabolism. Special attention to electrolyte imbalances and to calcium and phosphorus ratios in the blood are warranted during this period. Patients are given a daily multivitamin supplement.

Dietary Management. With any method, a careful dietary intake record must be maintained to measure progress toward the increased nutrition goals. Oral feedings are preferred if they are well tolerated and if they allow nutrition needs to be met. Concentrated liquids with added protein or amino acids and commercial formulas such as Ensure may be used as added interval nourishment. Solid foods given on the basis of individual preferences are usually tolerated by the second week. However, hypermetabolic states and poor appetite make oral feedings difficult for patients with major burns.

Either enteral or parenteral methods of feeding may be used to meet crucial nutrient demands when oral intake is inadequate, which is defined as less than 75% of goal intake for more than 3 days. When enteral feedings are impossible because of associated injuries or complications, parenteral feeding can provide essential nutrition support. Studies evaluating early (i.e., within 24 hours) versus delayed (i.e., after 48 hours) enteral nutrition support indicate that initiating nutrition support soon after the burn injury may stimulate protein retention and reduce the hypermetabolic response, but this has not been associated with an improved recovery rate and thus remains inconclusive.[23]

Follow-Up Reconstruction. Continued nutrition support is essential to maintain tissue strength for successful skin grafting or reconstructive plastic surgery. Patients need the physical rebuilding of body resources that surgery requires as well as personal support to rebuild their will and spirit, because disfigurement and disability are quite possible. Optimal physical stamina that is gained through persistent and supportive medical, nutrition, and nursing care helps patients to rebuild the personal resources that they need to cope.

SUMMARY

▪ Before surgery, the tasks are to correct any existing deficiencies and to build nutrition reserves to meet surgical demands. After surgery, the tasks are to replace losses and to support recovery. The additional task of encouraging eating is often necessary during this period of healing.

▪ Postsurgical feedings are given in a variety of ways, and the oral route is always preferred. However, the inability to eat or damage to the intestinal tract may require enteral tube feedings or parenteral feedings.

Special formulas are used for such alternate means of nourishment, and these are designed to meet individual needs.

▪ For patients who are undergoing surgery of the GI tract, special diets are modified in accordance with the surgical procedure being performed.

▪ For patients with massive burns, increased nutrition support is necessary in successive stages in response to the burn injury and to the continuing requirements of tissue rebuilding.

CRITICAL THINKING QUESTIONS

1. Describe the consequences of nutrient imbalances (specifically with protein, energy, vitamins, minerals, and fluid) on the preoperative, immediate postoperative, and long-term postoperative periods.
2. Describe appropriate medical nutrition therapy for patients who are undergoing gastric resection, cholecystectomy, and rectal surgery.
3. How do an ileostomy and a colostomy differ? What are the dietary needs for each?
4. Outline the nutrition care of a burn patient from treatment for immediate shock through recovery and tissue reconstruction.

CHAPTER CHALLENGE QUESTIONS

True-False

Write the correct statement for each statement that is false.

1. *True or False:* Nothing is given by mouth for at least 8 hours before surgery to avoid food aspiration during anesthesia.
2. *True or False:* The most common nutrient deficiency related to surgery is protein.
3. *True or False:* Vitamin C is essential for wound healing, because it is involved in building strong connective tissue.
4. *True or False:* Regardless of the type, oral liquid feedings usually provide little nourishment.
5. *True or False:* Tube feedings can only be successfully prepared from complete commercial preparations.
6. *True or False:* After gastrectomy, a patient can return to regular eating habits within a few days.
7. *True or False:* After a diseased gallbladder is surgically removed, a patient can freely tolerate any foods that contain high amounts of fat.
8. *True or False:* A careful diet record of the total food and liquid intake is important for a burn patient to ensure that increased nutrient and energy demands are met.

Multiple Choice

1. Postsurgical edema develops at the wound site as a result of
   a. decreased plasma protein levels.
   b. excess water intake.
   c. excess sodium intake.
   d. a lack of early ambulation and physical exercise.
2. In a postoperative orthopedic patient's diet, protein is essential to
   a. provide the extra energy that is needed to regain strength.
   b. provide a matrix to anchor mineral matter and to form bone.
   c. control the basal metabolic rate.
   d. give more taste to the diet, thereby increasing appetite.
3. Complete high-quality protein is essential to wound healing, because it
   a. supplies the essential amino acids that are needed for tissue synthesis.
   b. is used to meet the body's increased energy demands.
   c. is a source of glucose for the body.
   d. provides the most concentrated source of kilocalories.
4. A diet for postgastrectomy dumping syndrome should include which of the following? *(Circle all that apply.)*
   a. Small, frequent meals
   b. No liquid with meals
   c. No milk, sugar, sweets, or desserts
   d. A high protein content
5. For a burn patient, a diet that is high in protein and energy is essential to do which of the following? *(Circle all that apply.)*
   a. To replace the extensive loss of tissue protein at burn sites
   b. To provide essential amino acids for extensive tissue healing
   c. To counteract the negative nitrogen balance from a loss of lean body mass
   d. To meet the added metabolic demands of infection or fever

⊖volve Please refer to the Students' Resource section of this text's Evolve Web site for additional study resources.

REFERENCES

1. Kaiser MJ, Bauer JM, Rämsch C, et al. Frequency of malnutrition in older adults: a multinational perspective using the mini nutritional assessment. *J Am Geriatr Soc.* 2010;58(9):1734-1738.
2. Corish CA. Pre-operative nutritional assessment. *Proc Nutr Soc.* 1999;58(4):821-829.
3. Sullivan DH, Bopp MM, Roberson PK. Protein-energy undernutrition and life-threatening complications among the hospitalized elderly. *J Gen Intern Med.* 2001;17(12):923-932.
4. Joosten KF, Hulst JM. Prevalence of malnutrition in pediatric hospital patients. *Curr Opin Pediatr.* 2008;20(5):590-596.
5. Thorpe MP, Evans EM. Dietary protein and bone health: harmonizing conflicting theories. *Nutr Rev.* 2011;69(4):215-230.
6. Loenneke JP, Balapur A, Thrower AD, et al. Short report: relationship between quality protein, lean mass and bone health. *Ann Nutr Metab.* 2010;57(3-4):219-220.
7. Sun LC, Shih YL, Lu CY, et al. Randomized, controlled study of branched chain amino acid-enriched total parenteral nutrition in malnourished patients with gastrointestinal cancer undergoing surgery. *Am Surg.* 2008;74(3):237-242.

8. Grocott MP, Mythen MG, Gan TJ. Perioperative fluid management and clinical outcomes in adults. *Anesth Analg.* 2005;100(4):1093-1106.

9. Food and Nutrition Board, Institute of Medicine. *Dietary reference intakes for energy, carbohydrate, fiber, fat, fatty acids, cholesterol, protein, and amino acids.* Washington, DC: National Academies Press; 2002.

10. Wilson JX. Mechanism of action of vitamin C in sepsis: ascorbate modulates redox signaling in endothelium. *Biofactors.* 2009;35(1):5-13.

11. Long CL, Maull KI, Krishnan RS, et al. Ascorbic acid dynamics in the seriously ill and injured. *J Surg Res.* 2003;109(2):144-148.

12. Rümelin A, Humbert T, Lühker O, et al. Metabolic clearance of the antioxidant ascorbic acid in surgical patients. *J Surg Res.* 2005;129(1):46-51.

13. Ellinger S, Stehle P. Efficacy of vitamin supplementation in situations with wound healing disorders: results from clinical intervention studies. *Curr Opin Clin Nutr Metab Care.* 2009;12(6):588-595.

14. Lansdown AB, Mirastschijski U, Stubbs N, et al. Zinc in wound healing: theoretical, experimental, and clinical aspects. *Wound Repair Regen.* 2007;15(1):2-16.

15. Leistra E, Willeboordse F, van Bokhorst-de van der Schueren MA, et al. Predictors for achieving protein and energy requirements in undernourished hospital patients. *Clin Nutr.* 2011;30(4):484-489.

16. Ha L, Hauge T, Spenning AB, Iversen PO. Individual, nutritional support prevents undernutrition, increases muscle strength and improves QoL among elderly at nutritional risk hospitalized for acute stroke: a randomized, controlled trial. *Clin Nutr.* 2010;29(5):567-573.

17. Bankhead R, Boullata J, Brantley S, et al; A.S.P.E.N. Board of Directors. Enteral nutrition practice recommendations. *JPEN J Parenter Enteral Nutr.* 2009;33(2): 122-167.

18. Whelan K, Schneider SM. Mechanisms, prevention, and management of diarrhea in enteral nutrition. *Current Opin Gastroenterol.* 2011;27(2):152-159.

19. O'Keefe SJ. Tube feeding, the microbiota, and *Clostridium difficile* infection. *World J Gastroenterol.* 2010;16(2): 139-142.

20. Strohmayer E, Via MA, Yanagisawa R. Metabolic management following bariatric surgery. *Mt Sinai J Med.* 2010; 77(5):431-445.

21. American Dietetic Association. *ADA nutrition care manual.* American Dietetic Association; 2010.

22. American Burn Association. Burn incidence and treatment in the United States: 2011 fact sheet (website): www.ameriburn.org/resources_factsheet.php?PHPSESSID=4b52270c2 10bae604542f5b77e9827c6. Accessed November 16. 2011.

23. Wasiak J, Cleland H, Jeffery R. Early versus late enteral nutritional support in adults with burn injury: a systematic review. *J Hum Nutr Diet.* 2007;20(2):75-83.

FURTHER READING AND RESOURCES

American Burn Association. www.ameriburn.org

American Society for Parenteral and Enteral Nutrition. www.nutritioncare.org

Burn Foundation. www.burnfoundation.org

Ferreira LG, Anastacio LR, Correia MI. The impact of nutrition on cirrhotic patients awaiting liver transplantation. *Curr Opin Clin Nutr Metab Care.* 2010;13(5):554-561.

Koch TR, Finelli FC. Postoperative metabolic and nutritional complications of bariatric surgery. *Gastroenterol Clin North Am.* 2010;39(1):109-124.

CHAPTER 23

Nutrition Support in Cancer and AIDS

KEY CONCEPTS

- Environmental agents, genetic factors, and weaknesses in the body's immune system can contribute to the development of cancer.
- The strength of the body's immune system relates to its overall nutritional status.
- Nutrition problems affect the nature of the disease process and the medical treatment

methods for patients with cancer or acquired immunodeficiency syndrome (AIDS).
- The progressive effects of the human immunodeficiency virus (HIV) through its three stages of white T-cell destruction have many nutrition implications and often require aggressive medical nutrition therapy.

W ith the accumulating environmental problems and changing lifestyles of the past several decades, cancer has become a more prevalent health problem in the United States. Because cancer is generally associated with aging, increases in life expectancy have somewhat contributed to this growing incidence. Although cancer and HIV/AIDS share a direct relationship with the body's immune system and basic nutrition needs, their courses and fatal outcomes are distinct.

This chapter looks at nutrition support in relation to both cancer and HIV/AIDS. Both diseases have important nutrition connections for prevention and therapy.

SECTION I **CANCER**

PROCESS OF CANCER DEVELOPMENT

The Nature of Cancer

Multiple Forms

One of the problems with the study and treatment of cancer is that it is not a single problem: it has a highly variable nature, and it expresses itself in multiple forms. Cancer is a major health problem in the United States. It

is currently the second leading cause of death, and it affects 6.1% of all adults who are older than 18 years old.[1] The general term *cancer* is used to designate a malignant tumor or *neoplasm*, which is a term that refers to new growth. The many forms of cancer vary in prevalence worldwide and change as populations migrate to different environments. The Cultural Considerations box entitled "Types and Incidence of Cancer in American Populations" outlines the prevalence of cancer in the United States on the basis of various characteristics.

CULTURAL CONSIDERATIONS

TYPES AND INCIDENCE OF CANCER IN AMERICAN POPULATIONS

The prevalence of cancer at any given time has many variables. The National Center for Health Statistics has reported the prevalence of cancer by race, education level, and family income[1]:

Characteristic	Percentage of Population with any form of Cancer, Aged 18 Years Old and Older
Race	
White	6.2%
Black or African American	4.3%
Native American or Alaska Native	5.4%
Asian	3.0%
Hispanic or Latino	3.6%
Mexican	3.3%
Education	
No high school diploma or general educational development tests	6.1%
High school diploma or general educational development tests	6.4%
Some college or more	7.1%
Percent of Poverty Level	
Less than 100%	6.2%
100% to 199%	6.0%
200% to 399%	5.5%
400% or more	6.0%

The confounding factors associated with cancer risk are complicated and multifactorial. A health care trend toward the prevention of cancer is a goal of the Healthy People 2020 national objectives. With a continued dedication to research, ideally prevention instead of treatment will become the norm. Identifying high-risk patients and encouraging regular physical examinations are important aspects of general health care as well as a valuable prevention tools.

1. National Center for Health Statistics. *Health, United States, 2010: with special feature on death and dying.* Hyattsville, Md: U.S. Government Printing Office; 2011.

The Cancer Cell

The continuous process of cell division is guided by the genetic code that is contained in the deoxyribonucleic acid (DNA) of the cell nucleus. This orderly process can be lost as the result of a mutation, particularly when the mutation occurs in a regulatory gene. Cell growth may form malignant tumors when normal gene control is lost. Thus, the misguided cell and its tumor tissue represent normal cell growth that has gone wrong. Cancer tumors are identified by their primary site of origin, their stage or tumor size and the presence of metastasis, and their grade (i.e., how aggressive the tumor is).

Carcinogenesis is often described as having three phases: initiation, promotion, and progression. *Initiation* is the point at which a mutagen causes irreversible damage to the DNA. *Promotion* is caused by an agent that triggers the mutated cell to grow and reproduce. *Progression* is the phase during which the cancer cells advance and become a malignant tumor that is capable of metastasizing.

neoplasm any new or abnormal cellular growth, specifically one that is uncontrolled and aggressive.

mutation a permanent transmissible change in a gene.

metastasis the spread to other tissue.

carcinogenesis the development of cancer.

Causes of Cancer Cell Development

The underlying cause of cancer is the fundamental loss of cell control over normal cell reproduction. Several factors may contribute to this loss and change a normal cell into a cancer cell, including chemical carcinogens, radiation, oncogenic viruses, epidemiologic factors (e.g., race, region, age, heredity, occupation), psychologic stress, and dietary factors. Many aspects of cancer are outside of the scope of this text and will not be addressed in detail here. The discussion here will focus on the nutritional aspects of cancer development and treatment.

Dietary Factors

Nutrition and cancer care focus on the following two fundamental areas:

- *Prevention,* in relation to the environment and the body's natural defense system
- *Therapy,* in relation to nutrition support for medical treatment and rehabilitation

The association between diet and cancer is complex. Although it has been the subject of much research, many questions are still unanswered. Foods contain both carcinogenic and anticarcinogenic compounds. Studies have found conflicting results regarding the protective role of specific nutrient intakes as well as total fruit and vegetable consumption in relation to cancer risk.[2] A general consensus links micronutrient deficiency or toxicity with an increased risk of DNA damage and cancer.[3,4] Thus, a well-balanced diet that includes the ample intake of fruits, vegetables, whole grains, and fiber is the general recommendation for health promotion and disease prevention.

The Body's Defense System

The body's defense system is remarkably efficient and complex. Special cells protect the body from external invaders such as bacteria and viruses and from internal aliens such as cancer cells.

Defensive Cells of the Immune System

Two major cell populations provide the immune system's primary "search and destroy" defense for detecting and killing non-self substances that carry potential disease. These two populations of lymphocytes, which are special types of white blood cells, develop early during life from a common stem cell in the bone marrow. The two types are T cells, which are derived from thymus cells, and B cells, which are derived from bursal intestinal cells (Figure 23-1). A major function of T cells is to activate the phagocytes, which are the cells that destroy invaders and kill

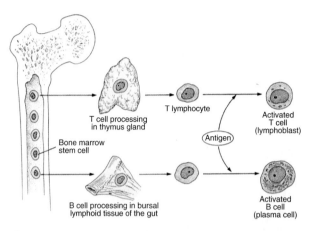

Figure 23-1 The development of the T and B cells, which are the lymphocyte components of the body's immune system. (Courtesy Eileen Draper.)

disease-carrying antigens. A major function of B cells is to produce proteins known as *antibodies*, which also kill antigens.

Relation of Nutrition to Immunity and Healing

Immunity. Balanced nutrition is necessary to maintain the integrity of the human immune system. Severe malnutrition compromises the capacity of the immune system as a result of the atrophy of the organs and tissues that are involved in immunity (e.g., liver, bowel wall, bone marrow, spleen, lymphoid tissue). Nutrition is also fundamental for combating sustained attacks of diseases such as cancer. The core of the immune system is made up of the internally derived *antibodies.* A direct and simple example of the important role of nutrition in immunity is the link between protein energy malnutrition and the subsequent suppression of immune function.

Healing. The strength of any body tissue is maintained through the constant building and rebuilding of

---

antigen any foreign or non-self substances (e.g., toxins, viruses, bacteria, foreign proteins) that trigger the production of antibodies that are specifically designed to counteract their activity.

antibody any of numerous protein molecules produced by B cells as a primary immune defense for attaching to specific related antigens.

atrophy tissue wasting.

tissue protein. Such strong tissue is a front line of the body's defense. This process of tissue building and healing requires optimal nutrition intake. Specific nutrients that include protein, essential fatty acids, and key vitamins and minerals must be constantly supplied in the diet. The wise and early use of vigorous medical nutrition therapy (MNT) for patients with cancer speeds the recovery of normal nutritional status after surgery; this includes immunocompetence, which improves a patient's response to therapy as well as his or her prognosis.[5,6]

NUTRITION COMPLICATIONS OF CANCER TREATMENT

Three major forms of therapy are used today as medical treatment for cancer: surgery, radiation, and chemotherapy. Each requires nutrition support. Drug-nutrient interactions are also a complication that may happen with any form of treatment.

Surgery

Any surgery requires nutrition support for the healing process (see Chapter 22). This requirement is particularly true for patients with cancer, because their general condition is often weakened by the disease process and its drain on the body's resources. With early diagnosis and sound nutrition support both before and after surgery, many tumors can be successfully removed. Nutrition intervention has specifically been shown to improve postoperative outcomes and to reduce the complications of patients with cancer of the gastrointestinal tract.[6,7] MNT also includes any needed modifications in food texture or specific nutrients, depending on the site of the surgery or the function of the organ involved. Various methods of feeding patients after surgery are covered in Chapter 22.

Radiation

Radiation therapy is often used by itself or in conjunction with surgery. This type of therapy involves treatment with high-energy radiography that is targeted to the cancer site to kill or shrink cancerous cells. Radiation may be administered to the body by an external machine (Figure 23-2) or by implanted radioactive materials at the cancer site. Although the goal is for only the cancer cells to die, other cells within close proximity to the target site and rapidly growing cells often die as well.

The site and intensity of the radiation treatment determine the nature of the nutrition problems that the patient may encounter. For example, radiation of the head, neck, or esophagus affects the oral mucosa and salivary

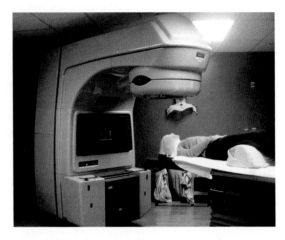

Figure 23-2 A radiation treatment machine. (Courtesy Jormain Cady, Virginia Mason Medical Center, Seattle, Wash. In: Lewis SM, Heitkemper MM, Dirksen SR, et al, eds. *Medical-surgical nursing: assessment and management of clinical problems.* 7th ed. St Louis: Mosby; 2007.)

secretions, thereby affecting taste sensations and sensitivity to food texture and temperature. Means of enhancing the appetite through food appearance and aroma as well as texture must be explored. Similarly, radiation to the abdominal area affects the intestinal mucosa, causing a loss of villi and possibly nutrient malabsorption. Ulcers, inflammation, obstructions, or fistulas may also develop as a result of tissue breakdown, and these conditions interfere with the normal functioning of the involved tissue. General malabsorption within the gastrointestinal (GI) tract may be further compounded by a lack of food intake as a result of anorexia and nausea.

Chemotherapy

Chemotherapeutic agents destroy rapidly growing cancer cells. Unlike radiation therapy, chemotherapy is administered to the general circulation by the blood,

immunocompetence the ability or capacity to develop an immune response (i.e., antibody production or cell-mediated immunity) after exposure to an antigen.

villi small protrusions from the surface of a membrane; finger-like projections that cover the mucosal surfaces of the small intestine that further increase the absorbing surface area; these are visible through a regular microscope.

fistulas from the Latin word for "pipe," an abnormal opening or passageway within the body or to the outside.

and it courses through the entire body. Because chemotherapeutic medications are highly toxic, they also affect normal, healthy cells. This accounts for their side effects on rapidly growing tissues (e.g., bone marrow, GI tract, hair follicles) as well as the problems that they cause for nutrition management. General complications include the following:

- *Bone marrow:* Interference with the production of specific blood factors causes a reduced red blood cell count and anemia, a reduced white blood cell count and lowered resistance to infections, and a reduced blood platelet level that results in bleeding.
- *GI tract:* Numerous problems may develop that interfere with food tolerance, such as nausea and vomiting, a loss of normal taste sensations, anorexia, diarrhea, ulcers, malabsorption, and mucositis.
- *Hair follicle:* Interference with normal hair growth results in general hair loss.

DRUG-NUTRIENT INTERACTIONS

Many medications used in cancer treatment have a high potential for drug-nutrient interactions. Problems may relate to the use of pretreatment antidepressant drugs such as monoamine oxidase inhibitors. These drugs may cause a hypertensive crisis if they are used when an individual consumes tyramine-rich foods. Therefore, a tyramine-restricted diet is indicated for patients who are taking monoamine oxidase inhibitors[8] (Table 23-1). Other antineoplastic drugs have known drug-nutrient interactions that should be addressed with patients on an individual basis. In addition, many patients experiment with herbs that are thought to have a protective role in cancer treatment or prevention. Some of the more commonly used herbs have food-drug interactions that may adversely affect the patient. Careful questioning will reveal herb use, and any negative potential interactions should be discussed. See the Drug-Nutrient Interaction box entitled "Drug-Nutrient Interactions With Commonly Used Drugs and Herbs in Patients With Cancer" for information about some possible interactions.

MEDICAL NUTRITION THERAPY IN THE PATIENT WITH CANCER

Nutrition Problems Related to the Disease Process

General feeding problems pose a great challenge to the clinical dietitian and the nurse who are planning and

TABLE 23-1 **TYRAMINE-RESTRICTED DIET**

High-Tyramine Foods to Avoid	
Meats	Fermented/dry sausage, pepperoni, salami, mortadella sausage, Chinese dried duck, and chicken liver (aged 9 days)
	All casseroles, lasagnas, pizzas, and breads made with these meats
	Improperly stored meat, fish, and poultry
	Improperly stored pickled herring
Cheeses	Mature or aged cheeses: English Stilton, bleu cheese, gruyere, Emmenthaler, Brie, camembert, processed American, gorgonzola, and cheddar (particularly New York State cheddar)
	All casseroles, lasagnas, breads, crackers, and pizzas made with these cheeses
Fruits and vegetables	Banana peels, sauerkraut, kim chee, fava beans, snow peas, and broad bean pods
Beverages	All tap beers, Chianti wine, and sherry
Soybean products	Fermented soy bean, soy bean paste, tofu, fermented bean curd, soy sauce, soy condiments, and miso soup
Concentrated yeast extracts	Marmite and vegemite

This diet was designed for patients who are taking monoamine oxidase inhibitors. These drugs have been reported to cause hypertensive crises when they are used with tyramine-rich foods, which are foods in which aging, protein breakdown, and putrefaction are used to increase flavor. In addition, foods that are old or that have not been properly refrigerated should not be consumed. Food sources of other pressor amines (e.g., histamine, dihydroxyphenylalanine, hydroxytyramine) should also be limited. All of the foods that are listed should be avoided. Limited amounts of foods with a lower tyramine amount (e.g., yeast bread) may be included in a specific individual's diet.
Over-the-counter drugs such as decongestants, cold remedies, and antihistamines should be avoided.
From the American Dietetic Association. *ADA nutrition care manual.* Chicago: American Dietetic Association; 2010.

providing care. These problems relate to the overall systemic effects of cancer as well as to the specific individual responses to the type of cancer involved.

General Systemic Effects

Cancer generally causes the following three basic systemic effects with regard to nutrition status:

- *Anorexia,* or loss of appetite, which results in poor food intake

---

mucositis an inflammation of the tissues around the mouth or other orifices of the body.

DRUG-NUTRIENT INTERACTION

DRUG-NUTRIENT INTERACTIONS WITH COMMONLY USED DRUGS AND HERBS IN PATIENTS WITH CANCER

DRUG OR NUTRIENT	POSSIBLE INTERACTIONS
Antineoplastic Drugs[1]	
Bexarotene (Targretin)	Grapefruit juice may increase drug concentration and toxicities
Methotrexate (Folex, Rheumatrex)	Alcohol may increase hepatotoxicity
Plicamycin (Mithracin)	Supplements that contain calcium and vitamin D may decrease effectiveness
Procarbazine (Matulane)	A mild monoamine oxidase inhibitor; a low-tyramine diet should be followed
Temozolomide (Temodar)	Food may decrease drug rate and absorption
Herbs	
Black cohosh	May increase the antiproliferative effect obtained with tamoxifen[2]
Chamomile	May increase bleeding when used with anticoagulants; may increase the sedative effect of benzodiazepines[3,4]
Dong quai	May increase the effects of warfarin[5]
Garlic	May increase bleeding time with aspirin, dipyridamole, and warfarin; may increase the effects and adverse effects of hyperglycemic agents[5]*
Ginkgo biloba	May increase bleeding time with aspirin, dipyridamole, and warfarin; may increase blood pressure when used with thiazide diuretics[5]*
Ginseng	May adversely affect platelet adhesiveness and blood coagulation; may increase hypoglycemia with insulin; may interfere with antipsychotic drugs through the inhibition of cytochrome p450[6]; may cause hypertension when used for the long term with caffeine; may increase the risk of hepatotoxicity when used with imatinib (Gleevec)[7]
Kava kava	May increase central nervous system depression when used with alcohol and sedatives; may cause hepatotoxicity[5]
Ma huang (ephedra)	Increases in toxicity when taken with β-blockers, monoamine oxidase inhibitors, caffeine, and St. John's wort[5]
St. John's wort	May cause serotonin syndrome when used with antidepressants and drugs that include the p450 microsomal enzyme for metabolism[8]
Yohimbe	Decreases the effects of antidepressants, antihypertensives, hyperglycemic agents, monoamine oxidase inhibitors, and St. John's wort[5]

*Caution only. There is limited evidence to support this interaction.

1. National Cancer Institute. *Nutrition in cancer care: other nutrition issues* (website): www.cancer.gov/cancertopics/pdq/supportivecare/nutrition/HealthProfessional/page5. Accessed April 2011.
2. Roberts H. Safety of herbal medicinal products in women with breast cancer. *Maturitas*. 2010;66:363-369.
3. Segal R, Pilote L. Warfarin interaction with *Matricaria chamomilla*. *CMAJ*. 2006;174(9):1281-1282.
4. Block KI, Gyllenhaal C, Mead MN. Safety and efficacy of herbal sedatives in cancer care. *Integr Cancer Ther*. 2004;3:128-148.
5. National Center for Complementary and Alternative Medicine. *Herbs at a glance* (website): http://nccam.nih.gov/health/herbsataglance.htm. Accessed May, 2011.
6. Wanwimolruk S, Wong K, Wanwimolruk P. Variable inhibitory effect of different brands of commercial herb supplements on human cytochrome P-450 CYP3A4. *Drug Metabol Drug Interact*. 2009;24(1):17-35.
7. Bilgi N, Bell K, Ananthakrishnan AN, Atallah E. Imatinib and Panax ginseng: a potential interaction resulting in liver toxicity. *Ann Pharmacother*. 2010;44:926-928.
8. Gurley BJ. Clinical pharmacology and dietary supplements: an evolving relationship. *Clin Pharmacol Ther*. 2010;87(2):235-238.

- *Increased metabolism,* which results in increased nutrient and energy needs
- *Negative nitrogen balance,* which results in more catabolism (i.e., the breaking down of body tissues)

The extent of these effects may vary widely from a mild response to an extreme form of debilitating cachexia as is seen with advanced disease. Extreme weight loss and weakness are caused by an inability to ingest or use nutrients, which results in the patient's body feeding off of its

cachexia a specific profound syndrome that is characterized by weight loss, reduced food intake, and systemic inflammation.

own tissue protein.[9,10] Approximately half of all patients with cancer experience some level of cachexia-associated weight loss, and up to 20% of all cancer deaths are attributed directly to this debilitating syndrome. The prevalence of cachexia varies with tumor site, and it is more prevalent in patients with gastric and pancreatic cancer compared with other forms of the disease.[11] An involuntary weight loss of more than 5% of the premorbid weight within a 6-month period is indicative of cachexia. The best way to treat cancer-related cachexia is to alleviate the cancer and the metabolic abnormalities associated with it. However, because this is not always an immediate possibility, aggressive MNT is the next best option.

Specific Effects Related to the Type of Cancer

In addition to the primary nutrition problems that are caused by the disease process itself, secondary problems with eating or nutrient metabolism result from tumors that cause obstructions or lesions in the GI tract or the surrounding tissue. Such conditions limit food intake and digestion as well as the absorption of nutrients. Depending on the nature and location of the tumor as well as the medical treatment of choice, a variety of individual nutrition problems may occur and require personal attention.

Basic Objectives of the Nutrition Plan

The fundamental principles of identifying needs and planning care on the basis of those needs underlie all sound patient care (see Chapter 17).

Nutrition Screening and Assessment

Determining and monitoring the nutritional status of each patient is the primary responsibility of the clinical dietitian. Various members of the health care team may take part in body measurements and the calculations of body composition, laboratory tests and the interpretation of their results, physical examination and clinical observations, and dietary analysis. Weight can change rapidly in these patients; therefore, accurate measurements must be taken instead of relying on self-reported or estimated values. Severe alterations in weight may change medication dosages and indicate nutrition problems.

Nutrition Intervention

The basic objectives of the nutrition intervention plan for patients with cancer are as follows[12]:

- Prevent weight loss, even among overweight patients.

- Maintain lean body mass.
- Prevent unintentional weight gain, particularly in certain groups of patients (e.g., those with hormone-related cancers such as prostate or breast cancer, those taking long-term high-dose steroids).
- Identify and manage treatment-related side effects.

Nutrient specifics of the plan are outlined in the Medical Nutrition Therapy section later in this chapter.

Prevention of Catabolism. Every effort is made to meet the increased metabolic demands of the disease process in an effort to prevent extensive catabolic effects in tissue breakdown. Maintaining nutrition from the beginning is far more efficient than rebuilding the body after extensive malnutrition. The nutrition intervention recommendations for patients with or at risk for cancer-related cachexia are to maximize the oral intake of nutrient-dense foods while liberalizing any diet restrictions and encouraging small, frequent meals. Dietary supplements that include branched-chain amino acids and protein powders may benefit the patient and help him or her to meet nutrient needs.

A variety of drugs are currently in use to increase appetite, decrease nausea, spare protein degradation, and improve caloric intake. Some examples include megestrol acetate (Megace), corticosteroids, cyproheptadine, ghrelin, glucocorticoids, branched-chain amino acids, eicosapentaenoic acid, and cannabinoids, all of which have limitations.[13] See the Drug-Nutrient Interaction box entitled "Cannabis (Medical Marijuana) as a Treatment for Anorexia" for information about the controversies that surround the use of cannabis for combating unintended weight loss in patients who suffer from cancer-related cachexia. For patients who are unable to meet their metabolic needs orally, enteral or parenteral feedings should be initiated.[12]

Relief of Symptoms. The symptoms of cancer and the side effects of treatment can be devastating for a patient. Stress management, pain management, relaxation techniques, psychologic support, and physical activity (as tolerated) are important aspects of overall patient care, and they can improve a patient's quality of life.

Although the clinical dietitian and the physician have the primary responsibility for planning and managing the MNT program, a tremendous contribution is made by the nursing staff and other health care personnel with regard to day-to-day support and counseling to help patients meet their nutrient requirements. This kind of constant care and support often differentiates combating the course of the disease and ensuring the comfort and well-being of the patient.

DRUG-NUTRIENT INTERACTION

CANNABIS (MEDICAL MARIJUANA) AS A TREATMENT FOR ANOREXIA

Both sides of the debate for the legalization of medical marijuana have genuine concerns. Proponents argue in favor of the effectiveness that marijuana has on relieving the nausea caused by cancer treatment, the wasting effects of acquired immunodeficiency syndrome, and the pain of glaucoma. Critics cite studies that indicate the addictiveness of marijuana and that link it to cancer and lung damage.

Dronabinol, which is sold under the brand name Marinol, is a capsule form of marijuana that has been approved by the U.S. Food and Drug Administration. It contains tetrahydrocannabinol, which is the active ingredient found in the plant marijuana; thus, the drug has similar side effects[1]:

- Dizziness
- Euphoria

- Paranoid reaction
- Somnolence (sleepiness)

Dronabinol is indicated for the treatment of anorexia associated with weight loss in patients with acquired immunodeficiency syndrome and for the nausea and vomiting associated with cancer chemotherapy in patients who have not adequately responded to conventional antiemetic treatments.[2]

The dosage should be tightly regulated by the physician, because each patient responds to dronabinol differently. Because this drug can be habit forming, the lowest dose needed to produce the desired result is recommended.

Sara Harcourt

1. Goldman L. Cannabis and clinical RDs: why you need to know about medical marijuana. *ADA Times.* 2007;4(3):5.
2. Seamon MJ, Fass JA, Maniscalco-Feichtl M, Abu-Shraie NA. Medical marijuana and the developing role of the pharmacist. *Am J Health Syst Pharm.* 2007;64(10):1037-1044.

Nutrition Monitoring and Evaluation

On the basis of detailed information that is gathered about each patient, including his or her living situation and other personal and social needs, the clinical dietitian (in consultation with the physician) develops a personal MNT plan for each patient. This plan should be evaluated for efficacy on a regular basis with the patient and his or her family. The plan should be changed as needed to meet the nutrition demands of the patient's condition as well as his or her individual desires and tolerances.

Medical Nutrition Therapy

Guidelines for MNT will vary depending on the cancer site, the stage of disease, the treatment modality, and the current nutritional status of the patient. Although individual needs vary, guidelines for MNT must meet specific nutrient needs and goals related to the accelerated metabolism and protein-tissue synthesis.

Energy

The hypermetabolic nature of cancer and its healing requirements place great energy demands on the patient. Sufficient fuel from carbohydrate and, to a lesser extent, fat must be available to spare protein for vital tissue building. An adult patient with good nutritional status needs between 25 to 30 kcal/kg of body weight for maintenance requirements. More kilocalories may be needed in accordance with the degree of individual stress, the amount of tissue synthesis that is taking place, and physical activity.

A malnourished patient may require significantly more energy intake, depending on the degree of malnutrition or the extent of tissue injury.

Protein

Essential amino acids and nitrogen are necessary for tissue building and healing and to offset the tissue breakdown that is caused by the disease. Efficient protein use depends on an optimal protein-to-energy ratio to promote tissue building and to prevent tissue catabolism. An adult patient with good nutritional status needs from 0.8 to 1.2 g/kg/day of protein to meet maintenance requirements, with an emphasis on high-quality protein sources. A malnourished patient needs additional protein to replenish deficits and to restore a positive nitrogen balance.

Vitamins and Minerals

Key vitamins and minerals help to control protein and energy metabolism through their coenzyme roles in specific cell enzyme pathways, and they also play important roles in building and maintaining strong tissue (see Chapters 7 and 8). Therefore, an optimal intake of vitamins and minerals (at least to the Dietary Reference Intake standards and sometimes to higher therapeutic levels) is needed. Vitamin and mineral supplements are often indicated to ensure dietary intake (see the Drug-Nutrient Interaction box, "Antiestrogens and Breast Cancer"). However, the unsubstantiated megadosing of dietary supplements (specifically those that contain antioxidants) may be counterproductive to the health of the patient

DRUG-NUTRIENT INTERACTION

ANTIESTROGENS AND BREAST CANCER

Tamoxifen citrate is an antiestrogenic drug that is used to treat breast cancer. Some common symptoms of interactions with this drug that are related to nutrition include the following:

- Nausea
- Bone pain
- Fluid retention
- Hot flashes
- Hypercalcemia

Estrogen is needed for bone formation along with vitamin D, calcium, and magnesium. With low levels of estrogen, calcium is taken from the bone, and bone resorption may result. Calcium and magnesium supplements can help to reduce resorption, but they should be taken separately from the tamoxifen citrate by at least 2 hours. Grapefruit juice should be avoided, because it can interfere with absorption, as can soy supplements and soy-based foods because of their estrogenic effect. Soy products do not contain estrogen, but they do contain compounds that are similar in structure to estrogen. Because of the similarity, these estrogen-like compounds may fit into the active site of the drug and therefore act as decoys to the true target estrogen.

Sara Harcourt

(see the Drug-Nutrient Interaction box, "Antioxidants and Chemotherapy").

The Academy of Nutrition and Dietetics Nutrition Care Manual indicates a potential benefit from the supplementation of the following nutrients for patients with specific types of cancer[12]:

- *Vitamin E*: patients with breast cancer who are receiving radiation; patients with head and neck cancer
- *Omega-3 fatty acid supplements*: patients with pancreatic cancer
- *Arginine*: patients with breast cancer; patients with head and neck cancer
- *Eicosapentaenoic acid*: patients with oral and laryngeal cancer
- *Honey*: patients who are receiving head or neck radiation
- *Glutamine*: patients undergoing hematopoietic cell transplantation
- *Antioxidants at levels higher than the Tolerable Upper Intake Level*: patients with non–small-cell lung cancer who are receiving chemotherapy

Fluid

Adequate fluid intake must be ensured for the following reasons:

- To replace GI losses from fever, infection, vomiting, or diarrhea
- To help the kidneys dispose of metabolic breakdown products from destroyed cancer cells and from the drugs that are used in chemotherapy

Some chemotherapeutic drugs (e.g., cyclophosphamide [Cytoxan]) require as much as 2 to 3 L of forced fluids daily to prevent hemorrhagic cystitis.

Nutrition Management

Achieving these nutrition objectives and needs in the face of frequent food intolerance, anorexia, or the inability to eat presents a great challenge for the nutrition support team and patient. The specific method of feeding depends on the patient's condition. The dietitian and the physician may manage a patient's nutrition care with the use of high-calorie nutritional supplements (e.g., Ensure, Boost) or with enteral or parenteral nutrition support (see Chapter 22).

Enteral: Oral Diet With Nutrient Supplementation

An oral diet with supplementation is the most desired form of feeding, when tolerated. A personal food plan must include adjustments in food texture and temperature, food choices, and tolerances, and it should provide as much energy and nutrient density as possible in smaller volumes of food (see the Clinical Applications box, "Strategies for Improving Food Intake in Patients With Cancer or Acquired Immunodeficiency Syndrome"). Special attention is given to eating problems that are caused by a loss of appetite, oral complications, GI problems, and pain (Table 23-2).

Loss of Appetite. Anorexia is a major problem in patients with cancer, and it curtails food intake when it is needed most. Anorexia often sets up a vicious cycle that can lead to the gross malnutrition of cancer-related cachexia, as discussed previously. A vigorous program of eating that does not depend on appetite for stimulus must be planned with the patient and his or her family. The overall goal is to provide food with as much nutrient density as possible so that every bite counts.

DRUG-NUTRIENT INTERACTION

ANTIOXIDANTS AND CHEMOTHERAPY

Complementary and alternative medicine is best described as diverse health care systems, products, and practices that are not generally considered part of conventional medicine. This type of treatment includes dietary supplement use, acupuncture, massage, herbal medicines, and mind-body medicine. The use of complementary and alternatively medicine—and most notably dietary supplement use—is highly prevalent in patients with cancer. In one community clinic study, 73% of cancer patients reported using vitamin, mineral, or other dietary supplements, but only 47% of those patients actually disclosed that information to their medical care providers.[1] Antioxidant supplements, particularly vitamin C, are often used by cancer patients in an effort to boost their immune system or to improve general health.[2] This practice may not be helpful, and it can in fact be harmful for patients who are being treated for certain types of cancer.

Tumor cells are characterized by their rapid rate of division, but normal, healthy cells such as skin cells and the cells that line the digestive tract divide quickly as well. Antineoplastic drugs, which are used to treat cancer, target the rapidly dividing cells and produce free radicals that cause oxidative damage. Patients often take vitamin C, which is a potent antioxidant, to reduce the unpleasant side effects

that are caused by the medications. Although vitamin C supplementation may help to alleviate the side effects of chemotherapy, it may also reduce the effectiveness of the anticancer treatment. Even at typical supplemental doses of 500 mg per day, vitamin C has been shown to prevent the cytotoxic effects of antineoplastic agents from killing tumor cells, not just healthy cells.[3]

Several studies have investigated whether the benefits of antioxidant supplements during chemotherapy offset the potential risks, but the results are still controversial.[4] Resveratrol is a phytochemical that has been found to have anticancer as well as antioxidant activity. In some studies, resveratrol shows promise in sensitizing tumor cells to chemotherapy, but the effect on healthy cells is not clear. Resveratrol may protect healthy cells, or it may increase their sensitivity to the harmful effects of antineoplastic agents.[5] This research is still in its infancy, and general recommendations cannot be made regarding dietary supplements of resveratrol during cancer treatment. To ensure safety during chemotherapy, patients should carefully discuss their use of supplemental vitamin C or other potent dietary antioxidants with their health care providers.

Kelli Boi

1. Rausch SM, Winegardner F, Kruk KM, et al. Complementary and alternative medicine: use and disclosure in radiation oncology community practice. *Support Care Cancer*. 2011;19(4):521-529.
2. van Tonder E, Herselman MG, Visser J. The prevalence of dietary-related complementary and alternative therapies and their perceived usefulness among cancer patients. *J Hum Nutr Diet*. 2009;22(6):528-535.
3. Heaney ML, Gardner JR, Karasavvas N, et al. Vitamin C antagonizes the cytotoxic effects of antineoplastic drugs. *Cancer Res*. 2008;68(19):8031-8038.
4. Lawenda BD, Kelly KM, Ladas EJ, et al. Should supplemental antioxidant administration be avoided during chemotherapy and radiation therapy? *J Natl Cancer Inst*. 2008;100(11):773-783.
5. Gupta SC, Kannappan R, Reuter S, et al. Chemosensitization of tumors by resveratrol. *Ann N Y Acad Sci*. 2011;1215:150-160.

CLINICAL APPLICATIONS

STRATEGIES FOR IMPROVING FOOD INTAKE IN PATIENTS WITH CANCER OR ACQUIRED IMMUNODEFICIENCY SYNDROME

Tips for Increasing Energy and Protein Intake
- Fortify foods with high-calorie condiments, sauces, and dressings.
- Add extra ingredients such as dry milk and cream during food preparation.
- Use high-calorie protein drinks between meals for added nutrients.
- Use regular-calorie foods and beverages rather than low-calorie or diet substitutes.
- Prepare favorite foods and freeze leftovers in small serving sizes for snacks.
- Eat by the clock: have a meal or snack every 1 or 2 hours.

- Eat more when the appetite is good.
- Enjoy meals with pleasant surroundings, company, and music.
- Keep a supply of easy-to-prepare and convenient foods on hand.
- Try mild exercise according to physical status.
- If the mouth is sore, use soft foods, avoid hot and cold temperature extremes, and discuss with a physician or nurse a topical anesthetic mouth rinse to use before eating.

TABLE 23-2 **DIETARY MODIFICATIONS FOR NUTRITION-RELATED SIDE EFFECTS OF CANCER, HUMAN IMMUNODEFICIENCY VIRUS, AND ACQUIRED IMMUNOEFICIENCY SYNDROME**

Symptom	Suggestions
Anorexia	Plan a menu in advance that involves small, frequent meals and snacks and that includes high-calorie, high-protein, and nutrient-dense foods.
	Consume high-protein foods first.
	Prepare and store small portions of favorite foods.
	Experiment with different foods, and seek foods that appeal to the sense of smell.
	Arrange for help with purchasing and preparing food and meals.
	Consume one third of the daily protein and calorie requirements at breakfast.
	Snack between meals.
	Be creative with desserts.
	Perform frequent mouth care to relieve symptoms and to decrease aftertastes.
Nausea and vomiting	Avoid spicy foods, greasy foods, and foods with strong odors.
	Eat dry, bland, soft, and easy-to-digest foods such as crackers, breadsticks, and toast throughout the day; avoid heavy meals.
	Remain upright for at least 1 hour after eating.
	Avoid eating in areas with strong cooking odors or that are too warm.
	Consume liquids between meals.
	Rinse out the mouth before and after eating.
	Suck on hard candies (e.g., peppermints, lemon drops) if there is a bad taste in the mouth.
Taste and smell alterations	Use herbs and seasonings to enhance flavors.
	Try new foods when feeling best.
	Use plastic utensils if foods taste metallic, and use gum or mints when experiencing a bitter taste in the mouth.
	Substitute poultry, fish, eggs, tofu, and cheese for red meat.
	Eat small, frequent meals and healthy snacks.
	Plan meals that include favorite foods.
	Have others prepare the meal.
	A vegetarian or Chinese cookbook can provide useful meatless, high-protein recipes.
	Add spices and sauces to foods.
	Eat meat with something sweet, such as cranberry sauce, jelly, or applesauce.
Xerostomia	Drink plenty of fluids (25 to 30 mL/kg per day), and use a straw to drink liquids.
	Eat moist foods with extra sauces and gravies.
	Perform oral hygiene at least four times per day, but avoid rinses that contain alcohol; brush dentures after each meal.
	Use hard candy, frozen desserts, chewing gum, and ice pops between meals to moisten the mouth.
	Consume very sweet or tart foods and beverages, which may stimulate saliva production.
	Drink fruit nectar instead of juice.
Diarrhea	Avoid greasy foods, hot and cold liquids, and caffeine.
	Drink at least 1 cup of liquid after each loose bowel movement.
	Limit gas-forming foods and beverages such as soda, cruciferous vegetables, legumes and lentils, chewing gum, and milk (if not well tolerated).
	Limit the use of sorbitol.
	Drink plenty of fluids throughout the day; room-temperature fluids may be better tolerated.
Constipation	Gradually increase fiber consumption to 25 to 30 g/day.
	Drink 8 to 10 cups of fluid each day.
	Maintain regular physical activity.
Mucositis and stomatitis	Eat foods that are soft, easy to chew and swallow, and nonirritating.
	Moisten foods with gravy, broth, or sauces.
	Avoid known irritants such as acidic, spicy, salty, and coarse-textured foods.
	Cook foods until they are soft and tender, or cut foods into small bites.
	Eat foods at room temperature.
	Supplement meals with high-calorie, high-protein drinks.
	Maintain good oral hygiene.
	Numb the mouth with ice chips or flavored ice pops.

Continued

TABLE 23-2　**DIETARY MODIFICATIONS FOR NUTRITION-RELATED SIDE EFFECTS OF CANCER, HUMAN IMMUNODEFICIENCY VIRUS, AND ACQUIRED IMMUNOEFICIENCY SYNDROME—cont'd**

Symptom	Suggestions
Neutropenia*	Check expiration dates on food; do not buy or use if the food is out of date.
	Do not buy or use food in cans that are swollen, dented, or damaged.
	Thaw foods in the refrigerator or microwave; never thaw foods at room temperature.
	Cook foods immediately after thawing.
	Refrigerate all leftovers within 2 hours of cooking, and eat them within 24 hours.
	Keep hot foods hot and cold foods cold.
	Avoid old, moldy, or damaged fruits and vegetables.
	Avoid tofu in open bins or containers.
	Cook all meat, poultry, and fish thoroughly; avoid raw eggs and fish.
	Buy individually packaged foods.
	Avoid salad bars and buffets when eating out.
	Limit exposure to large groups of people and people with infections.
	Practice good hygiene, and wash hands often.
Dehydration	Drink 8 to 12 cups of liquids a day, regardless of thirst.
	Add soup, flavored ice pops, and other sources of fluid to the diet.
	Limit caffeine.
	Drink most fluids between meals.
	Use antiemetics for relief from nausea and vomiting.

*Neutropenia involves a low white blood cell count and an increased risk of infection.
Modified from National Cancer Institute. *Nutrition in cancer care: nutrition implications of cancer therapies* (website): www.cancer.gov/cancertopics/pdq/supportivecare/nutrition/HealthProfessional/page4. Accessed April 2011.

Oral Complications. Various problems that contribute to eating difficulties may stem from a sore mouth, mucositis, or altered taste and smell acuity. Decreased saliva and sore mouth often result from radiation to the head and neck area or from chemotherapy. Spraying the mouth with artificial saliva is helpful. Good oral care habits are important to avoid infection and to prevent dental caries, both of which could further inhibit healthy eating. Basic mouth care includes the following:

- Visiting the dentist before treatment begins
- Examining the mouth daily for sores or irritation
- Brushing and flossing regularly with a soft-bristled toothbrush
- Ensuring that dentures fit correctly
- Using mouthwash that does not contain alcohol, which dries out the mouth

Frequent small snacks are often better accepted than traditional meals. The treatment may alter the tongue's taste buds, thereby causing taste distortion, taste blindness, and the inability to distinguish sweet, sour, salt, or bitter, thereby resulting in more food aversions. Strong food seasonings (for those who can tolerate them) and high-protein liquid drinks may be helpful. Because the treatment may also alter salivary secretions, foods with a high liquid content are favored. Solid foods may be swallowed more easily with the use of sauces, gravies, broth, yogurt, or salad dressings. A food processor or blender can turn foods into semisolid or liquid forms for easier

swallowing. Any dental problems should be corrected to help with chewing.

Gastrointestinal Problems. Chemotherapy often causes nausea and vomiting, which require special individual attention (see Table 23-2). Food that is hot, sweet, fatty, or spicy sometimes exacerbates nausea and should be avoided in accordance with individual tolerances. Small and frequent feedings of soft to liquid cold foods that are eaten slowly with rests in between may be helpful. The physician's use of antinausea drugs (e.g., prochlorperazine [Compazine, Zofran, Kytril]) may help with food tolerances. Surgical treatment that involves the GI tract requires related dietary modifications (see Chapter 22). Chemotherapy and radiation treatment can affect the mucosal cells that secrete lactase and thus induce lactose intolerance. In such cases, a soy-based nutrient supplement (e.g., Ensure [Ross Products, Columbus, Ohio]) may be helpful.

Pain and Discomfort. Patients are more able to eat if severe pain is controlled and if they are positioned as comfortably as possible. The current medical consensus is to administer pain-controlling medication as needed in close consultation with the patient and his or her family and then to carefully monitor patient responses. This is especially important for children with cancer who are undergoing painful treatments. Constipation is a common side effect of several pain medications. Preventive therapy to avoid additional discomfort from constipation is important and should focus on adequate fluids, soluble fiber, and regular physical activity (even short walks can help).

Enteral: Tube Feeding

When the GI tract can still be used but the patient is unable to eat and requires more assistance to achieve essential intake goals, tube feeding may be indicated. The following are indications for enteral nutrition[12]:

- Inadequate oral intake
- Oral intake is contraindicated
- Comatose
- Proximal bowel obstructions (e.g., esophageal obstructions)
- Oropharyngeal dysphagia
- Limited absorptive capacity
- Perioperative nutrition support with severe malnutrition

However, many patients have negative feelings about tube feeding, especially the use of a nasogastric tube. Alternatively, some highly motivated patients are able to place their small-caliber tubes themselves. In some instances, patients can be fed by pump-monitored slow drip during the night and be free from the tube during the day. Bolus feedings with percutaneous endoscopic gastrostomy tubes are often used for patients who require long-term nutrition support (i.e., more than 4 weeks), and they have the benefit of closely resembling normal meal patterns. The use of special formulas and delivery-system equipment has also made home enteral nutrition possible and practical.

Parenteral Feeding

When the GI tract cannot be used and nutrition support is vital, parenteral feedings must be initiated. The following are indications for parenteral nutrition support[12]:

- Nonfunctioning gastrointestinal tract
- Moderate to severe malnourishment with the anticipation of no enteral intake for at least 7 days
- Preoperative support for patients with severe malnutrition (i.e., weight loss of more than 10% to 15% or a serum albumin level of less than 2.8 g/dL) when surgery can be delayed for 7 to 14 days
- Aggressive oncologic treatment when the GI tract cannot be utilized

Peripheral Vein Feeding. For brief periods in cases that require less-concentrated intakes of energy and nutrients, solutions of dextrose, amino acids, vitamins, and minerals with the concurrent use of lipid emulsions may be fed into smaller peripheral veins. The use of smaller peripheral veins carries less risk than the use of a larger central vein, and it can supply necessary support when nutrient needs are not excessive.

Central Vein Feeding. When nutrition needs are greater and must continue over an extended period, central vein feeding often provides a life-saving alternative. The total parenteral nutrition process requires the surgical placement of the feeding catheter along with careful assessment, monitoring, and administration. Although total parenteral nutrition carries risks and thus requires skilled team management, this hyperalimentation process provides a significant means of turning the metabolic status of patients with cancer from catabolism to anabolism, thereby avoiding the serious development of cancer-related cachexia. Details of enteral and parenteral methods of feeding are discussed in Chapter 22.

CANCER PREVENTION

On the basis of the most current information about cancer research and prevention, the American Cancer Society has issued guidelines to encourage healthy lifestyle choices to reduce the risk of cancer.[14] These guidelines are established by a national panel of experts, and they are updated every 5 years. The World Cancer Research Fund and the American Institute for Cancer Research recently published an expert panel report regarding the global perspective of food, nutrition, and physical activity as they are related to cancer prevention.[15] The combined recommendations from these two reports are outlined in the next section of this chapter. In addition, the U.S. Food and Drug Administration (FDA) has defined specific food-labeling guidelines for linking certain foods and nutrients to decreased cancer risk.[16] A variety of other government and privately funded research studies are ongoing in the hopes of identifying a more specific cause of and cure for cancer.

American Cancer Society, World Cancer Research Fund, and American Institute for Cancer Research: Guidelines for Cancer Prevention

The most recent expert panel publications recommend the following lifestyle factors to reduce the risk of cancer[14,15]:

1. Be as lean as possible within the normal range of body weight through the following actions:
   - Balance caloric intake with physical activity.
   - Avoid excessive weight gain. Excess weight is believed to increase the risk of several types of cancer (Box 23-1).

2. Adopt a physically active lifestyle.
   - Children and adolescents: participate in at least 60 minutes per day of moderate to vigorous physical activity at least 5 days per week.
   - Adults: engage in at least 30 minutes of moderate to vigorous physical activity every day; 45 to 60 minutes of intentional physical activity is preferable.
   - Examples of moderate activity include walking, skating, yoga, softball or baseball, downhill skiing, garden maintenance, and lawn care. Vigorous activities include running, aerobics, fast bicycling, circuit weight training, soccer, singles tennis, basketball, cross-country skiing, and heavy manual labor.
3. Consume a healthy diet that has an emphasis on plant sources.
   - Become familiar with standard serving sizes and read food labels to become more aware of actual servings consumed.
   - Limit the consumption of salty foods and foods that are processed with sodium.
   - Limit the consumption of energy-dense foods, particularly processed foods that are high in added sugar, low in fiber, or high in fat. Avoid sugary drinks.
   - Eat five or more servings of vegetables and fruits every day.
   - Choose whole grains instead of processed (refined) grains and sugars.
   - Choose fish, poultry, and beans as alternatives to beef, pork, and lamb. Select lean cuts and small portions, and prepare the meat by baking, broiling, or poaching rather than frying. Avoid processed meats.
4. If alcoholic beverages are consumed, limit their intake. Limit alcohol intake to two drinks per day for men and one drink per day for women. One drink is defined as 12 oz of beer, 5 oz of wine, or 1.5 oz of 80-proof distilled spirits.
5. Aim to meet nutritional needs through diet alone; do not rely on supplements.

Dietary choices and physical activity are the most modifiable risk factors for cancer prevention. One third of all cancer deaths in the United States are attributed to poor diet and physical inactivity, including overweight and obesity.[14] Thus, following the preceding guidelines could make a significant difference in the lives of many individuals.

U.S. Food and Drug Administration Health Claims

Health claims approved for use on food labels are regulated by the FDA (see Chapter 13). The qualified health claims about cancer risk for use on food labels in the United States link the following nutrients with reduced risk[17]:

- *Dietary fat (lipids) and cancer.* Example claims approved for use include the following:
  - Development of cancer depends on many factors. A diet low in total fat may reduce the risk of some cancers.
  - Eating a healthful diet low in fat may help reduce the risk of some types of cancers. Development of cancer is associated with many factors, including a family history of the disease, cigarette smoking, and what you eat.
- *Fiber-containing grain products, fruits, vegetables, and cancer.* Example claims approved for use include the following:
  - Low fat diets rich in fiber-containing grain products, fruits, and vegetables may reduce the risk of some types of cancer, a disease associated with many factors.
  - Development of cancer depends on many factors. Eating a diet low in fat and high in grain products, fruits, and vegetables that contain dietary fiber may reduce your risk of some cancers.
- *Fruits and vegetables and cancer.* Example claims approved for use include the following:
  - *Example for use on broccoli:* Low fat diets rich in fruits and vegetables (foods that are low in fat and may contain dietary fiber, vitamin A, and vitamin C) may reduce the risk of some types of cancer, a disease associated with many factors. Broccoli is high in vitamins A and C, and it is a good source of dietary fiber.
  - *Example for use on oranges:* Development of cancer depends on many factors. Eating a diet low in fat

and high in fruits and vegetables, foods that are low in fat and may contain vitamin A, vitamin C, and dietary fiber, may reduce your risk of some cancers. Oranges, a food low in fat, are a good source of fiber and vitamin C.

On the basis of these consistent and strong associations, the Centers for Disease Control and Prevention (CDC) has developed a program to encourage Americans to eat five or more servings of fruits and vegetables every day, which is one of the nation's health promotion and disease prevention objectives.[18] The Fruits and Veggies Matter program (www.fruitsandveggiesmatter.gov) is partnered with the National Cancer Institute, the Department of Health and Human Services, and USA.gov. The CDC works closely with the Association of State and Territorial Public Health Nutrition Directors (www.astphnd.org), which is comprised of nutrition coordinators (formerly known as "5-A-Day" coordinators).

Ongoing Cancer Research

Research that links specific elements of the diet with the risk for cancer is difficult to do and complicated to interpret. Some studies have shown that diets that are low in fat and high in fiber, fruits, and vegetables, which are major sources of micronutrients and phytochemicals, are associated with decreased incidences and mortality rates of various cancers. The exact mechanisms by which such diets are protective against cancer are not yet clearly defined for each association and are still under investigation. Some examples of recent findings include the following:

- *Breast cancer:* Body fatness, alcohol consumption, and saturated fat intake were all risk factors.[19,20] A Mediterranean diet and fish-oil supplementation were associated with a reduced risk.[21]

- *Gastric cancer:* A Mediterranean diet was particularly protective as compared with the typical Western diet. The intake of carotenoids, retinol, α-tocopherol, and cereal fiber were protective. The intake of total meat, red meat, and processed meat were risk factors.[20]
- *Colorectal cancer:* Serum vitamin D concentration and the consumption of dietary fiber, calcium, and fish were protective. Red meat and processed meat intake, abdominal obesity, high body mass index, and alcohol consumption were risk factors.[20]
- *Prostate cancer:* Dairy protein and calcium from dairy products were associated with increased risk.[20]

Many other associations have been investigated, with some controversy. The article by Murthy and colleagues listed in the Further Reading and Resources section at the end of this chapter provides a review of the dietary factors that are associated with additional types of cancer and some anticarcinogenic properties of certain food and lifestyle choices.

The CDC hosts many programs that are aimed at preventing and controlling cancers as well as researching cause-and-effect relationships, including the National Comprehensive Cancer Control Program; the National Breast and Cervical Cancer Early Detection Program; the National Program of Cancer Registries; and the Colorectal Cancer Control Program. In addition to these programs, there are several initiatives that focus on education and awareness campaigns and research activities that are aimed at lung, prostate, and gynecologic cancers and cancer survivorship.[22] Many of these programs have nutrition-related objectives.

SECTION 2 **ACQUIRED IMMUNODEFICIENCY SYNDROME**

PROCESS OF ACQUIRED IMMUNODEFICIENCY SYNDROME DEVELOPMENT

This section looks at AIDS and compares its relationship to the body's immune system and course of development with that of cancer. According to the National Center for

Health Statistics, about 43,000 people are infected with HIV every year in the United States alone (see the Cultural Considerations box, "Types and Incidence of Human Immunodeficiency Virus and Acquired Immunodeficiency Syndrome in American Populations"). The most recent data reports indicate that 73% of the population infected with HIV is male.[23]

CULTURAL CONSIDERATIONS

TYPES AND INCIDENCE OF HUMAN IMMUNODEFICIENCY VIRUS AND ACQUIRED IMMUNODEFICIENCY SYNDROME IN AMERICAN POPULATIONS

More than 1 million cases of human immunodeficiency virus (HIV) have been diagnosed in the United States from the beginning of the epidemic to 2009.[1] The largest percentage of new HIV infections each year occur as a result of male-to-male sexual contact. Injection drug use and high-risk heterosexual contact are the next most common causes of HIV transmission. Acquired immunodeficiency syndrome (AIDS) is the sixth leading cause of death among people between the ages of 25 and 44 years.[2]

The percentage of new HIV infections according to race is disproportionate to the total U.S. population. For example, African Americans make up approximately 12% of the total U.S. population, but 45% of new HIV infection cases occur among African Americans.

The Centers for Disease Control and Prevention has reported the race and ethnicity of people with HIV/AIDS who were diagnosed during 2009 as follows:

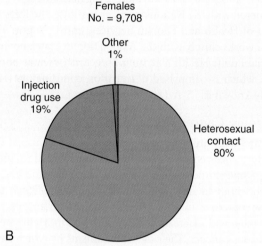

Transmission categories of adults and adolescents with HIV/AIDS who received the diagnosis during 2009 on the basis of data from 40 states with long-term, confidential, name-based reporting.[1]

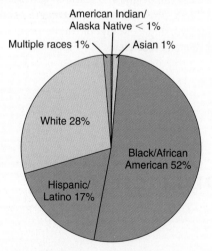

Race or ethnicity of people with HIV/AIDS who received the diagnosis during 2009 on the basis of data from 40 states with long-term, confidential, name-based reporting.[1]

Because no cures or vaccines for HIV are currently available, prevention is the only means of protection, regardless of race or gender.

With contribution from Jennifer Schmidt

1. Centers for Disease Control and Prevention. *Diagnoses of HIV infection and AIDS in the United States and dependent areas, 2009, HIV surveillance report, Volume 21* (website): www.cdc.gov/hiv/surveillance/resources/reports/2009report/. Accessed May 2011.
2. National Center for Health Statistics. *Health, United States, 2010: with special feature on death and dying.* Hyattsville, Md: U.S. Government Printing Office; 2011.

Evolution of Human Immunodeficiency Virus

The earliest known case of AIDS was identified in a blood sample collected in 1959 from a Bantu man living in what is currently the Democratic Republic of Congo, an area from which the current world epidemic is believed to have originated.[24] Early during the 1960s in the African country of Uganda, strange deaths began to occur from simple common infections such as pneumonia that did not respond to the usual antibiotic drugs. By the late 1970s and early 1980s, the same strange deaths were occurring in Europe and America. Similar reports of unexplained immune system failure increased rapidly in various parts of the world, and the pandemic spread. These early cases came from people with diverse social and medical backgrounds, including heterosexual and homosexual men, intravenous drug users, and recipients of transfused blood and blood products (e.g., patients with hemophilia, medical and surgical patients). After feverish research, the underlying infectious agent was finally discovered in May 1983. The French scientist Luc Montagnier, a leading pioneer in AIDS research, reported that he and his team at the Pasteur Institute in Paris had isolated the viral cause, which is now known as *HIV*.

Parasitic Nature of the Virus

No virus can have a life of its own. As a result of their structure and reproductive nature, viruses are the ultimate parasites. They are mere shreds of genetic material, a small packet of genetic information encased in a protein coat. Viruses only contain a small chromosome of nucleic acids (RNA or DNA), usually with fewer than five genes. They can live only through a host that they invade and infect, and they hijack the host's cell machinery to make a multitude of copies of themselves. Scientists agree that HIV, which is genetically similar to viruses found in African primates (e.g., simian immunodeficiency virus), was probably transmitted to human beings in an earlier age as hunters accidentally cut themselves while butchering their kills for food. The deadly strength of HIV results from its aggressive growth within an increasing number of hosts. Worldwide, 33.3 million people are living with HIV/AIDS; the majority of these individuals are in sub-Saharan Africa[25] (Figure 23-3).

Transmission and Stages of Disease Progression

HIV is transmitted from an infected person to another person through sexual contact (i.e., oral, anal, or vaginal),
through the sharing of needles or syringes, or through mother-to-child transmission. Blood, tissue, and organ donations are now very closely screened for HIV antibodies in most countries, thereby reducing this form of transmission. The primary mode of HIV transmission is sexual contact, which accounts for more than 80% of new cases.[25]

The individual clinical course of HIV infection varies substantially, but the following three distinct stages mark the progression of the disease:

- Primary HIV infection and extended latent period of viral incubation
- HIV-related diseases
- AIDS

There are two classification systems that are used for staging HIV: the CDC classification system and the World Health Organization Clinical Staging and Disease Classification System. The CDC classification system assesses HIV stages on the basis of the lowest documented helper T white blood cell count (i.e., CD4 cell count categories 1, 2, and 3) and the presence of specific HIV-related conditions (i.e., clinical categories A, B, and C).[26] The World Health Organization staging system is generally used in areas where laboratory values of CD4 cell counts are unavailable. This system relies on clinical manifestations to stage the severity of HIV. The CDC classification system is used in the United States and is discussed here.

CD4 T-Lymphocyte Categories

Laboratory values of CD4+ T lymphocytes are defined as follows:

- Category 1: 500 cells/µL or more
- Category 2: 200 to 499 cells/µL
- Category 3: less than 200 cells/µL

Clinical Categories

Category A: Asymptomatic or Acute HIV. Approximately 2 to 4 weeks after initial exposure and infection, a mild flu-like episode may occur. This brief (i.e., days to weeks) and mild response reflects the initial development of antibodies to the viral infection. Any subsequent HIV testing is positive. For a number of years,

---

pandemic a widespread epidemic distributed throughout a region, a continent, or the world.

parasite an organism that lives in or on an organism of another species, known as the *host*, from whom all nourishment is obtained.

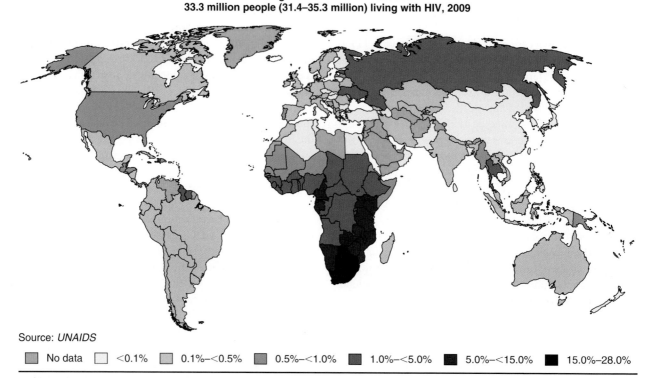

2010: a global view of HIV infection
33.3 million people (31.4–35.3 million) living with HIV, 2009

Source: *UNAIDS*

No data | <0.1% | 0.1%–<0.5% | 0.5%–<1.0% | 1.0%–<5.0% | 5.0%–<15.0% | 15.0%–28.0%

To calculate the adult HIV prevalence rate, we divided the estimated number of adults (15–49) living with HIV in 2009 by the 2009 population aged 15–49.

Depending on the reliability of the data available, there is more or less certainty surrounding any one estimate. Therefore we present ranges, called "plausibility bounds" around the estimates. The wider the bound, the more uncertainty there is surrounding the country's estimate. The extent of uncertainty depends mainly on the type of epidemic, and the quality, coverage and consistency of a country's surveillance system and in generalized epidemics, whether or not a population-based survey with HIV testing was conducted. A full description of the methods used to develop plausibility bounds can be found in *Sexually Transmitted Infections, 2010, 86 (Suppl. 2)*.

The designation employed and the presentation of the material in this map, including tables and colouring of country areas, do not imply the expression of any opinion whatsoever on the part of UNAIDS or WHO concerning the legal status of any country, territory, city or area of or its authorities, or concerning the delimitation of its frontiers or boundaries.

The *UNAIDS Report on the Global Aids Epidemic 2010* revises the estimate of the number of people living with HIV in 2008 of 33.4 million (31.1 million–35.8 million), published in *AIDS epidemic update: November 2009*, to 32.8 million (30.9 million–34.7 million), which is within the uncertainty range of the previous estimate. This revision is based on additional data becoming available for many countries, including data from population-based surveys such as in Mozambique.

AIDS Epidemic Update: November 2009 included Mexico in Latin America. The *UNAIDS Global Report 2010* includes Mexico in North America and categorizes the rest of Latin America as Central and South America. This report presents trend analysis based on the new definition of these regions.

Source: *UNAIDS Report on the Global AIDS Epidemic, 2010.*

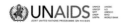

Figure 23-3 Global prevalence of human immunodeficiency virus infection. (From the Joint United Nations Programme on HIV/AIDS. *UNAIDS report on the global AIDS epidemic, UNAIDS/ONUSIDA, 2010, HIV prevalence map* [website]: www.unaids.org/globalreport/HIV_prevalence_map.htm. Accessed November 21, 2011.)

the person typically feels well. This long well period is deceptive, however, because it is a critical stage of viral incubation. The virus is hiding in lymphoid tissues (e.g., lymph nodes, spleen, adenoid glands, tonsils), where it rapidly multiplies as part of its parasite life cycle within the host, taking over more and more of the host's CD4 cells and gaining strength. Researchers emphasize the crucial nature of this incubation period and the importance of early medical treatment intervention after a positive HIV test. Early treatment may slow the viral

strengthening time while drugs and vaccines are developed to combat its steady progression.

Category B: Symptomatic Conditions. After the extended "well" HIV-positive stage, associated infectious illnesses begin to invade the body. This period of opportunistic illnesses is so named because, at this point, the HIV infection has killed enough host-protective T lymphocytes to damage the immune system severely and to lower the body's normal disease resistance so that even the most common everyday infections have an

BOX 23-2 **COMMON TYPES OF OPPORTUNISTIC INFECTIONS IN PATIENTS INFECTED WITH HUMAN IMMUNODEFICIENCY VIRUS**

CLINICAL CATEGORY B
- Bacillary angiomatosis
- Candidiasis, oropharyngeal (thrush)
- Candidiasis, vulvovaginal; persistent, frequent, or poorly responsive to therapy
- Cervical dysplasia (moderate or severe), cervical carcinoma in situ
- Constitutional symptoms, such as fever (38.5° C/101.3°F) or diarrhea lasting longer than 1 month
- Hairy leukoplakia, oral
- Herpes zoster (shingles) involving at least two distinct episodes or more than one dermatome
- Idiopathic thrombocytopenic purpura
- Listeriosis
- Pelvic inflammatory disease, particularly if complicated by tubo-ovarian abscess
- Peripheral neuropathy
- Salmonella septicemia, recurrent
- Toxoplasmosis of brain
- Wasting syndrome from human immunodeficiency virus

From the Centers for Disease Control and Prevention. 1993 revised classification system for HIV infection and expanded surveillance case definition for AIDS among adolescents and adults. *MMWR Recomm Rep* 1992;41:1-19.

opportunity to take root and grow (Box 23-2). Common symptoms during this period include persistent fatigue, mouth sores from thrush (i.e., oral *Candida albicans*), night sweats, diarrhea that lasts more than 1 month, a fever of more than 100° F, unintentional weight loss, remarkable headaches, shingles, cervical dysplasia or carcinoma, new or unusual cough, unusual bruises or skin discoloration, and peripheral neuropathy.

Category C: AIDS-Indicator Conditions. The terminal stage of HIV infection, which is designated as *AIDS,* is marked by rapidly declining T-lymphocyte counts and the presence of AIDS-indicator conditions (Box 23-3). Kaposi's sarcoma is the most common AIDS-associated cancer, and it is characterized by malignant and rapidly growing tumors of the skin and mucous linings of the GI and respiratory tracts; these tumors may cause severe internal bleeding. Low-dose radiation therapy or anticancer drugs may be used to slow the spread of tumors.

During severe immunodeficiency, protozoan parasites (i.e., primitive single-celled organisms) appear and infect a number of body organs. At lymphocyte counts of less than 50/mm³, cytomegalovirus (i.e., a herpes virus that causes lesions on the mucous linings of body organs) and lymphoma (i.e., any cancer of the lymphoid tissue) can flourish. This series of HIV effects on the body brings marked changes in body weight in both men and women (i.e., wasting syndrome), with women losing disproportionately more body fat. Other common conditions include infection with *Mycobacterium tuberculosis, Pneumocystis jiroveci* pneumonia, AIDS dementia complex, and progressive multifocal leukoencephalopathy.

When the virus kills enough white cells to overwhelm the immune system's weakened resistance to the disease complications, death follows.

MEDICAL MANAGEMENT OF THE PATIENT WITH HUMAN IMMUNODEFICIENCY VIRUS/ ACQUIRED IMMUNODEFICIENCY SYNDROME

Initial Evaluation and Goals

The initial medical evaluation of a person who has been newly diagnosed with HIV is critical to provide guidelines for ongoing comprehensive care by the HIV/AIDS team. This professional team includes medical, nutrition, nursing, and psychosocial health care specialists. Box 23-4 outlines an initial evaluation guide that emphasizes special coordinated medical care and the importance of nutrition, nursing, and psychosocial support.

The medical management of HIV infection is constantly evolving as a result of intensive medical research. Basic current goals are to achieve the following:
- Delay the progression of the infection and boost the immune system.
- Prevent opportunistic illnesses.
- Recognize the infection early and provide rapid treatment for complications, including infections and cancer.

Drug Therapy

Developing effective drugs is difficult because of the highly evolved nature of the virus. One of the earliest findings in the drug research for HIV has been a group of compounds called *nucleoside/nucleotide reverse transcriptase inhibitors* (NRTIs) that inhibit the virus's necessary enzyme for copying itself, thereby effectively preventing viral increase. Multiple toxic side effects have

BOX 23-3 **COMMON TYPES OF OPPORTUNISTIC INFECTIONS IN PATIENTS INFECTED WITH HUMAN IMMUNODEFICIENCY VIRUS**

CLINICAL CATEGORY C
- Candidiasis of the bronchi, trachea, or lungs
- Candidiasis, esophageal
- Cervical cancer, invasive
- Coccidioidomycosis, disseminated or extrapulmonary
- Cryptococcosis, extrapulmonary
- Cryptosporidiosis, chronic intestinal (longer than 1 month in duration)
- Cytomegalovirus disease (other than liver, spleen, or nodes)
- Cytomegalovirus retinitis with loss of vision
- Encephalopathy, related to human immunodeficiency virus
- Herpes simplex: chronic ulcers (longer than 1 month in duration); bronchitis, pneumonitis, or esophagitis
- Histoplasmosis, disseminated or extrapulmonary
- Isosporiasis, chronic intestinal (longer than 1 month in duration)
- Kaposi's sarcoma
- Lymphoma, Burkitt's (or equivalent term)
- Lymphoma, immunoblastic (or equivalent term)
- Lymphoma, primary, of brain
- *Mycobacterium avium* complex or *Mycobacterium kansasii,* disseminated or extrapulmonary
- *Mycobacterium tuberculosis,* pulmonary or extrapulmonary
- *Mycobacterium,* other species or unidentified species, disseminated or extrapulmonary
- *Pneumocystis jiroveci* pneumonia
- Pneumonia, recurrent
- Progressive multifocal leukoencephalopathy

From the Centers for Disease Control and Prevention. 1993 revised classification system for HIV infection and expanded surveillance case definition for AIDS among adolescents and adults. *MMWR Recomm Rep.* 1992;41:1-19.

BOX 23-4 **INITIAL EVALUATION OF PATIENTS WHO HAVE BEEN NEWLY DIAGNOSED WITH HUMAN IMMUNODEFICIENCY VIRUS**

- General history
  - History of present illness
  - Medical history
  - Current prescription and nonprescription medicines
  - Vaccination history
  - Partner information for disclosure of human immunodeficiency virus (HIV) status
  - Occupational history
  - Allergies
  - Reproductive history
- HIV treatment and staging
  - HIV exposure history
  - Most recent viral load and CD4 count
  - Current and previous antiretroviral regimens
  - Previous adverse antiretroviral drug reactions
  - Opportunistic infections
- Mental health and substance use history
- Sexual history
- Review of systems (including questions about common symptoms related to HIV infection)
- Comprehensive physical examination
  - Vital signs and pain assessment
  - Ophthalmologic assessment
  - Oral examination
  - Head, ears, nose, and throat examination
  - Dermatologic examination
  - Lymph node examination
  - Endocrinologic examination
  - Pulmonary and cardiac examination
  - Abdominal examination
  - Genital examination
  - Rectal examination
  - Musculoskeletal examination
  - Neuropsychological examination
- Diagnostic and laboratory assessment
  - Immunologic and virologic assessment
  - Tuberculosis evaluation
  - Screening for sexually transmitted infections
  - Hematologic assessment
  - Renal and hepatic assessment
  - Metabolic assessment

From the U.S. Department of Health and Human Services, Agency for Healthcare Research and Quality. *National Guideline Clearinghouse: guideline summary: primary care approach to the HIV-infected patient* (website): www.guideline.gov/content.aspx?id=34268&search=primary+care+approach+to+the+hiv-infected+patient%5c. Accessed May 2011.

been reported (Table 23-3), but some of these (e.g., nausea) may be helped by dietary modifications. Other types of antiretroviral drugs approved by the FDA and currently in use in the United States are non-NRTIs (NNRTIs), protease inhibitors, fusion inhibitors, entry inhibitors, and HIV integrase strand-transfer inhibitors.[27] NNRTIs prevent the reproduction of the viral cells by inhibiting reverse transcriptase. Protease inhibitors help to stop HIV by inhibiting the basic enzyme protease, which is essential to HIV's development. Unfortunately, the virus is capable of mutation in response to some drugs (specifically protease inhibitors) and thus becomes resistant to treatment.[28] Fusion inhibitors prevent the infection of healthy cells by binding to HIV. A combination of these medications, which is referred to as *highly active*

antiretroviral therapy (HAART), is the primary drug treatment regimen that is used to help slow the progression of HIV.

In addition to these antiretroviral drugs, many other drugs have been approved by the FDA to prevent or treat AIDS-related illnesses.

TABLE 23-3 **INITIAL ANTIRETROVIRAL THERAPY AND MAJOR TOXIC EFFECTS AND CAUTIONS**

Drug	Major Toxic Effects And Cautions	Drug	Major Toxic Effects And Cautions
Nucleoside Reverse Transcriptase Inhibitors		Etravirine/ Intelence	Rash Hypersensitivity reactions Nausea
Tenofovir disoproxil fumarate/ Viread, Atripla, Truvada	Renal insufficiency Osteomalacia Weakness, headache, diarrhea, nausea, vomiting, and flatulence	**Protease Inhibitors**	
		Atazanavir/ Reyataz	Indirect hyperbilirubinemia Hyperglycemia Fat maldistribution Possible increased bleeding in hemophilia patients Nephrolithiasis Skin rash Serum transaminase elevations Hyperlipidemia
Zidovudine/ Retrovir	Headache, nausea, and insomnia Bone marrow suppression: macrocytic anemia or neutropenia Lipoatrophy Lactic acidosis or severe hepatomegaly with hepatic steatosis Hyperlipidemia Insulin resistance Myopathy		
		Darunavir/Prezista	Skin rash Hepatotoxicity Diarrhea, nausea, and headache Hyperlipidemia Serum transaminase elevation Hyperglycemia Fat maldistribution Possible increased bleeding in hemophiliac patients
Abacavir/Ziagen	Hypersensitivity reactions (Human leukocyte antigen screening should be performed before initiation.)		
Didanosine/Videx EC	Pancreatitis Peripheral neuropathy Retinal changes Lactic acidosis with hepatic steatosis Nausea and vomiting Insulin resistance	Fosamprenavir/ Lexiva	Skin rash Diarrhea, nausea, and vomiting Headache Hyperlipidemia Serum transaminase elevation Hyperglycemia Fat maldistribution Possible increased bleeding in hemophiliac patients Nephrolithiasis
Emtricitabine/ Emtriva	Skin discoloration		
Stavudine	Peripheral neuropathy Lipoatrophy Pancreatitis Lactic acidosis or severe hepatomegaly with hepatic steatosis Hyperlipidemia Insulin resistance Rapidly progressive ascending neuromuscular weakness (rare)	Indinavir/Crixivan	Nephrolithiasis Gastrointestinal intolerance and nausea Hepatitis Indirect hyperbilirubinemia Hyperlipidemia Headache, weakness, blurred vision, dizziness, rash, metallic taste, thrombocytopenia, alopecia, and hemolytic anemia Hyperglycemia Fat maldistribution Possible increased bleeding in hemophiliac patients
Lamivudine/Epivir	Minimal toxicity		
Non-Nucleoside Reverse Transcriptase Inhibitors			
Efavirenz/Sustiva	Rash Neuropsychiatric symptoms Increased transaminase levels Hyperlipidemia Potentially teratogenic	Lopinavir + ritonavir	Gastrointestinal intolerance, nausea, vomiting, and diarrhea Pancreatitis Weakness Hyperlipidemia Serum transaminase elevation Hyperglycemia Insulin resistance Fat maldistribution Possible increased bleeding in hemophiliac patients
Nevirapine	Rash Symptomatic hepatitis, including fatal hepatic necrosis Avoid in women with >250 CD4 cells/μL and in men with >400 CD4 cells/μL		
Delavirdine/ Rescriptor	Rash Increased transaminase levels Nausea and headache		

Continued

TABLE 23-3 **INITIAL ANTIRETROVIRAL THERAPY AND MAJOR TOXIC EFFECTS AND CAUTIONS—cont'd**

Drug	Major Toxic Effects And Cautions	Drug	Major Toxic Effects And Cautions
Nelfinavir/Viracept	Diarrhea Hyperlipidemia Hyperglycemia Fat maldistribution Possible increased bleeding in hemophiliac patients Serum transaminase elevation	**Integrase Inhibitor** Raltegravir/ Isentress	Nausea Headache Diarrhea Pyrexia Creatine phosphokinase elevation, muscle weakness, and rhabdomyolysis
Ritonavir/Norvir	Gastrointestinal intolerance, nausea, and vomiting Paresthesias (circumoral and extremities) Hyperlipidemia Hepatitis Weakness Altered taste Hyperglycemia Fat maldistribution Possible increased bleeding in hemophiliac patients	**Fusion Inhibitor** Enfuvirtide/ Fuzeon **CCR5 Antagonist** Maraviroc/ Selzentry	Injection site reaction Increased bacterial pneumonia Hypersensitivity reaction Abdominal pain Cough Dizziness Musculoskeletal symptoms Pyrexia Rash Upper respiratory tract infections Hepatotoxicity Orthostatic hypotension
Saquinavir/ Invirase	Gastrointestinal intolerance, nausea, and diarrhea Headache Serum transaminase elevation Hyperlipidemia Hyperglycemia Fat maldistribution Possible increased bleeding in hemophiliac patients		
Tipranavir/Aptivus	Hepatotoxicity Skin rash Intracranial hemorrhage (rare) Hyperlipidemia Hyperglycemia Fat maldistribution Possible increased bleeding in hemophiliac patients		

Modified from the Panel on Antiretroviral Guidelines for Adults and Adolescents. *Guidelines for the use of antiretroviral agents in HIV-1-infected adults and adolescents* (website): www.aidsinfo.nih.gov/ContentFiles/AdultandAdolescentGL.pdf. Accessed April 2011.

Vaccine Development

A successful HIV vaccine would train the body's immune system to identify and destroy the virus. The development and testing of vaccines takes several years. After a potential vaccine is identified, it must go through the following three phases of testing and be determined to be effective before the FDA can approve it for public use:

- *Phase I:* The vaccine is tested in small groups of healthy, low-risk participants. This phase lasts 12 to 18 months.
- *Phase II:* The vaccine is tested in hundreds of high- and low-risk participants. This phase can last up to 2 years.
- *Phase III:* Thousands of high-risk participants are tested for both the safety and effectiveness of the vaccine. This phase usually lasts an additional 3 to 4 years.

Thailand became the first country to begin a phase III HIV vaccine trial. The two-vaccine combination was considered safe and somewhat effective for the prevention of HIV infection (the vaccine efficacy was 31% one year after vaccination).[29] The CDC and the National Institutes of Health are involved in coordinating vaccine research in the United States, and they are working in conjunction with other agencies worldwide to expedite the development of a more effective vaccine. Current challenges to the development of an effective vaccine include the degree of diversity of the virus, the ability of the virus to evade the hosts' immunity, and a lack of appropriate animal models.[30] More information about preventative and therapeutic vaccines can be found at http://aidsinfo.nih.gov.

MEDICAL NUTRITION THERAPY

Assessment

A comprehensive nutrition assessment provides the baseline information that is necessary for starting and continuing nutrition care. The clinical dietitian on the multidisciplinary care team conducts this assessment. The assessment should include the typical ABCD nutrition evaluations: *a*nthropometric, *b*iochemical, *c*linical, and *d*ietary parameters.[31] Further person-centered nutrition care necessary for all HIV-infected patients is evident in the ABCDEFs of nutrition assessment (see the Clinical Applications box, "The ABCDEFs of Nutrition Assessment for Patients With Acquired Immunodeficiency Syndrome").

Intervention

This portion of the nutrition care process includes planning, implementing, and documenting appropriate patient-specific interventions. There are no specific macronutrient or micronutrient recommendations for the patient with HIV, other than meeting his or her general needs. The key MNT objective is to reduce or eliminate malnutrition and to correct nutrition problems that are identified in the nutrition assessment.[12] Suggestions for nutrition-related symptom management are outlined in Table 23-2.

Dietitians can help to plan a patient-specific diet so that energy, protein, fluid, and micronutrient needs are met while not interfering with medication schedules. Food and water safety are important for all patients with compromised immunity, especially patients with HIV. Thus, the prevention of food-borne illness through appropriate cooking and storing food methods should be discussed during nutrition counseling. Complications from medications and comorbidities should also be addressed. Common comorbidities include cardiovascular risk (e.g., hyperlipidemia), liver disease, diabetes, and metabolic changes that lead to malnutrition.

Wasting Effects of Human Immunodeficiency Virus Infection on Nutritional Status

Severe Malnutrition and Weight Loss

Patients with HIV typically have a decreased appetite and an insufficient energy intake coupled with an elevated resting energy expenditure. Major weight loss follows and eventually leads to cachexia that is similar to that seen in patients with cancer. Malnutrition suppresses cellular immune function, thereby perpetuating the onset of opportunistic infections, which is the primary cause of death in patients with AIDS. The chronic and relentless body wasting of AIDS is so striking that in Africa it is called "slim disease." This wasting process plays a major role in the patients' decreased quality of life, the associated debilitating weakness and fatigue, and the progression of the disease.

CLINICAL APPLICATIONS

THE ABCDEFS OF NUTRITION ASSESSMENT FOR PATIENTS WITH HIV/AIDS

The initial nutrition assessment visit with a patient infected with human immunodeficiency virus (HIV) is a vital encounter serving both informational and relational functions. It provides the necessary baseline information for planning practical, individual nutrition support. More importantly, however, the initial visit establishes the essential provider/patient relationship, which is the human context in which continuing nutrition care and support are provided. The basic ABCDs of nutrition assessment (*a*nthropometry, *b*iochemical tests, *c*linical observations, and *d*ietary evaluations) provide a practical guide (see Chapter 17), with two more points added for HIV-infected patients.

*E*nvironmental, behavioral, and psychological assessment
- Living situation, personal support
- Food environment, types of meals, eating assistance needed

*F*inancial Assessment
- Medical insurance
- Income, financial support through caregivers
- Ability to afford food, enteral supplements, additional vitamins or minerals

Causes of Body Wasting

The characteristic body wasting of HIV infection may result from any of the following processes, either alone or in combination:

- *Inadequate food intake:* An important factor in the profound weight loss seen in these patients is severe anorexia. This state is related to the patient's life-changing situation as well as the body's physiologic changes from the disease and drug-nutrient interactions. In addition to anorexia, food insecurity complicates the lives of many individuals who are living with HIV, especially in developing countries.[32]

- *Malabsorption of nutrients:* Diarrhea and malabsorption are common symptoms that are related to drug-diet interactions and to the progressive effects of HIV infection. The viral infection causes the blunting of the intestinal villi and the secretion of abnormal intestinal enzymes. During the later stages of AIDS, the damaged intestinal tissues are open to opportunistic organisms, which results in severe diarrhea and malabsorption.[33] Probiotics may be beneficial for preserving gut function and reducing inflammation in some patients.[34]

- *Disordered metabolism:* During the final stage of weight loss in patients with AIDS, changes in metabolism (e.g., hypermetabolism, altered energy metabolism) occur. The progressive depletion of lean body mass and an increased resting energy expenditure also result.

- *Lean tissue wasting:* A decreased level of physical activity and exercise is common among terminally ill patients who are undergoing extensive medical therapy with a multitude of negative side effects. Disuse coupled with systemic inflammation and hypercortisolemia exacerbate muscle wasting and increase mortality. Providing extra protein and energy in the diet helps to preserve fat mass but not muscle mass.[35] Resistance training, appropriate nutrition, and the administration of human growth hormone appear to be effective for preventing lean tissue losses in some conditions of muscle wasting, but they have not been fully evaluated for HIV-associated lean tissue wasting.[36]

Lipodystrophy

Lipodystrophy is not well defined or objectively diagnosed; however, it is described as a disproportionate gaining of fat mass in the neck and abdomen with a concurrent loss of body fat in the face, buttocks, arms, and legs.[37] Patients with lipodystrophy continue to lose lean tissue while unbalanced changes in fat mass are taking place. The combined effects contribute to the abnormal body composition changes seen in patients with AIDS.

The most well understood causative factor for lipodystrophy is treatment with antiretroviral therapy (see the For Further Focus box, "Highly Active Antiretroviral Therapy and Lipodystrophy"). Other possible risk factors include age, sex, body mass index, ethnicity, genetic factors, CD4 count, viral load, and duration of HIV infection.[37]

FOR FURTHER FOCUS

HIGHLY ACTIVE ANTIRETROVIRAL THERAPY AND LIPODYSTROPHY

Lipodystrophy in patients with human immunodeficiency virus (HIV) involves lipoatrophy (i.e., body fat reduction) in the limbs and face and lipohypertrophy (i.e., increased fat mass) around the abdomen and the back of the neck. This redistribution of fat is associated with metabolic abnormalities and an increased risk for chronic conditions such as hyperlipidemia, hypertension, and insulin resistance.[1]

The introduction of antiretroviral drugs was an important step in the treatment of HIV and acquired immunodeficiency syndrome. Since that time, mortality and morbidity from HIV has significantly declined. Although HIV itself can lead to lipodystrophy, many body fat changes are the result of antiretroviral drugs themselves. Nucleoside reverse transcriptase inhibitors are associated with lipoatrophy,

non-nucleoside reverse transcriptase inhibitors are associated with lipohypertrophy, and protease inhibitors are associated with hyperlipidemia and insulin resistance.[2]

There is no cure for lipodystrophy; however, diet and exercise are key interventions to manage hyperlipidemia, insulin resistance, and central adiposity related to HIV-associated lipodystrophy. The dietary management of these patients is similar to that of patients without HIV who have cardiovascular risk factors. A diet that is low in saturated and trans fats, rich in fruits, vegetables, and whole grains, and adequate in protein, in combination with daily exercise, can reduce cardiovascular risk.[2]

Kelli Boi

1. Barbaro G. Heart and HAART: two sides of the coin for HIV-associated cardiology issues. *World J Cardiol.* 2010;2(3):53-57.
2. Pirmohamed M. Clinical management of HIV-associated lipodystrophy. *Curr Opin Lipidol.* 2009;20(4):309-314.

Nutrition Counseling, Education, and Supportive Care

Education and counseling are important factors of MNT and should focus on the following[12]:

- Appropriate and adequate food intake
- Food behaviors
- Symptoms that may affect appropriate food intake
- Benefits and risks of supplemental nutrients
- A review of nutritional strategies for symptom management to reduce the effects of disease and medication intolerance

Counseling Principles

The basic goal of nutrition counseling is to make the least amount of changes necessary in a person's lifestyle and food patterns to promote optimal nutritional status while providing maximal comfort and quality of life.

In this person-centered care process, the following counseling principles are particularly important:

- *Motivation:* Changes in behavior in any area require the motivation, desire, and ability to achieve one's goals. HIV/AIDS is no exception. Until a patient perceives food patterns and behaviors as appropriate goals, wait for a better time, and start with establishing a general supportive climate in which to continue working together. Any specific obstacle that is raised by the patient (e.g., time, physical limitations, money, increased anxiety) can be met with related suggestions to consider.
- *Rationale:* Any diet or food behavior change with possible benefits or risks must be clearly explained to the patient. Patients with HIV/AIDS are more vulnerable to the lure of unproven therapies.
- *Provider-patient agreement:* When the patient is ready, any change must involve an agreement, and it must fit daily routines and include caregivers as needed.
- *Manageable steps:* All information and actions should proceed in manageable steps that are as small as necessary and in order of complexity and difficulty. Do the simple and easy things first; information overload can discourage anyone. Clinicians should also keep in mind any cognitive or central nervous system decline in the patient. Such decline may contribute to memory loss and the inability to follow nutrition advice. Include individuals from the patient's support group in consultations.

Personal Food Management Skills

The patient's living situation and general practical skills with regard to planning, purchasing, and preparing food must be considered. The need for information and guidance when developing these skills or locating sources of help should be addressed. It is the responsibility of the registered dietitian to establish patient-specific meal plans that support the patient's medication regimens; this may include individualized plans for meal timing, macronutrient and micronutrient modulations, and symptom management.[31]

Community Programs

Information about available community food programs (e.g., Meals on Wheels for the delivery of prepared meals when the patient is too ill to shop for food or prepare it) may be needed. Information about food-assistance programs (e.g., the Supplemental Nutrition Assistance Program [SNAP] or food commodities [see Chapter 13]), for which lower-income patients may qualify, may be warranted.

Psychosocial Support

In the final analysis, every aspect of care provided should be given in a form and manner that provide genuine psychosocial support. All health care providers who work with patients with HIV/AIDS must be particularly sensitive to the psychologic and social issues that confront these patients. Major stress areas include issues related to autonomy and dependency, a sense of uncertainty and fear of the unknown, grief, change and loss, fear of symptoms and abandonment, and spiritual questions that arise when confronting a life-threatening disease. Common emotions are hostility, denial, withdrawal, depression, anxiety, guilt, and confusion. Health care providers must always be aware of how the patient and his or her caregivers relate to the disease and make use of the assistance of social workers and clinical psychologists as needed. Stress-reduction groups and activities—including exercise training—are helpful, as they are for other life-threatening conditions.

Health care workers must also examine their own stresses, values, and fears about sexual orientation and behavior, intravenous drug use, and fear of HIV transmission. Preconceived judgments are easily sensed by patients and threaten the provider-patient relationship. Before they can be effective with patients, all health care workers must first deal with their own fears and prejudices and learn to let go of any judgmental behavior.

SUMMARY

- The general term *cancer* is given to various abnormal malignant tumors in different tissue sites. The cancer cell is derived from a normal cell that loses control over its growth and reproduction. Cancer cell development occurs as a result of the mutation of regulatory genes, and it is influenced by environmental chemical carcinogens, radiation, and viruses. Other lifestyle factors associated with an increased risk for cancer include poor diet, excessive alcohol use, and smoking as well as physical and psychologic stress.
- Cell integrity is mediated by the body's immune system, primarily through its two types of white blood cells: T cells that kill invading agents that cause disease and B cells that make specific antibodies to attack these agents.
- Cancer therapy primarily consists of surgery, radiation, and chemotherapy. Supportive nutrition care must be highly individualized in accordance with the patient's body's responses to the disease and its treatment. This care is based on nutrition assessment and provided by the oral, enteral, or parenteral route.
- The nutrition care of patients with HIV/AIDS must be built on knowledge and compassion, with a sensitivity and concern for individual patient needs. The current worldwide spread of HIV and its fatal consequences have reached epidemic proportions, and they are still growing.
- The overall disease progression of HIV/AIDS follows the three distinct stages: (1) HIV infection; (2) symptomatic disease with opportunistic infection and illnesses; and (3) symptomatic AIDS with complicating diseases that lead to death.
- The medical management of HIV infection involves the supportive treatment of associated illnesses and diseases. During the terminal AIDS stage, the virus eventually gains enough strength to destroy the host's immune system, and death follows.
- Nutrition management centers on providing individual nutrition support to counteract the severe body wasting and malnutrition that are characteristic of the disease. The process of nutrition care involves a comprehensive nutrition assessment, the evaluation of personal needs, the planning of care with patient and caregivers, and the meeting of food needs.

CRITICAL THINKING QUESTIONS

1. In what two main ways does nutrition relate to cancer? Give examples of each.
2. Describe the types of defense cells that are the major components of the body's immune system. How does nutrition relate to immunity?
3. Describe the nutrition problems associated with each of the three medical treatments of cancer. Outline the general procedure for the nutrition management of a patient with cancer.
4. List and describe the reasoning behind each of the guidelines for cancer prevention.
5. Outline the basic parts of the comprehensive initial nutrition assessment of a patient with HIV infection, and describe the reasons for each piece of information and its evaluation.
6. Describe the general process of planning nutrition care on the basis of patient assessment information and the main types of nutrition problems of patients with HIV.

CHAPTER CHALLENGE QUESTIONS

True-False
Write the correct statement for each statement that is false.
1. *True or False:* Cancer-causing mutant genes may be inherited, thereby making a person more susceptible to the influence of some carcinogenic environmental agent.
2. *True or False:* Antigens are specialized protein components of the immune system that protect an individual from disease.
3. *True or False:* Cachexia is a muscle-wasting syndrome that occurs only in patients with HIV/AIDS.
4. *True or False:* Unlike patients with cancer, individuals with HIV/AIDS do not require nutrition support.
5. *True or False:* Lipodystrophy is the abnormal fat redistribution syndrome that is characteristic in some patients with HIV/AIDS who have protein wasting and body fat gain, often in abnormal places.
6. *True or False:* Individuals with HIV/AIDS have severely weakened immune systems; infections caused by parasites and bacteria that are not normally lethal could result in death in these patients.

Multiple Choice

1. Special blood cells that are major components of the immune system are
   a. erythrocytes.
   b. lymphocytes.
   c. neurotransmitters.
   d. platelets.

2. Side effects of cancer chemotherapy that reflect the toxic effect of the drugs on rapidly reproducing cells include
   a. severe headaches.
   b. GI symptoms.
   c. increased urination.
   d. increased appetite.

3. An adequate amount of high-quality protein is essential in the diet of a patient with cancer to
   a. prevent catabolism.
   b. meet increased energy demands.
   c. prevent anabolism.
   d. stimulate hypermetabolism.

4. Small amounts of which of the following types of food would most likely help to treat the nausea that is caused by cancer chemotherapy?
   a. Hot liquids
   b. Dry, spicy foods
   c. Warm, fat-seasoned foods
   d. Soft, cold foods

5. Which of the following is not a method by which HIV can be transmitted?
   a. Sexual contact
   b. Social kissing
   c. Sharing needles
   d. Blood transfusions

6. An individual with HIV infection is said to have AIDS when
   a. he or she loses 10 pounds.
   b. he or she has a rapid increase in helper T lymphocytes.
   c. he or she starts taking medications such as protease inhibitors.
   d. he or she has a rapid decrease in helper T lymphocytes.

7. Body wasting in the patient with HIV/AIDS is usually a result of which of the following?
   a. Inadequate food intake
   b. Malabsorption of nutrients
   c. Disordered metabolism
   d. All the above

⊖volve **Please refer to the Students' Resource section of this text's Evolve Web site for additional study resources.**

REFERENCES

1. National Center for Health Statistics. *Health, United States, 2010: with special feature on death and dying.* Hyattsville, Md: U.S. Government Printing Office; 2011.
2. Key TJ. Fruit and vegetables and cancer risk. *Br J Cancer.* 2011;104(1):6-11.
3. Ames BN, Wakimoto P. Are vitamin and mineral deficiencies a major cancer risk? *Nat Rev Cancer.* 2002;2(9):694-704.
4. Schmid HP, Fischer C, Engeler DS, et al. Nutritional aspects of primary prostate cancer prevention. *Recent Results Cancer Res.* 2011;188:101-107.
5. Xu J, Zhong Y, Jing D, Wu Z. Preoperative enteral immunonutrition improves postoperative outcome in patients with gastrointestinal cancer. *World J Surg.* 2006;30(7):1284-1289.
6. Chen Y, Liu BL, Shang B, et al. Nutrition support in surgical patients with colorectal cancer. *World J Gastroenterol.* 2011;17(13):1779-1786.
7. Wang X, Pan L, Zhang P, et al. Enteral nutrition improves clinical outcome and shortens hospital stay after cancer surgery. *J Invest Surg.* 2010;23(6):309-313.
8. Wimbiscus M, Kostenko O, Malone D. MAO inhibitors: risks, benefits, and lore. *Cleve Clin J Med.* 2010;77(12):859-882.
9. Bosaeus I. Nutritional support in multimodal therapy for cancer cachexia. *Support Care Cancer.* 2008;16(5):447-451.
10. Tisdale MJ. Cancer cachexia. *Curr Opin Gastroenterol.* 2010;26(2):146-151.
11. Tan BH, Fearon KC. Cachexia: prevalence and impact in medicine. *Curr Opin Clin Nutr Metab Care.* 2008;11(4):400-407.
12. American Dietetic Association. *ADA nutrition care manual.* Chicago: American Dietetic Association; 2010.
13. Tisdale MJ. Mechanisms of cancer cachexia. *Physiol Rev.* 2009;89(2):381-410.
14. Kushi LH, Byers T, Doyle C, et al; American Cancer Society 2006 Nutrition and Physical Activity Guidelines Advisory Committee. American Cancer Society Guidelines on Nutrition and Physical Activity for cancer prevention: reducing the risk of cancer with healthy food choices and physical activity. *CA Cancer J Clin.* 2006;56(5):254-281; quiz 313-314.
15. Wiseman M. The second World Cancer Research Fund/American Institute for Cancer Research expert report. Food, nutrition, physical activity, and the prevention of cancer: a global perspective. *Proc Nutr Soc.* 2008;67(3):253-256.
16. U.S. Food and Drug Administration. *Qualified health claims* (website): www.fda.gov/Food/LabelingNutrition/LabelClaims/QualifiedHealthClaims/default.htm. Accessed November 21, 2011.
17. U.S. Food and Drug Administration. *Health claims meeting significant scientific agreement (SSA)* (website): www.fda.gov/Food/LabelingNutrition/LabelClaims/HealthClaimsMeetingSignificantScientificAgreementSSA/default.htm#Approved_Health_Claims. Accessed November 21, 2011.

18. U.S. Department of Health and Human Services. *Healthy people 2020*. Washington, DC: U.S. Government Printing Office; 2010.

19. Patterson RE, Cadmus LA, Emond JA, Pierce JP. Physical activity, diet, adiposity and female breast cancer prognosis: a review of the epidemiologic literature. *Maturitas*. 2010; 66(1):5-15.

20. Gonzalez CA, Riboli E. Diet and cancer prevention: contributions from the European Prospective Investigation into Cancer and Nutrition (EPIC) study. *Eur J Cancer*. 2010; 46(14):2555-2562.

21. Hauner H, Hauner D. The impact of nutrition on the development and prognosis of breast cancer. *Breast Care (Basel)*. 2010;5(6):377-381.

22. Centers for Disease Control and Prevention. *Chronic disease prevention and health promotion: cancer* (website): www.cdc.gov/nccdphp/publications/aag/dcpc.htm. Accessed May 2011.

23. Centers for Disease Control and Prevention. *Diagnoses of HIV infection and AIDS in the United States and dependent areas, 2009, HIV surveillance report, Volume 21* (website): www.cdc.gov/hiv/surveillance/resources/reports/2009report/. Accessed May 2011.

24. Zhu T, Korber BT, Nahmias AJ, et al. An African HIV-1 sequence from 1959 and implications for the origin of the epidemic. *Nature*. 1998;391(6667):594-597.

25. Joint United Nations Programme on HIV/AIDS. UNAIDS report on the global AIDS epidemic, 2010 (website): www.unaids.org/globalreport/default.htm. Accessed November 2011.

26. Centers for Disease Control and Prevention. 1993 revised classification system for HIV infection and expanded surveillance case definition for AIDS among adolescents and adults. *MMWR Recomm Rep*. 1992;41(RR-17):1-19.

27. U.S. Food and Drug Administration. *Antiretroviral drugs used in the treatment of HIV infection* (website): www.fda.gov/ForConsumers/byAudience/ForPatientAdvocates/HIVandAIDSActivities/ucm118915.htm. Accessed November 2011.

28. Garriga C, Pérez-Elías MJ, Delgado R, et al; Spanish Group for the Study of Antiretroviral Drug Resistance. Mutational patterns and correlated amino acid substitutions in the HIV-1 protease after virological failure to nelfinavir- and lopinavir/ritonavir-based treatments. *J Med Virol*. 2007; 79(11):1617-1628.

29. Rerks-Ngarm S, Pitisuttithum P, Nitayaphan S, et al; MOPH-TAVEG Investigators. Vaccination with ALVAC and AIDSVAX to prevent HIV-1 infection in Thailand. *N Engl J Med*. 2009;361(23):2209-2220.

30. Gamble LJ, Matthews QL. Current progress in the development of a prophylactic vaccine for HIV-1. *Drug Des Devel Ther*. 2010;5:9-26.

31. Fields-Gardner C, Campa A; American Dietetic Association. Position of the American Dietetic Association: nutrition intervention and human immunodeficiency virus infection. *J Am Diet Assoc*. 2010;110(7):1105-1119.

32. Ivers LC, Cullen KA, Freedberg KA, et al. HIV/AIDS, undernutrition, and food insecurity. *Clin Infect Dis*. 2009; 49(7):1096-1102.

33. Georgiou NA, Garssen J, Witkamp RF. Pharma-nutrition interface: the gap is narrowing. *Eur J Pharmacol*. 2011; 651(1-3):1-8.

34. Hummelen R, Vos AP, van't Land B, et al. Altered host-microbe interaction in HIV: a target for intervention with pro- and prebiotics. *Int Rev Immunol*. 2010;29(5): 485-513.

35. Evans WJ. Skeletal muscle loss: cachexia, sarcopenia, and inactivity. *Am J Clin Nutr*. 91(4):1123S-1127S, 2010.

36. Glover EI, Phillips SM. Resistance exercise and appropriate nutrition to counteract muscle wasting and promote muscle hypertrophy. *Curr Opin Clin Nutr Metab Care*. 2010;13(6): 630-634.

37. Moreno S, Miralles C, Negredo E, et al. Disorders of body fat distribution in HIV-1-infected patients. *AIDS Rev*. 2009; 11(3):126-134.

FURTHER READING AND RESOURCES

AIDS information, treatment, and action. www.aids.org

AIDS, the official journal of the International AIDS Society. www.aidsonline.com

AIDS.gov. www.aids.gov

American Cancer Society. www.cancer.org

Centers for Disease Control and Prevention. Cancer prevention and control. www.cdc.gov/cancer

Centers for Disease Control and Prevention. National Center for HIV/AIDS, Viral Hepatitis, STD, and TB Prevention. www.cdc.gov/nchhstp

Joint United Nations Programme on HIV/AIDS. www.unaids.org

National Cancer Institute. www.cancer.gov

The National Institute of Allergy and Infectious Diseases. HIV/AIDS vaccines. www.niaid.nih.gov/topics/hivaids/research/vaccines/Pages/default.aspx

Fields-Gardner C, Campa A. Position of the American Dietetic Association: nutrition intervention and human immunodeficiency virus infection. *J Am Diet Assoc*. 2010;110(7):1105-1119.

McCullough ML, Patel AV, Kushi LH, et al. Following cancer prevention guidelines reduces risk of cancer, cardiovascular disease and all-cause mortality. *Cancer Epidemiol Biomarkers Prev*. 2011;20(6):1089-1097.

Murthy NS, Mukherjee S, Ray G, Ray A. Dietary factors and cancer chemoprevention: an overview of obesity-related malignancies. *J Postgrad Med*. 2009;55(1): 45-54.

APPENDIX A

Cholesterol Content of Select Foods

Item	Serving Size	Cholesterol (mg/Serving)	Cholesterol (mg/100 g)
Beef			
Ground, 80% lean meat and 20% fat, crumbled, cooked, pan browned	3 oz (85 g)	76	89
Tenderloin, steak, separable lean and fat, trimmed to ⅛″ fat, prime, cooked, broiled	3 oz (85 g)	73	86
Smoked sliced beef, Carl Buddig	2 oz (57 g)	38	67
Butter, without salt	1 Tbsp (14.2 g)	31	215
Cheese			
Cheddar	1 oz (28.35 g)	30	105
Cottage, low fat, 1% milk fat	½ cup (113 g)	5	4
Cream	1 Tbsp (14.5 g)	16	110
Parmesan, hard	1 oz (28.35 g)	19	68
Chicken			
Broilers or fryers, breast, meat only, cooked, roasted	3 oz (85 g)	72	85
Broilers or fryers, breast, meat and skin, cooked, roasted	3 oz (85 g)	72	84
Broilers or fryers, breast, meat only, cooked, fried	3 oz (85 g)	77	91
Broilers or fryers, dark meat, meat only, cooked, roasted	3 oz (85 g)	79	93
Cream, whipping, heavy	1 Tbsp (15 g)	21	137
Cream, sour, cultured	2 Tbsp (24 g)	12	52
Egg			
Whole, raw, fresh	1 large (50 g)	186	372
White only, raw, fresh	1 large (33 g)	0	0
Fish			
Halibut, Atlantic and Pacific, cooked, dry heat	3 oz (85 g)	51	60
Salmon, Atlantic, wild, cooked, dry heat	3 oz (85 g)	60	71
Tuna, light, canned in water, drained solids	3 oz (85 g)	26	30
Frozen yogurts, vanilla, soft-serve	½ cup (73 g)	1	2
Ice cream			
Chocolate, rich	½ cup (73 g)	44	60
Chocolate, light	½ cup (73 g)	21	28
Lamb, domestic, leg, whole (shank and sirloin), lean meat only, trimmed to ¼″ fat, choice, cooked, roasted	3 oz (85 g)	76	93
Liver			
Chicken, all classes, cooked, simmered	3 oz (85 g)	479	563
Beef, pan fried	3 oz (85 g)	324	381
Margarine	1 Tbsp (14.2 g)	0	0
Milk			
Buttermilk, fluid, cultured, low fat	1 cup (245 g)	10	4
Canned, evaporated	1 cup (252 g)	73	29
Reduced fat, fluid, 2% milk fat	1 cup (244 g)	20	8
Nonfat (skim)	1 cup (245 g)	5	2
Whole, 3.25% milk fat	1 cup (244 g)	24	10

Item	Serving Size	Cholesterol (mg/Serving)	Cholesterol (mg/100 g)
Pork			
Cured, bacon, cooked, pan fried	3 slices (23.7 g)	27	113
Fresh, enhanced, loin, top loin (chops), boneless, separable lean and fat, cooked, broiled	3 oz (85 g)	45	53
Ham, sliced, regular (approximately 11% fat)	2 slices (56 g)	32	57
Fresh, loin, tenderloin, separable lean and fat, cooked, broiled	3 oz (85 g)	80	94
Sausage, fresh, cooked	1 oz (28 g)	24	84
Shellfish			
Crustaceans, crab, Dungeness, cooked, moist heat	3 oz (85 g)	65	76
Crustaceans, shrimp, mixed species, cooked, moist heat	3 oz (85 g)	179	211
Crustaceans, spiny lobster, mixed species, cooked, moist heat	3 oz (85 g)	76	90
Mollusks, clam, mixed species, cooked, moist heat	3 oz (85 g)	57	67
Mollusks, oyster, Pacific, cooked, moist heat	3 oz (85 g)	85	100
Turkey			
Fryer-roasters, breast, meat and skin, cooked, roasted	3 oz (85 g)	76	90
Fryer-roasters, dark meat, meat only, cooked, roasted	3 oz (85 g)	95	112
Fryer-roasters, light meat, meat only, cooked, roasted	3 oz (85 g)	73	86
Veal, composite of trimmed retail cuts, lean and fat, cooked	3 oz (85 g)	97	114

From the U.S. Department of Agriculture Agricultural Research Service. *Nutrient data laboratory* (website): www.nal.usda.gov/fnic/foodcomp/search/. Accessed April 2011.

APPENDIX B

Dietary Fiber in Selected Plant Foods

Food	Serving Size	Total Dietary Fiber /Serving (g)	Total Dietary Fiber/100 g
Apple juice	1 cup (248 g)	0.5	0.2
Apples, raw, with skin	1 medium (182 g)	4.4	2.4
Banana	1 medium (118 g)	3.1	2.6
Beans, navy, canned	½ cup (131 g)	6.7	5.1
Beans, kidney, canned	½ cup (128 g)	6.9	5.4
Beans, lima, frozen, baby	1 cup (180 g)	10.8	6.0
Beans, pinto,	½ cup (120 g)	5.5	4.6
Beans, soy, green, raw	1 cup (256 g)	10.8	4.2
Beans, snap, green, frozen, cooked, boiled, drained, without salt	1 cup (135 g)	4.0	3.0
Bread, white	1 slice (25 g)	0.6	2.4
Bread, multigrain	1 slice (26 g)	1.9	7.4
Broccoli, boiled, drained	1 cup (156 g)	5.1	3.3
Brussels sprouts, boiled, drained	1 cup (156 g)	4.1	2.6
Cabbage, boiled, drained	1 cup (150 g)	2.9	1.9
Carrots, raw	1 cup (122 g)	3.4	2.8
Cauliflower, boiled, drained	1 cup (124 g)	2.9	2.3
Cereal, ready-to eat, General Mills, Whole Grain Total	¾ cup (30 g)	2.7	9.1
Cereal, ready-to-eat, Kellogg, Corn Flakes	1 cup (28 g)	0.7	2.5
Cereal, ready-to-eat, General Mills, Fiber One, Raisin Bran Clusters	1 cup (55 g)	11.6	21.0
Cereal, ready-to-eat, Malt-O-Meal, Puffed Wheat Cereal	1 cup (15 g)	1.1	7.3
Cereal, ready-to-eat, Kellogg, Rice Krispies	1¼ cup (33 g)	0.3	0.8
Cereal, ready-to-eat, Post, Shredded Wheat, bite-size	1 cup (52 g)	5.0	9.6
Cereal, ready-to-eat, Post, Cocoa Pebbles	¾ cup (30 g)	0.5	1.6
Cereal, oatmeal, prepared with water	1 cup (234 g)	4.0	1.7
Cherries, sweet, raw	½ cup (77 g)	1.6	2.1
Cookies, oatmeal	1 large (18 g)	0.5	2.8
Corn, sweet, yellow	1 ear (102 g)	2.0	2.0
Corn, canned	1 cup (256 g)	4.4	1.7
Flour, rice, brown	1 cup (158 g)	7.3	4.6
Flour, rice, white	1 cup (158 g)	3.8	2.4
Flour, wheat, white, all purpose, enriched	1 cup (125 g)	3.4	2.7
Flour, wheat, whole grain	1 cup (120 g)	12.8	10.7
Grapes, red or green	½ cup (75.5 g)	0.7	0.9
Lentils, boiled	½ cup (99 g)	7.8	7.9
Lettuce, iceberg, raw	1 cup, chopped	0.7	1.2
Lettuce, green leaf, raw	1 cup, shredded	0.5	1.3
Onions, raw	1 medium (110 g)	1.9	1.7
Orange, raw, navel	1 medium (140 g)	3.1	2.2
Peach, raw	1 medium (150 g)	2.2	1.5
Peanuts, raw	1 oz (28.35 g)	2.4	8.5

Food	Serving Size	Total Dietary Fiber /Serving (g)	Total Dietary Fiber/100 g
Peanut butter, creamy	2 Tbsp (32 g)	1.9	6.0
Pear, raw	1 medium	5.5	3.1
Peas, canned	1 cup (85 g)	3.5	4.1
Peas, edible-podded, boiled, drained	1 cup (160 g)	4.5	2.8
Plums, dried (prunes)	¼ cup (43.5 g)	3.1	7.1
Potato, sweet, baked with skin	1 medium (114 g)	3.8	3.3
Potato, russet, baked with skin	1 medium (173 g)	4.0	2.3
Potato, russet, without skin	1 medium (156 g)	2.3	1.5
Raisins	1 oz (28.35 g)	1.0	3.7
Strawberries, raw	½ cup	1.4	2.0
Tomato, raw	1 medium (123 g)	1.5	1.2
Tomato, canned, drained	½ cup (120 g)	1.2	1.0

From the U.S. Department of Agriculture Agricultural Research Service. *Nutrient data laboratory* (website): www.nal.usda.gov/fnic/foodcomp/search/. Accessed April 2011.

Suggestions for Salt-Free Seasoning

FISH

Breaded, battered fillets
   Dry mustard, onion, oregano, basil, garlic, thyme
Broiled steaks or fillets
   Chili or curry powder, tarragon
Fillets in butter sauce
   Thyme, chervil, dill, fennel
Fish soup
   Italian seasoning, bay leaf, thyme, tarragon
Fish cakes
   Tarragon, savory, dry mustard, white pepper, red pepper, oregano

BEEF

Swiss steak
   Rosemary, black pepper, bay leaf, thyme, clove
Roast beef
   Basil, oregano, bay leaf, nutmeg, tarragon, marjoram
Beef stew
   Chili powder, bay leaf, tarragon, caraway, marjoram
Meatballs
   Garlic, thyme, basil, oregano, onion, black pepper, dry mustard
Beef stroganoff
   Red pepper, onion, garlic, nutmeg, curry powder

POULTRY AND VEAL

Fried chicken
   Basil, oregano, garlic, onion, dill, sesame seed, nutmeg
Roast chicken or turkey
   Ginger, garlic, onion, thyme, tarragon
Chicken croquettes
   Dill, curry, chili, cumin, tarragon, oregano
Veal patties
   Italian seasoning, tarragon, dill, onion, sesame seeds
Barbecue chicken
   Garlic, dry mustard, clove, allspice, basil, oregano

GRAVIES AND SAUCES

Barbecue
   Bay leaf, thyme, red pepper, cinnamon, ginger, allspice, dry mustard, chili powder
Brown
   Chervil, onion, bay leaf, thyme, nutmeg, tarragon
Chicken
   Dry mustard, ginger, garlic, marjoram, thyme, bay leaf
Cream
   White pepper, dry mustard, curry powder, dill, onion, paprika, tarragon, thyme

SOUPS

Chicken
   Thyme, savory, ginger, clove, white pepper, allspice
Clam chowder
   Basil, oregano, nutmeg, white pepper, thyme, garlic powder
Mushroom
   Ginger, oregano, thyme, tarragon, bay leaf, black pepper, chili powder
Onion
   Curry, caraway, marjoram, garlic, cloves
Tomato
   Bay leaf, thyme, Italian seasoning, oregano, onion, nutmeg
Vegetable
   Italian seasoning, paprika, caraway, rosemary, thyme, fennel

SALADS

Chicken
   Curry or chili powder, Italian seasoning, thyme, tarragon
Coleslaw
   Dill, caraway, poppy seeds, dry mustard, ginger

Fish or seafood
  Dill, tarragon, ginger, dry mustard, red pepper, onion, garlic
Macaroni
  Dill, basil, thyme, oregano, dry mustard, garlic
Potato
  Chili powder, curry, dry mustard, onion

PASTA, BEANS, AND RICE

Baked beans
  Dry mustard, chili powder, clove, onion, ginger
Rice and vegetables
  Curry, thyme, onion, paprika, rosemary, garlic, ginger
Spanish rice
  Cumin, oregano, basil, Italian seasoning
Spaghetti
  Italian seasoning, nutmeg, oregano, basil, red pepper, tarragon
Rice pilaf
  Dill, thyme, savory, black pepper

VEGETABLES

Asparagus
  Ginger, sesame seeds, basil, onion
Broccoli
  Italian seasoning, marjoram, basil, nutmeg, onion, sesame seeds
Cabbage
  Caraway, onion, nutmeg, allspice, clove
Carrots
  Ginger, nutmeg, onion, dill
Cauliflower
  Dry mustard, basil, paprika, onion
Tomatoes
  Oregano, chili powder, dill, onion
Spinach
  Savory, thyme, nutmeg, garlic, onion

APPENDIX D

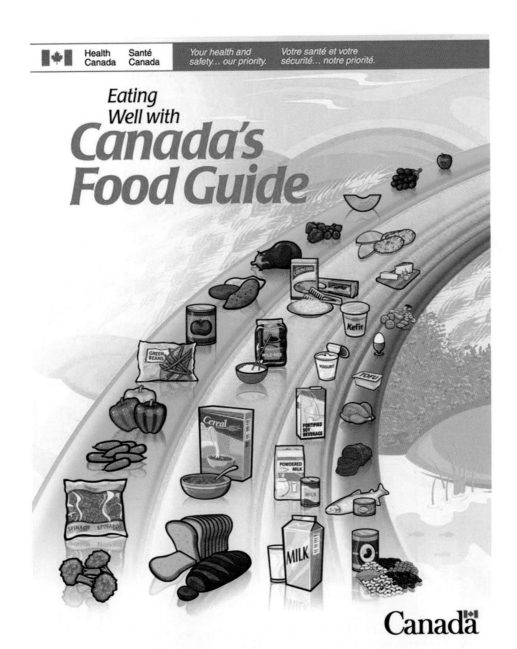

Recommended Number of *Food Guide Servings* per Day

Age in Years	Children			Teens		Adults			
	2-3	4-8	9-13	14-18		19-50		51+	
Sex	Girls and Boys			Females	Males	Females	Males	Females	Males
Vegetables and Fruit	4	5	6	7	8	7-8	8-10	7	7
Grain Products	3	4	6	6	7	6-7	8	6	7
Milk and Alternatives	2	2	3-4	3-4	3-4	2	2	3	3
Meat and Alternatives	1	1	1-2	2	3	2	3	2	3

The chart above shows how many Food Guide Servings you need from each of the four food groups every day.

Having the amount and type of food recommended and following the tips in *Canada's Food Guide* will help:

- Meet your needs for vitamins, minerals and other nutrients.
- Reduce your risk of obesity, type 2 diabetes, heart disease, certain types of cancer and osteoporosis.
- Contribute to your overall health and vitality.

What is One Food Guide Serving?
Look at the examples below.

Fresh, frozen or canned vegetables
125 mL (½ cup)

Leafy vegetables
Cooked: 125 mL (½ cup)
Raw: 250 mL (1 cup)

Fresh, frozen or canned fruits
1 fruit or 125 mL (½ cup)

100% Juice
125 mL (½ cup)

Bread
1 slice (35 g)

Bagel
½ bagel (45 g)

Flat breads
½ pita or ½ tortilla (35 g)

Cooked rice, bulgur or quinoa
125 mL (½ cup)

Cereal
Cold: 30 g
Hot: 175 mL (¾ cup)

Cooked pasta or couscous
125 mL (½ cup)

Milk or powdered milk (reconstituted)
250 mL (1 cup)

Canned milk (evaporated)
125 mL (½ cup)

Fortified soy beverage
250 mL (1 cup)

Yogurt
175 g
(¾ cup)

Kefir
175 g
(¾ cup)

Cheese
50 g (1½ oz.)

Cooked fish, shellfish, poultry, lean meat
75 g (2 ½ oz.)/125 mL (½ cup)

Cooked legumes
175 mL (¾ cup)

Tofu
150 g or
175 mL (¾ cup)

Eggs
2 eggs

Peanut or nut butters
30 mL (2 Tbsp)

Shelled nuts and seeds
60 mL (¼ cup)

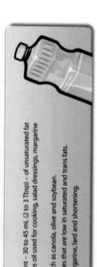

Oils and Fats

- Include a small amount – 30 to 45 mL (2 to 3 Tbsp) – of unsaturated fat each day. This includes oil used for cooking, salad dressings, margarine and mayonnaise.
- Use vegetable oils such as canola, olive and soybean.
- Choose soft margarines that are low in saturated and trans fats.
- Limit butter, hard margarine, lard and shortening.

Make each Food Guide Serving count...
wherever you are – at home, at school, at work or when eating out!

▸ **Eat at least one dark green and one orange vegetable each day.**
- Go for dark green vegetables such as broccoli, romaine lettuce and spinach.
- Go for orange vegetables such as carrots, sweet potatoes and winter squash.

▸ **Choose vegetables and fruit prepared with little or no added fat, sugar or salt.**
- Enjoy vegetables steamed, baked or stir-fried instead of deep-fried.

▸ **Have vegetables and fruit more often than juice.**

▸ **Make at least half of your grain products whole grain each day.**
- Eat a variety of whole grains such as barley, brown rice, oats, quinoa and wild rice.
- Enjoy whole grain breads, oatmeal or whole wheat pasta.

▸ **Choose grain products that are lower in fat, sugar or salt.**
- Compare the Nutrition Facts table on labels to make wise choices.
- Enjoy the true taste of grain products. When adding sauces or spreads, use small amounts.

▸ **Drink skim, 1%, or 2% milk each day.**
- Have 500 mL (2 cups) of milk every day for adequate vitamin D.
- Drink fortified soy beverages if you do not drink milk.

▸ **Select lower fat milk alternatives.**
- Compare the Nutrition Facts table on yogurts or cheeses to make wise choices.

▸ **Have meat alternatives such as beans, lentils and tofu often.**

▸ **Eat at least two Food Guide Servings of fish each week.***
- Choose fish such as char, herring, mackerel, salmon, sardines and trout.

▸ **Select lean meat and alternatives prepared with little or no added fat or salt.**
- Trim the visible fat from meats. Remove the skin on poultry.
- Use cooking methods such as roasting, baking or poaching that require little or no added fat.
- If you eat luncheon meats, sausages or prepackaged meats, choose those lower in salt (sodium) and fat.

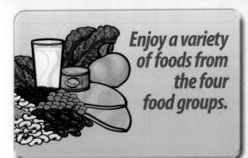

Enjoy a variety of foods from the four food groups.

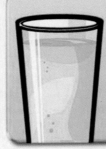

Satisfy your thirst with water!

Drink water regularly. It's a calorie-free way to quench your thirst. Drink more water in hot weather or when you are very active.

* Health Canada provides advice for limiting exposure to mercury from certain types of fish. Refer to www.healthcanada.gc.ca for the latest information.

Eat well and be active today and every day!

The benefits of eating well and being active include:

- Better overall health.
- Lower risk of disease.
- A healthy body weight.
- Feeling and looking better.
- More energy.
- Stronger muscles and bones.

Be active

To be active every day is a step towards better health and a healthy body weight.

Canada's Physical Activity Guide recommends building 30 to 60 minutes of moderate physical activity into daily life for adults and at least 90 minutes a day for children and youth. You don't have to do it all at once. Add it up in periods of at least 10 minutes at a time for adults and five minutes at a time for children and youth.

Start slowly and build up.

Eat well

Another important step towards better health and a healthy body weight is to follow Canada's Food Guide by:

- Eating the recommended amount and type of food each day.
- Limiting foods and beverages high in calories, fat, sugar or salt (sodium) such as cakes and pastries, chocolate and candies, cookies and granola bars, doughnuts and muffins, ice cream and frozen desserts, french fries, potato chips, nachos and other salty snacks, alcohol, fruit flavoured drinks, soft drinks, sports and energy drinks, and sweetened hot or cold drinks.

Read the label

- Compare the Nutrition Facts table on food labels to choose products that contain less fat, saturated fat, trans fat, sugar and sodium.
- Keep in mind that the calories and nutrients listed are for the amount of food found at the top of the Nutrition Facts table.

Limit trans fat

When a Nutrition Facts table is not available, ask for nutrition information to choose foods lower in trans and saturated fats.

Nutrition Facts Per 0 mL (0 g)	
Amount	**% Daily Value**
Calories 0	
Fat 0 g	0 %
Saturates 0 g	0 %
+ Trans 0 g	
Cholesterol 0 mg	
Sodium 0 mg	0 %
Carbohydrate 0 g	0 %
Fibre 0 g	0 %
Sugars 0 g	
Protein 0 g	
Vitamin A 0 %	Vitamin C 0 %
Calcium 0 %	Iron 0 %

Take a step today…

- Have breakfast every day. It may help control your hunger later in the day.
- Walk wherever you can – get off the bus early, use the stairs.
- Benefit from eating vegetables and fruit at all meals and as snacks.
- Spend less time being inactive such as watching TV or playing computer games.
- Request nutrition information about menu items when eating out to help you make healthier choices.
- Enjoy eating with family and friends!
- Take time to eat and savour every bite!

For more information, interactive tools, or additional copies visit Canada's Food Guide on-line at: www.healthcanada.gc.ca/foodguide

or contact:
Publications
Health Canada
Ottawa, Ontario K1A 0K9
E-Mail: publications@hc-sc.gc.ca
Tel.: 1-866-225-0709
Fax: (613) 941-5366
TTY: 1-800-267-1245

Également disponible en français sous le titre :
Bien manger avec le Guide alimentaire canadien

This publication can be made available on request on diskette, large print, audio-cassette and braille.

Advice for different ages and stages…

Children

Following Canada's Food Guide helps children grow and thrive.

Young children have small appetites and need calories for growth and development.

- Serve small nutritious meals and snacks each day.
- Do not restrict nutritious foods because of their fat content. Offer a variety of foods from the four food groups.
- Most of all... be a good role model.

Women of childbearing age

All women who could become pregnant and those who are pregnant or breastfeeding need a multivitamin containing folic acid every day. Pregnant women need to ensure that their multivitamin also contains iron. A health care professional can help you find the multivitamin that's right for you.

Pregnant and breastfeeding women need more calories. Include an extra 2 to 3 Food Guide Servings each day.

Here are two examples:

- Have fruit and yogurt for a snack, or
- Have an extra slice of toast at breakfast and an extra glass of milk at supper.

Men and women over 50

The need for vitamin D increases after the age of 50.

In addition to following Canada's Food Guide, everyone over the age of 50 should take a daily vitamin D supplement of 10 µg (400 IU).

How do I count Food Guide Servings in a meal?

Here is an example:

Vegetable and beef stir-fry with rice, a glass of milk and an apple for dessert

250 mL (1 cup) mixed broccoli, carrot and sweet red pepper	= 2 **Vegetables and Fruit** Food Guide Servings
75 g (2½ oz.) lean beef	= 1 **Meat and Alternatives** Food Guide Serving
250 mL (1 cup) brown rice	= 2 **Grain Products** Food Guide Servings
5 mL (1 tsp) canola oil	= part of your **Oils and Fats** intake for the day
250 mL (1 cup) 1% milk	= 1 **Milk and Alternatives** Food Guide Serving
1 apple	= 1 **Vegetables and Fruit** Food Guide Serving

Calculation Aids and Conversion Tables

A group of French scientists created the metric system of weights and measures called the Système International. Here are a few conversion factors to help you make transitions in your necessary calculations.

METRIC SYSTEM OF MEASUREMENT

The metric system is a simple decimal system that is based on units of 10. It is uniform, and it is used internationally.

Weight Units:

1 kilogram (kg) = 1000 grams (g or gm)
1 g = 1000 milligrams (mg)
1 mg = 1000 micrograms (mcg or μg)

Length Units:

1 meter (m) = 100 centimeters (cm)
1000 m = 1 kilometer (km)

Volume Units:

1 liter (L or l) = 1000 milliliters (ml or mL)
1 mL = 1 cubic centimeter (cc)

Temperature Units:

The Celsius (C) scale, which is based on 100 equal units between 0° C (the freezing point of water) and 100° C (the boiling point of water), is used in all scientific work.

Energy Units:

Kilocalorie (kcal) = Amount of energy required to raise 1 kg water by 1° C
Kilojoule (kJ) = Amount of energy required to move a 1-kg mass 1 m with a force of 1 newton
1 kcal = 4.184 kJ

AMERICAN SYSTEM OF MEASUREMENT

The American system of measurement is not a decimal system but rather a collection of different units. Its roots are primarily British, but it is now predominantly used in the United States only.

Weight Units:

1 pound (lb) = 16 ounces (oz)

Length Units:

1 foot (ft) = 12 inches (in)
3 ft = 1 yard (yd)

Volume Units:

3 teaspoons (tsp) = 1 tablespoon (Tbsp)
16 Tbsp = 1 cup
1 cup = 8 fluid ounces (fl oz)
4 cups = 1 quart (qt)
5 cups = 1 imperial quart (qt) (used in Canada)

Temperature Units:

The Fahrenheit (F) scale is based on 180 equal units between 32° F (the freezing point of water) and 212° F (the boiling point of water) at standard atmospheric pressure.

CONVERSIONS BETWEEN MEASUREMENT SYSTEMS

Weight:

1 oz = 28.35 g
2.205 lb = 1 kg

509

Length:

1 in = 2.54 cm
1 ft = 30.48 cm
39.37 in = 1 m

Volume:

1.06 qt = 1 L
0.85 imperial qt = 1 L (used in Canada)

Temperature:

Boiling point of water = 100° C = 212° F
Body temperature = 37° C = 98.6° F
Freezing point of water = 0° C = 32° F

Interconversion Formulas:

Fahrenheit temperature (° F) = $\frac{9}{5}$ (° C + 32)
Celsius temperature (° C) = $\frac{5}{9}$ (° F − 32)

RETINOL EQUIVALENTS

The following internationally accepted definitions and equivalences are provided to calculate retinol-equivalent conversions.

Definitions:

International units (IU) and retinol equivalents (RE) are defined as follows:
1 IU = 0.3 μg retinol (0.0003 mg)
1 IU = 0.6 μg β-carotene (0.0006 mg)
1 RE = 6 μg retinol
1 RE = 6 μg β-carotene
1 RE = 12 μg other provitamin A carotenoids
1 RE = 3.33 IU retinol
1 RE = 10 IU β-carotene

Conversion Formulas:

On the basis of weight, β-carotene is half as active as retinol; on the basis of structure, the other provitamin carotenoids are one fourth as active as retinol. In addition, retinol is more completely absorbed in the intestines, whereas the provitamin carotenoids are much less efficiently used, with an average absorption of approximately one third. Therefore, with regard to overall activity, β-carotene is one sixth as active as retinol, and the other carotenoids are one twelfth as active. These differences in use provide the basis for the 1:6:12 relationship shown in the equivalences given and in the following formulas for calculating retinol equivalents from values of vitamin A, β-carotene, and other active carotenoids, which are expressed as either international units or micrograms.

If retinol and β-carotene are given in micrograms:
RE = Micrograms of retinol + (Micrograms of β-carotene/6)
If both are given as international units:
RE = (International units of retinol/3.33) + (International units of β-carotene/10)
If β-carotene and other carotenoids are given in micrograms:
RE = (Micrograms of β-carotene/6) + (Micrograms of other carotenoids/12)

APPROXIMATE METRIC CONVERSIONS

When You Know...	...Multiply By...	...To Find...
Weight		
Ounces	28	Grams
Pounds	0.45	Kilograms
Length		
Inches	2.5	Centimeters
Feet	30	Centimeters
Yards	0.9	Meters
Miles	1.6	Kilometers
Volume		
Teaspoons	5	Milliliters
Tablespoons	15	Milliliters
Fluid ounces	30	Milliliters
Cups	0.24	Liters
Pints	0.47	Liters
Quarts	0.95	Liters
Temperature		
Fahrenheit temperature	$\frac{5}{9}$ (after subtracting 32)	Celsius temperature

Cultural Dietary Patterns and Religious Dietary Practices

Foods that are specifically associated with certain cultural groups are noted. Individuals may consume typical American foods as well. Assumptions about dietary patterns cannot be made, but knowledge of these unique foods provides a common understanding of the range of possible food choices.

CULTURAL DIETARY PATTERNS

Ethnic Group	Bread, Cereal, Rice, and Pasta Group	Vegetable Group	Fruit Group	Milk, Yogurt, and Cheese Group	Meat, Poultry, Fish, Dry Beans, Eggs, and Nuts Group	Fats, Oils, And Sweets Group
Native American (Each tribe may have specific foods; commonly consumed foods are listed here.)	Blue corn flour (ground dried blue corn kernels) used to make cornbread, mush dumplings; fruit dumplings (walakshi); fry bread (biscuit dough deep fried); ground sweet acorns; tortillas; wheat or rye used to make cornmeal and flour	Cabbage, carrots, cassava, dandelion greens, eggplant, milkweed, onions, pumpkin, squash (all varieties), sweet and white potatoes, turnips, wild tullies (a tuber), yellow corn	Dried wild cherries and grapes; wild bananas, berries, and yucca	None	Duck, eggs, fish eggs (roe), geese, groundhog, kidney beans, lentils, nuts (all), peanuts, pine nuts, pinto beans, venison, wild rabbit	None
African American	Biscuits; cornbread as spoon bread, cornpone, or hush puppies; grits	Leafy greens including dandelion greens, kale, mustard greens, collard greens, turnips	None	Buttermilk	Pork and pork products, scrapple (cornmeal and pork), chitterlings (pork intestines), bacon, pig's feet, pig ears, souse, pork neck bones, fried meats and poultry, organ meats (kidney, liver, tongue, tripe), venison, rabbit, catfish, buffalo fish, mackerel, legumes (black-eyed peas, kidney beans, navy beans, chickpeas)	Lard
Japanese	Rice and rice products, rice flour (mochiko), noodles (comen, soba), seaweed around rice with or without fish (sushi)	Bamboo shoots (takenoko), burdock (gobo), cabbage (napa), dried mushrooms (shiitake), eggplant, horseradish (wasabi), Japanese parsley (seri), lotus root (renkon), mustard greens, pickled vegetables, seaweed (laver, nori, wakame, kombu), vegetable soup (mizutaki), white radish (daikon)	Pear-like apples (nasi), persimmons	None	Fish and shellfish including dried fish with bones, raw fish (sashimi), fish cake (kamaboko); soybeans as soybean curd (tofu), fermented soybean paste (miso), and sprouts; red beans (adzuki)	Soy and rice oil

Continued

Ethnic Group	Bread, Cereal, Rice, and Pasta Group	Vegetable Group	Fruit Group	Milk, Yogurt, and Cheese Group	Meat, Poultry, Fish, Dry Beans, Eggs, and Nuts Group	Fats, Oils, And Sweets Group
Chinese	Rice and related products (flour, cakes, noodles); noodles made from barley, corn, and millet; wheat and related products (breads, noodles, spaghetti, stuffed noodles [wonton], filled buns [bow])	Bamboo shoots; cabbage (napa); Chinese celery; Chinese parsley (coriander); Chinese turnips (lo bok); dried day lilies; dry fungus (black Judas ear); leafy green vegetables including kale, Chinese cress, Chinese mustard greens (gai choy), Chinese chard (bok choy), amaranth greens (yin choy), wolfberry leaves (gou gay), Chinese broccoli (gai lan); lotus tubers; okra; snow peas; stir-fried vegetables (chow yuk); taro root; white radish (daikon)	Kumquats	None	Fish and seafood (all kinds, dried and fresh); hen, legumes, nuts, organ meats, pigeon eggs, pork and pork products, soybean curd (tofu), steamed stuffed dumplings (dim sum)	Peanut, soy, sesame, and rice oil; lard
Filipino	Noodles, rice, rice flour (mochiko), stuffed noodles (wonton), white bread (pan de sal)	Bamboo shoots, dark green leafy vegetables (malunggay and salyot), eggplant, sweet potatoes (camotes), okra, palm, peppers, turnips, root crop (gabi)	Avocado, bitter melon (ampalaya), guavas, jackfruit, limes, mango, papaya, pod fruit (tamarind), pomelos, tangelo (naranghita)	Custards	Fish in all forms; dried fish (dilis); egg roll (lumpia); fish sauce (alamang, bagoong); legumes such as mung beans, bean sprouts, chickpeas; organ meats (liver, heart, intestines); pork with chicken in soy sauce (adobo); pork sausage; soybean curd (tofu)	None
Southeastern Asians (i.e., Laos, Cambodia, Thailand, Vietnam, the Hmong, and the Mien)	Rice (long and short grain) and related products such as noodles; Hmong cornbread or cake	Bamboo shoots, broccoli, Chinese parsley (coriander), mustard greens, pickled vegetables, water chestnuts, Thai chili peppers	Apple pear (Asian pear), bitter melon, coconut cream and milk, guava, jackfruit, mango	Sweetened condensed milk	Beef; chicken; deer; eggs; fish and shellfish (all kinds, both freshwater and saltwater); legumes including black-eyed peas, peanuts, kidney beans, and soybeans; organ meats (liver, stomach); pork; rabbit; soybean curd (tofu)	Lard, peanut oil

Ethnic Group	Bread, Cereal, Rice, and Pasta Group	Vegetable Group	Fruit Group	Milk, Yogurt, and Cheese Group	Meat, Poultry, Fish, Dry Beans, Eggs, and Nuts Group	Fats, Oils, And Sweets Group
Mexican	Corn and related products; taco shells (fried corn tortillas); tortillas (corn and flour); white bread	Cactus (nopales), chili peppers, salsa, tomatoes, yambean root (jicama), yucca root (cassava or manioc)	Avocado, guacamole (mashed avocado, onion, cilantro [coriander], chilies), papaya	Cheese, flan, sour cream	Black or pinto beans (rejoles); refried beans (frijoles refritos); flour tortilla stuffed with beef, chicken, eggs, or beans (burrito); corn tortilla stuffed with chicken, cheese, or beef topped with chili sauce (enchilada); Mexican sausage (chorizo)	Bacon fat, lard (manteca), salt pork
Caribbean persons (includes Puerto Rican and Cuban individuals)	Rice; starchy green bananas (plantains), usually fried	Beets, eggplant, tubers (yucca), white yams (boniato)	Tropical fruits, avocado, plantains, grapefruit, lemons, limes	Flan, hard cheese (queso de mano)	Chicken, fish (all kinds and preparations including smoked, salted, canned, fresh), legumes (all kinds, especially black beans), pork (fried), sausage (chorizo)	Olive and peanut oil, lard
Jewish (These foods reflect the religious and cultural customs of the Jewish people. Adherences to religious dietary patterns by followers of the different forms of Judaism [i.e., Orthodox, Conservative, Reform, and Reconstructionist] vary. Generally, Orthodox Jews and many Conservative Jews follow kosher dietary rules when eating at home and dining out. Others may only observe these rules when in their own homes. "Keeping kosher" rules are reviewed in the section that addresses religious dietary patterns.)	Bagels, buckwheat groats (kasha), dumplings made with matzoh meal (matzoh balls or knaidelach), egg bread (challah), noodle or potato pudding (kugel), crepes filled with farmer cheese and fruit (blintzes), unleavened bread or large crackers made with wheat flour and water (matzoh)	Potato pancakes (latkes); a vegetable stew made with sweet potatoes, carrots, prunes, and sometimes brisket (tzimmes); beet soup (borscht)	None	None	A mixture of fish formed into balls and poached (gefilte fish); smoked salmon (lox)	Chicken fat

Reprinted from Grodner M, Long S, Walkingshaw BC. *Foundations and clinical applications of nutrition.* 4th ed, St. Louis: Mosby; 2007.

RELIGIOUS DIETARY PRACTICES

	Seventh-Day Adventist	Buddhist	Eastern Orthodox	Hindu	Jewish	Mormon	Muslim	Roman Catholic
Beef	Avoided by most devout	Avoided by most devout		Prohibited or strongly discouraged				
Pork	Prohibited or strongly discouraged	Avoided by most devout		Avoided by most devout	Prohibited or strongly discouraged		Prohibited or strongly discouraged	
All meat	Avoided by most devout	Avoided by most devout	Permitted but some restrictions apply	Avoided by most devout	Permitted but some restrictions apply		Permitted but some restrictions apply	Permitted but some restrictions apply
Eggs, dairy	Permitted but avoided at some observances	Permitted but avoided at some observances	Permitted but some restrictions apply	Permitted but avoided at some observances	Permitted but some restrictions apply			
Fish	Avoided by most devout	Avoided by most devout	Permitted but some restrictions apply	Permitted but some restrictions apply	Permitted but some restrictions apply			
Shellfish	Prohibited or strongly discouraged	Avoided by most devout	Permitted but avoided at some observances	Permitted but some restrictions apply	Prohibited or strongly discouraged			
Meat and dairy at same meal					Prohibited or strongly discouraged			
Leavened foods					Permitted but some restrictions apply			
Ritual slaughter of animals					Practiced		Practiced	
Alcohol	Prohibited or strongly discouraged			Avoided by most devout		Prohibited or strongly discouraged	Prohibited or strongly discouraged	
Caffeine	Prohibited or strongly discouraged					Prohibited or strongly discouraged	Avoided by most devout	

Reprinted from Kittler PG, Sucher KP. *Food and culture.* 4th ed, Belmont, Calif: Brooks/Cole; 2004.

Glossary

1-α-hydroxylase the enzyme in the kidneys that catalyzes the hydroxylation reaction of 25-hydroxycholecalciferol (i.e., calcidiol) to calcitriol, which is the active form of vitamin D; 1-↑-hydroxylase activity is increased by parathyroid hormone when blood calcium levels are low.

absorption the process by which nutrients are taken into the cells that line the gastrointestinal tract.

acetone a major ketone compound that results from fat breakdown for energy in individuals with uncontrolled diabetes; persons with diabetes periodically take urinary acetone tests to monitor the status of their diabetes control.

achalasia a disorder of the esophagus in which the muscles of the tube fail to relax, thereby inhibiting normal swallowing.

acidic or alkaline diets diets based on the theory that diets high in acidic foods (e.g., animal protein, caffeine, simple sugars) will disrupt the body's normal pH balance, which is slightly alkaline.

acidosis a blood pH of less than 7.35; respiratory acidosis is caused by an accumulation of carbon dioxide (an acid); metabolic acidosis may be caused by a variety of conditions that result in the excess accumulation of acids in the body or by a significant loss of bicarbonate (a base).

adipocytes fat cells.

adipose tissue the storage site for excess fat.

adipose fat stored in the cells of adipose (fatty) tissue.

aerobic capacity a state in which oxygen is required to proceed; milliliters of oxygen consumed per kilogram of body weight per minute as influenced by body composition.

aldosterone a hormone of the adrenal glands that acts on the distal nephron tubule to stimulate the reabsorption of sodium in an ion exchange with potassium; the aldosterone mechanism is essentially a sodium-conserving mechanism, but it also indirectly conserves water, because water absorption follows sodium resorption.

aldosteronoma the excess secretion of aldosterone from the adrenal cortex; symptoms and complications include sodium retention, potassium wasting, alkalosis, weakness, paralysis, polyuria, polydipsia, hypertension, and cardiac arrhythmias.

alkalosis a blood pH of more than 7.45; respiratory alkalosis is caused by hyperventilation and an excess loss of carbon dioxide; metabolic alkalosis is seen with extensive vomiting in which a significant amount of hydrochloric acid is lost and bicarbonate (a base) is secreted.

allergens food proteins that elicit an immune system response or an allergic reaction; symptoms may include itching, swelling, hives, diarrhea, and difficulty breathing as well as anaphylaxis in the worst cases.

allergy a state of hypersensitivity to particular substances in the environment that works on body tissues to produce problems in the functioning of the affected tissues; the agent involved (i.e., the allergen) may be a certain food that is eaten or a substance (e.g., pollen) that is inhaled.

alpha-linolenic acid an essential fatty acid with 18 carbon atoms and three double bonds; found in soybean, canola, and flaxseed oil.

amenorrhea the absence of a menstrual period in a woman of reproductive age.

amenorrheic the absence or abnormal cessation of the menses.

amino acids the nitrogen-bearing compounds that form the structural units of protein; after digestion, amino acids are available for the synthesis of required proteins.

aminopeptidase a specific protein-splitting enzyme secreted by glands in the walls of the small intestine that breaks off the nitrogen-containing amino end (i.e., NH2) of the peptide chain, thereby producing smaller-chained peptides and free amino acids.

anabolism the metabolic process of building large substances from smaller parts; the opposite of catabolism.

anaerobic a microorganism that can live and grow in an oxygen-free environment.

anaphylaxis a severe and sometimes fatal allergic reaction that results from exposure to a protein that the body perceives as foreign and that elicits a systemic response that involves multiple organs.

anemia a blood condition that is characterized by a decreased number of circulating red blood cells, decreased hemoglobin, or both.

anencephaly a neural tube defect in which the brain does not form.

anencephaly the congenital absence of the brain that results from the incomplete closure of the upper end of the neural tube.

angina pectoris a spasmodic, choking chest pain caused by a lack of oxygen to the heart; this is a symptom of a heart attack, and it also may be caused by severe effort or excitement.

anorexia nervosa an extreme psychophysiologic aversion to food that results in life-threatening weight loss; a psychiatric eating disorder that results from a morbid fear of fatness in which a person's distorted body image is reflected as fat when the body is malnourished and extremely thin as a result of self-starvation.

anthropometric measurements the physical measurements of the human body that are used for health assessment, including height, weight, skinfold thickness, and circumference (i.e., of the head, hip, waist, wrist, and mid-arm muscle).

antibody any of numerous protein molecules produced by B cells as a primary immune defense for attaching to specific related antigens.

antidiuretic hormone a hormone of the pituitary gland that acts on the distal nephron tubule to conserve water by reabsorption; also called *vasopressin*.

antigen any foreign or non-self substances (e.g., toxins, viruses, bacteria, foreign proteins) that trigger the production of antibodies that are specifically designed to counteract their activity.

antioxidant a molecule that prevents the oxidation of cellular structures by free radicals

anuria the absence of urine production; anuria indicates kidney shutdown or failure.

appetite-regulating network a hormonally controlled system of appetite stimulation and suppression.

arteriole the smallest branch of an artery that connects with the capillaries.

ascites the accumulation of serous fluid (i.e., blood and lymph serum) in the abdominal cavity.

ascites fluid accumulation in the abdominal cavity

ascorbic acid the chemical name for vitamin C; the vitamin was named after its ability to cure scurvy.

atherosclerosis the underlying pathology of coronary heart disease; a common form of arteriosclerosis that is characterized by the formation of fatty streaks that contain cholesterol and that develop into hardened plaques in the inner lining of major blood vessels such as the coronary arteries.

atonic without normal muscle tone.

atopy patch test a diagnostic test that is used to assess for allergic reactions on the skin.

atrophy tissue wasting.

auscultation listening to the sounds of the gastrointestinal tract with a stethoscope.

azotemia an excess of urea and other nitrogenous substances in the blood.

baby bottle tooth decay the decay of the baby teeth as a result of inappropriate feeding practices such as putting an infant to bed with a bottle; also called *nursing bottle caries, bottle mouth,* and *bottle caries.*

basal energy expenditure (BEE) the amount of energy (in kcal) needed by the body for the maintenance of life when a person is at complete digestive, physical, mental, thermal, and emotional rest (i.e., 10 to 12 hours after eating and 12 to 18 hours after physical activity; measured immediately upon waking).

beriberi a disease of the peripheral nerves that is caused by a deficiency of thiamin (vitamin B1) and is characterized by pain (neuritis) and paralysis of legs and arms, cardiovascular changes, and edema.

bile an emulsifying agent produced by the liver and transported to the gallbladder for concentration and storage; it is released into the duodenum with the entry of fat to facilitate enzymatic fat digestion by acting as an emulsifier.

binge-eating disorder a psychiatric eating disorder that is characterized by the occurrence of binge eating episodes at least twice a week for a 6-month period.

blood urea nitrogen a test of nephron function that measures the ability to filter urea nitrogen, which is a product of protein metabolism, from the blood.

body composition the relative sizes of the four body compartments that make up the total body: lean body mass (muscle mass), fat, water, and bone.

body dysmorphic disorder an obsession with a perceived defect of the body.

body mass index (BMI) the body weight in kilograms divided by the square of the height in meters (i.e., kg/m^2).

body mass index the body weight in kilograms divided by the square of the height in meters (kg/m²); this measurement correlates with body fatness and the health risks associated with obesity.

bolus feeding a volume of feeding from 250 mL to 500 mL over a short period of time (usually 10 to 15 minutes) that is given via several feedings per day.

Bowman's capsule the membrane at the head of each nephron; this capsule was named for the English physician Sir William Bowman, who in 1843 first established the basis of plasma filtration and consequent urine secretion in the relationship of the blood-filled glomeruli and the filtration across the enveloping membrane.

branched-chain amino acids amino acids with branched side chains; three of the essential amino acids are branched-chain amino acids: leucine, isoleucine, and valine.

brush border the cells that are located on the microvilli within the lining of the intestinal tract; the microvilli are tiny hair-like projections that protrude from the mucosal cells that help to increase surface area for the digestion and absorption of nutrients.

bulimia nervosa a psychiatric eating disorder related to a person's fear of fatness in which cycles of gorging on large quantities of food are followed by compensatory mechanisms (e.g., self-induced vomiting, the use of diuretics and laxatives) to maintain a "normal" body weight.

cachexia a specific profound syndrome that is characterized by weight loss, reduced food intake, and systemic inflammation.

Cajun a group of people with an enduring tradition whose French-Catholic ancestors established permanent communities in the southern Louisiana coastal waterways after being expelled from Acadia (now Nova Scotia, Canada) by the reigning English during the late eighteenth century; they developed a unique food pattern from a blend of native French influence and the Creole cooking that was found in the new land.

calcitriol the activated hormone form of vitamin D.

calorie a measure of heat; the energy necessary to do work is measured as the amount of heat produced by the body's work; the energy value of a food is expressed as the number of kilocalories that a specified portion of the food will yield when it is oxidized in the body.

carboxypeptidase a protein enzyme that splits off the carboxyl group (i.e., –COOH) at the end of peptide chains.

carboxypeptidase a specific protein-splitting enzyme secreted as the inactive zymogen procarboxypeptidase by the pancreas; after it has been activated by trypsin, it acts in the small intestine to break off the acid (i.e., carboxyl) end of the peptide chain, thereby producing smaller-chained peptides and free amino acids.

carcinogenesis the development of cancer.

carotene a group name for three red and yellow pigments (↑-, ↓-, and ↖-carotene) that are found in dark green and yellow vegetables and fruits; ↓-carotene is most important to human nutrition because the body can convert it to vitamin A, thus making it a primary source of the vitamin.

carotenoids organic pigments that are found in plants; known to have functions such as scavenging free radicals, reducing the risk of certain types of cancer, and helping to prevent age-related eye diseases; more than 600 carotenoids have been identified, with ↓-carotene being the most well-known.

catabolism the metabolic process of breaking down large substances to yield smaller building blocks.

catabolism the metabolic process of breaking down large substances to yield smaller building blocks.

cellulitis the diffuse inflammation of soft or connective tissues (e.g., in the foot) from injury, bruises, or pressure sores that leads to infection; poor care may result in ulceration and abscess or gangrene.

cerebrovascular accident a stroke; a stroke is caused by arteriosclerosis within the blood vessels of the brain that cuts off oxygen supply to the affected portion of brain tissue, thereby paralyzing the actions that are controlled by the affected area.

chelator a ligand that binds to a metal to form a metal complex.

cholecalciferol the chemical name for vitamin D3 in its inactive form; it is often shortened to *calciferol*.

cholecystectomy the removal of the gallbladder.

cholecystitis acute gallbladder inflammation.

cholelithiasis gallstones.

cholesterol a fat-related compound called a *sterol* that is synthesized only in animal tissues; a normal constituent of bile and a principal constituent of gallstones; in the body, cholesterol is primarily synthesized in the liver; in the diet, cholesterol is found in animal food sources.

chronic dieting syndrome a cyclic pattern of weight loss by dieting followed by rapid weight gain; this abnormal psychophysiologic food pattern becomes chronic, changing a person's natural body metabolism and relative body composition to the abnormal state of a *metabolically obese* person of normal weight.

chronic kidney disease-mineral and bone disorder a clinical syndrome that develops as a systemic disorder of mineral and bone metabolism in patients with chronic kidney disease; results from abnormalities of calcium, phosphorus, parathyroid hormone, or vitamin D metabolism; causes abnormalities in bone turnover, mineralization, volume, linear growth, strength, and soft-tissue calcification.

chylomicron a lipoprotein formed in the intestinal cell that is composed of triglycerides, cholesterol, phospholipids, and protein; chylomicrons allow for the absorption of fat into the lymphatic circulatory system before entering the blood circulation.

chyme the semifluid food mass in the gastrointestinal tract that is present after gastric digestion.

chymotrypsin a protein-splitting enzyme secreted as the inactive zymogen chymotrypsinogen by the pancreas; after it has been activated by trypsin, it acts in the small intestine to continue breaking down proteins into shorter-chain polypeptides and dipeptides.

chymotrypsin one of the protein-splitting and milk-curdling pancreatic enzymes that is activated in the small intestine from the precursor chymotrypsinogen; it breaks specific amino acid peptide links of protein.

clinically severe or significant obesity a body mass index of 40 or more or a body mass index of 35 to 39 with at least one obesity-related disorder; also referred to as *extreme obesity* and *morbid obesity*.

cobalamin the chemical name for vitamin B12; this vitamin is found mainly in animal protein food sources; it is closely related to amino acid metabolism and the formation of the heme portion of hemoglobin; the absence of its necessary digestion and absorption agents in the gastric secretions, hydrochloric acid and intrinsic factor, leads to pernicious anemia and degenerative effects on the nervous system.

colloidal osmotic pressure (COP) the fluid pressure that is produced by protein molecules in the plasma and the cell; because proteins are large molecules, they do not pass through the separating membranes of the capillary walls; thus, they remain in their respective compartments and exert a constant osmotic pull that protects vital plasma and cell fluid volumes in these areas.

colostrum a thin yellow fluid that is first secreted by the mammary glands a few days after childbirth, preceding the mature breast milk; it contains up to 20% protein, including a large amount of lactalbumin, more minerals, and less lactose and fat than mature milk as well as immunoglobulins that represent the antibodies that are found in maternal blood.

competitive foods any food or beverage that is served outside of a federal meal program in a food-program setting, regardless of nutritional value.

complex carbohydrates large complex molecules of carbohydrates composed of many sugar units (polysaccharides); the complex forms of dietary carbohydrates are starch, which is digestible and provides a major energy source, and dietary fiber, which is indigestible (humans lack the necessary enzymes) and thus provides important bulk in the diet.

conditionally indispensable amino acids the six amino acids that are normally considered dispensable amino acids because the body can make them; however, under certain circumstances (e.g., illness), the body cannot make them in high enough quantities, and they become indispensable to the diet.

congestive heart failure a chronic condition of gradually weakening heart muscle; the muscle is unable to pump normal blood through the heart–lung circulation, which results in the congestion of fluids in the lungs.

continuous feeding an enteral feeding schedule with which the formula is infused via a pump over a 24-hour period.

coronary heart disease the overall medical problem that results from the underlying disease of atherosclerosis in the coronary arteries, which serve the heart muscle with blood, oxygen, and nutrients.

creatinine a nitrogen-carrying product of normal tissue protein breakdown; it is excreted in the urine; serum creatinine levels are an indicator of renal function.

Cushing's syndrome the excess secretion of glucocorticoids from the adrenal cortex; symptoms and complications include protein loss, obesity, fatigue, osteoporosis, edema, excess hair growth, diabetes, and skin discoloration.

dehiscence a splitting open; the separation of the layers of a surgical wound that may be partial, superficial, or complete and that involves total disruption and resuturing.

dialysate the cleansing solution used in dialysis: contains dextrose and other chemicals similar to those in the body.

dialysis the process of separating crystalloids (i.e., crystal-forming substances) and colloids (i.e., glue-like substances) in solution by the difference in their rates of diffusion through a semipermeable membrane; crystalloids (e.g., blood glucose, other simple metabolites) pass through readily, and colloids (e.g., plasma proteins) pass through slowly or not at all.

Dietary Reference Intakes (DRIs) the nutrient recommendations for each gender and age group that can be used for assessing and planning diets for healthy populations.

dietetics the management of the diet and the use of food; the science concerned with nutrition planning and the preparation of foods.

digestion the process by which food is broken down in the gastrointestinal tract to release nutrients in forms that the body can absorb.

dipeptidase the final enzyme in the protein-splitting system that produces the last two free amino acids.

dispensable amino acids the five amino acids that the body can synthesize from other amino acids that are supplied through the diet and thus do not have to be consumed on a daily basis.

diuresis the increased excretion of urine.

diuretic any substance that induces urination and subsequent fluid loss.

diverticulitis the inflammation of pockets of tissue (i.e., diverticula) in the lining of the mucous membrane of the colon.

dual-energy x-ray absorptiometry radiography that makes use of two beams (i.e., dual) that measure bone density and body composition.

dysphagia difficulty swallowing.

early-onset obesity a genetically associated obesity that occurs during early childhood.

eating disorders not otherwise specified subthreshold disordered eating that is not consistent with the diagnostic criteria for bulimia nervosa or anorexia nervosa (e.g., binge eating disorder)

edema an unusual accumulation of fluid in the interstitial compartments (i.e., the small structural spaces between tissue parts) of the body.

edema the excess accumulation of fluid in the body tissues.

element a single type of atom; a total of 118 elements have been identified, of which 94 occur naturally on Earth; elements cannot be broken down into smaller substances.

elemental formula a nutrition support formula composed of simple elemental nutrient components that require no further digestive breakdown and are thus readily absorbed (e.g., glucose, amino acids, medium-chain triglycerides).

elemental formula a nutrition support formula that is composed of simple elemental nutrient components that require no further digestive breakdown and are thus readily absorbed; these formulas include protein as free amino acids and carbohydrate as the simple sugar glucose.

emulsifier an agent that breaks down large fat globules into smaller, uniformly distributed particles; the action is chiefly accomplished in the intestine by bile acids, which lower the surface tension of the fat particles, thereby breaking the fat into many smaller droplets and thus greatly increasing the surface area of fat and facilitating contact with the fat-digesting enzymes.

enriched a word that is used to describe foods to which vitamins and minerals have been added back to a food after a refining process that caused a loss of some nutrients; for example, iron may be lost during the refining process of a grain, so the final product will be enriched with additional iron.

enteral a mode of feeding that makes use of the gastrointestinal tract through oral or tube feeding.

enteral a mode of feeding that makes use of the gastrointestinal tract through oral or tube feedings.

enterokinase an enzyme produced and secreted in the duodenum in response to food entering the small intestine; it activates trypsinogen to its active form of trypsin.

enzymes the proteins produced in the body that digest or change nutrients in specific chemical reactions without being changed themselves during the process, so their action is that of a catalyst; digestive enzymes in gastrointestinal secretions act on food substances to break them down into simpler compounds. (An enzyme usually is named after the substance [i.e., substrate] on which it acts, with the common word ending of *-ase*; for example, sucrase is the specific enzyme for sucrose, which it breaks down into glucose and fructose.)

ergocalciferol the chemical name for vitamin D2 in its inactive form; it is produced by some organisms (not humans) upon ultraviolet irradiation from the precursor ergosterol.

ergogenic the tendency to increase work output; various substances that increase work or exercise capacity and output.

erythropoietin hormone that stimulates the production of red blood cells in the bone marrow.

esophageal varices the pathologic dilation of the blood vessels within the wall of the esophagus as a result of liver cirrhosis; these vessels can continue to expand to the point of rupturing.

esophagitis inflammation of the esophagus

essential (or primary) hypertension an inherent form of high blood pressure with no specific identifiable cause; it is considered to be familial.

exogenous originating from outside the body.

expanded-criteria donors any brain-dead donor who is older than 60 years old or a donor who is older than 50 years old with two of the following conditions: history of hypertension, a terminal serum creatinine level of at least 1.5 mg/dL, or death from a cerebrovascular accident.

extrusion reflex the normal infant reflex to protrude the tongue outward when it is touched.

exudate various materials such as cells, cellular debris, and fluids that have escaped from the blood vessels and that are deposited in or on the surface tissues, usually as a result of inflammation; the protein content of exudate is high.

familial hypertriglyceridemia a genetic disorder that results in elevated blood triglyceride levels despite lifestyle modifications; it requires drug therapy.

fatty acids the major structural components of fats.

ferritin the storage form of iron.

fetal alcohol spectrum disorders a group of physical and mental birth defects that are found in infants who are born to mothers who used alcohol during pregnancy; the physical and mental disabilities vary in severity, and there is no cure.

fetal alcohol syndrome (FAS) a combination of physical and mental birth defects that are found in infants who are born to mothers who used alcohol during pregnancy; this is the most severe of the fetal alcohol spectrum disorders, and there is no cure.

filé powder a substance that is made from ground sassafras leaves; it seasons and thickens the dish into which it is put.

fistulas from the Latin word for "pipe," an abnormal opening or passageway within the body or to the outside.

fluorosis an excess intake of fluoride that causes the yellowing of teeth, white spots on the teeth, and the pitting or mottling of tooth enamel.

food neophobia the fear of new food.

galactosemia an autosomal recessive genetic disorder in which the liver does not produce the enzyme that is needed to metabolize galactose.

gastrin a hormone that helps with gastric motility, that stimulates the secretion of gastric acid by the parietal cells of the stomach, and that stimulates the chief cells to secrete pepsinogen.

gastroscopy an examination of the upper intestinal tract with a flexible tube with a small camera on the end; the tube is approximately 9 mm in diameter, and it takes color pictures as well as biopsy samples, if necessary.

glomerular filtration rate (GFR) the volume of fluid that is filtered from the renal glomerular capillaries into Bowman's capsule per unit of time; this term is used clinically as a measure of kidney function.

glomerulus the first section of the nephron; a cluster of capillary loops that are cupped in the nephron head that serves as an initial filter.

glucagon a hormone secreted by the ↑ cells of the pancreatic islets of Langerhans in response to hypoglycemia; it has an effect opposite to that of insulin in that it raises the blood glucose concentration and thus is used as a quick-acting antidote for a low blood glucose reaction; it also counteracts the overnight fast during sleep by breaking down liver glycogen to keep blood glucose levels normal and to maintain an adequate energy supply for normal nerve and brain function.

gluconeogenesis the formation of glucose from noncarbohydrate substances such as amino acids.

GLUT4 an insulin-regulated protein that is responsible for glucose transport into cells.

glycemic index the increase above fasting in the blood glucose level more than 2 hours after the ingestion of a constant amount of that food divided by the response to a reference food.

glycerides the chemical group name for fats; fats are formed from a glycerol base with one, two, or three fatty acids attached to make monoglycerides, diglycerides, and triglycerides, respectively; glycerides are the principal constituents of adipose tissue, and they are found in animal and vegetable fats and oils.

glycogen a complex carbohydrate found in animal tissue that is composed of many glucose units.

glycogen a polysaccharide; the main storage form of carbohydrate in the body, which is stored primarily in the liver and to a lesser extent in muscle tissue.

glycogenesis the anabolic process of creating stored glycogen from glucose.

glycolipid a lipid with a carbohydrate attached.

goiter an enlarged thyroid gland that is caused by a lack of enough available iodine to produce the thyroid hormone thyroxine.

gynecomastia the excessive development of the male mammary glands, frequently as a result of increased estrogen levels.

Hamwi method a formula for estimating the ideal body weight on the basis of gender and height.

health promotion the active engagement in behaviors or programs that advance positive well-being.

health a state of optimal physical, mental, and social well-being; relative freedom from disease or disability.

Heimlich maneuver a first-aid maneuver that is used to relieve a person who is choking from the blockage of the breathing passageway by a swallowed foreign object or food particle; to perform the maneuver, when standing behind the choking person, clasp the victim around the waist, place one fist just under the sternum (i.e., the breastbone), grasp the fist with the other hand, and then make a quick, hard, thrusting movement inward and upward to dislodge the object.

hematuria the abnormal presence of blood in the urine.

hemoglobin a conjugated protein in red blood cells that is composed of a compact, rounded mass of polypeptide chains that forms globin (the protein portion) and that is attached to an iron-containing red pigment called *heme*; hemoglobin carries oxygen in the blood to cells.

hemolytic uremic syndrome a condition that results most often from infection with *Escherichia coli* and that presents with a breaking up of red blood cells (i.e., hemolysis) and kidney failure.

hepatic encephalopathy a condition in which toxins in the blood lead to alterations in brain homeostasis as a result of liver disease; this results in apathy, confusion, inappropriate behavior, altered consciousness, and eventually coma.

hepatitis the inflammation of the liver cells; symptoms of acute hepatitis (i.e., of less than 6 months' duration) include flu-like symptoms, muscle and joint aches, fever, feeling sick or vomiting, diarrhea, headache, dark urine, and yellowing of the eyes and skin; symptoms of chronic hepatitis (i.e., of more than 6 months' duration) include jaundice, abdominal swelling and sensitivity, low-grade fever, and fluid retention (i.e., ascites).

homeostasis the state of relative dynamic equilibrium within the body's internal environment; a balance that is achieved through the operation of various inter-related physiologic mechanisms.

hypercalcemia a serum calcium level that is above normal.

hypercholesterolemia elevated blood cholesterol levels.

hyperemesis gravidarum a condition that involves prolonged and severe vomiting in pregnant women, with a loss of more than 5% of body weight and the presence of ketonuria, electrolyte disturbances, and dehydration.

hyperglycemia an elevated blood glucose level.

hyperhomocysteinemia the presence of high levels of homocysteine in the blood; associated with cardiovascular disease.

hyperkalemia a serum potassium level that is above normal.

hypernatremia a serum sodium level that is above normal.

hyperphosphatemia a serum phosphorus level that is above normal.

hypertension chronically elevated blood pressure; systolic blood pressure is consistently 140 mm Hg or more or diastolic pressure is consistently 90 mm Hg or more.

hypocalcemia a serum calcium level that is below normal.

hypoglycemia a low blood glucose level; a serious condition in diabetes management that requires immediate sugar intake to counteract, followed by a snack of complex carbohydrate (e.g., bread, crackers) and protein (e.g., lean meat, peanut butter, cheese) to maintain a normal blood glucose level.

hypoglycemia an abnormally low blood glucose level that may lead to muscle tremors, cold sweat, headache, and confusion.

hypokalemia a serum potassium level that is below normal.

hypomagnesemia a serum magnesium level that is below normal.

hyponatremia a serum sodium level that is below normal.

hypophosphatemia a serum phosphorus level that is below normal.

hypotension low blood pressure.

idiopathic of unknown cause.

immunocompetence the ability or capacity to develop an immune response (i.e., antibody production or cell-mediated immunity) after exposure to an antigen.

indispensable amino acids the nine amino acids that must be obtained from the diet because the body does not make adequate amounts to support body needs.

insulin a hormone that is produced by the pancreas, attaches to insulin receptors on cell membranes, and allows the absorption of glucose into the cell.

intrauterine growth restriction (IUGR) a condition that occurs when a newborn baby weighs less than 10% of predicted fetal weight for gestational age.

jambalaya a dish of Creole origin that combines rice, chicken, ham, pork, sausage, broth, vegetables, and seasonings.

ketoacidosis the excess production of ketones; a form of metabolic acidosis that occurs with uncontrolled diabetes or starvation from burning body fat for energy fuel; a continuing uncontrolled state can result in coma and death.

ketones the chemical name for a class of organic compounds that includes three keto acid bases that occur as intermediate products of fat metabolism.

ketosis the accumulation of ketones, which are intermediate products of fat metabolism, in the blood.

kilocalorie the general term *calorie* refers to a unit of heat measure, and it is used alone to designate the small calorie; the calorie that is used in nutrition science and the study of metabolism is the large Calorie or kilocalorie, which avoids the use of large numbers in calculations; a kilocalorie, which is composed of 1000 calories, is the measure of heat that is necessary to raise the temperature of 1000 g (1 L) of water by 1° C.

kinesiotherapist a health care professional who treats the effects of disease, injury, and congenital disorders through the application of scientifically based exercise principles that have been adapted to enhance the strength, endurance, and mobility of individuals with functional limitations or for those patients who require extended physical conditioning.

lactated Ringer's solution a sterile solution of calcium chloride, potassium chloride, sodium chloride, and sodium lactate in water that is given to replenish fluid and electrolytes; this solution was developed by the English physiologist Sidney Ringer (1835-1910).

laparoscopic fundoplication a surgery that is used to treat gastroesophageal reflux disease; the upper portion of the stomach (i.e., the fundus) is wrapped around the esophagus and sewn into place so that the esophagus passes through the muscle of the stomach; this strengthens the esophageal sphincter to prevent acid reflux.

life expectancy the number of years that a person of a given age may expect to live; this is affected by environment, lifestyle, gender, and race.

linoleic acid an essential fatty acid that consists of 18 carbon atoms and two double bonds; found in vegetable oils.

lipectomy the surgical removal of subcutaneous fat by suction through a tube that is inserted into a surface incision or by the removal of larger amounts of subcutaneous fat through a major surgical incision.

lipids the chemical group name for fats and fat-related compounds such as cholesterol and lipoproteins.

lipids the chemical group name for organic substances of a fatty nature; the lipids include fats, oils, waxes, and other fat-related compounds such as cholesterol.

lipiduria lipid droplets found in the urine that are composed mostly of cholesterol esters.

lipogenesis the anabolic process of forming fat.

lipoproteins chemical complexes of fat and protein that serve as the major carriers of lipids in the plasma; they vary in density according to the size of the fat load being carried (i.e., the lower the density, the higher the fat load); the combination package with water-soluble protein makes possible the transport of non–water-soluble fatty substances in the water-based blood circulation.

macrosomia an abnormally large baby.

macrosomia excessive fetal growth that results in an abnormally large infant; this condition carries a high risk for perinatal death.

major minerals the group of minerals that are required by the body in amounts of more than 100 mg/day.

masculinization a condition marked by the attainment of male characteristics (e.g., facial hair) either physiologically as part of male maturation or pathologically by either sex.

mechanical soft diet a meal plan that consists of foods that have been chopped, blended, ground, or prepared with extra fluid to make chewing and swallowing easier.

medical nutrition therapy a specific nutrition service and procedure that is used to treat an illness, injury, or condition; it involves an in-depth nutrition assessment of the patient, nutrition diagnosis, nutrition intervention (which includes diet therapy, counseling, and the use of specialized nutrition supplements), and nutrition monitoring and evaluation.

menopause the end of a woman's menstrual activity and capacity to bear children.

metabolic syndrome a combination of disorders that, when they occur together, increases the risk of cardiovascular disease and diabetes; it is also known as *syndrome X* and *insulin resistance syndrome.*

metabolism the sum of all chemical changes that take place in the body by which it maintains itself and produces energy for its functioning; products of the various reactions are called *metabolites.*

metabolism the sum of the vast number of chemical changes in the cell that ultimately produce the materials that are essential for energy, tissue building, and metabolic controls.

metastasis the spread to other tissue.

micelles packages of free fatty acids, monoglycerides, and bile salts; the non–water-soluble fat particles are found in the middle of the package, whereas the water-soluble part faces outward and allows for the absorption of fat into intestinal mucosal cells.

microalbuminuria low but abnormal levels of albumin in the urine.

microvilli extremely small, hair-like projections that cover all of the villi on the surface of the small intestine and that greatly extend the total absorbing surface area; they are visible through an electron microscope.

mucosal folds the large, visible folds of the mucous lining of the small intestine that increase the absorbing surface area.

mucositis an inflammation of the tissues around the mouth or other orifices of the body.

mutation a permanent transmissible change in a gene.

myocardial infarction (MI) a heart attack; a myocardial infarction is caused by the failure of the heart muscle to maintain normal blood circulation as a result of the blockage of the coronary arteries with fatty cholesterol plaques that cut off the delivery of oxygen to the affected part of the heart muscle.

MyPlate a visual pattern of the current basic five food groups—grains, vegetables, fruits, dairy, and protein—arranged on a plate to indicate proportionate amounts of daily food choices.

negative energy balance what occurs when more total energy is expended than consumed.

neoplasm any new or abnormal cellular growth, specifically one that is uncontrolled and aggressive.

nephrolithiasis the formation of a kidney stone.

nephron the functional unit of the kidney that filters and reabsorbs essential blood constituents, secretes hydrogen ions as needed to maintain the acid-base balance, reabsorbs water, and forms and excretes a concentrated urine for the elimination of wastes.

nephrosis degenerative lesions of the renal tubules of the nephrons and especially of the thin basement membrane of the glomerulus that helps to support the capillary loops; marked by edema, albuminuria, and a decreased serum albumin level.

nephrotoxic poisonous to the kidney.

niacin the chemical name for vitamin B3; this vitamin was discovered in relation to the deficiency disease pellagra, which is largely a skin disorder; it is important as a coenzyme factor in many cell reactions related to energy and protein metabolism.

nursing diagnosis "[a] clinical judgment about individual, family, or community responses to actual or potential health problems/life processes. Nursing diagnoses provide the basis for selection of nursing interventions to achieve outcomes for which the nurse is accountable," as defined by the North American Nursing Diagnosis Association.

nursing process the means by which nurses deliver care to patients; it includes the following steps: assessment, diagnosis, planning, implementation, and evaluation.

nutrition integrity as defined by the School Nutrition Association, "a level of performance that assures all foods and beverages available in schools are consistent with the Dietary Guidelines for Americans, and, when combined with nutrition education, physical activity, and a healthful school environment, contributes to enhanced learning and development of lifelong, healthful eating habits."

nutrition science the body of science, developed through controlled research, that relates to the processes involved in nutrition internationally, clinically, and in the community.

nutrition the sum of the processes involved with the intake of nutrients as well as assimilating and using them to maintain body tissue and provide energy; a foundation for life and health.

oliguria the secretion of small amounts of urine in relation to fluid intake (i.e., 0.5 mL/kg per hour or less).

organic farming the use of farming methods that employ natural means of pest control and that meet the standards set by the National Organic Program of the U.S. Department of Agriculture; organic foods are grown or produced without the use of synthetic pesticides or fertilizers, sewage sludge, genetically modified organisms, or ionizing radiation.

osmosis the passage of a solvent (e.g., water) through a membrane that separates solutions of different concentrations and that tends to equalize the concentration pressures of the solutions on either side of the membrane.

osmotic pressure hydrostatic pressure across a semipermeable membrane that is necessary to maintain the normal movement of fluid between the capillaries and the surrounding tissue.

osmotic pressure the pressure that is produced as a result of osmosis across a semipermeable membrane.

osteoblast cells that are responsible for the mineralization and formation of bone.

osteodystrophy an alteration of bone morphology found in patients with chronic kidney disease.

osteopenia a condition that involves a low bone mass and an increased risk for fracture.

osteoporosis a disease of the skeletal system that is characterized by a bone mineral density value that is more than 2.5 standard deviations below a 20-year-old sex-matched healthy person's average.

osteoporosis an abnormal thinning of the bone that produces a porous, fragile, lattice-like bone tissue of enlarged spaces that are prone to fracture or deformity.

pancreatic amylase a major starch-splitting enzyme that is secreted by the pancreas and that acts in the small intestine.

pancreatic lipase a major fat-splitting enzyme produced by the pancreas and secreted into the small intestine to digest fat.

pandemic a widespread epidemic distributed throughout a region, a continent, or the world.

pantothenic acid a B-complex vitamin that is found widely distributed in nature and that occurs throughout the body tissues; it is an essential constituent of the body's main activating agent, coenzyme A; this special compound has extensive metabolic responsibility for activating a number of compounds in many tissues, and it is a key energy metabolism substance in every cell.

parasite an organism that lives in or on an organism of another species, known as the *host*, from whom all nourishment is obtained.

parenteral a mode of feeding that does not involve the gastrointestinal tract but that instead provides nutrition support via the intravenous delivery of nutrient solutions.

parenteral a mode of feeding that does not make use of the gastrointestinal tract but that instead provides nutrition support via the intravenous delivery of nutrient solutions.

parotid glands the largest of the three pairs of salivary glands; the parotid glands lie, one on each side, above the angle of the jaw and below and in front of the ear; they continually secrete saliva, which passes along the duct of the gland and into the mouth through an opening in the inner cheek that is level with the second upper molar tooth; normal saliva flow facilitates the chewing and swallowing of food and prevents problems that occur with a dry mouth.

pellagra the deficiency disease caused by a lack of dietary niacin and an inadequate amount of protein that contains the amino acid tryptophan, which is a precursor of niacin; pellagra is characterized by skin lesions that are aggravated by sunlight as well as by gastrointestinal, mucosal, neurologic, and mental symptoms.

pepsin the main gastric enzyme specific for proteins; pepsin begins breaking large protein molecules into shorter chain polypeptides, and it is activated by gastric hydrochloric acid.

pepsin the main gastric enzyme specific to proteins; it begins breaking large protein molecules into shorter-chain polypeptides; gastric hydrochloric acid is necessary for its activation.

peritoneal cavity a serous membrane that lines the abdominal and pelvic walls and the undersurface of the diaphragm to form a sac that encloses the body's vital visceral organs.

pernicious anemia a form of megaloblastic anemia that is caused by destroyed gastric parietal cells that produce intrinsic factor; without intrinsic factor, vitamin B12 cannot be absorbed.

pharynx the muscular membranous passage that extends from the mouth to the posterior nasal passages, the larynx, and the esophagus.

pheochromocytoma a tumor of the adrenal medulla or the sympathetic nervous system in which the affected cells secrete excess epinephrine or norepinephrine and cause headache, hypertension, and nausea.

photosynthesis the process by which plants that contain chlorophyll are able to manufacture carbohydrate by combining carbon dioxide and water; sunlight is used as energy, and chlorophyll is a catalyst.

phylloquinone a fat-soluble vitamin of the K group that is found primarily in green plants.

plasma protein any of a number of protein substances that are carried in the circulating blood; a major one is *albumin*, which maintains the fluid volume of the blood through colloidal osmotic pressure.

polarity the interaction between the positively charged end of one molecule and the negative end of another (or the same) molecule.

polydipsia excessive thirst and drinking.

polymeric formula a nutrition support formula that is composed of complete protein, polysaccharides, and fat as medium-chain fatty acids.

polypharmacy the use of multiple medications by a patient.

polypharmacy the use of multiple medications by the same patient.

polyuria an excess water loss through urination.

portal hypertension high blood pressure in the portal vein

portal an entrance or gateway; for example, the portal blood circulation designates the entry of blood vessels from the intestines into the liver; it carries nutrients for liver metabolism, and it then drains into the body's main systemic circulation to deliver metabolic products to body cells.

pregnancy-induced hypertension the development of hypertension during pregnancy after the twentieth week of gestation.

probiotic a food that contains live microbials, which are thought to benefit the consumer by improving intestinal microbial balance (e.g., lactobacilli in yogurt).

proenzyme an inactive precursor (i.e., a forerunner substance from which another substance is made) that is converted to the active enzyme by the action of an acid, another enzyme, or other means.

prohormone a precursor substance that the body converts to a hormone; for example, a cholesterol compound in the skin is first irradiated by sunlight and then converted through successive enzyme actions in the liver and kidney into the active vitamin D hormone, which then regulates calcium absorption and bone development.

proteinuria an abnormal excess of serum proteins (e.g., albumin) in the urine.

pulmonary edema an accumulation of fluid in the lung tissues.

pyridoxine the chemical name of vitamin B6; in its activated phosphate form (i.e., B2PO4), pyridoxine functions as an important coenzyme factor in many reactions in cell metabolism that are related to amino acids, glucose, and fatty acids.

Ramadan the ninth month of the Muslim year, which is a period of daily fasting from sunrise to sunset.

Recommended Dietary Allowances (RDAs) the recommended daily allowances of nutrients and energy intake for population groups according to age and gender with defined weight and height.

refeeding syndrome a potentially lethal condition that occurs when severely malnourished individuals are fed high-carbohydrate diets too aggressively; a sudden shift in electrolytes and fluid retention and a drastic drop in serum phosphorus levels cause a series of complications that involves several organs.

registered dietitian (RD) a professional dietitian accredited with an academic degree from an undergraduate or graduate study program who has passed required registration examinations administered by the Commission on Dietetic Registration.

rennin the milk-curdling enzyme of the gastric juice of human infants and young animals (e.g., calves); rennin should not be confused with renin, which is an important enzyme produced by the kidneys that plays a vital role in the activation of angiotensin.

resistant hypertension the presence of high blood pressure despite treatment with three antihypertensive medications

resorption the breaking down and releasing of minerals from bones.

resorption the destruction, loss, or dissolution of a tissue or a part of a tissue by biochemical activity (e.g., the loss of bone, the loss of tooth dentin).

resting energy expenditure (REE) the amount of energy (in kcal) needed by the body for the maintenance of life at rest over a 24-hour period; this is often used interchangeably with the term *basal energy expenditure*, but in actuality it is slightly higher.

retinol the chemical name of vitamin A; the name is derived from the vitamin's visual functions related to the retina of the eye, which is the back inner lining of the eyeball that catches the light refractions of the lens to form images that are interpreted by the optic nerve and the brain and that makes the necessary light–dark adaptations.

riboflavin the chemical name for vitamin B2; this vitamin was discovered in relation to an early vitamin deficiency syndrome called *ariboflavinosis* that is mainly evidenced in the breakdown of skin tissues and resulting infections; it also has a role as a coenzyme factor in many cell reactions related to energy and protein metabolism.

rickets a disease of childhood that is characterized by the softening of the bones from an inadequate intake of vitamin D and insufficient exposure to sunlight; it is also associated with impaired calcium and phosphorus metabolism.

saccharide the chemical name for sugar molecules; may occur as single molecules in monosaccharides (glucose, fructose, galactose), two molecules in disaccharides (sucrose, lactose, maltose), or multiple molecules in polysaccharides (starch, dietary fiber, glycogen).

salivary amylase a starch-splitting enzyme in the mouth that is secreted by the salivary glands and that is commonly called *ptyalin* (from the Greek word *ptyalon,* meaning "spittle").

saturated the state of being filled; the state of fatty acid components being filled in all their available carbon bonds with hydrogen, thus making the fat harder and more solid; such solid food fats are generally from animal sources.

school breakfast and lunch programs federally assisted meal programs that operate in public and nonprofit private schools and residential child-care institutions; these programs provide nutritionally balanced, low-cost, or free meals to children each school day.

scurvy a hemorrhagic disease caused by a lack of vitamin C that is characterized by diffuse tissue bleeding, painful limbs and joints, thickened bones, and skin discoloration from bleeding; bones fracture easily, wounds do not heal, gums swell and tend to bleed, and the teeth loosen.

secondary hypertension an elevated blood pressure for which the cause can be identified and which is a symptom or side effect of another primary condition.

senescence the process or condition of growing old.

simple carbohydrates sugars with a simple structure of one or two single-sugar (saccharide) units; a monosaccharide is composed of one sugar unit, and a disaccharide is composed of two sugar units.

sorbitol a sugar alcohol that is often used as a nutritive sugar substitute; it is named for where it was discovered in nature, in ripe berries of the *Sorbus aucuparia* tree; it also occurs in small quantities in various other berries, cherries, plums, and pears.

speech-language pathologist a specialist in the assessment, diagnosis, treatment, and prevention of speech, language, cognitive communication, voice, swallowing, fluency, and other related disorders.

spina bifida a congenital defect in the embryonic fetal closing of the neural tube to form a portion of the lower spine, which leaves the spine unclosed and the spinal cord open to various degrees of exposure and damage.

spina bifida a neural tube defect in which the lower end of the neural tube does not close properly and the spinal cord may protrude through the spinal column.

state land grant universities an institution of higher education that has been designated by the state to receive unique federal support as a result of the Morrill Acts of 1862 and 1890.

steatorrhea fatty diarrhea; excessive amount of fat in the feces, which is often caused by malabsorption diseases.

stillbirth the death of a fetus after the twentieth week of pregnancy.

stoma the opening that is established in the abdominal wall that connects with the ileum or the colon for the elimination of intestinal wastes after the surgical removal of diseased portions of the intestines.

sugar alcohols nutritive sweeteners that provide 2 to 3 kcal/g; examples include sorbitol, mannitol, and xylitol; these are produced in food-industry laboratories for use as sweeteners in candies, chewing gum, beverages, and other foods.

teratogen a drug or substance that causes a birth defect.

thermic effect of food an increase in energy expenditure caused by the activities of digestion, absorption, transport, and storage of ingested food; a meal that consists of a usual mixture of carbohydrates, protein, and fat increases the energy expenditure equivalent to approximately 10% of the food's energy content (e.g., a 300-kcal piece of pizza would elicit an energy expenditure of 30 kcal to digest the food).

thiamin the chemical name of vitamin B1; this vitamin was discovered in relation to the classic deficiency disease beriberi, and it is important in body metabolism as a coenzyme factor in many cell reactions related to energy metabolism.

thyroid-stimulating hormone (TSH) an anterior pituitary hormone that regulates the activity of the thyroid gland; also known as *thyrotropin.*

thyrotropin-releasing hormone (TRH) a hormone that is secreted by the hypothalamus and that stimulates the release of thyroid-stimulating hormone by the pituitary.

thyroxine (T_4) an iodine-dependent thyroid gland hormone that regulates the metabolic rate of the body.

thyroxine (T_4) thyroid prohormone; the active hormone form is T3; it is the major controller of basal metabolic rate.

tocopherol the chemical name for vitamin E, which was named by early investigators because their initial work with rats indicated a reproductive function; in people, vitamin E functions as a strong antioxidant that preserves structural membranes such as cell walls.

trace minerals the group of elements that are required by the body in amounts of less than 100 mg/day.

transferrin a protein that binds and transports iron through the blood.

transport the movement of nutrients through the circulatory system from one area of the body to another.

triglycerides the chemical name for fats in the body or in food; three fatty acids attached to a glycerol base.

trypsin a protein-splitting enzyme produced in the pancreas and released into the small intestine; the inactive precursor trypsinogen is activated by enterokinase.

trypsin a protein-splitting enzyme secreted as the inactive proenzyme trypsinogen by the pancreas and that is activated and works in the small intestine to reduce proteins to shorter-chain polypeptides and dipeptides.

ultrasonography an ultrasound-based diagnostic imaging technique that is used to visualize the muscles and internal organs; also referred to as *sonography.*

urea the chief nitrogen-carrying product of dietary protein metabolism; urea appears in the blood, lymph, and urine.

vagotomy the cutting of the vagus nerve, which supplies a major stimulus for gastric secretions.

vasculitis the inflammation of the walls of blood vessels.

villi small protrusions from the surface of a membrane; finger-like projections that cover the mucosal surfaces of the small intestine and that further increase the absorbing surface area; they are visible through a regular microscope.

villi small protrusions from the surface of a membrane; finger-like projections that cover the mucosal surfaces of the small intestine that further increase the absorbing surface area; these are visible through a regular microscope.

VO₂max the maximal uptake volume of oxygen during exercise; this is used to measure the intensity and duration of exercise that a person can perform.

waist circumference the measurement of the waist at its narrowest point widthwise, just above the navel; waist circumference is a rough measurement of abdominal fat and a predictor of risk factors for cardiovascular disease; this risk factor increases with a waist measurement of more than 40 inches in men and of more than 35 inches in women.

weaning the process of gradually acclimating a young child to food other than the mother's milk or a bottle-fed substitute formula as the child's natural need to suckle wanes.

Wilson's disease an autosomal recessive genetic disorder in which copper accumulates in tissue and causes damage to organs.

xerostomia a dryness of the mouth from a lack of normal secretions.

xerostomia the condition of dry mouth that results from a lack of saliva; saliva production can be hindered by certain diseases (e.g., diabetes, Parkinson's disease) and by some prescription and over-the-counter medications.

zymogen an inactive enzyme precursor.

Index

Page numbers followed by "f" indicate figures, "t" indicate tables, and "b" indicate boxes.